Neurological Differential Diagnosis

Springer
London
Berlin
Heidelberg
New York
Barcelona
Budapest
Hong Kong
Milan
Paris
Santa Clara
Singapore
Tokyo

JOHN PATTEN

Neurological Differential Diagnosis

2nd Edition

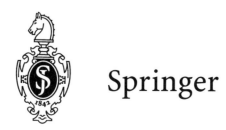

Springer

John Philip Patten, BSc, MB, BS, FRCP
Consultant Neurologist, King Edward VII Hospital
Midhurst, Sussex GU29 0BL, UK

Formerly: Consultant Neurologist to South West Thames
Regional Health Authority; Visiting Assistant Professor,
University of Texas Medical Branch, Galveston; Resident Medical
Officer, National Hospital for Nervous Diseases, Queen Square, London

ISBN 3–540–19937–3 Springer-Verlag Berlin Heidelberg New York

British Library Cataloguing in Publication Data
Patten, John
  Neurological Differential Diagnosis.–
  2 Rev. ed
  I. Title
  616.80475
  ISBN 3–540–19937–3

Library of Congress Cataloging-in-Publication Data
Patten, John, 1935–
  Neurological differential diagnosis/John Patten. – 2nd ed.
    p.   cm.
  Includes bibliographical references and index.
  ISBN 3–540–19937–3 (alk. paper)
  1. Nervous system – Diseases – Diagnosis.   2. Diagnosis, Differential.   I. Title.
  [DNLM: 1. Nervous System Diseases – diagnosis.   WL 141 P316n   1995]
RC348.P37   1995
616.8′0475 – dc20
DNLM/DLC
for Library of Congress   95–14336

Typeset by EXPO Holdings, Malaysia
Printed by Bell & Bain Ltd, Glasgow, UK
28/3830-543210 Printed on acid-free paper

*To my patients, whose courage, suffering and trust
have served as a constant source of inspiration.
To my family past and present, whose love and support
have made everything possible.*

Preface to the First Edition

The majority of doctors are ill at ease when confronted by a patient with a neurological problem. Candidates for qualifying examinations and higher diplomas dread that they will be allocated a neurological 'long case'.

This is a serious reflection on the adequacy of training in neurology. It is still possible in some medical schools for a student to go through the entire clinical course without an attachment to the neurological unit. Increasing competition for teaching time has led to the situation where in most US medical schools, and at least one new medical school in the UK, a two-week clinical attachment to the neurology service is considered adequate. Those fortunate enough to attend a postgraduate course find a minimum of 3 months' intensive training is necessary before any confidence in tackling a neurological problem is achieved.

Unfortunately, neurological textbooks seldom seem to recognize the intensely practical nature of the subject. There are many short texts that achieve brevity by the exclusion of explanatory material; these are difficult to read and digest. At the opposite extreme are the neurological compendia, often unbalanced by excessive coverage of rare diseases and all based on the assumption that patients announce on arrival that they have a demyelinating, heredofamilial, neoplastic etc. disorder. These texts are useful only to those who already have a good working knowledge of neurological diseases.

Patients present with symptoms that need careful evaluation before physical examinations which in turn should be firmly based on the diagnostic possibilities suggested by the history. Understanding neurological symptoms and signs requires a good knowledge of the gross anatomy of the nervous system, its blood supply and supporting tissues; and yet an almost universal feature of neurological texts is the paucity of instructive diagrams. Most students readily admit that this is an insoluble problem, as their poorly remembered neurological anatomy is often both inadequate and inappropriate to the clinical situation.

The present text is a personal approach to this complex and fascinating subject, and basically reflects the way the author coped with this difficulty. The subject matter is dealt with in two ways:

1. Symptomatic, regional anatomical basis for those areas where local anatomy determines symptoms and signs, allowing what might otherwise be regarded as 'small print' anatomy to be understood and appreciated;

2. Full discussion of the historical diagnostic clues in those conditions that are diagnosed almost exclusively on symptoms such as headache, face pain and loss of consciousness.

Throughout, an attempt has been made to preserve the 'common things are common' approach which is widely rumoured to be the secret of passing examinations, and is also the basis of good clinical practice. Rare disorders are discussed briefly, but it is important that beginners realize that rare diseases are usually diagnosed when it becomes apparent that the disorder does *not* fit into any of the common clinical pictures. The first aim therefore should be to gain a very good grasp of the common disorders rather than attempting to learn long lists of very rare diseases.

The text is profusely illustrated, and although anatomical accuracy has been preserved, artistic licence has been taken whenever necessary to illustrate an important point. Each diagram is drawn from a special angle of view that enables the reader to visualize the area under discussion in situ in the patient. It is easy to construct a 'diagram' so remote from actual anatomy that it becomes incomprehensible. It is hoped that this problem has been avoided.

Neurological terms are defined whenever they occur and neurological 'jargon' is explained, although the beginner is well advised to keep to factual statements until he is very sure of himself. As an example of the incorrect use of jargon the following is abstracted from a report by a physician. The patient actually had a left sixth nerve palsy and a mild hemiparesis due to cerebal metastases:

He has the spastic dystonic gait of the multiple sclerotic. Also he has a third nerve paraplegia with ocular movements to the left and with nystagmus. He has cogwheel rigidity of the upper extremities and an absence of patellar reflexes. His speech is beginning to slur and there is the mask facies of the multiple sclerotic ... I do not believe ... further studies to be necessary as the clinical signs are all too obvious!

Specific references are not given; this book is intended for the novice who wishes to develop a 'feel' for the subject and in the author's opinion references are unnecessary. This is not intended to indicate that the writer claims originality for all the information provided. The knowledge contained in this text is a distillate of wisdom gained from many teachers and, indeed, generations of teachers, who have passed on their own observations. The personal part of this text is the attempt to organize this information around the anatomy of the nervous system to reinforce this knowledge and make the subject less intimidating to the beginner. In particular I would like to acknowledge my debt to my first teacher, Dr Swithin Meadows, who aroused my enthusiasm for the subject and then inspired me to attempt to emulate his skill as a clinical neurologist.

I am also indebted to many undergraduate students at Westminster Medical School, University College Hospital and the University of Texas Medical Branch, and postgraduates at the National Hospital for Nervous Diseases, whose questions, suggestions and enthusiasm originally encouraged me to bring this approach to a wider audience.

Dr John R. Calverley, Associate Professor of Neurology in the University of Texas Medical Branch at Galveston, provided enormous encouragement in the early development of this project and allowed me to try the format on several generations of postgraduate students in his department.

I would like to express my thanks to him and his colleagues for making my stay so instructive and enjoyable. Dr M. J. Harrison read the original manuscript and made many useful suggestions which have been incorporated into the text. I am very grateful for his help and encouragement.

I would like to thank my wife and family for their continued support during the years this text has been in preparation, and Miss Gillian Taylor for typing the often illegible manuscript.

John Patten
(1975)

Preface to the Second Edition

Since this book was first published 19 years ago, I have often been asked what prompted me to write it and who had done the illustrations. The answers to these questions are intimately related in reverse order. The book actually evolved around the collection of illustrations that I had drawn and constantly revised to improve my own knowledge of neuroanatomy, ever since my preclinical training began in 1954. My art master at school was upset that I would not transfer to art college at the age of 14 and my father was upset that I resisted his attempts to persuade me to study architecture, but I was allowed to study art as an extra subject until my A-level examinations.

I eventually realized that my attempts were successfully clarifying the often incomprehensible illustrations in most neurology textbooks of the time. These usually consisted of blobs and lines, with little or no structural form to relate them to the brain, spinal cord or any position inside the person. The book therefore developed around some of these key illustrations. They started to take final shape while I was teaching at the University of Texas Medical Branch in Galveston, between 1968 and 1971. I had the opportunity to run an evening course in advanced neurology and each 2-hour lecture was based on a single hand-out diagram of the area under consideration, and this proved extremely popular and a sound basis for discussion of differential diagnosis.

The then available textbooks were very heavy on ponderous prose and very light on practical diagnosis and management, and almost bereft of illustrations to both lighten the text and provide clarification. The main motivation, therefore, was to write the textbook that I wished had been available to me when I started in neurology. The temerity to attempt to write such a book at a relatively early stage in my career came from the feeling that it was essential to do this before I became too remote from the initial learning process and had forgotten the problems that had caused me the most difficulty. I was only too aware of this because I was so often 'fobbed off' by my own teachers when I asked for an explanation of some unusual feature in a case, and was asked to accept 'because it happens' as an adequate explanation. I realized that they had either forgotten or had never understood the underlying anatomical basis of some of the more bizarre but well-known peculiarities of the behaviour of neurological disease processes.

The actual format of the book, which was unique at that time, was undoubtedly influenced by three widely differing textbooks that had made a dramatic impression on me. The first was *Biological drawings* by Maud Jepson (1938), an ancillary textbook for advanced-level zoology and botany studies which first brought to my attention just how much information can be conveyed from a carefully constructed illustration, with detailed annotations rather than labels. The second was *Bedside diagnosis* by Charles Seward, which was the first short textbook in any subject that made it clear that thumbnail sketches of specific illnesses could convey vast amounts of information, without becoming telegraphic meaningless sentences. Finally, as a house physician, the only textbook on my first ward was a copy of Frank Walsh's original textbook *Clinical neuro-ophthalmology* (1947). This was a massive tome where the text was both lightened and enhanced by little case reports of variable length that not only put immediate meat on the skeleton of information under discussion but also seemed to leave it indelibly printed on the memory, in a way that I had not encountered previously. Any merit the present book has undoubtedly owes a lot to these formative influences.

Neuroanatomical illustration requires an admixture of representational artwork, line illustrations and modified technical drawing techniques, including exploded sections of the diagram to make special points. Drawings of all these types are to be found in the original volume. In this latest version, my son Graham, who actually modelled for the childhood Duchenne dystrophy in the first edition and is now a graduate in scientific illustration and head of design and advanced applications at Virtuality PLC, has assisted me and the overall improvement in the quality of illustrations owes everything to his advice and skill and his own redrawing of several of my originals. I hope that if a third edition becomes possible, our joint efforts, perhaps using advanced technology to provide a back-up to the text, may produce an even better result.

In this revision very much more time was spent on the text than was originally envisaged, because of the total transformation of the speciality in the last 15 years by imaging techniques and neuro-physiological advances. When the first edition was completed, CT scanning was in its infancy, visual-evoked responses had only just been standardized and the main investigational techniques were still lumbar puncture, angiography, myelography and air encephalography. All these procedures have potentially serious drawbacks and are even potentially lethal if incorrectly applied. It became apparent that a surprising amount of the previous text was concerned with information designed to avoid these complications and facilitate diagnosis on clinical grounds, using minimal investigations to confirm or refute the diagnosis, with the least risk to the patient. Unfortunately it is also true that there are many parts of the world where neurologists still have no access to the full range of modern investigational techniques, and even in the developed areas limited access and expense may preclude their use.

The investigational agenda may have altered but the practical importance of making a sound clinically based diagnosis *before* embarking on investigations remains the same. All the available techniques have limitations, and even the final interpretation of the significance of MRI scan findings often requires consideration of the clinical features in the case before final resolution. A 'scan first and think later' philosophy has little to commend it, and yet threatens to take over as both an expensive, and in many instances ineffectual, method of working. At least 75% of neurological practice does not deal with diseases where there is a simple solution that can be revealed by scanning.

There is also the risk of an attitude gaining ground that the 'scans are normal therefore there can be nothing wrong', and this is an inevitable consequence of practising sloppy, short-cut neurology. For this reason, the main content of this textbook, which is firmly based on detailed analysis of patients' symptomatology and the careful search for possibly associated physical findings, should not be the dying gasp of clinical neurology as my generation knew it. I think this information will have to be learned again if this hardwon knowledge is lost as a result of the neurological consultation becoming shortened to 5 minutes without examining the patient, the only decision taken being which part of the body to scan. This type of approach ignores the fact that at least half the patients referred will not have a neurological disease, or indeed any disease at all, and these patients in particular can only be effectively identified by a very detailed analysis of their symptoms and always take more time than patients with clear-cut and easily identifiable neurological disease.

The success of the previous edition was surprising: numerous foreign language versions, multiple reprints, and friendly reviews and kind unsolicited comments from many colleagues, have all been a source of great satisfaction, and its continuing popularity many years after much of the inves-tigational detail was long out of date is reassuring. Unfortunately, for various personal reasons there has been no possibility of rewriting or updating until recently.

Many of the original reviews commented on the quality and value of the simple clinical information contained, and this is now expanded and honed as a result of my seeing over 2000 new outpatients and 400 emergency admissions per annum over the last 20 years. The first 8 years were in a unit without neurosurgery on site and without the advantage of CT scanning, which was regarded by the NHS as an expensive luxury, as was MRI scanning, until several years after their establishment as important new investigational techniques. Their advent has more than adequately demonstrated that the hardwon clinical skills of several generations of neurologists are precise and valuable. There is much pleasure to be derived from seeing a scan reveal exactly what the clinical picture had sug-gested. Until scanning became available, important instant management decisions had to be taken purely on the basis of clinical experience.

This new edition is therefore offered in the hope that it will help a new generation of aspiring neurologists to get a head start in the specialty, armed with the clinical core knowledge that will enhance their enjoyment of their work and be of benefit to those who seek their advice.

I would like to put on record my appreciation of the help I have received in my clinical practice over the past 20 years, and the advice and encouragement from others during the preparation of this volume. I have been very fortunate in having Dr Tony Broadbridge as my neuroradiologist during most of that period when we had to continue practising 20th century neurology without the advantage of CT scanning. His skill in the old fashioned techniques of myelography, angiography and air encephalography was unsurpassed, and his subsequent skill in CT scan interpretation underpinned my clinical practice. In recent years I have also had the advantage of being able to call upon the radiological skills of Dr B. J. Loveday, Dr R. Hoare and Dr E. Burrows with their special skills in MRI techniques and interpretation, which has undoubtedly helped me to improve my own diagnostic skills.

I have been able to call upon the neurosurgical skills of Mr David Uttley, Professor David Thomas, Mr Sean O'Laoire and, latterly, Mr Henry Marsh. All have brought their expertise to bear on my patients, with great skill and success. My former neurophysiologist colleague, Dr Sam Bayliss, and the dedication and hard work of his senior technicians, Miss Kathy Spink and Miss Cindy Brayshaw, also deserve mention. I must also thank Dr Mary Hill for her interest and ability in the field of clinical neuropsychology. Much of my enormous workload has been shared by my clinical assistant of 14 years, Dr Jane Thompson, and her special interest in the care of the young chronic sick and patients with epilepsy has been much appreciated. The friendship and support of Dr William Gooddy during some difficult times in recent years has been invaluable.

I was originally asked to undertake this revision by the late Michael Jackson of Springer-Verlag, whose friendship and guidance were invaluable. Dr Gerald Graham took on his role and finally persuaded me, and now Dr Andrew Colborne has the thankless task of urging me to finish. Roger Dobbing and the production team at Springer have been outstanding in their attention to detail, ensuring the best possible location of the illustrations, tables and radiographs in the text. I am delighted with the end result.

Finally I must put on record my indebtedness to my wife, who in the last difficult 22 years has underwritten my efforts to continue coping with an almost impossible workload, as indeed have my children. I am delighted to say we have survived the experience!

John Patten

Contents

1. History-Taking and Physical Examination

By tradition, the first chapter in any textbook on CNS diseases deals with and stresses the vital importance of history-taking, and this necessity appears inescapable. Yet in neurology the history can be so critical, in indicating both the probable site and the possible nature of the lesion, that comprehensive coverage is impossible in a single chapter. The features of the clinical history appropriate to each region will be emphasized and will form a major part of each of the subsequent chapters. At this stage discussion will be confined to some broad generalizations.

The secret of good history-taking is to be a good listener. However rushed you may be, it is vital that the patient feels that he has the whole of your time and attention during the interview. You must also be constantly aware that the majority of patients are extremely frightened, even though their outward bahaviour may range from 'tongue-tied' tremulous anxiety to the blustering type who insists that he only came because his wife was worried about him! The patients requiring most care and caution are those who are self-effacing and apologetic for wasting your time, as with remarkable regularity these are the ones who actually do have a serious disease.

It is also essential to avoid the presumption that because the patient is in the neurological clinic they must have a disease and it must be neurological. This is an attitude that often prevails in medical schools, where not only is the impression given that every patient has a disease but that it is also likely to be a rare one. I doubt that any student will recollect ever being shown an interesting patient who had nothing wrong with them, even though a great many lessons can be learned from such patients.

The first consideration should be to determine whether the patient's symptoms suggest any particular disease. If the patient reads numerous unrelated symptoms from a three-page checklist the likelihood of serious disease rapidly diminishes, but every symptom must be analysed in detail. One of them may be significant, and surprisingly often it is the one considered least important by the patient.

Every effort should be made to put the patient at ease. Repeatedly looking at the clock, not looking up from the notes, avoiding eye contact or continually interrupting all put the patient at a disadvantage and reduce the chances of obtaining a coherent history. Several minutes spent discussing the weather, the news of the day, the patient's work or pastimes, may seem to be time-wasting to the uninitiated but the relaxation and the insight gained into the patient's mood, their reaction to the consultation and their intellectual ability is often better than can be obtained from several minutes of more formal testing or direct questioning embarked upon before the patient has had time to settle into the consultation.

When the patient is relaxed and talking freely, discussion of the actual symptoms can begin. The referral letter may be of help in guiding the questioning, but it is always important to ask the patient to relate the entire history again. Otherwise, half-digested views expressed by others may intrude into the history as facts rather than suppositions. Cross-checking the history with a relative or friend can be important. In diseases affecting the patient's consciousness or intellect the history may be confused or impossible to obtain without the help of a third party. If the patient wishes to have a friend or relative in the consultation with them, this should be welcomed. Their presence may not only improve the relaxed atmosphere but can lead to additional information of major importance. There is, however, a risk that the third party may become too involved, and if this gets out of hand you may feel more like a referee than a participant.

Patients may also understate the duration and severity of their disability, and a completely different story may emerge from enquiries made of the accompanying relative. These supplementary interviews may be best conducted in another room, while the patient is undressing. In the case of epileptic attacks in children parents are often loth to reveal the details of the ictal behaviour in front of the child, although I personally prefer to have the child in the room as they need to understand what happens to them: they are the ones that have to live with the problem, not the parents. Peculiar behavioural traits at any age clearly cannot be readily discussed in front of the patient, and a private interview with relatives, fellow employees and others in contact with the patient can be very instructive. Great difficulty occurs when relatives phone or write in advance of the consultation to reveal important facts that they would not be prepared to mention in front of the patient, with the proviso that under no circumstances must the patient find out what they have done. This may require the doctor to behave as if clairvoyant during the consultation, in an effort not to reveal prior knowledge while formulating appropriate questions to elicit the same information direct from the patient. This presents legal as well as ethical difficulties, when for example a patient suffering from epilepsy denies that they are having episodes, so that they can regain their driving licence, and relatives secretly reveal that they continue to have attacks.

In all cases an accurate sequential history of the entire course of the illness is essential. The diagnostic difference between weakness of an arm coming on overnight, over a week or over several months is so important that vague statements such as 'gradually' should never be accepted at face value. A clerk with a radial nerve palsy present on waking one Sunday morning was asked if he had been drinking. With considerable embarrassment he admitted that he had become drunk for the first time in his life the night before this occurred. Yet with this single question one could exclude a stroke (the diagnosis made elsewhere), and explain both the aetiology and the excellent prognosis of a 'Saturday night radial nerve palsy' to the relieved patient.

In other patients bizarre historical events may be deliberately concealed for fear of embarrassment or of moral judgements being made by the doctor. The onset of symptoms during sexual activity or related to alcohol over indulgence are frequently suppressed for this reason, and only direct questions may elicit the truth.

A consultant surgeon underwent two **normal** lumbar punctures and then four-vessel angiography rather than reveal that intercourse in his office during his lunch-break was the cause of his severe benign exertional migraine headache and not a subarachnoid haemorrhage – the diagnosis he preferred not to challenge! Similarly, the family of an elderly patient with periodic confusion and amnesia, who had been extensively investigated elsewhere with negative findings, was asked about her drinking habits. Initial angry denial was later retracted after a family conference, with the admission that her wardrobe was full of empty sherry bottles! Considerable tact is called for in such instances, and yet these personal matters must be pursued if unnecessary investigations and an incorrect diagnosis are to be avoided.

In neurological medicine, in addition to making the initial diagnosis, in many instances the doctor's role will be to help the patient accept and cope with what may prove to be a lifelong or even a progressive disability. Establishing a friendly, confident relationship at the first interview will help ensure a useful supportive role in the future. Some neurologists may feel that this role should be delegated to other carers, such as counsellors or trained nurses. It is difficult to see how this apparent lack of interest in following the patient will enable the novice neurologist to develop a soundly based knowledge of the natural history of the diseases in which they claim expertise. At a more practical level following patients in the clinic also reduces the chances of perpetuating a diagnostic error.

When the comment 'hopeless historian' is seen on the notes it is as much a comment on the doctor taking the history as it is on the patient. The interview must be tailored to suit the patient and the skill to do this can only be acquired, it cannot be taught. The ability to sit back and listen does not come easily to many, but it is only the eventual acceptance that one cannot force the pace of an interview without losing much of value that eventually leads to the realization that this is the only way to take a good history. Even the most anxious and inarticulate historian can be persuaded to divulge a wealth of useful information if sympathetically handled. An overt 'my time is valuable' attitude will lessen, rather than improve, the chances of obtaining a useful history and, even worse, produce a very dissatisfied and angry patient. Patients do not expect to be hectored or lectured when they have come for help, and the consultation should not be allowed to degenerate into a confrontation.

The circumlocutory historian and the patient who insists on including irrelevant detail can be the most trying of all. Any attempt to alter the line of questioning will start another chain of irrelevances. A good example is when the exact circumstances in which an event occurred lead to controversy as to which aunt was present and exactly which shop the patient was in when it happened! It is best to sit and listen and wait for the useful pieces of information to emerge. These are often the facts regarded as the least important by the patient.

Considering how infinitely variable symptoms can be, it is amazing how often patients eventually describe their feelings and symptoms in almost identical phrases. The diagnosis of several classic syndromes depends on typical symptom descriptions. For example, the 'red-hot needle' jabs of pain in tic douloureux; the 'déjà vu' associated with temporal lobe attacks, or the 'icy-cold bandage around the waist or legs' described by patients with spinal cord lesions. Some of these feelings are so bizarre that the patient hesitates to mention them for fear of being accused of imagining things, and the risk of asking somewhat leading questions must be accepted, when attempting to establish exactly what the patient is trying to describe. During medical training such emphasis is placed on avoiding leading questions that the ability to do so is seriously flawed, and yet unless such questions are asked the whole history of a patient referred with headache may finally consist of 'the patient has a pain in the head' as the sole information. If the patient has difficulty describing the quality of their symptoms it is perfectly acceptable to offer a selection of adjectives, in no particular order and with no particular emphasis, to see if they can select an appropriate description. Great care has been taken in all chapters to include the terminology actually used by patients, rather then the scientific terms used to describe symptoms. These can be utilized in history-taking and, as an example, the patient should be asked whether they have 'pins and needles' rather than whether they have 'paraesthesiae'.

Extremely disconcerting is the patient who prefaces every statement with 'to be absolutely truthful', which conveys the impression that they spend a lot of their time telling lies and that the history that they are giving has been carefully vetted and they will only disclose what they think is relevant and important, and that certain areas are 'off limits' for exploration. These patients also tend to avoid eye contact; such consultations can be time consuming and unrevealing and leave a definite feeling that there is a 'hidden agenda' which only time will reveal. An elderly cleric's wife with a 30-year history of atypical facial pain, gave such an impression. In view of the psychological basis of this disorder, attempts were made to see if there were any stresses that preceded or had operated over this enormous period of time. At the first consultation she admitted that there were and that all might be revealed in the future. Following a dramatic improvement with appropriate medication, on her third visit she revealed that her marriage had been a sham since her wedding day, when her husband revealed that he was an active homosexual and had only married her because that had been a requirement for his future in the church.

Perhaps the most intimidating of all is the patient who has made 'a few notes' to assist the interview and then produces a bundle of papers from a dauntingly large briefcase, which only the patient is allowed to read. Even the most relaxed doctor will find their eyes straying to the clock at frequent intervals. Listening intently, or insisting on being allowed to read the list oneself, and resigning oneself to the inevitable log-jam created in the clinic by the time the patient finally leaves the room, is the only possible approach to this difficult problem. Any attempt to divert the patient from their script will prove disastrous as they will not be deflected and you will only have to start again if you attempt to alter the course of the proceedings.

The above suggestions may not appeal to those who think that doctors ought not to adopt a passive role,

and who see themselves as too busy and much too important to be slowed down by vague patients. Such a person would be ill advised to embark on a career in neurology, where history-taking is the major skill.

A useful rule in neurology is that the more bizarre and unusual a symptom, the more likely it is to be organic. An arrogant approach, assuming that a symptom which is not known to the examiner must be functional or imaginary, is very likely to lead to misdiagnosis. It is dangerous to presume universal knowledge. While taking the history, a mental note should be made, as different features emerge, as to exactly how you will tailor the subsequent examination, to further evaluate the significance of that part of the history. Are there any signs that would confirm or refute that any particular symptom is significant?

Having exhausted the history of the present complaint and possibly yourself in the process, there are several further direct questions to be asked. These include the previous medical history, previous occupational history and the family history. The latter is of major importance in neurology, as the speciality encompasses an extraordinary range of inherited diseases which in many instances may not present until the patient is well into adulthood.

The past medical history should include any surgical procedures, with special attention to possible malignancy. Sometimes the patient was not told or has forgotten the malignant nature of their tumour or, even worse, the relatives know but not the patient. The treatment given may also be significant. Some patients who had deep X-ray therapy for seminoma 25 years ago are now presenting with a delayed myelopathy syndrome which mimics motor neuron disease. Delayed metastases up to 20 years after apparently successful surgery are not uncommon in lesions as diverse in their behaviour as malignant melanoma and thyroid carcinoma.

General medical conditions such as arterial disease obviously have neurological implications, and diabetes and the collagen vascular diseases can be associated with a multitude of complications, both of the disease itself and of its treatment, particularly in the latter instance with steroids and immunosuppressants. There are very few medical or surgical conditions that have not been associated with neurological complications. In the past, a previous history of venereal disease was extremely important because of the protean manifestations of neurosyphilis. These days the history must include details of the patient's sexual orientation when differential diagnosis indicates that this may be important, owing to the advent of AIDS, which has an even wider range of direct and indirect complications than was ever encountered with syphilis.

Any drugs used to treat any condition in the past may be significant. Two classic examples relate to the use of phenothiazines. Tardive dyskinesia may occur 20 years after the use of a major tranquillizer for an acute psychotic breakdown, and elderly patients with apparent idiopathic Parkinson's disease may be found to be taking prochlorperazine for 20 years, to prevent any recurrence of 'dizziness'.

Occupational exposure is perhaps of less importance now that the use of potentially hazardous substances in the workplace is more carefully regulated, but surprisingly brief periods of exposure may be forgotten and of significance. Previous asbestos exposure is one good example, and nasopharyngeal carcinoma related to wood dust has been correlated with only 6 months' employment in a furniture factory. Therefore, any occupation, however brief, should be included.

It has always been traditional to include alcohol and tobacco consumption in the routine questioning; sadly it is now necessary to include the illicit use of so-called 'recreational drugs', as both the type of agent and the method of administration may have neurological implications.

The family history is very important. The cause of death in deceased relatives, especially the parents, should be obtained. One of my patients, when asked the cause of death in her parents, said, 'I am not sure doctor, but I know it was nothing serious'. This is best defined as 'natural causes'! In those inherited diseases that present in childhood, such as Duchenne muscular dystrophy and Friedreich's ataxia, there are often living affected relatives, leaving little doubt. In conditions such as Huntington's chorea, which may begin in the 40s or 50s, the affected parent may have died many years previously, with the cause of death being concealed by the rest of the family; or the embarrassing possibility that the affected person was illegitimate may be revealed. Occasionally the recognition of an inherited disorder in one patient may lead to the discovery that several other affected family members around the country have had a variety of other incorrect diagnoses attached to their disability.

It is only at the stage of the physical examination that the full value of a careful history becomes apparent. If a full neurological examination were performed on every patient it would take up to an hour for its completion and would prove extremely boring, which increases the risk of missing a subtle physical sign. The history serves to indicate those parts of the examination that should be performed with special care, skill and finesse. Few would perform exactly the same physical examination on a patient complaining of headache as they would on one presenting with pain in the leg, and yet the ability to tailor the examination to suit the situation is based entirely on the history.

If a confident diagnosis of the site and probable nature of the lesion has not been made by the completion of the history, it is very unlikely that the diagnosis will suddenly become apparent during subsequent physical examination. Paradoxically, the most complete overall examination of the CNS is needed in those patients whose history suggests that it is unlikely that they have a neurological disease. This view must be supported by a careful comprehensive exclusory examination.

Having made a provisional diagnosis based on the history, the physical examination should be performed in a similar considerate way. A warm room with reasonable privacy is essential for a neurological examination. Although the doctor is accustomed to the sight of a tendon hammer and tuning fork, he must remember that the patient may not have seen either before. The anxious glances that patients always make towards the examination equipment as they climb on to the couch is graphic evidence of their level of anxiety. Always explain to the patient what is to be done before doing it. Suddenly flashing a light at the patient's eyes or sticking a pin into a limb without warning will not inspire confidence or cooperation. When eliciting plantar responses warn the patient that it will hurt. Patients will tolerate considerable discomfort if invited to do so, but do not take kindly to unannounced aggression! Elicitation of both the supinator and ankle jerks is quite painful for the patient, and yet some doctors repeatedly strike the tendons and wonder why the patient will not relax. Notes such as 'patient will not relax' or 'plantars impossible' usually indicate poor examination technique rather than an adverse comment on the patient's cooperation.

The best methods of performing the various parts of the neurological examination will be detailed in the following chapters. This will always be in the setting of diseases that will actually cause abnormalities that can be confirmed, or perhaps refuted, by the appropriate test.

The only way to understand the mechanism and correct elicitation of physical signs is in relation to situations where correct technique actually matters. For example, in a patient with backache correct testing of the corneal response may not be critical, but in a patient with a giddy attack, facial weakness or face pain, the sign must be understood and elicited correctly, as depression or absence of the corneal response may be the only physical sign of an underlying lesion in the cerebellopontine angle.

Throughout this volume emphasis will be placed on the recognition of the diagnostic features in the history, and the planning of the subsequent clinical examination to confirm or refute the provisional diagnosis at the bedside. The ultimate objective is to arrive at the correct diagnosis in the least number of moves. Even the advent of advanced imaging techniques has not diminished the importance of the history and clinical examination, as what to scan and how to interpret the findings still depends on the clinical diagnosis, which has been made purely on the basis of the history and the signs. Hence the dismay of neuroradiologists when asked to comment on an investigation without adequate clinical detail. However dramatic the advances in imaging and the use of databanks, it is unlikely that neurological skills will become extinct in the immediate future.

2. The Pupils and Their Reactions

Because of the long intracranial, intracerebral and extracranial courses of the nerve pathways that control the size and reactions of the pupils, lesions in many areas may cause pupillary abnormalities. Important differential diagnostic information may easily be overlooked by a cursory examination of the pupils, or unnecessary investigations may be performed when a physiological or pharmacological inequality in pupil size is mistaken for a physical sign. In the unconscious patient the size and reactions of the pupils are of paramount importance in both diagnosis and minute-to-minute management.

Basic Examination Technique

1. The size, shape and symmetry of the pupils in moderate lighting conditions should be noted.

2. The direct and indirect responses of the pupils to a bright light should be elicited. An inadequate light source is the most frequent cause of absence of the light reflexes: modern high-intensity flashlights should be used. The direct light reflex is the constriction of the pupil that occurs when it is directly illuminated. The indirect response or consensual light reflex is the simultaneous constriction of the opposite pupil. Make sure that the patient is looking into the distance to avoid the accommodation reflex constricting the pupils, and where appropriate close the blinds to lower the ambient lighting level.

3. The accommodation reaction should be tested. This is the constriction of the pupil that automatically occurs as the patient attempts to converge the eyes. Failure of this response is usually due to the patient's failure to converge. Convergence is most readily achieved if the patient tries to look at the end of their own nose, or at the examiner's finger brought in from below the level of the nose. The majority of people find it much easier to converge while looking downwards. It is helpful if the examiner holds the patient's eyelids so that the pupils can be easily observed (Fig. 2.1).

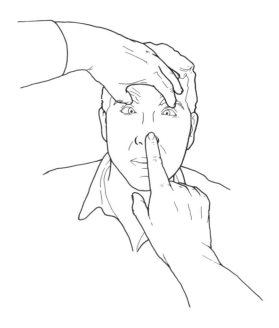

2.1   Correct technique for testing accommodation.

General Considerations

1. It is important to establish whether any drops have been put into the patient's eyes. Many patients have been investigated for what later proved to be pharmacological pupillary inequality because of a failure to observe this simple rule. It is also important to establish whether any drugs that may influence pupil size are being taken, either medically or illicitly. Previous surgical procedures on the eye may produce eccentric, dilated or small pupils.

2. If the pupils are unequal it is important to decide which one is abnormal. A frequent mistake is to investigate for the cause of a dilated pupil on one side, because the larger pupil is always the more impressive, when the patient actually has a constricted pupil on the other side due to a Horner's syndrome.

3. If the pupils are unequal in size there are two additional features that should help establish the cause:

- If there is ptosis of the eyelid on the side of the small pupil the patient has a Horner's syndrome on that side.
- If there is ptosis on the side of the large pupil the patient has a partial third nerve lesion on that side.

The light reflex and accommodation reflexes will be normal in a Horner's syndrome and impaired in a partial third nerve lesion. In the absence of ptosis if both pupils react normally to light and accommodation the patient probably has 'physiological anisocoria' and there has always been pupillary inequality. Many otherwise normal people have slight asymmetry in the size of the pupils, which only becomes of significance when they are examined by a neurologist.

4. Whenever a patient is found to have a widely dilated pupil that is fixed to light and accommodation without accompanying ptosis, the possibility that they have deliberately instilled atropine drops into the eye should always be considered. I have encountered this situation twice and both the patients were nurses. Instilling 1% pilocarpine drops into both eyes will confirm this. The pharmacologically blocked pupil will not constrict. Accidental scopolamine introduction into the eye from antinausea patches and splashed into the eyes of veterinary nurses has also occurred. The introduction of plants of the genus *Datura* (known in the USA as Jimson weed) into British gardens has provided a rich source of anticholinergic substances capable of causing fixed dilated pupils, as well as serious toxic confusional states in small children who accidentally come into contact with any part of the plant or eat the seeds.

5. Pupils are usually small in infancy, become larger in adolescence and are 'normal' size in adulthood. In old age they again become small and the light reaction increasingly difficult to see, especially in people with dark brown eyes. Many elderly patients have been incorrectly diagnosed as having Argyll Robertson pupils because of this normal change in pupil size with age, which is called 'senile miosis' (miosis = pupillary constriction; mydriasis = pupillary dilation).

6. The pupils of many patients show a phasic constriction and dilatation to light of constant intensity. This phenomenon is called 'hippus' and has no known pathological significance.

Pupil Size and Reactions

Pupil size is controlled by a circle of constrictor fibres innervated by the parasympathetic nervous system and a ring of radially arranged dilator fibres controlled by the sympathetic nervous system. The resting size of the pupil is governed by the amount of light falling on the eye and depends on the integrity of the parasympathetic nerves. Increased activity in the sympathetic nerves is reflected in slight pupillary dilatation, as occurs in an anxious patient. It is unusual for changes in pupil size to affect vision, so that the majority of pupillary abnormalities are asymptomatic. A fully dilated pupil on one side will not focus close up, and will cause blurring on attempted reading. Small pupils aid close focusing and are usually asymptomatic.

Parasympathetic Pathways (Fig. 2.2)

The neural activity related to the intensity of light falling on the retina is conveyed in the optic nerve to the optic chiasm. The impulses then decussate and are conveyed in **both** optic tracts to **both** lateral geniculate bodies. Only some 10% of the fibres reaching the geniculate bodies subserve the light reflex and are relayed in the periaqueductal grey to both Edinger–Westphal nuclei, and therefore light falling on either eye inevitably excites both nuclei, and causes constriction of both pupils – the anatomical basis of the consensual light reflex.

The Edinger–Westphal nuclei are also stimulated by activity in the adjacent third nerve nuclear mass, which controls the medial rectus muscles. Therefore when both medial rectus muscles are activated as the eyes converge, the Edinger–Westphal nuclei become active and constrict the pupils, further aided by the simultaneous contraction of the ciliary muscle. This is the basis of the accommodation reflex, which is a much more powerful stimulus to pupilloconstriction than the light reflex.

The parasympathetic fibres are carried in the third nerve to the orbit. They lie in a superficial and dorsal position on the nerve, which may explain the variable abnormalities of the pupil in third nerve palsies (to be discussed later; Fig. 2.2a).

The final relay of the parasympathetic pathway is in the ciliary ganglion, which lies in the posterior orbit on the branch of the third nerve to the inferior oblique muscle. The ganglion gives origin to eight to ten short ciliary nerves, which subdivide into 16–20 branches that pass around the eye to reach the sphincter pupillae. Only 3% of these fibres supply the pupillary musculature; the rest supply the ciliary muscle, which alters the shape of the lens for focusing.

Abnormalities of the Parasympathetic Pathway

1. The light reflex and the resting size of the pupil depend on adequate light perception by at least one eye. There is no direct light reaction in a completely blind eye, but the resting pupil size will be the same as that in the intact eye. If both eyes are blind both pupils will be dilated and fixed to light if the cause is located anterior to the lateral geniculate bodies.

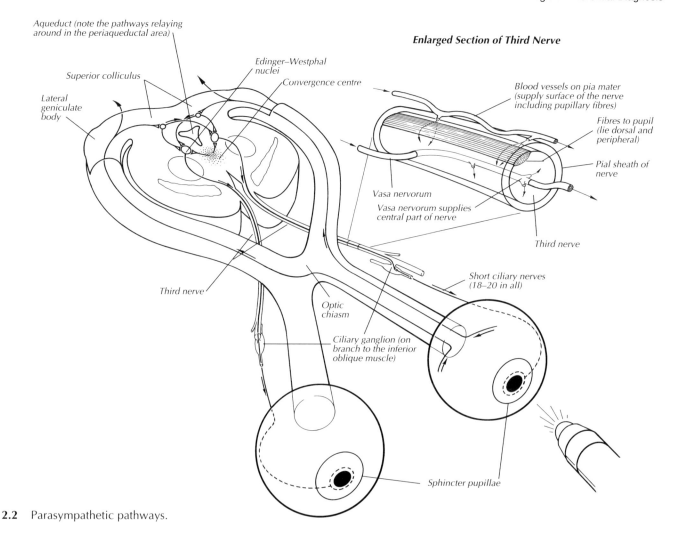

Aqueduct (note the pathways relaying around in the periaqueductal area)

Superior colliculus

Edinger–Westphal nuclei

Convergence centre

Enlarged Section of Third Nerve

Lateral geniculate body

Blood vessels on pia mater (supply surface of the nerve including pupillary fibres)

Fibres to pupil (lie dorsal and peripheral)

Pial sheath of nerve

Vasa nervorum

Vasa nervorum supplies central part of nerve

Third nerve

Third nerve

Short ciliary nerves (18–20 in all)

Optic chiasm

Ciliary ganglion (on branch to the inferior oblique muscle)

Sphincter pupillae

2.2   Parasympathetic pathways.

If bilateral blindness is the result of destruction of the occipital cortex the light reflex pathways will be intact. Therefore, it is possible for a patient to be completely blind and still have preserved light reflexes in both eyes. Furthermore, if there is any perception of light in an eye that is for practical purposes blind, the light reaction may well be preserved.

Minor lesions of the retina, optic nerve and chiasm and the optic tract, and in particular optic nerve damage due to multiple sclerosis, cause what is called an 'afferent pathway lesion'. This results in an abnormal pupillary response known as the Marcus–Gunn pupil. When the normal eye is stimulated by a bright light there is no abnormality; the pupil constricts and stays constricted. When the affected eye is stimulated the reaction is slower, less complete, and so brief that the pupil may start to dilate again while it is still illuminated. This is called the pupillary escape phenomenon. The reaction is best seen if the light is rapidly alternated from one eye to the other, each stimulus lasting about 2 or 3 seconds, with a second between. The normal pupil is seen to constrict and stay small, the abnormal pupil dilates instead of constricting as the

light falls on it. The is called the swinging light test. The reaction is thought to be due to a further reduction in the small number of fibres subserving the light reflex on the affected side, and can also occur in macular degeneration in the nearly blind eye.

2. A lesion of one optic tract does not affect the resting size of the pupil because of the consensual nature of the light reflex, but in this situation a better light reflex may be seen if the light is shone on the intact half of the retina (see Chapter 3 for details of the field defect). This is called the Wernicke pupil reaction. It is very difficult to elicit this sign owing to the inevitable dispersion of light within the eye.

3. Lesions compressing or infiltrating the tectum of the midbrain (the area of the superior collicular bodies) will interfere with the decussating light reflex fibres in the periaqueductal area. This results in pupils that are semidilated and fixed to light. This is often coupled with loss of upward gaze, and is then known as the Parinaud syndrome (see Chapter 7).

4. The Argyll Robertson pupil is also traditionally attributed to damage in the periaqueductal area and is a classic sign of neurosyphilis. When associated with

tabes dorsalis it is characteristically complicated by severe bilateral ptosis and marked overaction of the frontalis muscle to compensate. This produces a classic facial appearance. The typical Argyll Robertson pupil is small, irregular and fixed to light but reactive to accommodation. It is the latter feature that suggests that the light pathways leading to the Edinger–Westphal nuclei are damaged, but this cannot explain the small size of the pupil or its irregularity. It is also worth recalling that accommodation is a much stronger stimulus to pupilloconstriction than light, as there are many more fibres serving the accommodation reflex than the light reflex and the apparent dissociation may merely reflect very minimal pupil reactivity. It has been suggested that a local lesion of the iris might be responsible.

Other causes of what are perhaps incorrectly called Argyll Robertson pupils are pinealomas, diabetes, brainstem encephalitis, multiple sclerosis and Wernicke's encephalopathy. These conditions usually cause fixed semidilated pupils and sometimes unequal pupils; only a **small, irregular, fixed pupil** should be attributed to neurosyphilis. The Argyll Robertson pupil cannot be dilated by atropine, which supports the view that local factors are important in determining pupil size. This sign has become a neurological curiosity, as untreated syphilis is now so rare (Fig. 2.3). Other causes of small pupils that are apparently fixed to light include senile miosis and the use of pilocarpine or ß-blocker drops in the treatment of glaucoma.

5. Epidemic encephalitis lethargica, which last occurred in the 1920s, caused many cases of parkinsonism associated with loss of convergence. This disability resulted in pupils that reacted to light but not to accommodation, simply because the eyes could not converge. This 'reversed Argyll Robertson pupil' has become a clinical rarity, as there have been no epidemics in the last 70 years, although sporadic cases are occasionally reported.

6. Lesions affecting the third nerve may or may not involve the pupillary fibres. The pupillomotor fibres lie dorsally in the first segment of the nerve, rotate medially as the nerve passes through the cavernous sinus, and assume an inferior position as the nerve enters the orbit. They always lie superficially. Whether or not the pupil is involved is of great differential diagnostic value, and this will be discussed in detail in Chapter 5. At this point it is sufficient to note that if the nerve trunk itself is infarcted the superficially placed pupillary fibres may well be spared, as their blood supply is derived from the overlying pia mater.

As a general rule, if the pupil is affected the cause is surgical (i.e. compressive); and if spared, the cause is more likely to be medical (diabetes, cranial arteritis, arteriosclerosis, meningovascular syphilis or, particularly in the younger age groups, migraine). The whole

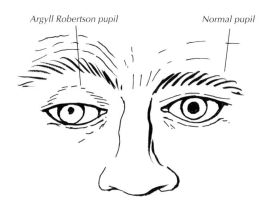

Argyll Robertson pupil　　　*Normal pupil*

Note: Ptosis, pupil is small, irregular, does not react to light but does to accommodation.

With 1% atropine solution in both eyes

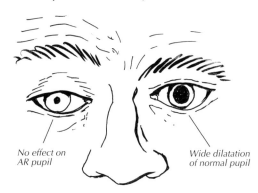

No effect on AR pupil　　　*Wide dilatation of normal pupil*

2.3 Argyll Robertson pupil. (For illustrative purposes, patient's left pupil is shown as normal. AR pupils are usually bilateral, although they can be asymmetrical.)

investigative approach to the patient with a third nerve lesion is influenced by the state of the pupil.

7. Degeneration of the nerve cells in the ciliary ganglion causes a Holmes–Adie or 'tonic' pupil. The cause of this condition is unknown, but a viral basis has been suggested. It is often associated with loss of knee jerks and impairment of sweating. Blurred vision for close work or eye pain in bright light commonly occurs. The Holmes–Adie pupil is a widely dilated circular pupil that may react very slowly, if at all, to very bright light and shows a more definite response to accommodation. This dissociation demonstrates the greater constrictive effect of accommodation. Both reactions are minimal and thought to be produced by a combination of slow inhibition of the sympathetic and partial reinnervation by parasympathetic fibres. The onset may be surprisingly acute, and a unique situation demonstrated this very graphically.

CASE REPORT I

A 41-year-old research scientist, specializing in visual pathway mechanisms, was involved in experimentation on his own eyes on a daily basis. He arrived at his laboratory one morning having developed a classic Holmes–Adie pupil overnight. The nature of his studies precluded any possibility that this had developed slowly.

The Holmes–Adie pupil is at first unilateral and more frequently found in females. It is often unnecessarily confused with Argyll Robertson pupils, which are small, irregular and usually bilateral. Chronic bilateral Holmes–Adie pupils may become progressively smaller and apparently fixed to light, but remain circular.

Congenital syphilis can cause fixed dilated pupils, but these are bilateral and other signs of congenital neurosyphilis will usually be found. Confirmation of the diagnosis of a Holmes–Adie pupil can be made by the pupillary response to 2.5% methacholine drops. This chemical is too rapidly hydrolysed by acetylcholine-sterase to have any effect in the normal eye. In the denervated pupil, denervation hypersensitivity (due to enzyme depletion) allows the pupilloconstrictor effect to be seen. However, 80% of diabetic patients react to methacholine in this way and 8% of normal subjects also show a response, and the test cannot be regarded as entirely specific for the Holmes–Adie pupil (Fig. 2.4). Furthermore, the solution has to be freshly made and is not readily available and this test has now been replaced by the use of 1.8% pilocarpine drops, which

Holmes–Adie pupil   *Normal*

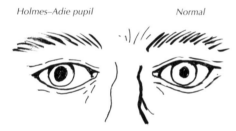

Note: No ptosis, pupil is large, regular, does not react to light (other than prolonged exposure) but may show some response to accommodation)

2.5% methacholine (mecholyl) in both eyes

The sensitized H–A pupil promptly constricts   *No effect on normal eye*

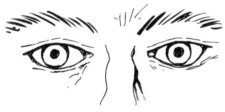

Holmes–Adie pupils are usually unilateral: another feature to distinguish them from the AR pupil

1.8% pilocarpine drops in affected eye
Pupil constricts   *Pupil constricts*

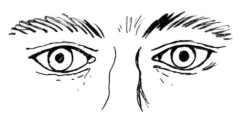

2.4   Holmes–Adie pupil.

are easier to obtain and produce the same response. If any doubt remains, slit lamp examination of the pupil will reveal wriggling and undulating movements of the edge of the iris in bright light.

8. Blunt trauma to the iris may disrupt the fine short ciliary nerve filaments in the sclera, causing an irregularly dilated pupil with impairment of the light reaction. A history of trauma is diagnostic. This is called post-traumatic iridoplegia (paralysis of the iris).

9 Diphtheria is now a rare cause of pupillary dilatation due to damage to the ciliary nerves. It usually occurred in the second and third weeks of the illness and was often combined with palatal paralysis. The pupillary abnormality usually recovered.

Confusing Causes of Ptosis

In assessing pupil size we have stressed the importance of ptosis as a parallel physical sign. In all instances where ptosis is detected it is important to remember some other causes of ptosis that may alter the significance of the finding.

1. Oedema of the eyelid due to infection, venous obstruction or allergy such as an insect bite, will all produce ptosis. This is best detected by looking at the thickness of the eyelid from below.

2. The ptosis may be congenital. It is worth looking at old photographs of the patient, because if it is long-standing and mild no-one may have ever commented on it. Passport photographs, being full-face, are best for this purpose.

3. The ptosis may be familial. Family photographs may be instructive, often revealing whole families sitting with their eyes half closed and looking down their noses at the photographer.

4. Myasthenia gravis should produce variable ptosis and should not affect the pupil, but in some instances the ptosis is remarkably static and occasionally unresponsive to an Edrophonium (tensilon) test, leaving diagnostic doubts until other features of the condition develop (see Chapter 18).

Sympathetic Pathways

The course of the cervical sympathetic pathway is shown in Figure 2.5. Although the pathway apparently starts in the hypothalamus there is a considerable degree of ipsilateral cortical control. A lesion anywhere in the pathway on the right side will affect the right pupil.

There are three neurons. The first passes from the hypothalamus to the lateral grey in the cervicothoracic spinal cord at levels C8 and T1, to the intermediomedial and intermediolateral cells, the ciliospinal centre of Budge. The second passes from the spinal cord to the superior cervical ganglion via the white rami of nerve roots C8 and T1. The third neuron, from the superior

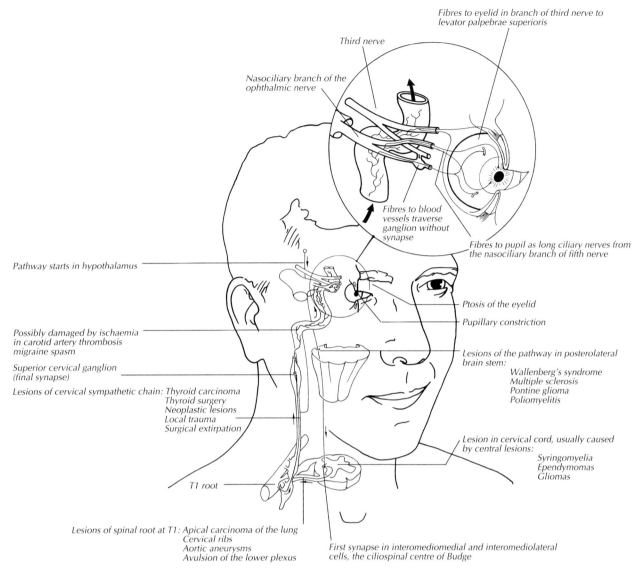

Fibres to eyelid in branch of third nerve to levator palpebrae superioris

Third nerve

Nasociliary branch of the ophthalmic nerve

Fibres to blood vessels traverse ganglion without synapse

Fibres to pupil as long ciliary nerves from the nasociliary branch of fifth nerve

Pathway starts in hypothalamus

Ptosis of the eyelid

Pupillary constriction

Possibly damaged by ischaemia in carotid artery thrombosis migraine spasm

Lesions of the pathway in posterolateral brain stem:
  Wallenberg's syndrome
  Multiple sclerosis
  Pontine glioma
  Poliomyelitis

Superior cervical ganglion (final synapse)

Lesions of cervical sympathetic chain: Thyroid carcinoma
  Thyroid surgery
  Neoplastic lesions
  Local trauma
  Surgical extirpation

Lesion in cervical cord, usually caused by central lesions:
  Syringomyelia
  Ependymomas
  Gliomas

T1 root

Lesions of spinal root at T1: Apical carcinoma of the lung
  Cervical ribs
  Aortic aneurysms
  Avulsion of the lower plexus

First synapse in interomediomedial and interomediolateral cells, the ciliospinal centre of Budge

2.5   Cervical sympathetic pathway. Showing the complete course of the sympathetic and pathological lesions and their sites of occurrence.

cervical ganglion, supplies the pupil and the blood vessels of the eye. The fibres enter the cranial cavity on the surface of the carotid artery and reach the eye and eyelid as follows:

1. Fibres carried in the third nerve innervate the superior and inferior tarsus muscles of Muller and orbitalis. These muscles assist eye opening by attachment to the tarsal plates, opposing the action of orbicularis. When paralysed, the upper lid is ptosed and the lower lid pulls up – so-called 'upside down' ptosis – narrowing the palpebral fissure and producing an apparent enophthalmos.

2. Vasomotor fibres in the nasociliary branch of the fifth nerve traverse the ciliary ganglion without synapse to supply the blood vessels of the eye.

3. Pupillodilator fibres on the nasociliary nerve continue by passing around the eye as the long ciliary nerves to innervate the pupil.

Abnormalities of the Sympathetic Pathway

A single physical sign results from damage to the cervical sympathetic pathway and is known as Horner's syndrome. Associated physical signs will often allow the location of the causative lesion in the long pathway to be identified. Horner's syndrome can be extremely subtle and is perhaps the most often missed sign; it is readily overlooked by the less than obsessional examiner. The features are as follows:

1. The affected pupil is slightly smaller than its fellow, owing to reduced pupillodilator activity. This asymmetry is minimal in a bright light and exaggerated in darkness. The pupil reacts normally to light and accommodation, but over a reduced range. It also redilates more slowly than the unaffected pupil.

2. There is a variable degree of ptosis of the eyelid. In severe cases the lid may reach to the edge of the pupil; in other patients the ptosis may be barely detectable and may vary from time to time during the day, owing to hypersensitivity to circulating catecholamines. On up gaze a full range of movement of the lid will be achieved by the intact third nerve-innervated musculature.

3. The eye may appear slightly bloodshot owing to a loss of vasoconstrictor activity to the vessels of the bulbar conjunctiva.

4. Sweating over the forehead or forequarter of the body may be impaired, depending on the site of the lesion (see later).

5. In congenital Horner's syndrome the iris on the affected side fails to pigment and remains a blue-grey colour. This is called heterochromia.

6. Enopthalmos (sunken eye) is not a detectable feature of Horner's syndrome in man: it is an optical illusion produced by the narrowed palpebral fissure.

Horner's Syndrome

Hemisphere Lesions

Hemispherectomy, massive infarction of one hemisphere or haemorrhage into the thalamus may all cause a Horner's syndrome on the same side.

Brainstem Lesions

The sympathetic pathways in the brain stem lie adjacent to the spinothalamic tract throughout its course. Therefore, Horner's syndrome due to a brainstem lesion is nearly always associated with pain and temperature loss on the opposite side of the body. Vascular lesions, multiple sclerosis, pontine gliomas and brainstem encephalitis may all cause a Horner's syndrome at this level (see Chapter 11). It is also likely to be associated with anhydrosis over the whole upper forequarter of the body.

Cervical Cord Lesions

Owing to the central position of the pathway in the lateral grey column at C8 and T1 level the sympathetic pathway is often involved in central cord lesions such as syringomyelia, glioma, ependymomas or the central cord syndrome following cervical cord trauma. These conditions will also cause loss of pain sensation in the arms, loss of arm reflexes and sometimes bilateral

Horner's syndrome. This can be very hard to detect because it is usually the ptosis that draws attention to the condition, the pupils being small but symmetrical and normally reactive to light and accommodation (see Chapter 15). Anhydrosis of the ipsilateral upper limb and face is often present with lesions at this level. The Horner's syndrome in these post-traumatic spinal cord lesions may vary from time to time and even alternate from side to side. The mechanism is uncertain.

Root Lesions at T1

The intraspinal T1 root is rarely affected by simple disc lesions or degenerative disc disease because this is a relatively non-mobile segment of the spinal column. The root outside the spinal canal lies on the apical pleura as it passes laterally, and is vulnerable to damage by primary or metastatic malignant disease. The classic syndrome of Pancoast, usually due to a carcinoma of the lung apex, consists of severe nocturnal pain in the shoulder and axilla, wasting of the small hand muscles and a Horner's syndrome, all on the same side. Other causes include cervical rib (usually in young females) and avulsion of the lower brachial plexus (Klumpke's paralysis) following traction injuries of the arm (see Chapter 16.) Aneurysms of the aortic arch and subclavian artery may damage the sympathetic at this level.

The Sympathetic Chain

Throughout its course in the neck the sympathetic chain may be damaged by neoplastic infiltration, during surgical procedures on the larynx, pharynx, thyroid, parathyroid, or surgically extirpated for a number of indications. Numerous carotid artery lesions may damage the sympathetic fibres lying on its surface. These include occlusion of the carotid artery, carotid artery dissection and during the course of migraine attacks, especially in cluster headache (see Chapter 20). Malignant disease in the jugular foramen at the skull base causes various combinations of Horner's syndrome with lesions of cranial nerves IX, X, XI and XII (see Chapter 6). Anhydrosis is rarely a feature of lesions at this level.

Miscellaneous Causes

Congenital Horner's syndrome has been described above. Lesions in the cavernous sinus or orbit usually damage both the sympathetic and the parasympathetic pathways simultaneously producing a semidilated pupil that is fixed to light, combined with other extraocular nerve palsies (see Chapter 5).

Other Features of Horner's Syndrome

The associated physical signs or history usually leave little doubt as to the site and cause of Horner's syndrome. There are some other useful diagnostic pointers. Central lesions usually affect sweating over the entire head, neck, arm and upper trunk on the same side. Lesions in the lower neck affect sweating over the entire face. Lesions above the superior cervical ganglion may not affect sweating at all, as the main outflow to the facial blood vessels and sweat glands is below the superior cervical ganglion.

The presence of three neurons in the pathway leads to some useful pharmacological tests based on the phenomenon of denervation hypersensitivity. The decrease in amine oxidase at the nerve endings caused by a lesion at or beyond the superior cervical ganglion sensitizes the pupil to adrenaline 1:1000, which has no effect on the normal pupil. The effect of cocaine on the pupil depends on its blocking effect on noradrenaline reuptake, therefore cocaine has no effect on a sympathetically denervated pupil at any level because no noradrenaline is available.

Both these tests have now been superseded by the instillation of 1% hydroxyamphetamine drops which release noradrenaline. If the lesion is preganglionic, noradrenaline is available, is released and the pupil dilates. If the lesion is postganglionic there is no noradrenaline and no response is seen. The pattern of responses is summarized in Figure 2.6.

It is worth stressing that Horner's syndrome with no demonstrable cause, even after extensive investigation and prolonged follow-up, is fairly common and the cause in 30% of cases remains obscure. Transient

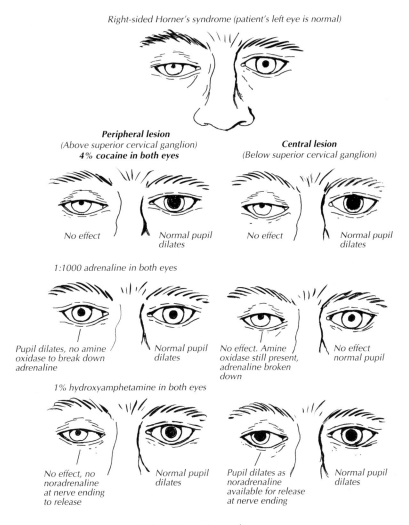

Right-sided Horner's syndrome (patient's left eye is normal)

Peripheral lesion
(Above superior cervical ganglion)
4% cocaine in both eyes

No effect   *Normal pupil dilates*

Central lesion
(Below superior cervical ganglion)

No effect   *Normal pupil dilates*

1:1000 adrenaline in both eyes

Pupil dilates, no amine oxidase to break down adrenaline   *Normal pupil dilates*

No effect. Amine oxidase still present, adrenaline broken down   *No effect normal pupil*

1% hydroxyamphetamine in both eyes

No effect, no noradrenaline at nerve ending to release   *Normal pupil dilates*

Pupil dilates as noradrenaline available for release at nerve ending   *Normal pupil dilates*

2.6 Horner's syndrome.

Horner's syndrome during ordinary migraine and cluster headache is very common and under-recognized.

Pupillary Abnormalities in the Unconscious Patient

The management of head injuries and the unconscious patient is fully discussed in Chapter 23. It is appropriate to consider the pupillary responses at this stage.

Normally Reacting Equal Pupils

In an unconscious patient normal pupils are a reassuring sign indicating that no life-threatening changes have occurred that require immediate surgical action. In the absence of a history of head trauma an immediate search for metabolic or pharmacological causes of coma should be initiated. Seventy per cent of unconscious patients have not had an intracranial catastrophe but are in diabetic coma, hypoglycaemic coma, other metabolic coma, or have taken a drug overdose. Normal pupillary reactions are an important pointer to these possibilities.

Unequal Pupils

This is the single most important physical sign in the unconscious patient. Until proved otherwise a dilated pupil indicates that a herniated temporal lobe is stretching the third nerve on that side and prompt treatment with steroids and/or mannitol is necessary while CT scanning and urgent surgical referral is arranged. Diagnostic problems can occur if the affected eye has been directly damaged in the injury, or if someone has unwisely put mydriatic drops in the eye in a fruitless search for papilloedema – fruitless because patients with acute head injury will die long before papilloedema appears. Any drops instilled into the patient's eye should be clearly documented in the notes. An immediate note of the exact pupil size and shape when the patient is first examined should be made routinely. This will be of vital importance in the subsequent monitoring of the patient's condition.

Bilateral Dilated Pupils

The final stage of progressive tentorial herniation is heralded by progressive dilatation of the previously unaffected pupil. The chances of the patient recovering if this stage is reached are poor. This is also one of the signs of irreversible cerebral damage following cardiac arrest. In spite of the poor prognosis in such cases full medical measures to lower intracranial pressure should be initiated, while scanning is used to determine whether any further useful action can be taken.

Pharmacological causes include glutethamide, anticholinergic and amphetamine-like agents. The following is an interesting and possibly unique example of autopharmacological fixed dilated pupils.

CASE REPORT II

At a time when some neurologists routinely treated head injuries by neuromuscular blockade and assisted respiration, an 11-year-old child was admitted following a head injury and treated in this way by a neurologist who happened to be in the hospital. Four hours later the neurologist on call was summoned to see the patient for the first time because the child had developed fixed dilated pupils and a blood pressure of 230/140. The intensive care unit had diagnosed coning. The odd feature was that the child's pulse was 160, which is not consistent with this diagnosis. It was suggested that the neuromuscular blockade be reversed because it seemed more likely that the child had regained consciousness and that the physical findings represented massive adrenaline outpouring in a terrified child. By the time the on-call neurologist arrived at the hospital 15 minutes later, the child was fully conscious, the pupils were reactive and the blood pressure was 120/80. Fortunately the child had no recollection of these events and made an uncomplicated recovery and was discharged from hospital in 48 hours.

Bilateral Pinpoint Pupils

This finding is the hallmark of another lethal neurological situation: a massive intrapontine haemorrhage. This is usually characterized by sudden collapse and the development of pinpoint pupils, deep coma and a spastic tetraparesis with brisk reflexes. Opiates produce similar pupillary abnormalities but cause depressed reflexes. In the elderly unconscious patient the possibility that pilocarpine drops have been instilled as treatment for glaucoma should also be considered, in view of the hopeless prognosis if intrapontine haemorrhage has occurred. If pilocarpine has been used other causes of coma should be rapidly excluded. This can normally be achieved by CT scanning, as such haemorrhages are readily detectable.

Pupillary Change due to Drug Intoxication

1. Small miotic pupils: narcotics, phenothiazines, alcohol and barbiturates may all cause small and therefore inevitably poorly reactive pupils, unless a very bright light and a lens are used for the examination.
2. Large mydriatic pupils: atropine, scopolamine, amphetamines, marijuana, LSD, Ecstasy, cocaine and glutethamide may all cause dilated pupils and altered mental state. As noted earlier, atropine poisoning from datura plants, poisonous mushrooms or belladonna should be considered in children with a toxic confusional state and fixed dilated pupils, which is the diag-

nostic clue to these conditions. In any confused, unconscious or behaviourally abnormal patient drug intoxication should always be considered, and the state of the pupils may be the most important clue as to the type of substance involved.

The pupils should always be examined with the special problems of the particular patient in mind. In this way there is less risk of a subtle abnormality being overlooked and the risk of unnecessary investigation of physiological variations is greatly reduced. As an aide mémoire to diagnosis Table 2.1 details the major pupillary abnormalities and likely causes.

Table 2.1 Pupillary abnormalities

Reaction	Small (miotic) pupils	Large (mydriatic) pupils
Non-reactive to light	Argyll Robinson pupils (usually irregular)	Holmes–Adie (will slowly react to (very bright light)
	Pontine haemorrhage – may react with very bright light (observed by using magnifying lens)	Post-traumatic iridoplegia
		Mydriatic drops
		Atropine drops
	Opiates	Overdose
	Pilocarpine drops	Glutethamide
		Amphetamine
		Cocaine or derivatives
		Poisoning
		Belladonna
		Datura (jimson weed)
		Brain death
Reactive to light	Old age	Childhood
	Holmes–Adie pupil (in constricted phase)	Anxiety states
	Horner's syndrome	Physiological anisocoria
	Anisocoria (physiologically smaller)	
	Inflammatory disease of the iris (usually irregular)	

3. Vision, the Visual Fields and the Olfactory Nerve

The visual pathways extend from the retina to the occipital pole. Part of their course is extracerebral and part in the substance of the hemisphere. Due to the complex but constant decussations and rotations of nerve fibres in the visual pathways, visual field defects can provide very accurate localizing information. Patients tend to notice abrupt visual deterioration and may present with a detailed description of their defect, whereas defects of insidious onset often develop unnoticed.

CASE REPORT I

A 43-year-old headmaster of an approved school in Kenya presented after two accidents where he had run into pedestrians walking by the road on his left-hand side. He had insidiously developed a left homonymous hemianopia which proved to be due to a right temporal lobe glioma, and he died following biopsy.

CASE REPORT II

A 63-year-old woman was arrested by the police following three road traffic accidents in a 2 week period during which she had struck parked vehicles on her left-hand side. She had been unaware of these collisions and had wondered who had damaged her car. A witness to one of these events reported her to the police. A left homonymous macular splitting hemianopia was detected and found to be due to an occipital lobe glioma. She unfortunately died 6 months later, following excision and radiotherapy.

A routine examination of the optic fundus, visual acuity and visual fields should be made in all patients with neurological disease. It is unwise to assume that the patient's visual fields are normal because no visual symptoms have been noted. At the opposite extreme, patients' with seriously impaired vision require very careful field testing, however difficult this may be to perform.

CASE REPORT III

A 70-year-old man had been attending the eye clinic with progressive visual failure over 1 year. Because of the severity of the visual failure his visual fields had not been documented at the early attendances. He was finally referred for a neurologi-

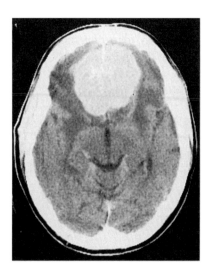

CRIII. *Meningioma compressing the optic chiasm.*

cal opinion when vision was less than 6/60 in both eyes. In spite of poor visual acuity, confrontation field testing revealed a bitemporal hemianopia. Investigation revealed an enormous subfrontal meningioma compressing the optic chiasm. Successful removal unfortunately produced only minimal recovery of visual function. However, a dramatic improvement in his personality, which had altered considerably over several years, was noticed.

In any part of the neurological examination signs are more readily detected if the examiner has some idea as to what he might find, or what he must exclude. The technique and use of confrontation field testing at the bedside is therefore described in detail later, in relation to the various clinical situations in which field defects may be anticipated.

It is also appropriate to consider the olfactory nerve in this setting. Its close proximity to the roof and medial wall of the orbit, its close relationship to the optic nerve and chiasm and its final division just above the optic tract, means that organic lesions of the olfactory pathway have a high likelihood of also affecting the pregeniculate visual pathway. The course, relations and clinical disorders of the olfactory nerve are therefore included at the end of this chapter.

Visual Acuity

Visual acuity is documented in Europe as 6/6–6/60, where the test distance is 6 m. In the USA it is documented as 20/20–20/200, reflecting the test distance of 20 feet. The size of the print is arranged so that each letter subtends an angle of 1° of an arc at that distance. The letters in the 6/60 line are therefore ten times larger than the letters of the 6/6 line. Patients with field defects or scotomas (blind areas) may need to move their eye around to identify individual letters. Provided that they ultimately identify the letter correctly with that eye, this is permissible. The smallest line that the patient can read is documented as the visual acuity, and if at least half the letters on a line are correctly identified it should be recorded as 'part'; for example '6/12 pt' shows that the patient successfully identified at least four letters on the 6/12 line. Whether or not the patient was wearing glasses and whether refractive error was excluded by reading the chart through a pinhole should be documented. Sequential documentation of the visual acuity provides very accurate evidence of improvement or deterioration in vision, and should be recorded routinely at all subsequent visits

Colour Vision

Colour vision is especially important in neuro-ophthalmology in the detection of pregeniculate pathway lesions. For reasons that are not clear, the visual field to a red object is strikingly affected by damage in these pathways. If a patient with impaired visual acuity can still detect a red object a pregeniculate nerve pathway lesion is unlikely. Conversely, the earliest evidence of a pituitary lesion may be a bitemporal hemianopia, specifically to a red object. Similarly an optic tract lesion may produce an incongruous hemianopic defect to red (see later). To detect other abnormalities of colour vision Ishihara colour plates remain the standard test, those patterns requiring accurate perception of red being of particular value to the neurologist.

Visual Fields

Confrontation Testing of the Visual Fields

The results of confrontation testing are often recorded in clinical notes somewhat disparagingly as 'fields grossly normal', as if the test were a poor substitute for more accurate testing. In skilled hands confrontation testing can be as accurate as screen or perimeter testings, and in some situations may be the only way the fields can be tested. These situations include the examination of patients with a seriously disturbed mental state, physical disability preventing the patient from sitting at the apparatus, or a dense central field defect that prevents the patient fixing a target object, which is necessary to keep the eye still during field testing.

When testing patients with greatly reduced visual acuity qualitative tests of the fields utilizing hand movements and finger counting can **only** be performed by confrontation methods. The standard shorthand for documenting these findings on a field chart is HM (hand movements only detected) and CF (count fingers in affected area). These abbreviations are used on the illustrations in this chapter.

The Technique (Fig. 3.1)

For accurate field testing red and white hatpins of 5 mm and 10 mm diameter are ideal. Routine screening is usually performed with a 10 mm white pin. The smaller pins are useful for detecting small scotomata (small field defects in the centre of the visual fields). The red pins are especially useful in testing visual fields where a compressive lesion of the optic nerve, optic chiasm or optic tract is suspected.

1. The examiner should sit opposite the patient, ideally in a chair but, where circumstances demand, leaning across the bed in front of the patient. Each eye is tested individually, and if the examiner routinely holds the patient's other eye shut with his hand held at arm's length, a constant examiner–patient distance is established. An idea if the size of the normal field at this distance is readily acquired and skill in detecting early peripheral field defects is quickly achieved.

2. Throughout the test the patient is asked to look straight at the examiner's eye (the right eye when testing the patient's left eye, and vice versa). This ensures that the patient holds the eye still during testing. If the patient cannot see the examiner's eye, they are asked to stare in the direction of the examiner's face while an assessment of the peripheral visual field is made. The examiner is in the ideal position to see if the patient has to move his eye to find the test object.

3. The test pin, usually the 10 mm white one, is brought in along a series of arcs to a point some 18 inches in front of the patient's eye. If an arc from behind were not used the patient's temporal field would extend to infinity if the test object was large enough. The pin should be brought in from 'round the corner' of the patient's field from four directions, NE, SE, SW and NW. This will be bound to pick up any field defect in either the upper or the lower temporal or nasal fields. The object should be moved in quite quickly. If it is moved too slowly very few patients can resist the temp-

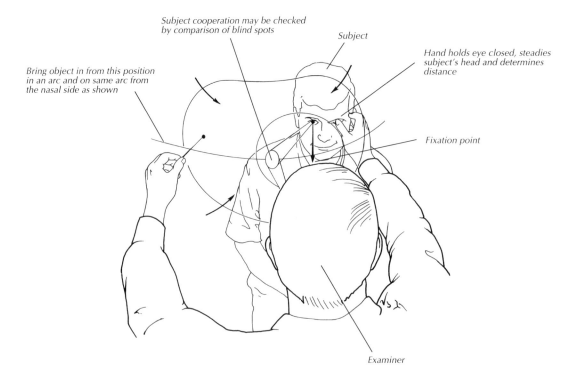

Subject cooperation may be checked by comparison of blind spots

Subject

Hand holds eye closed, steadies subject's head and determines distance

Bring object in from this position in an arc and on same arc from the nasal side as shown

Fixation point

Examiner

3.1   Visual field testing by confrontation.

tation to shift their gaze to look for it as they anticipate its likely location.

4. The close control that the examiner has over the whole proceedings enables quick repeat testing to be performed, and 'pseudo' field defects due to bushy eyebrows, ptosis of the eyelid or a large nose are easily identified. Quite often field defects due to such problems are accidentally recorded on a standard perimeter. Merely tilting the patient's head from the line of the obstructing organ will solve this problem.

5. If any defect is difficult to interpret on an organic basis, as a cross-check on the patient's cooperation and reliability the patient's blind spot can be found and directly compared with the examiner's own blind spot. With practice it should be possible to identify the patient's blind spot and confirm that in both its lateral and vertical extent it is identical to that of the examiner.

The results of confrontation testing are conventionally recorded as seen by the patient, which means reversing the defect as seen by the examiner during confrontation testing. To further avoid confusion the right and left fields should be clearly indicated and a factual note added as to the nature of the field defect discovered, such as a right homonymous hemianopia, or a bitemporal upper quadrantic hemianopia. The correct use of the different terms is illustrated in Figure 3.2.

More sophisticated tests, which are time-consuming and not possible at the bedside, are available and are mainly used in ophthalmology, these include:

- Amsler chart – best for detecting defects due to macular or retinal disease. This consists of a geometric grid which is placed in front of the patient's eye. In retinal disease the vertical and horizontal lines distort (metamorphopsia), in optic nerve disease part of the grid will disappear or become blurred.

- Tangent (Bjerrum) screen testing – best for identifying defects in the central 25° of vision and the method of most value to neurologists. Its use is discussed in detail in the next section.

- Goldman perimeter – a highly sophisticated illuminated dome with projected coloured light dots giving a highly accurate delineation of unusual defects such as arcuate scotomata; essential in neuro-ophthalmological practice but beyond the scope of the present volume.

Tangent Screen Test (Bjerrum Screen)

The tangent screen is a black cloth screen marked like a target with rings subtending 5° at 2 m (or 6 feet). Each eye is tested separately. An assortment of coloured discs – white and red being the most import-

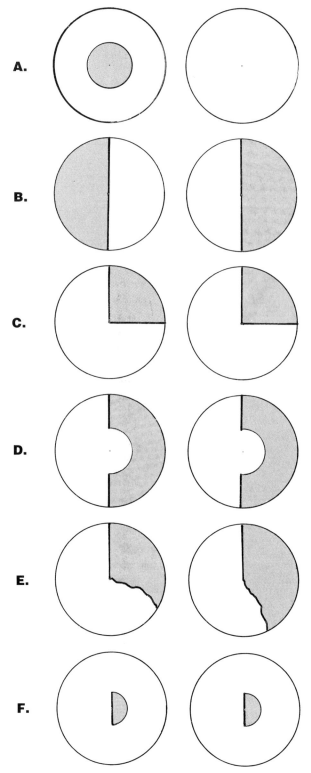

A. *Left central scotoma (optic nerve nerve lesion)*
B. *Bitemporal hemianopia (chiasmal lesion)*
C. *Right upper quadrantic hemianopia (left temporal lobe lesion)*
D. *Macula-sparing hemianopia (left calcarine cortex lesion)*
E. *Incongruous right hemianopia (lesion of optic tract)*
F. *Right homonymous hemianopic scotoma (lesion of tip of occipital pole)*

3.2   Field defect nomenclature.

ant in neurology – of differing diameters are mounted on a black wand. If the patient's visual acuity permits, they are asked to stare at a white spot in the centre of the target. This is the first disadvantage of this technique, as testing is almost impossible if the patient cannot fix, although a more substantial object may be substituted at the centre of the target if necessary.

The object is then brought in from the edge of the screen, or taken out from the centre, to explore the visual field in all directions from fixation (the centre of the visual field). The size of the object can be increased or decreased, making it possible to demonstrate whether the defect is relative or complete. A complete defect will be steep-sided and no object, however large, is seen within the area marked; this can be marked on the screen with chalk. A slope-sided defect will demonstrate a zone around the edge of the defect where a progressively smaller object can be detected before the field becomes normal. In post-geniculate lesions a steep-sided instant transition edge of the defect will be found. In pregeniculate lesions a slope-sided defect that is more marked to a red object may be found.

Accurately documented on a standard recording sheet, sequential studies of the tangent screen visual fields can form a valuable permanent record of changes in the visual fields. This is still of value where a small pituitary lesion has been detected and surgery has been deferred until visual difficulties are encountered. This is cheap and easily reproducible, and may reduce the need for frequent and more expensive scanning. This is of particular value with prolactin-secreting tumours, where the other symptoms can be controlled pharmacologically and the only definite indication for surgery is progressive visual impairment. The beginnings of a bitemporal defect to red can be more definitive in taking this decision than scanning.

Application of Confrontation Testing to Specific Clinical Situations

The Patient Who Has Noticed a 'Hole' in His Vision

Small scotomas are often noticed by accident when the patient is reading a notice or looking at a clock (a scotoma is a small patch of visual loss within the visual field). The onset always appears to be abrupt, as it is noticed suddenly by the patient. An exception occurs when an embolus impacts in the central retinal artery and then moves peripherally. Abrupt blindness followed by a diminishing deficit can usually be described on a minute-to-minute basis by an intelligent patient, which leaves no doubt as to both the acuteness of onset and the nature of the problem. When evaluating a patient with this symptom it is best to allow the patient to find the defect himself by moving the white pin about in his own visual field. Once the position is found the size and shape of the defect can be established by moving the pin in and out of the blind area.

Special attention should be paid to whether:

1. The defect crosses the horizontal meridian. Retinal lesions due to a vascular occlusion cannot do so
2. The defect extends to the blind spot. Defects due to B_{12} deficiency, toxins or glaucoma usually extend into it. This is called a caecocentral scotoma
3. The defect crosses the vertical meridian. Organic visual field defects due to pathway damage have a sharp vertical edge at the midline.

In all cases it is vital to check that there is not an identical defect in the opposite eye that the patient has not noticed. As a general rule patients are much more likely to notice the defect in their temporal field than that in the much smaller nasal field. Homonymous hemianopic scotomas may be missed unless this rule is followed.

The Patient with 'Blurred Vision in One Eye'

The examiner should ask the patient to look in the general direction of his eye if the patient's visual acuity is too poor to actually see it. Then, working outwards from the defect with a 10 mm white pin, the examiner should try to establish the size and shape of the scotoma. If the pin is not seen at all, two or three fingers held still should be tried, and finally, if all else fails, a moving hand should be brought in from the periphery. If the examiner can establish that there is a rim of intact peripheral vision, however poor it is, then the patient has a central scotoma, usually implying either retrobulbar neuritis or optic nerve compression (see below). Once a central scotoma in one eye is detected it is essential to test the peripheral field of the other eye, looking for a defect in the upper temporal field. If such a defect is present, it is highly likely that the optic nerve is compressed (see Fig. 3.11 for explanation) the central $5°$ circle of vision is responsible for the 6/6 acuity. The peripheral retina can only see 6/60, hence the dramatic effect on vision of an apparently small central scotoma.

The Patient with Sudden Visual Deterioration in Both Eyes

Acute bilateral inflammation of the optic nerve (retrobulbar neuritis) may occur but is unusual. The two important conditions to be excluded are severe bilateral papilloedema due to any cause, or the rapidly progressive phase of visual deterioration in a patient with optic chiasmal compression.

Papilloedema alone should not affect central vision, but if a haemorrhage or exudate occurs into the macula area of the retina rapid visual failure will occur. This possibility can be readily excluded by fundal examination.

If sudden deterioration occurs in the course of an ongoing visual failure ophthalmoscopy will often reveal the presence of optic atrophy. If optic atrophy is found to be already present when the patient first notices visual impairment, it implies some degree of chronicity and, however poor the visual acuity, the fields must be carefully tested.

Chiasmal compression may be misdiagnosed as retrobulbar neuritis or tobacco amblyopia if field testing is omitted. Patients with chiasmal compression often develop severe but unrecognized bitemporal field defects and seek advice only when central vision becomes acutely impaired. If a bitemporal field defect is detected urgent investigation to exclude a lesion compressing the optic chiasm is mandatory. The following is a good example of this situation.

CASE REPORT IV

A 36-year-old woman had been investigated for infertility and subsequently became pregnant following the use of clomiphen. During the pregnancy she became toxaemic, with a blood pressure as high as 200/120. In the 34th week she developed rapidly progressive visual failure thought to be due to the hypertension. On neurological examination both optic discs were pale but there was no suspicion of papilloedema or haemorrhage into the maculae. Although visual acuity was less than 6/60, using hand movements and finger counting it was obvious that there was dense bitemporal hemianopia indicating chiasmal compression. The child was delivered by caesarean section immediately and the chiasm explored the next day. The remnants of a pituitary tumour were found admixed with blood clots. Following decompression her vision became normal and the premature infant developed normally. Any delay in recognition of the clinical situation could have resulted in permanent blindness. This patient was seen in 1973, before scanning was available.

Testing for a bitemporal field defect involves the standard routine except that the use of a red pin is particularly helpful. The ultimate typical defect resulting from damage to the chiasm is a bitemporal hemianopia. In the early stages this may be a defect to a red object only. The patient may describe the red pin as appearing to be grey in the affected half field, changing to red as it crosses into the intact nasal half field. It is important to be aware that most normal people notice that the red pin is a duller red in the temporal field and that it is appreciably brighter in the nasal field; this is a physiological variation without significance. In the early stages of chiasmal compression the temporal defect to a red pin may only affect the upper or lower quadrant, depending on the direction of compression (see below). Later in the course of the disease the defect will extend to include not only loss of vision for a red pin in the affected half field, but also progressive loss of appreciation of a white pin in the temporal fields, and finally finger and even hand movements will not be detected, as the defect becomes complete.

Even at this late stage, if the chiasm is compressed from below by a pituitary lesion the upper half of the temporal field may be completely lost, but some hand movements may be detected in the lower half field, or conversely in the case of chiasmal compression from above and behind by a craniopharyngioma (see Figs. 3.6 and 3.13 for explanation). This was the situation in the third case report at the beginning of this chapter, a meningioma compressing the chiasm from above.

The Patient Who Complains of 'Difficulty in Reading' or 'Bumps into Things on One Side'

Quite often patients attend hospital aware that something is wrong with their vision but unaware that they have a dense homonymous field defect. Many of these patients insist they are blind in one eye because they cannot see to that side, and persist in attempts to get glasses to improve vision in their 'bad' eye, long after detailed attempts to explain the binocular nature of their defect to them have failed to convince them that glasses will not help. Blindness in one eye causes impairment of distance perception but the good eye provides a full field of vision to both sides and they do not bump into things (see Case report later).

Patients complain bitterly that they cannot read if the visual defect splits the midline. If they have a left-sided field defect they cannot find the beginning of the next line, or if the defect is on the right side reading may prove impossible as they cannot scan along the line to the next word. At a more serious level, repeated traffic accidents may occur before the problem is recognized.

In general, if the patient is aware of his visual defect it is likely that the defect is macular splitting as it bisects the central field. If the patient is unaware of a deficit and merely bumps into things, he may have a macular sparing hemianopia or an attention hemianopia. The latter is not an absolute defect but an inability to see in one half field when vision is distracted by an object in the other half field.

Testing for a homonymous hemianopia should involve three phases:

1. The examiner should test for an attention field defect. The examiner sits in front of the patient, who should keep both eyes open; each of the examiner's hands should be held about 1 foot to the side and 18 inches in front of each of the patient's eyes. The patient is then asked to point to either hand when he

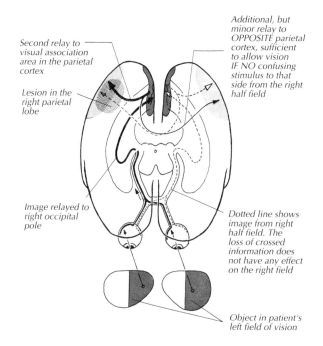

Second relay to visual association area in the parietal cortex

Lesion in the right parietal lobe

Image relayed to right occipital pole

Additional, but minor relay to OPPOSITE parietal cortex, sufficient to allow vision IF NO confusing stimulus to that side from the right half field

Dotted line shows image from right half field. The loss of crossed information does not have any effect on the right field

Object in patient's left field of vision

3.3   Possible explanation of attention hemianopia.

sees the fingers move. At first just one hand at a time should be moved. If the patient consistently fails to see the hand on one side he may well have a full hemianopia, but if he sees the fingers move on one hand when they are moved alone, but consistently fails to see them when both hands are moved simultaneously, he has an attention hemianopia. The anatomical basis for this finding is shown in Figure 3.3. Further information may be gained from the spinning drum test to demonstrate optokinetic nystagmus (see also Chapter 7). This is the same as so-called 'railway nystagmus', where the eye follows an object until it goes out of range and then quickly moves back to pick up the next object, producing a form of pursuit nystagmus. It depends on the integrity of the parietal lobe and is often abolished in a parietal lobe lesion. A drum with a series of vertical black lines on a white background is rotated in front of the patient's eyes. If the patient has a right parietal lesion the nystagmus will be absent when the drum is rotating to the right and intact when rotating to the left. It is an ipsilateral phenomenon.

2. Formal testing of the whole field in each eye by the standard confrontation technique using a white pin should then be performed to establish whether the patient has a homonymous field defect on one side or the other.

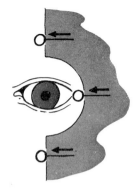

"Macular-Sparing"

Note that the pin is seen to the side of the mid-line when the macular is spared

The pin is brought in from the blind field. This prevents the patient shifting gaze to follow the pin, making it difficult to detect the midline position

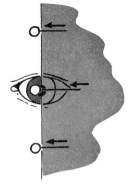

"Macular-Splitting"

If the patient and examiner are exactly aligned the pinhead comes into view exactly in the midline of the pupil as shown

3.4   Detection of macular sparing during confrontation field testing.

3. The field must then be re-evaluated to see if the defect is 'macular splitting' or 'macular sparing'. This is of considerable diagnostic and prognostic importance. Basically, one is looking for a small 5° circle of retained vision in the centre of the hemianopic field. The pin is brought across the midline above and below the centre of vision to detect the midline of the field. Then the pin is brought across on the central meridian. If the pin is detected on the same line as the first two points then the defect splits the macula . If it is about 1.5–2 inches to the side of the midline then the macula is spared (Fig. 3.4). The importance of this distinction is discussed later and is of major diagnostic significance. Confrontation testing will establish the basic defect. If there is any doubt about the central field, further field testing using the tangent screen or an arc or bowl perimeter, is necessary.

Visual Evoked Responses (VER)

In the investigation of visual pathway disease VERs have proved a major advance in demonstrating and quantifying pathway lesions. The simplest and most used technique is for the patient to sit 1 m from a chequerboard pattern, the black and white squares alternating every 1–2 seconds. Potentials are recorded over the occipital area by three electrodes over a 300 m.sec time base and the resulting potential is averaged from 100 or more stimuli. A large biphasic slow wave is recorded and the latency to the first wave, the P100, and its amplitude are measured. There is no universal standardization and norms have to be estab-

lished for each apparatus. The P100 is usually between 95 and 110 m.sec, any prolongation indicating delay, mainly in the pregeniculate pathway. The shape and size of the potential can be compared side to side and with established norms.

The investigation has proved to be a relatively inexpensive, reproducible and reliable technique, and until the advent of MRI scanning was the linch pin investigation in the diagnosis of multiple sclerosis, having the advantage of detecting residual evidence of an optic nerve lesion that occurred many years before. It provided confirmation where there was suspected 'disc pallor' which was so often used as evidence of an additional lesion elsewhere in the nervous system in suspected multiple sclerosis. This sometimes had unfortunate consequences when spinal cord compression was missed because of this unconfirmed suspicion. Abnormal VERs gave sufficiently reliable support to avoid myelography. The importance of VERs has been somewhat reduced since the advent of MRI scanning where it is available. They can also be of value in confirming non-organic visual loss. If the patient looks in the direction of the screen and flash stimuli are used normal responses will be deteched if vision is intact.

Anatomy of the Visual Pathways

To understand field defects one must understand the apparently intricate anatomy of the pathways. Yet the course of the pathways makes considerable sense once understood, and the details become easy to remember.

1. The macula of the retina (the most important group of retinal cells, responsible for central vision) is situated to the temporal side of the optic nerve head (it is not the nerve head itself, which is a popular misconception). The fibres from the macula have to shift sideways en masse to get into the appropriate position in the optic nerve. This causes the macular fibres to crowd into the temporal half of the disc (Fig. 3.5).

2. The macular fibres gradually move centrally into the optic nerve and complete the shift to the centre of the nerve as it joins the chiasm. The optic nerve is then effectively split down the middle. The lateral fibres go straight back into the optic tract on the same side and the medial fibres cross (decussate) to the other side. They do so in a specific pattern, which is fully discussed later. The function of the chiasm is to bring the information from the halves of each retina that look to the right and the halves that look to the left together in the same optic tract (Fig. 3.6).

3. When the information derived exclusively from the left or right side of vision arrives in the optic tract it is

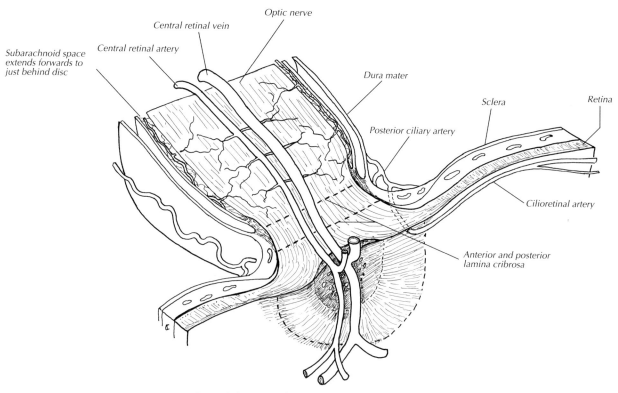

Subarachnoid space extends forwards to just behind disc

Central retinal artery

Central retinal vein

Optic nerve

Dura mater

Sclera

Retina

Posterior ciliary artery

Cilioretinal artery

Anterior and posterior lamina cribrosa

3.5 Schematic diagram to show the optic nerve head.

initially conveyed in the inner and outer halves of the tract, duplicating the pattern in the optic nerves. Information from the same point on each retina must be relayed to immediately adjacent parts of the visual cortex. This process starts with the rotation of the fibres in the optic tract inwards through 90°. This brings the fibres from the lower and upper fields together in the medial and lateral halves of the tract respectively. Then in the posterior tract the fibres fan out towards the six layers of the geniculate body, as shown in Figure 3.6, allowing the adjacent fibres from each retina to interdigitate. The crossed fibres enter layers 1, 4 and 6 and the uncrossed fibres enter layers 2, 3 and 5. The macula fibres occupy a big central wedge of the geniculate body, with the lower fields represented medially and the upper fields laterally.

4. The resultant fibres then sweep out into the hemisphere in two fan-shaped projections, which later come together to reach the occipital cortex as shown in Figure 3.7. The lower fibres sweep forward into the anterior temporal lobe as Meyer's loop. The upper fibres take a more direct route back into the parietal lobe. Although this course is almost impossible to indicate diagrammatically, the fibres all sweep back towards the occipital cortex deep in the substance of the hemisphere. They do not run straight back just under the medial surface. Therefore, a lesion at area 5

in Figure 3.7 does not damage the fibres to the macular area, which lie deep in the substance of the brain at this point.

5. The calcarine or visual cortex lies astride the calcarine fissure. The cells subserving the peripheral fields lie anteriorly, and those subserving macular vision are concentrated at the extreme tip: the upper fields represented in the lower half and the lower fields in the upper half of the cortex. The longitudinal extent of the calcarine cortex is important in permitting strikingly localized visual defects to occur as a result of vascular lesions in this area.

Visual Defects Due to Lesions at Pregeniculate Level

Retinal Lesions

The retina consists of the retinal nerve cells lying on the choroid at the back of the eye. The nerve fibres from these cells come straight forward and then angle sharply to run on the surface of the retina towards the optic nerve head. They do so in an orderly way, as shown in Figure 3.5. The most critical part of the retina is the very densely packed mass of cells known as the macula. The fibres from this area form the papillomacu-

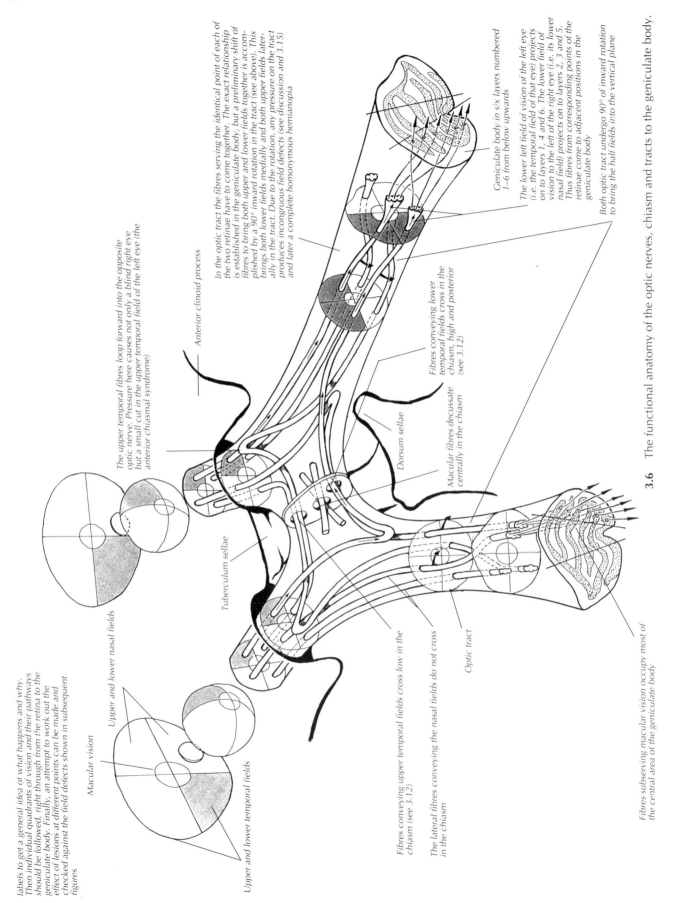

labels to get a general idea of what happens and why. Then individual quadrants of vision and their pathways should be followed, right through from the retina to the geniculate body. Finally, an attempt to work out the effect of lesions at different points can be made and checked against the field defects shown in subsequent figures

Macular vision

Upper and lower nasal fields

Upper and lower temporal fields

The upper temporal fibres loop forward into the opposite optic nerve. Pressure here causes not only a blind right eye but a small cut in the upper temporal field of the left eye (the anterior chiasmal syndrome)

Anterior clinoid process

Tuberculum sellae

Dorsum sellae

Fibres conveying upper temporal fields cross low in the chiasm (see 3.12)

The lateral fibres conveying the nasal fields do not cross in the chiasm

Macular fibres decussate centrally in the chiasm

Fibres conveying lower temporal fields cross in the chiasm, high and posterior (see 3.12)

Optic tract

Fibres subserving macular vision occupy most of the central area of the geniculate body

In the optic tract the fibres serving the identical point of each of the two retinae have to come together. The exact relationship is established in the geniculate body, but a preliminary shift of fibres to bring both upper and lower fields together is accomplished by a 90° inward rotation in the tract (see above). This brings both lower fields medially and both upper fields laterally in the tract. Due to the rotation, any pressure on the tract produces incongruous field defects (see discussion and 3.15) and later a complete homonymous hemianopia

Geniculate body in six layers numbered 1–6 from below upwards

The lower left field of vision of the left eye (i.e. the temporal field of that eye) projects on to layers 1, 4 and 6. The lower field of vision to the left of the right eye (i.e. its lower nasal field) projects on to layers 2, 3 and 5. Thus fibres from corresponding points of the retinae come to adjacent positions in the geniculate body

Both optic tract undergo 90° of inward rotation to bring the half fields into the vertical plane

3.6 The functional anatomy of the optic nerves, chiasm and tracts to the geniculate body.

5. Anterior visual cortex lesion (*one of the most frequently encountered defects*)

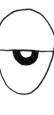
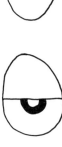

The area shown is supplied by the posterior verebral artery. The tip (marked 6) is thought to be supplied by a branch from the middle cerebral. This classical field defect, a macula sparing homonymous hemianopia, is very typical of a posterior cerebral artery occlusion

6. Macular cortex lesion

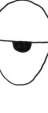

Damage to the tip of the occipital pole (direct trauma, head injury, bullet wound) produces homonymous macular defects. These may be incomplete but are always exactly congruous

7. Intermediate visual cortex lesion

Damage in this area which spares both peripheral and the macular field produces homonymous ring scotoma. It is due to infarction of the distal reaches of the posterior cerebral artery territory and produces a very disconcerting field defect which is readily missed. The patient has difficulty reading but the visual acuity will be normal because of preserved central vision and the peripheral field would be intact

4. Main radiation lesion

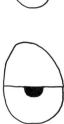

Seen with extensive parietotemporal gliomas or complete middle cerebral artery occlusions (the middle cerebral supplies the entire radiation at this level). Causes a complete homonymous hemianopia

3. Parietal radiation lesion (*very rare in pure form*)

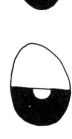
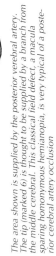

Affects all fibres (macula and peripheral) causing an inferior quadrantic homonymous hemianopia

2. Lesions of the optic peduncle

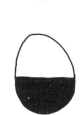

The fibres pass from the lateral geniculate below and behind the lenticular nucleus and the internal capsule. This area is supplied by the thalamogeniculate branches of the posterior cerebral artery and the geniculate body, by the anterior choroidal artery. A complete homonymous hemianopia results from occlusions (the associated findings are discussed in a later chapter on 'Strokes')

1. Temporal radiation lesion

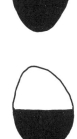

The fibres carrying the upper temporal fields sweep forward into the temporal lobe (called Meyer's loop). Lesions here, usually tumours, classically produce an upper congruous quadrantic homonymous hemianopia

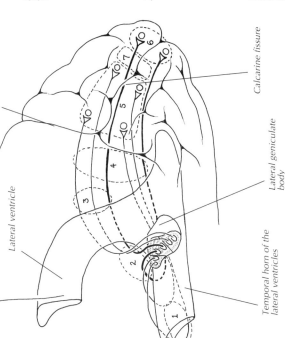

Parieto-occipital fissure

Lateral ventricle

Lateral geniculate body

Temporal horn of the lateral ventricles

Calcarine fissure

3.7 Visual radiations and field defects.

lar bundle as they enter the optic nerve. These nerve cells are especially sensitive to a variety of toxins and, if damaged, a caecocentral scotoma results (Fig. 3.8). The commonest toxins are tobacco and alcohol. Vitamin B_1 and B_{12} deficiencies also cause caecocentral scotomas. Ethambutol, amiodarone, isoniazid, chloramphenicol and iodoquinol may all be toxic to these cells and nerve fibres.

Several neurological disorders are associated with retinitis pigmentosa (see Chapter 4). This usually begins as a peripheral retinal cell degeneration, causing night blindness (hemeralopia) but ultimately leading to optic atrophy associated with perhaps the most dramatic narrowing of the retinal vessels seen. It is thought that this may play a prime role in causing the optic atrophy and severe visual failure.

Choroidoretinitis, due to local patches of inflammation of the retina, causes scotomas of shape and size appropriate to the area of damage. The retinal appearance is quite characteristic: the normal pink retina disappears and the pigment layer peels back, exposing the underlying white sclera. This produces typical little rounded white patches with a black rim in the middle of a normal retina. A very severe form is juxtapapillary choroidoretinitis, where the lesion occurs adjacent to the optic disc and damages incoming nerve fibres, leading to a more serious field defect with an arcuate scotoma radiating out from the blind spot, typical of a nerve bundle lesion (Fig. 3.10). The severity of visual impairment will depend on the exact location of the inflammatory lesions. The commonest cause of choroidoretinitis is previous infection with cytomegalovirus or toxoplasmosis.

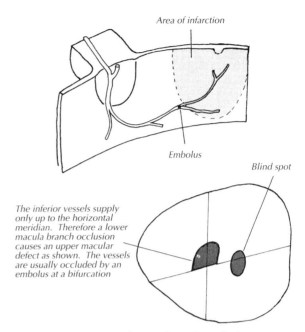

3.9   Retinal artery branch occlusion.

The retinal circulation is derived from the central retinal artery, which divides into upper and lower branches on the disc supplying the retina above and below the horizontal meridian of the eye. Branch occlusion, usually due to an embolus, causes a defect in the appropriate area that extends only to the horizontal meridian because of the strict distribution of the vessels above and below the horizontal line (Fig. 3.9).

Optic Disc Lesions

Developmental defects of the disc (colobomata) and hyaline masses that develop during life (drusen) may both cause central scotomas, or if they damage nerve fibre bundles in the optic nerve head arcuate scotomas result. Glaucoma always damages retinal nerve fibres on the disc margins owing to the stretching effect of raised intraocular pressure which produces arcuate scotomas radiating from the blind spot often initially extending upwards. This is called a Seidel scotoma, which later extends from below the blind spot until it forms complete ring called a Bjerrum scotoma (Fig. 3.10).

Papilloedema (swelling of the optic nerve head) may cause field defects in several ways:

• Enlargement of the blind spot due to the oedema affecting retinal cells directly adjacent to the disc

• Haemorrhage or exudate into the macula itself, which may cause abrupt visual failure

• Transient visual obscuration during any movement or change of position which further raises intracranial pressure, such as bending, straining or standing up suddenly

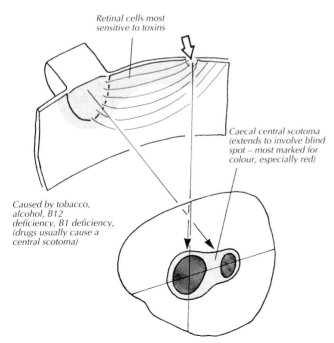

3.8   Toxic amblyopia.

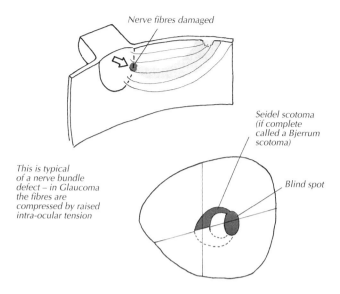

Nerve fibres damaged

Seidel scotoma (if complete called a Bjerrum scotoma)

Blind spot

This is typical of a nerve bundle defect – in Glaucoma the fibres are compressed by raised intra-ocular tension

3.10   Glaucoma effect of nerve bundle lesion.

- Chronic papilloedema may cause progressive gliosis (scarring) of the optic nerve head. Eventually progressive visual failure occurs, producing peripheral field constriction. This is due to damage to the nerve fibres crossing the swollen disc margin.

- If the papilloedema is due to hydrocephalus (distension of the ventricular system) the dilated third ventricle may splay the chiasm, causing a binasal hemianopia due to lateral pressure from the carotid siphon on each side. This is an extremely rare field defect (see later)

- If the cerebral hemisphere herniates on one side, the posterior cerebral artery may be stretched across the tentorial edge causing a macular sparing hemianopia. This can be a false localizing sign (see Chapter 23)

- Visual defects may also be found related to the location of the underlying lesion causing the papilloedema.

Optic Nerve Lesions

Acute Retrobulbar Neuritis

This is really the universal response of the optic nerve to a variety of toxic and metabolic insults. An attack of retrobulbar neuritis is not necessarily synonymous with an attack of multiple sclerosis. The number of patients with retrobulbar neuritis who go on to develop other manifestations of multiple sclerosis ranges from 35% to 75%, with females twice as likely to develop other symptoms within the next 15 years. Conversely, VER evidence shows that some 90% of patients with known

multiple sclerosis have evidence of previous, sometimes asymptomatic, retrobulbar neuritis.

Symptomatically the patient complains that central vision is acutely impaired by a 'fluffy ball', a 'puff of smoke', a 'steamed-up window' or a sensation as if 'looking through ground glass', and often claim that if they could 'see round it' vision would be normal. The visual acuity is usually impaired down to 6/60 or 6/36 (20/200 in the USA). There is usually discomfort in the eye, especially provoked by movement, and this may be severe. Very severe eye pain with blurred vision can also occur in migrainous neuralgia, and this can readily mimic an attack of retrobulbar neuritis. Conversely, very brief attacks of retrobulbar neuritis may be misdiagnosed as a migraine attack.

The majority of patients with acute retrobulbar neuritis recover satisfactory vision within 10–20 days, although VERs usually remain abnormal in those cases due to demyelinating disease.

Ischaemic optic neuritis due to vascular disease is of increasingly recognized importance. It is a specific complication of cranial arteritis but may occur in patients who only have arteriosclerotic vascular disease. It does not recover. In the acute phase haemorrhages and oedema of the optic disc are the rule, and these features are uncommon in idiopathic retrobulbar neuritis.

Optic neuritis has also been seen in association with autoimmune abnormalities and malignancy elsewhere in the body, and it is a classic complication of syphilis. With the recent resurgence of this disorder it should again enter into the differential diagnosis. A variety of opportunistic infections in patients who have AIDs may also produce optic neuritis and retinitis. These include cytomegalovirus, varicella and cryptococcosis. Lyme disease includes optic neuritis among its many neurological manifestations.

In cases due to toxic causes recovery may not occur. Optic nerve damage due to ethambutol used in the treatment of tuberculosis is dose related and the risk is especially high in patients with renal failure. The blood level should always be monitored in patients receiving the drug. Amiodarone has been reported to cause permanent bilateral visual loss, possibly related to ischaemia of the optic nerve. Isoniazid has been reported as causing optic nerve damage but this is extremely rare. In children chloramphenicol may cause irreversible blindness due to optic neuritis. Iodoquinol used in the treatment of amoebiasis may cause optic neuritis if the maximum permissible dose is exceeded.

The classic resulting field defect due to retrobulbar neuritis is a central scotoma, and although a full recovery of the visual field usually occurs a defect to a red pin may persist. A few patients are left with a sensation of decreased luminescence in the affected eye and note that colours look 'washed out' or desaturated, owing to persistent impairment of red perception. In the acute stage the optic disc appears normal unless the inflammation is just behind the nerve head, when 'papillitis' with swelling of the nerve head may be seen. This is distinguished from papilloedema by the accompanying severe loss of visual acuity, as vision remains normal in papilloedema unless specific complications occur as described earlier. The main differential diagnosis of acute retrobulbar neuritis is optic nerve compression.

Leber's Hereditary Optic Neuropathy

Leber's hereditary optic neuropathy is an uncommon disorder due to a defect in mitochondrial DNA. It is always a maternally transmitted disorder, mainly affecting young men aged between 20 and 25 years of age. It is of sudden painless onset and unilateral, the other eye becoming involved a few weeks or months later. There is rapidly progressive loss of vision and visual field testing reveals a caecocentral scotoma. After 6–8 weeks the condition subsides and some 30% of patients may regain some vision, but all are left with optic atrophy and telangiectatic vessels in the periphery of the retina on examination.

Optic Nerve Compression (Fig. 3.12)

The papillomacular bundle conveying central vision is very vulnerable to extrinsic compression. Hence a com-

pressive lesion also tends to cause a central scotoma rather than a field defect spreading in from the periphery, as might be anticipated on purely anatomical grounds. The central defect may develop so slowly that

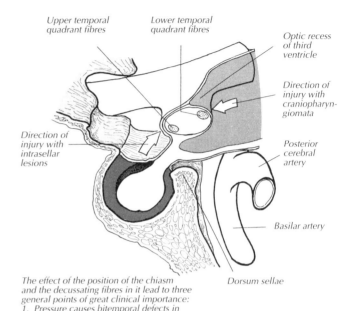

The effect of the position of the chiasm and the decussating fibres in it lead to three general points of great clinical importance:
1. Pressure causes bitemporal defects in vision
2. Lesions arising in the sella cause a defect starting in upper quadrants
3. Lesions arising behind or above the sella cause defects starting in lower quadrants

3.11 Relationship of the optic chiasm to the third ventricle and hypophysis cerebri.

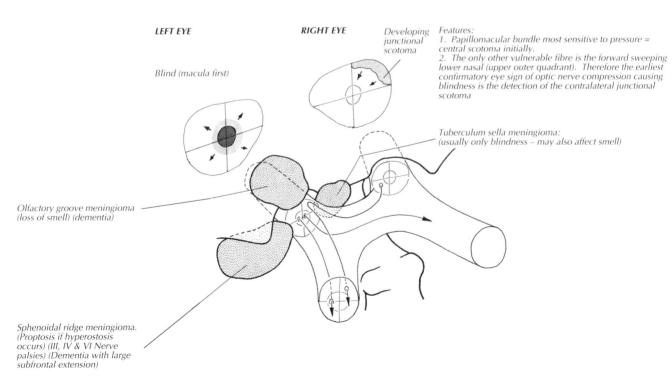

3.12 Intracranial optic nerve compression and anterior chiasmal lesions.

the patient discovers the loss of vision by accident, as when grit or soap gets into the good eye. A useful distinction from retrobulbar neuritis is that on fundal examination in such a case there is often well-marked optic atrophy already present when the visual deficit is first discovered, whereas in acute retrobulbar neuritis optic atrophy usually takes several weeks to appear.

CASE REPORT V

A 28-year-old Italian chef living in London went to Italy on holiday. He borrowed a friend's motor scooter and was riding along without protective goggles. Some grit flew into his left eye. He put his hand up to his eye and noticed he could not see. He had accidentally discovered that he had become blind in the right eye. This proved to be due to optic nerve compression by a neurofibroma arising on the first division of the fifth nerve.

Any central scotoma that is discovered accidentally or any 'acute retrobulbar neuritis' that does not recover as anticipated should be regarded as being due to optic nerve compression until proved otherwise. An important part of the initial and follow-up examinations is a search for an early field cut in the opposite eye due to damage to the decussating fibres that loop forward into the optic nerve. This is known as the anterior chiasmal syndrome of Traquair.

In all cases of unilateral visual loss the sense of smell, the functioning of cranial nerves III, V, VI, and the corneal reflex should be carefully tested.

MRI scanning is the most sensitive technique for investigating lesions in the orbit and optic foramen.

Optic Nerve Tumours

Malignant tumours, usually pilocytic astrocytomas in the optic nerve, optic chiasm or optic tract, occur mainly in children or in patients with neurofibromatosis. The visual defect produced by a glioma in the optic nerve is usually a 'hole' in vision, which may occur anywhere in the field. Optic atrophy is usually well established by the time that the defect is noticed and straight X-rays of the orbit may reveal evidence of enlargement of one or both optic foramina. Tumours in the optic chiasm or optic tract produce field defects typical of lesions in these areas (see below).

Metastatic Disease

The optic nerve may be secondarily involved by local or remote malignant disease, including the malignant lymphomas. Malignant disease in the orbit tends to produce proptosis rather than field defects and, paradoxically, the optic nerve seems very resistant to damage which is simply due to stretching.

Optic Chiasm Lesions

The internal anatomy of the chiasm has already been indicated in detail in Figure 3.6. From a practical point of view four anatomical features are important: (Fig. 3.11).

1. The optic chiasm does not lie on the tuberculum sellae as is often thought, but is usually situated above and behind the pituitary gland and the dorsum sellae. There is some anatomical variation in the exact position, which is described as a pre-fixed or post-fixed location, which may cause some variations in the resulting field defect. The position, which is described and discussed below, is that most frequently observed.

2. The central papillomacular bundle seems to be less vulnerable to compression in the chiasm and visual defects usually spread in from the periphery to involve macular vision late in the course of the disease, in contrast to the effect of compression of the optic nerve in its short intracranial course.

3. The lower nasal fibres (upper temporal fields) cross low and anteriorly in the chiasm and are damaged by lesions arising in the pituitary fossa and extending upwards.

4. The upper nasal fibres (lower temporal fields) cross high and posteriorly in the chiasm and are damaged by lesions damaging the chiasm from above and behind, notably craniopharyngiomas.

Anterior Chiasmal Lesions (Fig. 3.12)

The junction of the optic nerve and the chiasm may be damaged from any direction. Meningiomas commonly arise from the densely adherent dura mater in this region and cause progressive visual failure in one eye, with loss of sense of smell and/or lesions of cranial nerves III, IV, V and VI. The visual field loss includes a peripheral defect in the opposite eye (the anterior chiasmal syndrome of Traquair). Some tumours may reach a massive size before detection, often producing unrecognized loss of sense of smell, and may even present as an acute dementing illness caused by frontal lobe damage or hydrocephalus.

Chiasmal Lesions (Figs. 3.13 and 3.14)

The basic field defect is a bitemporal hemianopia – the patient is in effect 'wearing blinkers'. The defect may develop very insidiously, with later abrupt visual failure as the presenting symptom when the macular pathways finally become involved. In both sexes endocrine dysfunction usually antedates visual symptoms by many years. In the male impotence and in the female secondary amenorrhoea are the main endocrine symptoms. This is now recognized to be due to hyper-

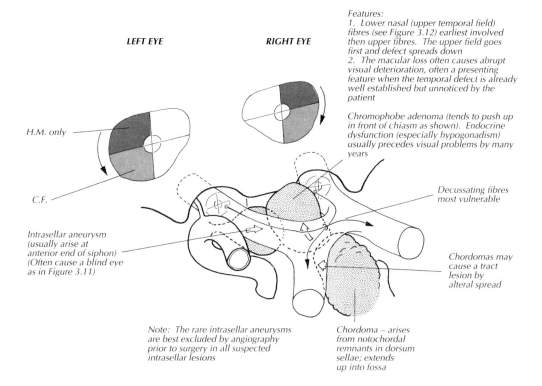

LEFT EYE   **RIGHT EYE**

Features:
1. Lower nasal (upper temporal field) fibres (see Figure 3.12) earliest involved then upper fibres. The upper field goes first and defect spreads down
2. The macular loss often causes abrupt visual deterioration, often a presenting feature when the temporal defect is already well established but unnoticed by the patient

Chromophobe adenoma (tends to push up in front of chiasm as shown). Endocrine dysfunction (especially hypogonadism) usually precedes visual problems by many years

H.M. only

Decussating fibres most vulnerable

C.F.

Intrasellar aneurysm (usually arise at anterior end of siphon) (Often cause a blind eye as in Figure 3.11)

Chordomas may cause a tract lesion by alteral spread

Note: The rare intrasellar aneurysms are best excluded by angiography prior to surgery in all suspected intrasellar lesions

Chordoma – arises from notochordal remnants in dorsum sellae; extends up into fossa

3.13   Chiasmal compression from below.

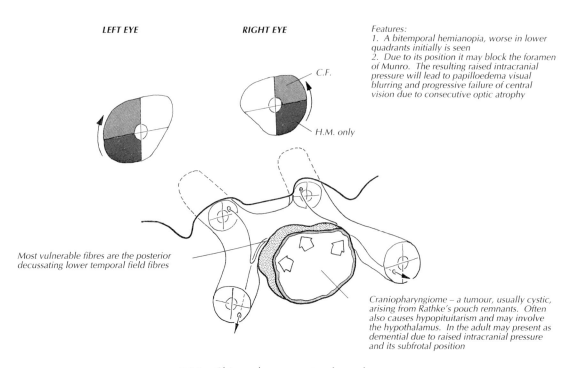

LEFT EYE   **RIGHT EYE**

Features:
1. A bitemporal hemianopia, worse in lower quadrants initially is seen
2. Due to its position it may block the foramen of Munro. The resulting raised intracranial pressure will lead to papilloedema visual blurring and progressive failure of central vision due to consecutive optic atrophy

C.F.

H.M. only

Most vulnerable fibres are the posterior decussating lower temporal field fibres

Craniopharyngiome – a tumour, usually cystic, arising from Rathke's pouch remnants. Often also causes hypopituitarism and may involve the hypothalamus. In the adult may present as demential due to raised intracranial pressure and its subfrotal position

3.14   Chiasmal compression from above.

prolactinaemia, and the recognition of both macro-adenomas and microadenomas secreting prolactin is one of the major advances in neuroendocrinology in recent years.

MRI scanning has enabled the identification of very small tumours that are best treated with bromocriptine, which blocks the secretion of prolactin. It is still not clear whether these lesions inevitably progress to macroadenomas. These tumours are chromophobe adenomas which were previously thought to be non-endocrinologically active.

Eosinophil adenomas (secreting growth hormone and causing acromegaly), aneurysms of the carotid syphon, and chordomas arising from notochord remnants in the dorsum sella may all produce an identical syndrome. All cause a bitemporal hemianopia which typically spreads down from the upper fields into the lower fields as it damages the chiasm from below.

Craniopharyngiomas which distort the chiasm from above and behind may cause any of three distinct syndromes in addition to the visual problem, which consists of a bitemporal hemianopia spreading up from the lower fields into the upper fields (see Fig. 3.14). These syndromes are:

1. In infancy the tumour may cause pituitary dwarfism
2. In adulthood progressive visual failure occurs, with variable pituitary dysfunction
3. In old age a craniopharyngioma may block the third ventricle, causing hydrocephalus and producing dementia.

Lateral Chiasmal Lesions (Fig. 3.15)

Lateral compression of the chiasm is quite rare. The most frequent cause is dilatation of the intracavernous part of an arteriosclerotic carotid artery. This condition occurs most frequently in elderly hypertensive females. The defect is usually unilateral but may become bilateral if the chiasm is pushed across against the opposite carotid artery. If the onset is abrupt the visual problem is usually combined with a bloodshot eye and extraocular nerve palsies (see Chapter 5). Another possible mechanism is dilatation of the third ventricle in association with chronic aqueductal stenosis or blockage of the fourth ventricle outflow. The chiasm is splayed laterally by the dilating third ventricle and is damaged by the pulsatile carotid arteries pressing against its lateral edges.

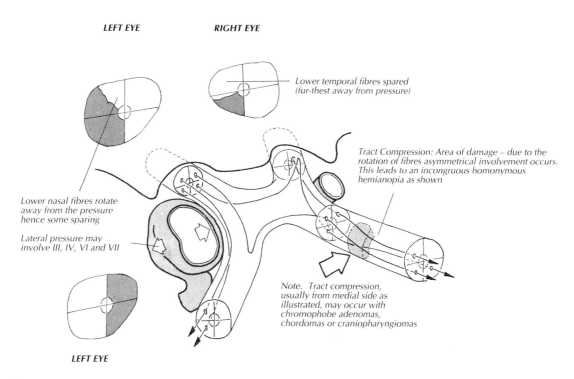

LEFT EYE   *RIGHT EYE*

Lower temporal fibres spared (fur-thest away from pressure)

Tract Compression: Area of damage – due to the rotation of fibres asymmetrical involvement occurs. This leads to an incongruous homonymous hemianopia as shown

Lower nasal fibres rotate away from the pressure hence some sparing

Lateral pressure may involve III, IV, VI and VII

Note. Tract compression, usually from medial side as illustrated, may occur with chromophobe adenomas, chordomas or craniopharyngiomas

LEFT EYE

Lateral Chiasmal Compression: Most often (and a very rare event anyway) due to an aneurysmal dilution of the terminal carotid artery as shown on the left. This produces a nasal field defect in the same eye. Occasionally the chiasm will be pushed across against the opposite carotid artery – leading to a binasal hemianopia

3.15 Lateral chiasmal and optic tract compression.

Optic Tract Lesions (Fig. 3.15)

Optic tract lesions produce very striking incongruous homonymous hemianopias [incongruous defects are those in which the shape of the defect is different in the two half fields (see Fig. 3.2E)]. Although incongruity can usually be established on confrontation testing, minor degrees are best demonstrated by formal screen testing. The importance of demonstrating incongruity is that a tract lesion or lateral geniculate lesion will be the cause, if incongruity is marked. Pituitary tumours, craniopharyngiomas, chordomas and meningiomas may all produce tract lesions by extending upwards, backwards and laterally. Often the cerebral peduncle on the same side is damaged and mild pyramidal signs in the opposite limb may be detected. Compressive lesions are usually the cause; multiple sclerosis can produce a tract lesion but this is quite uncommon.

Lateral Geniculate Body Lesions

Lateral geniculate body lesions are extremely rare and cause very marked incongruous homonymous hemianopic defects.

All pregeniculate visual pathway lesions cause variability in the density of the defect, with sloping sides and the possibility of progression from a simple field defect to a red pin, to a defect also to a white pin, and finally to the inability to detect even hand movements as the defect becomes complete. Detecting early defects requires considerable knowledge and some degree of skill but is extremely rewarding, as early diagnosis really does have value in these situations. Because the lesion is pregeniculate, an afferent pupillary defect to light and even atrophy may be detected if the lesion is longstanding.

When we consider lesions affecting the postgeniculate visual pathways the situation is quite different. With the exception of attention hemianopias the defects are steep-sided and usually absolute, but variable degrees of loss of vision are sometimes found. A 10 mm white pin is all that is necessary to document the defect. Such lesions do not affect visual acuity and will not cause pupillary defects or optic atrophy.

Lesions Affecting the Visual Radiations (see Fig. 3.7)

Optic Peduncle Lesions

Because the fibres emerging from the lateral geniculate body sweep over the trigone of the lateral ventricles, lying below and behind the capsular region (see also Chapter 9), field defects are not a constant feature of a simple capsular cerebral vascular accident. This region of the visual radiation is most often damaged by occlusion of one of the thalamo-perforating or thalamo-geniculate arteries arising from the posterior cerebral artery. This produces a clinical picture which includes a homonymous hemianopia with hemisensory loss (posterior thalamic damage) and a very mild motor deficit which usually recovers, presumably due to oedema of the adjacent motor pathways in the internal capsule. Lesions purely affecting the optic peduncle are extremely rare.

Temporal Lobe Lesions

The fibres conveying visual information from the opposite upper temporal fields sweep forwards and downwards into the temporal lobe in what is known as Meyer's loop. In the anterior loop there is some splaying of the fibres so that an incongruous defect can be produced, but this is usually of minimal degree and once the fibres have looped round to pass posteriorly, congruous defects are the rule. A congruous defect is one which, however bizarre, the shape is identical in both eyes. In patients suspected of harbouring a temporal lobe lesion careful evaluation of the upper visual fields is indicated.

Parietal Lobe Lesions

The part of the visual radiation lying in the anterior part of the parietal lobe conveys information from the lower visual fields. Therefore a lesion in the anterior parietal part of the radiation will produce a lower quadrantic hemianopia. This is an extremely rare field defect encountered on only one occasion by the author, the patient being an 8-year-old boy with a cerebral abscess. These fibres are quickly rejoined by the upper field fibres sweeping up from the temporal lobe, and more typically a parietal lesion damages all the fibres, causing a complete homonymous hemianopia. Attention hemianopias due to peripheral posterior parietal lesions were fully discussed earlier in this chapter.

Testing for visual field defects complicating parietal lobe lesions may prove difficult because of concurrent intellectual, agnostic or dysphasic difficulties due to the lesion responsible. In these situations testing the visual field to threat may be helpful.

Testing Visual Fields By Threat

When the patient is looking directly to you, sharply wave the flat of the hand towards the eye from outside the normal temporal field of vision. If the temporal field is intact, the patient should blink immediately the hand flashes into view. If the patient consistently fails to blink when threatened from one side, a hemianopic defect can be presumed. The only special point to watch is that the hand should not get near enough to set up a draught, which will provoke a corneal response simulating blinking to threat.

Lesions of the Anterior Visual Cortex

The peripheral visual fields are represented in the most anterior part of the calcarine cortex. The blood supply is derived from the posterior cerebral artery. Infarction of this area due to occlusion of this vessel produces a macular-sparing hemianopia. The other rare cause of this particular field defect is a meningioma of the tentorium cerebelli pressing against this area of the cortex. Vascular occlusions in this area occur quite commonly in migraine. Bilateral infarction of this area leads to tunnel vision, with a small ring of 2–5° of intact vision. This is extremely disabling, as patients can see only objects in the direct line of vision and cannot scan to an object in the peripheral fields, even though the visual acuity remains quite normal. This may follow cerebral air or fat embolism. Non-organic tunnel vision is encountered in hysteria and is discussed later.

CASE REPORT VI

A 72-year-old man was referred with suspected hysterical visual deficit. His visual acuities had been documented at 6/6 but he claimed he could not see, and when he attempted to walk continually fell over furniture and was even unable to eat a meal because of difficulty with his vision. His visual fields had not been tested. On examination he had total loss of the peripheral visual fields with only 1° or 2° of intact macular vision. The total loss of peripheral vision meant that he could only see in the direction of gaze. Changing his direction of gaze was extremely difficult because the lack of peripheral vision meant that he had no target to guide him. Everything he saw was seen by accident. His problem would be best appreciated by trying to walk around a room with 3-foot long cardboard tubes held to both eyes. CT scanning revealed bilateral posterior cerebral artery territory infarction with sparing of the macular cortex.

Lesions of the Macular Cortex

If the tip of one occipital pole is damaged a congruous, homonymous and extremely small hemianopia occurs. It is thought that the occipital pole has an independent blood supply derived from the middle cerebral artery, and that this accounts for the macular sparing in posterior cerebral arterial occlusions (see above). For the same reason small hemianopic field defects may result from failure of this separate blood supply. Patients usually notice the defect located in the temporal field in this situation, emphasizing the importance of looking

for an identical defect in the nasal field of the other eye to confirm that the defect is homonymous and that the scotoma noted by the patient is not due to an optic nerve or retinal lesion in one eye.

Lesions of the Intermediate Calcarine Cortex

These are extremely unusual but produce an interesting field defect consisting of a half ring of visual loss surrounding the intact macular and with preserved peripheral vision. Depending on its width, the patient may notice a frustrating hole halfway along a long word while reading, or even more disconcertingly when working on a column of figures. The less than conscientious examiner may completely miss such a defect and the patient may well be regarded as having non-organic disease, as unfortunately so often happens in neurology.

Cortical Blindness

Total destruction of the occipital cortex by infarction or trauma will result in cortical blindness. It is important to recognize that this is the only situation where blindness will be associated with preservation of the light reflexes, and the pupils will be of normal size and vary in size with the ambient lighting conditions. The situation may be further confused if the damage extends to the visual association areas, resulting in Anton's syndrome, where the patient is unaware that they are unable to see. This is also known as denial of cortical blindness.

CASE REPORT VII

A 56-year-old man was referred for impaired vision and clumsiness which had come on suddenly about 6 weeks earlier. He was shown into the room by a nurse, walked forwards towards the consultant's voice and fell over the patient's chair, apologizing profusely for his clumsiness. He continued to look straight ahead, by which time the consultant had moved round to his side to assist him and he only looked in the new direction when spoken to. This alerted suspicion and a hand waved in front of the patient's face was totally ignored. When asked if he could see anything, he said that there was a person in front of him and when asked if he could see the hand in front of his face, he confirmed that he could do so, even though no hand was offered. He continued to behave throughout the interview and examination as if he could see, and would only concede that his vision was 'blurred' in spite of overwhelming evidence to the contrary. There were no other abnormal physical findings. The lesion was presumed to be vascular. The patient was seen in the days before CT scanning was available to confirm the diagnosis.

Non-Organic Visual Field Defects

There are several types of visual field defect that are non-organically determined, and non-organic visual impairment is one of the commonest manifestations of hysteria or malingering.

Constricted Visual Fields

This is probably the most frequent simulated field defect. The patient demonstrates normal central vision but is unable to see anything in the periphery. The non-organic nature is best identified by demonstrating that the field defect remains exactly the same size, however far away the object is taken. Theoretically, the size of the target should also be doubled the further away the examiner. This defect never presents a serious difficulty for the patient who may have walked into the room and sat down without any evidence of their defect, such as walking into furniture in the blind part of their field, and will claim to have an intact field perhaps only 3 inches in diameter at normal reading distance. When the test is repeated with the examiner several yards away, the intact visual field remains exactly the same size. This is a physical impossibility, as the field subtends an arc and at double the distance the intact field should be double the size. This is more accurately called tubular vision (Fig. 3.16).

CASE REPORT VIII

A 12-year-old girl claimed visual difficulty and was shown to have such a field defect. The patient's parents were unwilling to accept a non-organic explanation in spite of more extensive investigations than were justified by the signs, and all tests were normal. After some acrimonious discussion and denial that there could be any possible background stresses the child was taken for a second opinion. One year later an enquiry of her general practitioner revealed that the child had eventually admitted a sexual assault by a relative.

Complete Blindness

Complete blindness due to non-organic causes is usually consequent upon some drama. The afflicted patient often continues to behave as if they can see while claiming total loss of vision, for example they do not walk into objects or door frames, or stumble and fall over minor undulations. The pupil reactions and VERs are normal, and if the patient can be taken unawares a blink to threat can usually be demonstrated.

CASE REPORT IX

A 10-year-old child was brought to the clinic claiming that she had been blind since a school friend slammed the car boot-lid on her head after they had put their satchels in the boot. There were no signs of organic disease and an expectant approach was adopted. Three months later the vision miraculously recovered. This was only after the girl who had slammed the lid had been made into a pariah at the school because she was responsible for the blindness. The patient subsequently admitted that this had been deliberate in order to create exactly that situation, because she was jealous of the other girl's popularity.

CASE REPORT X

A 42-year-old female had complained of near complete visual loss for several years and this was said to be due to multiple sclerosis. In spite of her difficulties she was still teaching at school, rode her bicycle and played her guitar. There were no organic ocular signs and her field defect was asymmetrical and spiral in type, strongly suggestive of non-organicity. The VERs were normal and certainly her abilities belied the severity of the claimed visual problem. She subsequently needed a D and C and was reviewed preoperatively; no signs of multiple sclerosis were found but she was aware that an attack might be triggered by surgery. On recovery from the anaesthetic she claimed total blindness. There were still no ocular signs and as an example of her retained abilities she was able to pick up and sprinkle salt and pepper on her meal with great accuracy in front of her family and attending physician. This did not arouse any comment from the family. This state persisted for over a year, and when her husband was appraised of the likelihood that this was not organic he insisted she returned to the hospital that had made the original diagnosis. Her vision miraculously recovered overnight. Further exploration as to the reasons for this episode, which had persisted for 4 years, was thought unwise!

Monocular Blindness

This condition also tends to follow dramatic incidents, such as trauma in or around the eye occurring in an emotional setting. It is characterized by no abnormality on examination, a normal direct and indirect light reflex, normal VERs and a positive response to the spinning drum test, as discussed earlier.

Modern investigational techniques have enabled non-organic disease to be identified with greater cer-

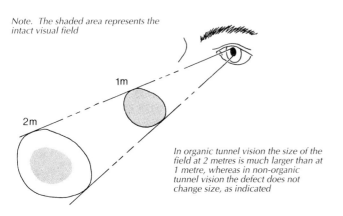

Note. The shaded area represents the intact visual field

In organic tunnel vision the size of the field at 2 metres is much larger than at 1 metre, whereas in non-organic tunnel vision the defect does not change size, as indicated

3.16   Non-organic tunnel vision.

tainty and this is particularly true of non-organic visual defects. Unfortunately, this has not improved our ability to help such patients, who will persist in their claims and their relatives and friends will persist in their belief that the doctors do not know what they are doing. They are quite willing, however, to accept that miracles occur when such patients make an equally dramatic recovery!

Visual Hallucinations

Damage to the visual pathways may cause irritative phenomena, appreciated by the patient as flashes of light or colour. More complicated visual images are usually the result of abnormal activity in visual association areas, in particular in the temporal lobes. Retinal damage is perhaps the most familiar, as in the universal experience of 'seeing stars' after a blow to the eye. Damage to or ischaemia of the retina causes hallucinations confined to one eye, consisting of unformed 'flashes' or 'speckles' of light, like stars on a dark background. This is often the last phase of the prodrome of a syncopal attack before loss of consciousness, and gives rise to the term 'blackout'.

Similar disturbances of vision in one eye may also occur at the onset of a migraine headache. Oedema of the retina due to central serous retinitis causes metamorphopsia (an undulating shape) and alterations in colour perception, but this is a visual aberration rather than a hallucination. Jaundice and digitalis overdose may alter colour perception so that everything appears yellow.

Optic nerve, chiasm and tract lesions do not cause visual hallucinations. Although complex visual hallucinations have been reported in patients with chiasmal lesions due to tumours, it seems likely that these were due to simultaneous damage to the hypothalamus or medial temporal lobes caused by the same lesion.

Visual hallucinations due to occipital pole ischaemia, or to seizures originating in this area, usually consist of unformed blobs of colour, usually in the red-orange end of the spectrum. Undoubtedly the most common cause is ischaemia of the occipital poles occurring during or preceding a migraine attack. It is also quite possible for a patient to have repeated attacks of this sort without necessarily developing the headache, and patients in this category should be kept under careful review or have a CT scan. Occipital lobe lesions can mimic migraine very convincingly.

CASE REPORT XI

*A 56-year-old woman suffered three epileptic attacks in the wake of visual hallucinations over a 4 year period. Many times a year, over that time, the visual hallucinations con-*sisted of alternating flashing yellow triangles, having an effect rather like flashing temporary roadworks indicators. If the yellow triangle remained upside down no fit would occur but on the three occasions when alternate triangles became upright, within 30 seconds of the change she convulsed. No underlying lesion could be demonstrated and all the symptoms disappeared when she was started on carbamazepine.*

Visual hallucinations in migraine may be monocular, hemianopic or bilateral and consist of zig-zag lines or circular lines on a dark background, like the plan of a castle, the hallucination that is also called 'fortification spectra'. Red and orange blobs that may alter in size and seem to explode are often described. Another variant is a sensation as if rain were running down a window pane in one half of vision. This may persist for several hours.

Formed visual images, still pictures like a tableau, or micropsia or macropsia, where the surroundings seem to become very small or very large, are a feature of temporal lobe epileptic phenomena or occur during migrainous vascular spasm, in which there is ischaemia of the medial temporal lobe. It has been suggested that the idea for 'Alice in Wonderland' was the result of macropsia during a migraine attack experienced by Lewis Carroll.

CASE REPORT XII

A 65-year-old woman who suffered lifelong migraine with visual phenomena, reported her most frightening experience. An attack had started conventionally with flickering lights, but after 20 minutes, when the headache began, her vision remained abnormal and started to distort. All the verticals in the room seemed to undulate and the door frame appeared much narrower at the top than at the bottom. To her horror, when she put her arm out to stroke the dog, her arm appeared to be about 12 feet long, tapering to a very small hand that she could see patting her dog, which looked like a small porcelain figurine. This distortion of vision lasted a further 20 minutes before clearing.

CASE REPORT XIII

A 35-year-old woman arrived at a junction controlled by traffic lights. She had a car full of children that she was taking to school. She had had a slight headache since waking that morning. As she pulled up, the scene seemed to change and suddenly the cars at the opposite side of the junction appeared to be a vast distance away and the oncoming vehicles became the size of toys. The lights changed in her favour but she was frightened to drive off as she thought she would never reach the other side of the junction. She sat terrified, surrounded by irate drivers, one of whom drove her car to the side of the road for her. She sat for another 15 minutes before her vision cleared. The headache then increased markedly and became typical of migraine. She had had no previous experiences of this sort and no further events occurred during a 6-month follow-up.

A static tableau type of hallucination is known as 'déjà vu'. This consists of an extremely brief feeling of familiarity with a scene that is abruptly 'frozen', like a still frame inserted into a moving picture. Typical attacks last a split second only and occur occasionally in normal people. Some patients with temporal lobe epilepsy may experience attacks many times a day, and sometimes they occur as a prodrome to a seizure.

More complicated and persisting visual hallucinations may occur as part of a temporal lobe attack, but are encountered more frequently in toxic confusional states or schizophrenia. The most frequently encountered hallucinatory state of this sort seen by neurologists is undoubtedly that occurring in patients on anti-parkinsonian medication. It is a feature of such hallucinations that they are silent. Several elderly people have mentioned that they did not mind the hallucinatory person sitting at the other end of their settee but they wished that they would answer when spoken to! These hallucinations usually involve animals or people, and may occasionally be abnormal in size.

CASE REPORT XIV

A 70-year-old man with long-standing Parkinson's disease started having mild visual hallucinations. However, on one memorable occasion, when his wife returned from shopping he met her at the gate and asked who all the people were who had come to the house for a party. The only unusual feature as far as he was concerned was that they were all only 3 feet tall.

CASE REPORT XV

A 65-year-old man with well-controlled Parkinson's disease took his dog for a walk and when he returned told his wife that the local common land was full of giant-sized people about 10 feet tall, and that all the trees had been bedecked with flags. The further course in this patient is detailed in Chapter 12 (case report VII). This improved only after his drugs were reduced.

A feature of visual hallucinosis is that there is no detectable field defect even during the attack. However, if the hallucinations occur during the onset of ischaemic damage a defect may be detectable after the episode. It is also characteristic that the patient can remember in vivid detail exactly what happened during the episode of visual hallucinosis.

The Olfactory Nerve and the Olfactory System

It is logical to follow the section on visual hallucinations with a discussion of the olfactory mechanisms, as in this system aberrations or hallucinations of smell sensation are an important component of the clinical features.

Anatomical Features (Fig. 3.17)

The receptor cells of the olfactory epithelium lie in the olfactory cleft in the upper 10 mm of the nasal septum, the roof of the nasal cavity and the lateral wall of the nose, to just above the origin of the superior concha. The epithelium is bathed in lipid-rich fluid produced by Bowman's glands, suggesting that lipid solubility is important in odour detection. The receptor cells are derived from ectoderm and are unique in being replaced from stem cells every 30 days. The cell bodies lie in the epithelium and the central fibres enter the cranial cavity via the cribriform plate as nonmyelinated axons without synapses. These fibres synapse with the mitral cells of the olfactory glomeruli. The axons of these mitral cells form the olfactory tract, which contains both centripetal and centrifugal fibres. The latter probably modulate activity in the glomeruli. This allows a relatively small number of receptor cells and fibres to distinguish an enormous variety of odours.

The olfactory tracts run posteriorly under the frontal lobes just above the optic nerves and chiasm and terminate in front of the anterior perforated substance as three striae. The destination of the medial striae is unknown. Many enter the opposite medial striae and may be the origin of the centrifugal fibres that go back down the opposite olfactory tract. The intermediate striae end in the olfactory tubercle but the further connections of the tubercle are unknown. The lateral olfactory striae synapse with the neurons of the anterior perforated substance, the lateral olfactory gyrus, the prepyriform cortex and the medial amygdaloid nuclei. This whole group constitutes the olfactory cortex in man. The olfactory pathway is also unique in being the only sensory pathway that has no relay in the thalamus.

The subsequent distribution of olfactory information in the limbic system (see Chapter 10) contributes to the pleasurable (or otherwise) features of olfaction, and the appropriate autonomic responses by way of the hypothalamus. This is controlled by relays in the secondary olfactory cortex of the entorhinal complex, which includes the uncus and the posterior orbitofrontal cortex. Descending pathways from these areas to the pontine reticular formation mediate reflex activity such as salivation.

Testing Smell Sensation

The patient's history will usually include observations such as the inability to smell burning, onions or petrol. They will also, almost always, mention that their taste sensation is also disordered, because most of the

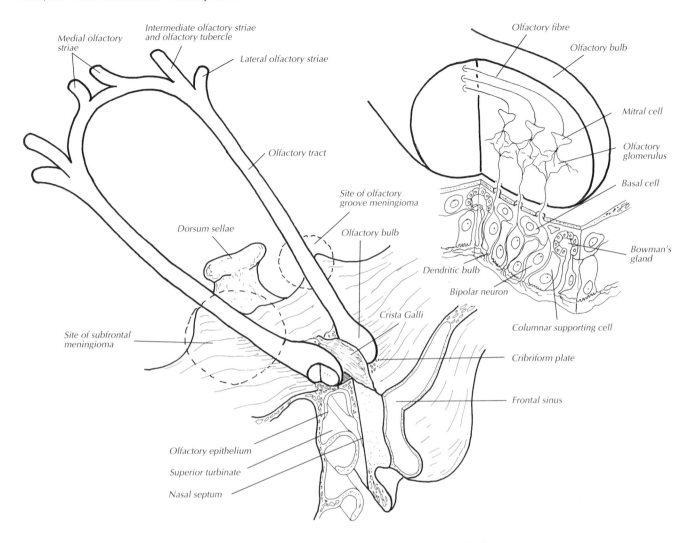

3.17 The olfactory pathways and olfactory bulb.

savour of food is derived from smell rather than taste. The standard odours used for testing are oil of peppermint, oil of cloves and asafoetida. For routine testing, oil of cloves or peppermint is probably sufficient. Asafoetida, an unpleasant smell, usually deteriorates in the test bottle and conventional smelling salts produce lacrimation and nasal discharge and so are unsuitable for testing. A few drops of oil of cloves or peppermint on a ball of cotton wool in a small bottle with a tight lid should be used. The odour should be presented to each nostril in turn, having established that the airway is clear and indeed that the smell is still detectable by the examiner. Loss of sense of smell in one nostril is of much greater potential significance than bilateral loss of smell, which may be related to one of the more general conditions discussed below.

Clinical disorders of Olfaction

Local trauma, dried-up airways, allergic rhinitis, polyps, foreign bodies and inflammatory disease such as

Wegener's granulomatosis may all cause loss of sense of smell by direct damage to the mucosa or by preventing air from reaching the olfactory epithelium.

Drugs and metabolic disease may interfere with the highly metabolically active cells of the nasal olfactory mucosa. Antihistamines, antibiotics, anti-metabolites, anti-inflammatories and anti-thyroid drugs may all interfere with cellular metabolism and therefore smell appreciation.

Head injury, particularly blows to the forehead or occiput, which set up fore-and-aft movements of the brain, are likely to shear off the nerve fibres as they pass through the cribriform plate. Loss of sense of smell complicates up to 30% of head injuries. If the dura is torn there is also the risk of CSF rhinorrhoea and subsequent meningitis. In some instances incomplete loss of smell may lead to bizarre aberrations where everything smells strange or scented or even foul, with a resulting dramatic effect on taste sensation and appetite. Unfortunately, such abnormalities following head injury are permanent.

Tumours, especially meningiomas, of the olfactory groove produce unrecognized unilateral anosmia and, if large, may result in dementia. Progressive loss of vision in the eye on the same side will eventually occur, hence the importance of testing smell in patients presenting with a blind eye and in all cases of dementia. Pituitary tumours and aneurysms in the anterior circulation may also damage the olfactory tract.

Olfaction deteriorates with age. It is the first sensory modality to be affected and may account for the tendency of elderly patients to lose their appetite and over spice their food.

Loss of sense of smell on a central basis has not been identified but aberration of sense of smell on a central basis is common. This may occur briefly in patients with complex partial seizures originating in the uncinate lobe, where sudden unpleasant smells of very brief duration constitute the olfactory aura. Burning rubber or rotting cabbage are the most frequent descriptions given. It is always unpleasant. The complaint of continual unpleasant smells or everything smelling awful is almost always of psychotic origin or a monosymptomatic depressive illness, and is very resistant to treatment. Ongoing unpleasant odours due to chronic suppurative sinus disease seems much less frequent than in the pre-antibiotic and pre-decongestant era.

Unilateral loss of sense of smell with no obvious local cause should always be investigated by scanning.

4. Examination of the Optic Fundus

A complete discussion of abnormal fundal appearances is beyond the scope of this text. However, it is essential that students examine the optic fundus in as many patients as possible to obtain a clear idea as to the range of normal appearances, and that every opportunity is taken to examine abnormal fundi. This is very much an acquired skill and so often fundal appearances are not clearly seen by students because of poor technique. Discussion will therefore be limited to technique, some normal variants that may be encountered and a description of some of the appearances seen in patients with neurological disorders.

Hints on Fundal Examination

1. Ideally the fundus should be examined in a darkened room, but complete darkness may make it difficult to find the patient! There is no need to dilate the pupils routinely as this might cause subsequent diagnostic confusion and there is a definite risk of precipitating glaucoma in the elderly.

2. The patient should be asked to fix their gaze on a distant object, straight ahead at eye level, both to help them hold the eye still and to dilate the pupil. They should be asked to keep their gaze fixed on that point even when the examiner's head gets in the line of vision, as it inevitably does. It is important to develop the ability to look at the patient's right eye with your right eye and their left eye with your left eye. Not only does this facilitate the patient's keeping the opposite eye looking into the distance but it can also avoid unpleasant proximity and nose-to-nose contact. It is also worth learning to examine the fundi upside down, leaning in over the patient's head, as a skill particularly useful in the emergency room and intensive care unit, where the more conventional approach may be made difficult by other procedures. Most unsuccessful ophthalmoscopy is caused by the patient trying to follow the ophthalmoscope light instead of holding the eye still.

3. The ideal line of approach should bring the optic disc straight into view. The examiner should look through the hole in the ophthalmoscope and then move in from about a foot away from the patient, keeping the pink-glowing pupil in view all the time. The light beam should then be aimed so that it would emerge from the back of the patient's head in the midline at eye level. The pale circle of the optic nerve head should immediately come into view if the patient continues looking straight ahead with the eye held still (Fig. 4.1).

4. If only blood vessels on a pink background are seen they should be followed backwards against the angle of any branches that are seen and the disc will eventually come into view (Fig. 4.2).

As a general hint on fundal examination, once some degree of skill has been achieved if the disc is found only with great difficulty, the patient may well have papilloedema: the pink disc has merged into the retina and the vessels end suddenly in oedema instead of on the disc. If the disc flashes into view like a new white tennis ball, the patient probably has primary optic atrophy, the disc pallor being accentuated against the normal retina. This simple observation can be extremely useful during the anxiety of the clinical examination for degrees and diplomas. The appearance of the normal optic disc is shown in Figure 4.3.

The Normal Optic Fundus

In childhood the optic disc and retina always appear wet and glistening and there are more prominent blood vessels than in the adult. This may simulate the early changes of developing papilleodema. Even in this age range the centre of the optic disc is always paler than the surrounding disc, and if this is the case early papilloedema is unlikely.

In the adult patient the disc colour varies from pale to fleshy, with a varying degree of vascularity. Where only the four main vessels traverse the disc its normal pale colour is striking. Where the vessels branch early, so

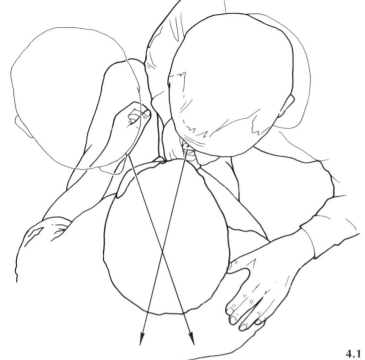

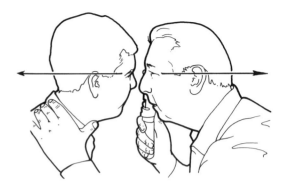

Note: The examiner's and the patient's eyes must be horizontal and the ophthalmoscope should be aimed towards the centre of the head, as shown. A common error is to try to look straight into the eye. The optic disc is displaced to the nasal side, as shown in Figure 4.2.

4.1   Examination of the eyes.

that a leash of vessels crosses the disc margin, it is more difficult to see the underlying disc and early disc swelling may be suspected.

The nasal edge of the disc is always less clearly demarcated than the temporal edge, an effect exaggerated if there is a little rim of pigment at the temporal margin, which is quite a common normal variant (see Fig. 4.8).

In the elderly the normally miotic pupil makes opthalmoscopy more difficult and the disc often assumes a yellow colour, making the margins less distinct. The vessels are often thinner than in younger patients. These appearances can simulate an ischaemic retina with ischaemic optic atrophy.

Common Fundal Abnormalities

Papilloedema

Some doctors think the neurological examination of the optic fundus involves purely the exclusion of papilloedema: Others believe the absence of papilloedema excludes raised intracranial pressure. Neither view is correct. Papilloedema due to raised intracranial pressure takes several weeks to develop, and a patient with rapidly rising intracranial pressure may die long before any disc swelling becomes apparent. In any clinical situation, if the history suggests rising intracranial pressure a normal disc does not mean that a lumbar puncture is without hazard (see also Chapter 15).

Because of the slow development of disc changes there is a sequence of findings that may indicate developing papilloedema. The sequence of events in acute papilloedema is as follows (Fig. 4.4):

1. Some increase in venous calibre and tortuosity. If this change is very marked without other abnormality,

4.2   Horizontal section of the eye, showing relative positions of the pupil, macula, optic disc and pupillary muscle fibres.

Central retinal vein

Central retinal artery

Optic disc   *Macula lutea*

Circular pupilloconstrictor fibres

Radial pupillodilator fibres

Lens

Ciliary body

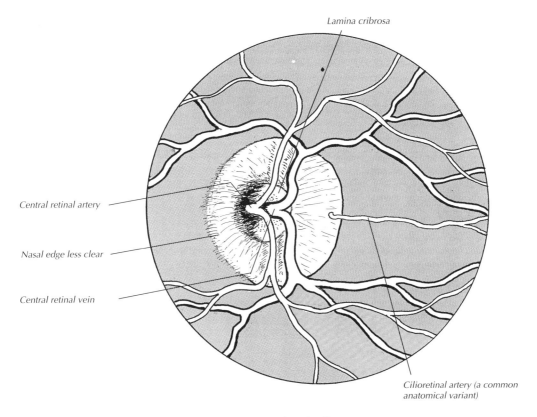

Lamina cribrosa

Central retinal artery

Nasal edge less clear

Central retinal vein

Cilioretinal artery (a common anatomical variant)

4.3   A normal optic disc.

heavy protein diseases such as macroglobulinaemia should be excluded.

2. The central area of the disc (the optic cup) is usually slightly pale compared to the rest of the disc and the vessels are usually seen to plunge into it. In early papilloedema this area becomes pinker and less distinct, the vessels seeming to disappear suddenly on the surface of the disc.

3. The disc margins start to blur. It is essential to be aware from the examination of many normal discs that the nasal edge is always less distinct than the temporal edge, and this blurring and even slight heaping is accentuated in those patients whose retinal vessels enter the disc more to the nasal side than usual. In true papilloedema the earliest swelling is seen at the upper and lower margins, where the entering fibres are most crowded, and then at the nasal edge. One of the most frequent 'false positive' signs in neurology is questionable blurring of the nasal disc margins.

4. Finally the whole disc becomes suffused, swollen and slightly elevated. The margins may disappear and the swelling completely conceals the vessel origins, the vessels seeming to emerge from a mushy pink swelling. Streaky perivenous haemorrhages occur and cottonwool spots – small round white blobs known as cytoid bodies – appear. This indicates that very severe axonal damage is occurring and irreversible changes in vision may already have occurred. In established papil-loedema, enlargement of the blind spot should be readily demonstrable if the technique of confrontation field testing has been mastered.

The early changes are very subjective and fluorescein retinal angiography has enabled the problem to be resolved in many cases, but the advent of CT scanning has reduced the need for expert opinions on the state of a disc in suspected papilloedema, which was in previous times one of the most appreciated skills of the neurologist. The absence of papilloedema should never be regarded as an absolute indication that intracranial pressure is not raised. Scanning has emphasized just how dangerously unreliable the presence or absence of papilloedema was in assessing such cases now that patients are regularly identified with gross displacement of intracranial structures without papilloedema. In the past many patients were undoubtedly harmed when a lumbar puncture was performed because there appeared to be no papilloedema.

Chronic papilloedema may be complicated by secondary changes in the macular area. The so-called macular star is oedema radiating out from the macula and seriously interfering with vision. These changes are more often seen in papilloedema due to 'benign' causes such as malignant hypertension, renal failure and benign intracranial hypertension (pseudotumour cerebri).

Conditions Simulating Papilloedema

An exceptionally deep optic cup or myelinated nerve fibres are common disc appearances often mistaken for papilloedema. These are illustrated in Figures 4.5 and 4.6.

The peculiar disc appearances in a patient with high myopia when examined with the opthalmoscope should be appreciated. It can be extremely difficult to focus the myopic disc, giving an impression of disc margin swelling and disc elevation. It is worth learning to look through the patient's own spectacles, which immediately resolves this problem. A rather small but perfectly normal disc should be seen.

Causes of Papilloedema (Table 4.1)

Although a full discussion of the causes of papilloedema is inappropriate to the discussion of fundal appearances, a list of common causes is given in Table 4.1.

It should be noticed that the causes are not exclusively neurological and that there are haematological and biochemical causes. Raised intracranial pressure due to any mass lesion in the brain has to be considered, but also conditions interfering with the circulation of the CSF, such as previous meningitis or subarachnoid haemorrhage interfering with CSF resorption. Blockage of CSF circulation due to aqueductal stenosis or congenital anomalies in the posterior fossa should also be considered.

There are a variety of other causes of papilloedema, in many of which the mechanism is obscure. In some cases a high CSF protein or altered blood products block CSF reabsorption by the arachnoid granulations. In some instances diffuse brain swelling is responsible and in others impaired venous drainage of the brain or of the retina itself is the cause. The common causes of central retinal vein thrombosis are therefore included in Table 4.1.

Secondary (Consecutive) Optic Atrophy

If the patient survives the cause of the papilloedema, further changes may appear in the optic disc following subsidence of the papilloedema. Occasionally general physicians may seek neurological advice if papilloedema has not resolved within a few days of a patient receiving effective antihypertensive therapy. This concern is quite unnecessary: several weeks will elapse before significant resolution is apparent. This is most easily confirmed by following the disc appearances in a patient under treatment for benign intracranial hypertension.

Even while disc swelling is still obvious, the nerve head may start to become a greyish white colour and

Table 4.1 Causes of papilloedema

Raised intracranial pressure due to mass lesions	Cerebral tumours
	benign
	malignant
	Intracranial haematoma
	extradural
	subdural
	intracerebral
	Cerebral abscess
	bacterial
	fungal
Raised intracranial pressure due to CSF circulatory block	Aqueductal stenosis
	Intraventricular tumours
	Fourth ventricle outflow block
Cerebral oedema	associated with intracranial tumour
	Post head injury
	Post cerebral anoxia
	Benign intracranial hypertension
	Lead poisoning
	Steroid withdrawal
	Vitamin A intoxication
Raised CSF protein or altered blood products causing impaired CSF resorption	Post subarachnoid haemorrhage
	Post meningitis
	Guillain–Barré Syndrome
	Hypertrophic polyneuritis
	Spinal cord tumours
Malignant phase of hypertension	
Metabolic disorders	Hypercapnia
	Hypocalcaemia (in childhood in particular)
	Malignant thyrotoxic exophthalmos
Disorders of the circulation	Central retinal vein thrombosis
	Lateral sinus thrombosis
	Jugular vein thrombosis
	Superior vena cava obstruction
	Polycythaemia rubra vera
	Multiple myelomatosis
	Macroglobulinaemia
	Diabetes mellitus
	Hyperlipidaemia
	Arteriosclerotic vessels in the retina
	Vasculitis including temporal arteritis

the patient may notice decreasing visual acuity. When the swelling finally subsides the patient may be left with a flat greyish-white nerve head with very indistinct edges. This scarring process – gliosis – in the nerve head may lead to further serious deterioration of vision long after raised intracranial pressure has been

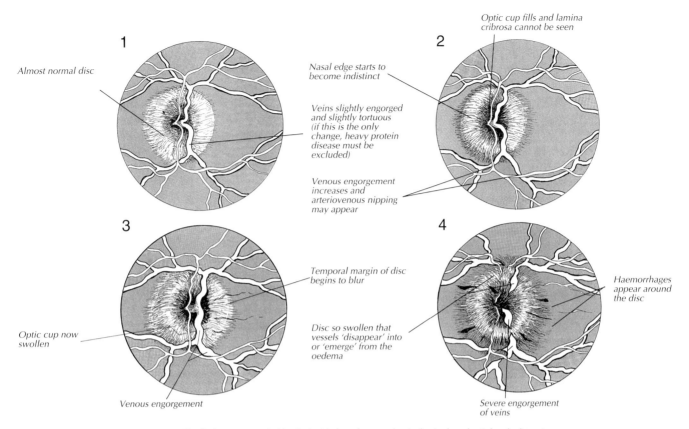

1 Almost normal disc

2 Optic cup fills and lamina cribrosa cannot be seen

Nasal edge starts to become indistinct

Veins slightly engorged and slightly tortuous (if this is the only change, heavy protein disease must be excluded)

Venous engorgement increases and arteriovenous nipping may appear

3 Optic cup now swollen

Venous engorgement

Temporal margin of disc begins to blur

Disc so swollen that vessels 'disappear' into or 'emerge' from the oedema

4 Haemorrhages appear around the disc

Severe engorgement of veins

The final appearance is identical with that of a central retinal vein thrombosis but the latter is unilateral and haemorrhages are usually a prominent feature

4.4 The sequence in developing papilloedema.

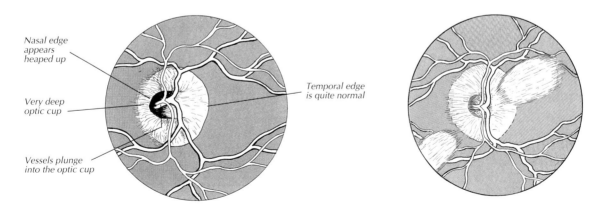

Nasal edge appears heaped up

Very deep optic cup

Vessels plunge into the optic cup

Temporal edge is quite normal

This appearance is very often mistakenly described as papilloedema. In papilloedema the cup is the first part of the disc to fill and become abnormal

Normally nerve fibres are bare beyond the lamina cribrosa. Sometimes they are myelinated on the disc or even on the retina as in this case. The appearance is typically flared and careful focussing will usually reveal the fibres traversing the area. This abnormality will produce a field defect as it obscures the retinal cells. The patient is unaware of the defect as it is present from birth

4.5 Deep optic cup simulating papilloedema.

4.6 Medullated nerve fibres.

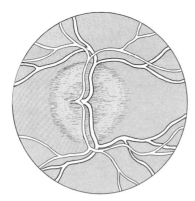

This is a late result of previous papilloedema. It is character-ized by attenuation of the blood vessels and a greyish flattened disc with unclear margins

4.7   Secondary optic atrophy.

relieved. This is called consecutive or secondary optic atrophy (Fig. 4.7). Typically there is progressive loss of the peripheral visual field, starting nasally and cul-minating in near-total blindness. The earliest possible relief of raised intracranial pressure is therefore indi-cated, but no confident prognosis for vision can be given to a patient who has evidence of optic atrophy or decreased acuity when first seen. The visual loss may continue to progress even when the pressure is effect-ively reduced. Papilloedema should always be regarded as an emergency, not just because of possible serious underlying disease but also because of its potential for causing blindness unless rapidly relieved by diuretics, steroids, mannitol or surgery where appropriate.

Primary Optic Atrophy

Following any toxic insult, injury, occlusion of the central retinal artery, compressive, infiltrative or demyelinating process affecting the optic nerve, the patient may develop primary optic atrophy. The nerve head becomes extremely pale and the lamina cribrosa becomes very distinct. This is a highly subjective

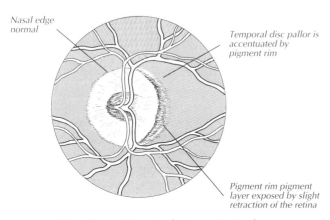

Nasal edge normal

Temporal disc pallor is accentuated by pigment rim

Pigment rim pigment layer exposed by slight retraction of the retina

4.8   Pigment rim simulating optic atophy.

appearance and doubtful cases are often recorded as 'slight pallor of discs'. In the past many patients were incorrectly diagnosed as suffering from multiple scler-osis using this highly subjective sign as corroborative evidence, a very unwise policy. The visual acuity and the visual field to red may be normal and do not alone disprove the diagnosis of primary optic atrophy. VERs should always be used to confirm that this suspected finding is abnormal.

The normal variations in disc colour are consider-able. The temporal edge of the disc is relatively avas-cular and always looks pale compared with the nasal half of the disc. The lamina cribrosa is often well marked and forms the very pale central area of the disc. The pallor of a normal disc may be accentuated by a rim of pigment that is often seen at the temporal edge of the disc due to the slight retraction of the retina that occurs developmentally (Fig. 4.8).

Miscellaneous Appearances

1. Patients with decreasing visual acuity may have macular degeneration and a close inspection of the macula (to be found two disc diameters from the tem-poral edge of the disc) is necessary. This requires dilatation of the pupil in most instances. The normal macula is a small pale-yellow spot in a slightly darker area of the retina, and expert ophthalmological advice is necessary for full evaluation of this region.

2. Patients with transient ischaemic attacks may have evidence of embolization of the retinal vessels. Small, highly refractile fragments of cholesterol may be seen blocking arterioles, usually at the bifurcations. Distally the vessels appear pale and empty.

3. Patients with night blindness and patients with a variety of inherited neurological disorders may have retinitis pigmentosa. This consists of spider like nets of pigment that are initially seen at the periphery of the retina (Fig. 4.9). This will later be associated with a severe degree of primary optic atrophy secondary to severe narrowing of the arterioles and destruction of the retinal cells. Peripheral constriction of the fields occurs with progressive diminution in visual acuity, cul-minating in blindness. The marked narrowing of the arterioles is an important diagnostic feature. Retinitis pigmentosa is associated with Lawrence–Moon–Beidl syndrome, abetalipoproteinaemia, Kearns–Sayre syn-drome and Refsum's disease.

4. Rapid loss of central vision, often described by the patient as if a red or orange ball were present in front of the eye, with persistent after-images, metamorphopsia or micropsia, is a feature of a disease known as central serous retinopathy. In this condition there may be marked oedema and heaping up of the retina, causing the distortion of vision. The condition occurs mainly in young males and responds to steroids.

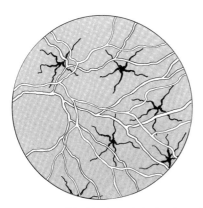

Striking attenuation of the blood vessels: both veins and arteries are extremely narrowed, with spider-like patches of pigment. Initially only found at the periphery, hence no optic disc shown in this view.

4.9 Retinitis pigmentosa.

5. Brief attacks of metamorphopsia, typically lasting 20–30 minutes, occur in migraine and attacks lasting seconds only may occur in complex partial seizures.

Other Unusual Disc Appearances

Prepapillary Arterial Loops

These may be found in 5% of patients. They usually project forwards about 1.5 mm from the centre of the disc as a little coiled loop that heads back on itself. In 75% of patients this is associated with the presence of a cilioretinal artery (Fig. 4.10). The loop usually arises from the inferior artery and may be covered with a glistening white sheath. Small venous loops may appear with raised venous pressure. These are smaller and do not arise on the disc itself.

Persistent Hyaloid Artery

This is a remnant of the artery that supplied the lens during development. It comes straight forward off the disc and ends blindly. It is not tortuous. It can occasionally be the source of a vitreous haemorrhage (Fig. 4.11).

Persistent Bergmeisters Papilla

Bergmeisters papilla is a sheet of glial cells that surround the hyaloid artery embryologically. This normally disappears at 7 months' gestational age. If remnants persist, a white sheet, like a veil or a ship's sail, projects forwards into the vitreous of the eye, arising from the disc. This is referred to as a persistent glial membrane (Fig. 4.12).

Colobomas of the Optic Disc

Colobomas are due to the persistence of the inferor embryonic cleft of the developing eyeball and produce

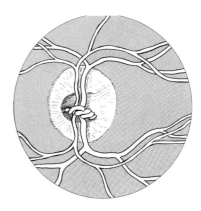

Various loops of the blood vessels on the disc may be encountered. The commonest are arterial, and careful focussing will usually reveal that the vessel is twisted on itself and heads back towards the disc before turning into the upper and lower division

4.10 Prepapillary arterial loops.

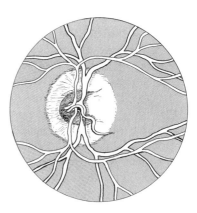

Embryologically the artery runs straight forwards towards the back of the lens in the hyaloid canal. A persistent remnant will project forward and has a snake-like appearance. Careful focussing will reveal its full extent

4.11 Persistent hyaloid artery.

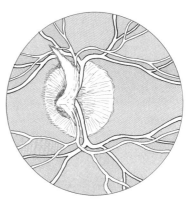

These are glial membrane remnants, usually originating on the disc and often attached to or partially sheathing the emerging vessels. They produce a white flare like a ship's sail

4.12 Bergmeister's papilla.

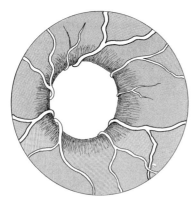

Colobomas are congenital malformations of the disc which produce a flat white cupped disc, the vessels seeming to emerge around the edges of a deep cup

4.13   Coloboma.

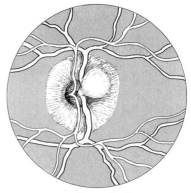

A fairly common congenital anomaly of uncertain origin. If they are in the centre of the disc they may simulate papill-loedema and tend to produce arcuate scotomas, mimicking the field defects of glaucoma. Careful focusing on the disc will often reveal their presence but fluorescein angiography may also be helpful in evaluating the appearance

4.14   Drusen.

a white hole in the retina. They can extend forward to produce a defect in the iris but if in the disc itself, produce an appearance as if a white saucer had been pushed into the optic nerve head (Fig. 4.13).

Drusen

These are developmental abnormalities in the optic nerve head producing a refractile mass that grows and may produce arcuate nerve bundle-type visual field defects. If embedded just behind the disc, the appearance may simulate papilloedema. Their exact nature is uncertain but they are quite common. Fluorescein angiography can be particularly helpful in resolving this diagnostic problem (Fig. 4.14).

Ophthalmoscopy requires a certain amount of skill. Once the skill is acquired a considerable degree of familiarity with normal fundal appearances is necessary to detect minor but possibly significant abnormalities. In many instances the interpretation of appearances is highly subjective, and it is wrong to place too much reliance on disputed appearances unless corroboratory evidence using field testing, fluorescein angiography or visually evoked potentials confirms the suspected abnormality.

5. The Third, Fourth and Sixth Cranial Nerves

This group of three cranial nerves controls the upper eyelid, eye movements and pupils. Each has a long intracranial course. Due to this they are subject to damage by a wide range of disease processes at various sites. A careful history and clinical examination will usually provide all the information necessary for accurate diagnosis. Difficulty in remembering the actions of the various extraocular muscles and their nerve supply is a universal problem, and therefore these aspects are covered extensively in this chapter.

The Extra Ocular Muscles

The names, positions and actions of the extra ocular muscles are illustrated and discussed in Figures 5.1–5.4. The main points to note are:

1. The medial rectus muscle of one eye and the lateral rectus muscle of the other work as a yoked pair to produce lateral eye movements. The central mechanisms responsible for synchronizing these actions are discussed in Chapter 7.
2. The vertically acting rectus muscles are at their most effective when the eye is abducted, that is, looking outwards, as in this position the line of pull of the muscles is along the vertical axis of the eye.
3. In the same way the oblique muscles are maximally effective when the eye is adducted, that is, looking inwards, as their line of pull is then along the vertical axis of the eye.

These are the most important points to remember when evaluating eye movements from a neurological standpoint. All the muscles have secondary actions and some have torsional effects. It is probably because these other movements are given such emphasis in anatomical textbooks that so few can understand or remember the simple facts needed for an adequate neurological examination!

Diplopia

The single symptom that often indicates damage to one or other of the three nerves under discussion is diplopia. This should not be taken to imply that diplopia is always due to a nerve lesion. A discussion of other causes of diplopia will be found at the end of this chapter.

Explanation of Diplopia

The eyes are normally positioned so that the image falls on exactly the same spot on the retina of each eye. The slightest displacement of either eye causes diplopia as the image is shifted to a different position on the retina of the displaced eye (confirm this by displacing one of your own eyes by gently pressing it through the eyelid). In the case of nerve lesions the weak muscle or muscles can usually be detected by direct observation of the eye movements. Occasionally, mild lesions or other diseases may cause diplopia in which the degree of weakness is too slight to be observed. In these situations the cover test is useful.

The Cover Test

This test is based on the fact that the separation of the two images becomes greatest as the eyes attempt to look in the direction of action of the weak muscle, because the disparity in eye movements is then maximal. The false image falls progressively further away from the macula of the lagging eye and is therefore always projected as the outer image of the two. If the examiner asks the patient to follow a stick until double vision is maximal, and then determines which eye he must cover to obliterate the outer image, the affected eye is identified. The weak muscle can then be determined from the direction of the gaze (Fig. 5.5).

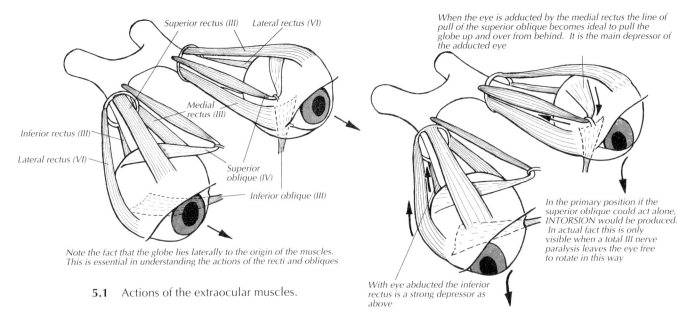

Note the fact that the globe lies laterally to the origin of the muscles.
This is essential in understanding the actions of the recti and obliques

5.1   Actions of the extraocular muscles.

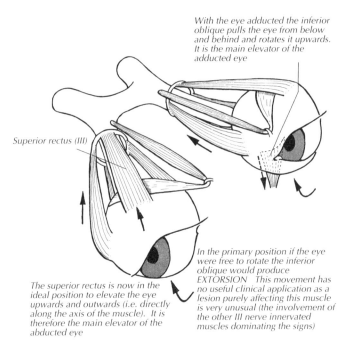

These muscles usually act as a pair in
conjugate gaze to either side. The
medial recti act together in
convergence. The central pathways
for these movements are discussed in
Chapter 7

5.2   Actions of the medial and lateral rectus muscles (lateral gaze to right side).

Clinical Manifestations of Extraocular Nerve Lesions

Third Nerve Palsy (Fig. 5.6)

A complete third nerve lesion causes total paralysis of the eyelid and therefore diplopia only occurs when the lid is held up. Severe diplopia then occurs in all directions, except on lateral gaze to the side of the third nerve lesion (because the lateral rectus muscle is intact).

When the lid is lifted the eye will be found deviated outwards (lateral rectus action) and downwards (secondary depressant action of the superior oblique muscle). The integrity of these muscles and hence their nerve supply should be carefully evaluated to be certain that the third nerve is the **only** nerve affected.

5.3   Action of vertically acting muscles in down gaze.

5.4   Action of vertically acting muscles in up gaze.

To do this the examiner should test lateral gaze in the affected eye and note the disappearance of diplopia in that direction. The normal downward movement produced by the superior oblique muscle cannot be tested because the paralysed medial rectus does not allow the eye to adduct. Instead the secondary action of the muscle is observed. The depressed position of the eye is usually already apparent. If the patient makes a further effort to look downwards the eye will rotate inwards (intorsion), as the superior oblique muscle pulls sideways across the eye when it is in this position.

(a L VI nerve palsy is illustrated)

On looking to the L. the L. eye remains static. As the object moves the image falls on the retina to the nasal side and is projected further and further into the temporal half field, away from the macula

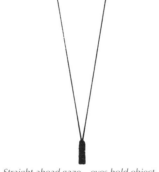

On gazing to the R. both eyes move sufficiently to keep the object on the macula of each eye

Straight ahead gaze – eyes hold object on the macula

The rules are:
   The false image is always the outer one
   The false image always comes from the affected eye

5.5   Mechanism of diplopia.

(The eyelid sags passively – the eye can be shut tightly via the VII nerve)

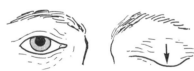

To show the position of the eye when the lid is lifted
The eye is abducted (intact VI) and slightly depressed (intact IV). The pupil is dilated

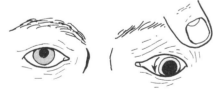

To confirm intact IV nerve; note the inward rotation (intorsion) of the eye when the patient attempts to look down. This is the rotary action of the superior oblique that occurs when the eye cannot be abducted

5.6   Ptosis in complete third nerve palsy.

Observation of this movement is the best evidence of an intact superior oblique muscle and hence the integrity of the fourth nerve.

The pupil may be normal or dilated and fixed to light. This important feature is fully discussed later. The lesion should be described as a pupil-sparing third nerve palsy if it reacts normally. This feature, and whether or not the onset was painful, is critical in the differential diagnosis.

Fourth Nerve Palsy (Fig. 5.7)

A fourth nerve lesion causes weakness of the superior oblique muscle, producing very subtle diplopia. The weakness of the muscle in the primary position, looking

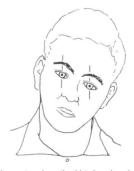

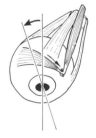

The patient has tilted his head to the L. to line up the image from the good eye with the outwardly rotated R. eye

Normally the superior oblique, by pulling across the top of the eye, slightly rotates it inwards. If paralysed the eye will rotate slightly outwards causing a slightly oblique image

5.7   Compensatory head tilt in a patient with a superior oblique paralysis of the right eye.

straight ahead, allows the eye to rotate slightly out-wards. This movement is known as extorsion and the unopposed pull of the ipsilateral inferior rectus muscle will slightly elevate the eye. The very slight slant of the image will make the patient tilt their head slightly away from the side of the affected eye to line up with the vertical image from the normal eye. In children this head tilt may be misdiagnosed as torticollis.

Frank diplopia occurs when the patient looks down and away from the side of the affected eye. This often leads to trouble going downstairs, as two treads are seen when the patient looks downwards and sideways, as one normally does while descending stairs. Similarly, diplopia may occur while reading a news-paper or a book.

A common error is to diagnose weakness of the superior rectus on the unaffected side, because the unaffected eye looks down when the patient is fixing with the affected eye. In bilateral fourth nerve lesions, which often complicate head injury, as the patient looks from side to side the outward-looking eye appears to drop down, producing an apparent alternating superior rectus palsy, which is in reality over action of the opposite inferior rectus muscle, the paired muscle of the paralysed superior oblique (Fig. 5.8).

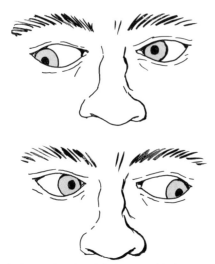

On looking to the right or left, the outward looking eye suddenly pulls down as the brain attempt to compensate for theweakness of the superior oblique as the eye looks inwards. The overaction of the paired inferior rectus muscle pulls the eye down. A striking finding which may be mistakenly diagnosed as bilateral weakness of the superior rectus.

5.8   Bilateral fourth nerve palsy (simulating bilateral superior rectus palsy.)

Sixth Nerve Palsy

A sixth nerve palsy (Fig. 5.9) causes the greatest problem for the patient, as there is no ptosis to obliter-

(The lid is not ptosed – the eye is tightly shut)

To show the position of the eye when open
The affected eye is deviated towards the nose. To prevent diplopia the patient may turn the head until the right eye is sufficiently abducted to give a single image

5.9   Voluntary eye closure to obliterate double vision with a sixth nerve palsy of the left eye.

ate the false image and disconcerting diplopia persists in nearly all directions of gaze except away from the affected side. Occasionally patients will deliberately shut the affected eye to prevent the diplopia, and this can be misinterpreted as ptosis. If the examiner holds the normal eyelid shut, the lid on the side of the 'pseudo ptosis' will open. At rest the affected eye is pulled medially by the unopposed action of the medial rectus muscle. The patient may compensate by turning his head towards the weak muscle to produce a single image which, at the same time, gives the patient a somewhat shifty look!

Intracranial Anatomy of the Third, Fourth and Sixth Cranial Nerves
(Fig. 5.10)

These nerves run a generally converging course towards the apex of the orbit from widely separate origins in the brain stem. The anatomy of the nuclei is described in greater detail in Chapter 7.

The Third Nerve (Oculomotor Nerve)

The third nerves emerge from the midbrain between the cerebral peduncles. They then splay out as they pass anteriorly, lying between the posterior cerebral arteries and the superior cerebellar arteries, and then run parallel to the posterior communicating arteries until they enter the cavernous sinus. They then lie between the two layers of dura that form the lateral wall of the sinus. The nerve enters the orbit through the superior orbital fissure and divides into two main branches. The upper branch supplies the eyelid and the superior rectus muscle. The lower branch supplies

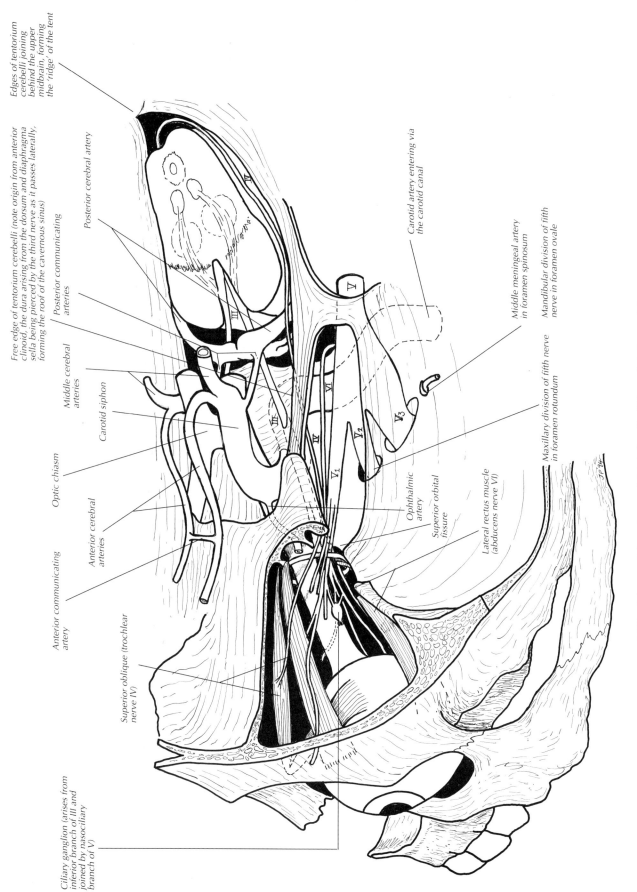

Edges of tentorium cerebelli joining behind the upper midbrain, forming the 'ridge' of the tent

Free edge of tentorium cerebelli (note origin from anterior clinoid, the dura arising from the dorsum and diaphragma sella being pierced by the third nerve as it passes laterally, forming the roof of the cavernous sinus)

Posterior communicating arteries

Posterior cerebral artery

Middle cerebral arteries

Carotid siphon

Optic chiasm

Anterior cerebral arteries

Anterior communicating artery

Superior oblique (trochlear nerve IV)

Ciliary ganglion (arises from inferior branch of III and joined by nasociliary branch of V)

Carotid artery entering via the carotid canal

Middle meningeal artery in foramen spinosum

Mandibular division of fifth nerve in foramen ovale

Maxillary division of fifth nerve in foramen rotundum

Ophthalmic artery

Superior orbital fissure

Lateral rectus muscle (abducens nerve VI)

5.10 Intracranial anatomy of third, fourth, fifth and sixth cranial nerves.

the medial rectus, inferior rectus and inferior oblique and, via the ciliary ganglion, the pupil (see Chapter 3).

The Fourth Nerve (Trochlear Nerve)

This nerve has several unusual features. The supranuclear control is entirely crossed. Its nucleus lies in the dorsum of the brain stem at the level of the inferior colliculus and the fibres decussate (cross over) around the periaqueductal grey and in the superior medullary velum, so that the right nerve originates in the left trochlear nucleus and vice versa. It is the only nerve that emerges on the dorsum of the brain stem. The nerve has a very long intracranial course from the posterior fossa, after encircling the brain stem and passing forwards on the opposite side to enter the cavernous sinus. It enters the roof of the orbit through the superior orbital fissure and actually crosses the third nerve in order to do so. It derives its name from the fact that the superior oblique, the only muscle it supplies, passes round a trochlea (pulley) in the anteromedial orbital roof just under the inner end of the eyebrow.

The Sixth Nerve (Abducent Nerve)

This nerve emerges from the front of the brain stem at the pontomedullary junction, deep in the posterior fossa. It ascends on the front of the brain stem and then angles sharply forwards over the tip of the petrous bone and into the canal under the petroclinoid ligament (Dorello's canal) to enter the back of the cavernous sinus. It lies free in the sinus, enters the orbit through the superior orbital fissure, and passes laterally to reach the lateral rectus muscle.

Causes of Extraocular Nerve Lesions

There are five main sites of potential damage to these nerves, as indicated in Figure 5.11.

Nuclear and Fascicular Lesions

These will be considered in detail in the chapter on brainstem lesions (Chapter 11). There are usually other evidences of brainstem damage to confirm that this is the site of the lesion, and several named syndromes involving these nerves have been described. Causes include brainstem vascular disease, multiple sclerosis, pontine gliomas, extrinsic compression, poliomyelitis, Wernicke's encephalopathy and congenital maldevelopment of the cranial nerve nuclei. Multiple sclerosis is the commonest cause of isolated sixth nerve lesions in the brain stem.

Lesions in the Basilar Area

All three nerves are subject to damage by basal meningeal disease processes. These include tuberculous, fungal and bacterial meningitis, carcinomatous meningitis, direct neoplastic invasion from the sinuses and nasopharynx, meningovascular syphilis, sarcoid, Guillain–Barre syndrome and herpes zoster. In many of these conditions there are multiple or bilateral nerve lesions to indicate a diffuse pathological process. Aneurysmal dilatation or ectasia of the basilar artery may also cause multiple nerve palsies.

Specific involvement of the third nerve in this area occurs in two critical ways, both requiring prompt action.

1. Direct compression by a posterior communicating artery aneurysm. The onset is usually acute with

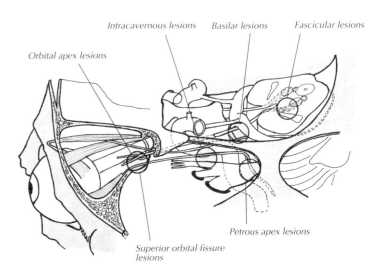

5.11 Anatomical basis of the various lesions.
Lesions as defined by sites in the text

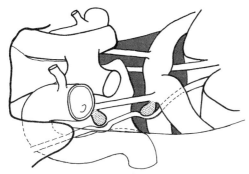

Aneurysms at either end (they typically occur at these sites) are likely to damage III nerve as the artery is immediately adjacent to it

5.12   Posterior communicating artery aneurysms.

severe pain, and the pupil is almost always affected and is dilated and fixed to light (Fig. 5.12).

2. The nerve may be progressively damaged by the prolapsing temporal lobe when the hemisphere is displaced by a mass. This is called a tentorial pressure cone. The patient becomes drowsy and the pupil on the affected side becomes dilated, ptosis develops, and finally a complete third nerve palsy ensues (Fig. 5.13). A third nerve palsy in this situation is very rarely false-localizing (see Chapter 23), and urgent CT scanning and neurosurgical intervention may be indicated.

The sixth nerve may also be affected in the basal area by increased intracranial pressure, although by a different mechanism. This is a situation usually encountered in children, because posterior fossa tumours are more common in childhood and this is often a false-localizing sign. This is because a tumour in the posterior fossa typically causes hydrocephalus – dilatation of the ventricles – and the whole brain tries to squeeze down through the tentorium. This pushes the entire brain stem downwards and the sixth nerve becomes stretched over the petrous tip. One or both nerves may be affected in this way by a lesion quite remote from the nerve itself (see Fig. 5.13).

Lesions at the Petrous Tip

The sixth nerve is clearly the only vulnerable nerve in this area and there are four main causes of damage.

1. Mastoiditis or middle ear infection may cause diffuse inflammation of the petrous bone and thrombosis of the overlying petrosal sinuses. This causes severe ear pain and a combination of sixth, seventh, eighth and occasionally fifth nerve lesions, and is known as Gradenigo's syndrome. This must be differentiated from Ramsay Hunt Syndrome (geniculate herpes zoster), in which there is a vesicular eruption in the ear and a seventh nerve palsy and occasionally other cranial nerve lesions (see also Chapter 6).

2. Lateral sinus thrombosis secondary to mastoiditis may lead to rapidly rising intracranial pressure due to impaired cerebral venous drainage. This may cause a direct or indirect sixth nerve palsy as discussed above. To differentiate this situation from a posterior fossa abscess used to be very difficult. CT scanning has transformed this situation. Previously CSF examination, including compression of the jugular vein, was the only way of making this diagnosis. If the lateral sinus was thrombosed, the normal venous pressure rise on jugular vein compression was not transmitted into the head and no rise in CSF pressure was seen when the affected vein was compressed. The danger was that if the clinical diagnosis was incorrect, the sudden increase in the already elevated intracranial pressure could have serious repercussions.

3. Carcinomas of the nasopharynx or the paranasal sinuses tend to infiltrate through the fissures of the skull base, and a sudden painless sixth nerve palsy may be the first evidence of malignant disease in these tissues.

4. Benign transient sixth nerve palsies may occur in children following mild infections. The advent of CT scanning has made management of this worrying situ-

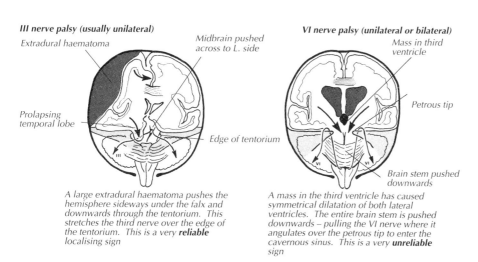

III nerve palsy (usually unilateral)

Extradural haematoma

Midbrain pushed across to L. side

Prolapsing temporal lobe

Edge of tentorium

*A large extradural haematoma pushes the hemisphere sideways under the falx and downwards through the tentorium. This stretches the third nerve over the edge of the tentorium. This is a very **reliable** localising sign*

VI nerve palsy (unilateral or bilateral)

Mass in third ventricle

Petrous tip

Brain stem pushed downwards

*A mass in the third ventricle has caused symmetrical dilatation of both lateral ventricles. The entire brain stem is pushed downwards – pulling the VI nerve where it angulates over the petrous tip to enter the cavernous sinus. This is a very **unreliable** sign*

5.13   The different mechanisms underlying third and sixth nerve palsies in patients with raised intracranial pressure (seen from front).

ation much easier. Previously the diagnosis was difficult to make and was only really confirmed by the subsequent recovery, which often took several weeks, during which time the child had to be kept under constant review.

Lesions in the Region of the Cavernous Sinus

1. Cavernous sinus thrombosis remains a very serious condition that usually occurs as a complication of sepsis of the skin over the upper face or in the paranasal sinuses, and is often lethal in diabetic patients. As the sixth nerve lies free in the sinus it is the most vulnerable nerve The sixth nerve palsy is coupled with severe pain, exophthalmos and oedema of the eyelids, which later involves the opposite eyelid as extension of the thrombosis to the opposite cavernous sinus is almost inevitable.

2. Intrasellar tumours such as chromophobe adenomas may extend laterally into the sinus and may damage the third nerve (Fig. 5.14).

3. Aneurysmal dilatation of the intracavernous portion of the carotid artery usually occurs in elderly

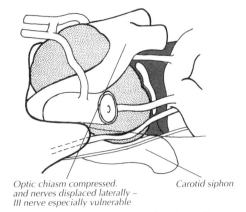

Optic chiasm compressed. and nerves displaced laterally – III nerve especially vulnerable   *Carotid siphon*

5.14   Intrasellar mass spreading laterally.

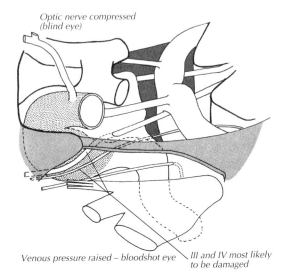

Optic nerve compressed (blind eye)

Venous pressure raised – bloodshot eye   *III and IV most likely to be damaged*

5.15   Intracavernous aneurysm (anterior type).

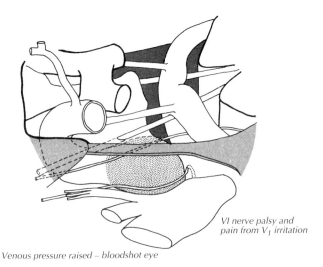

VI nerve palsy and pain from V₁ irritation

Venous pressure raised – bloodshot eye

5.16   Intracavernous aneurysm (posterior type).

hypertensive females. If the swelling of the artery is at the anterior end of the sinus, oedema of the eyelid, exophthalmos, blindness and a third nerve lesion may occur simultaneously, heralded by quite severe pain. If the dilatation is at the posterior end of the sinus, the first division of the fifth nerve may be irritated with severe pain over the fifth nerve distribution (ophthalmic division) and a sixth nerve palsy. The eye becomes suffused and proptosed (Figs. 5.15 and 5.16). If the vessel actually ruptures into the sinus it is rarely fatal as the cavernous sinus will contain the haemorrhage, but a severe unilateral and later bilateral pulsatile exophthalmos occurs. This is called a caroticocavernous fistula and may also follow a head injury if a basal fracture tears the carotid artery at its point of entry into the sinus. This is now treated by catheter embolization of the artery instead of direct surgery.

4. Primary tumours in the sinus are rare but meningiomas of the sphenoid wing may invade the sinus laterally. Tumours within the sphenoid sinus and mucocoeles related to infection in the sphenoid or ethmoid sinuses may spread into the sinus medially or from below. Chordomas of the basi sphenoid may extend up into the pituitary fossa or laterally into both cavernous sinuses, and craniopharyngiomas may behave similarly from above and behind. Secondary carcinomas in the sinus itself or in the skull base may occur, and carcinoma of the nasopharynx may extend directly into the sinus. This is one of the commonest presenting symptoms of carcinoma of the nasopharynx.

Lesions at the Superior Orbital Fissure and Orbit

There are numerous neoplasms that may arise in the posterior orbit and a fairly well-defined syndrome results. These lesions are listed in Table 5.1. Because all the nerves are relatively close together, palsies of the third, fourth and sixth nerves in various combina-

Table 5.1   Lesions arising in the orbit and optic foramina

Meningiomas	40%
Haemangiomas	10%
Gliomas	5%
Pseudotumour of the orbit	5%
Carcinoma of the lacrimal duct Neurofibroma Fibrous dysplasia of bone Sarcoma Epidermoid Melanoma Lipoma Hand–Schuller–Christian disease Tolosa–Hunt syndrome Arteriovenous malformations	40%

ttions may occur. Involvement of the fifth nerve may cause pain and later numbness in the distribution of the first division of the fifth nerve, with depression of the corneal response.

Some generalizations are possible:

1. Malignant infiltration of the orbit (by direct spread of carcinoma of the nasopharynx or remote spread from carcinomas in other sites) produces rapidly evolving extraocular nerve palsies and proptosis.

2. Benign tumours in the orbit may cause very slowly progressive but quite marked proptosis, with remarkably little visual loss or nerve palsies until quite late in the course of the disease. The diplopia is often purely the result of mechanical displacement of the globe.

3. Lesions in the superior orbital fissure or intracranial lesions just behind the fissure cause nerve palsies with little or no proptosis.

4. Lesions in the orbit tend to cause proptosis as an early sign. If, in addition, there is considerable pain and redness of the eye the condition known as 'pseudo tumour of the orbit' must be considered. This is usually associated with a high ESR and responds to steroids. It may well be a mild variant of the rare Tolosa–Hunt syndrome, in which a mass of granulomatous tissue is found behind the eye and in the orbital fissure. The possibility of unilateral proptosis with superior rectus muscle weakness being due to endocrine disease must always be excluded. Even in the absence of frank thyrotoxicosis, hyperthyroidism is the most common cause of unilateral proptosis.

5. Vascular tumours and arteriovenous malformations in the orbit may only cause proptosis when the patient is lying down, bending forwards or performing the Valsalva manoeuvre while passing a motion.

CASE REPORT I

A 64-year-old man with known carcinoma of the prostate with bony metastases presented with an incomplete right sixth

nerve palsy. This had occurred quite painlessly and examination revealed no evidence of proptosis or other extraocular nerve lesions. In view of the recent change in his hormonal therapy, which had successfully controlled pain in a known rib metastasis, it was decided to observe this conservatively and for 3 weeks there was no change in his condition. Suddenly, in the fourth week, the sixth nerve palsy became complete, although there was no other change in the symptomatology. A CT scan revealed extensive destruction of the basi sphenoid on the right-hand side, and the patient received radiotherapy to the affected area and fully recovered in 3 months.

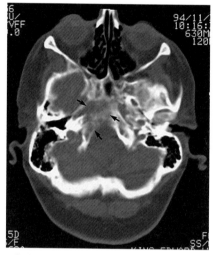

CRI. *Skull base destruction due to metastatic prostatic carcinoma.*

This case confirms the extreme vulnerability of the sixth nerve to infection and carcinoma, with its long course adjacent not only to the meninges but also to the skull base.

CT and MRI scanning have revolutionized the investigation of orbital lesions in what was previously a diagnostic minefield.

Miscellaneous Disease Processes Causing Extraocular Nerve Lesions

1. A number of medical diseases may cause painless acute extraocular nerve palsies. These are diabetes mellitus, meningovascular syphilis and arteriosclerosis A **painful** third nerve palsy with **pupil sparing** is nearly always due to diabetes. The presumed pathology is infarction of the nerve trunk, and hence in third nerve lesions due to these causes the pupil is usually spared (see Figure 2.4a for explanation). The prognosis in all instances is for complete recovery of function to occur over some 4–12 weeks. If recovery does not occur the diagnosis must be reconsidered.

In comparison, an extraocular palsy due to a surgical cause is almost **always** painful, and when the third nerve is involved **the pupil is also affected**. Another uncommon vascular cause of painful extraocular nerve palsy is cranial arteritis, a condition usually confined to patients over 60 years of age and accompanied by severe nocturnal headache and scalp tenderness (see also Chapter 20).

2. During acute migraine headaches transient extraocular nerve palsies or Horner's syndrome may occur. An incomplete third nerve palsy generally accompanied by a dilated pupil is the usual finding, but less typically a sixth nerve palsy may be seen. The transient nature of the palsy, repeated identical attacks and the characteristics of the headache should suggest the diagnosis. The first episode may prompt exclusion of an aneurysm. A long history of repeated attacks may allow a confident diagnosis to be made without further investigations.

3. Third and sixth nerve lesions may occur during acute herpes zoster ophthalmicus. The diagnosis is usually very obvious, with an extensive vesicular eruption over the forehead preceded by severe pain. The prognosis for recovery is good.

4. Fourth nerve lesions in isolation are quite rare. Diabetes is probably the most frequent medical cause. In children medulloblastomas which infiltrate the superior medullary velum may produce bilateral fourth nerve palsies. Trauma is the commonest surgical cause of unilateral or bilateral fourth nerve lesions. Apparent unilateral dysfunction of the superior oblique muscle may follow damage to the trochlea itself by trauma to the upper orbital margin. Extrinsic compression by tumours rarely causes fourth nerve lesions, as the nerve is long enough to move away from the lesion without being damaged.

CASE REPORT II

A 42-year-old woman was referred by an ophthalmologist for further investigation of a fourth nerve palsy that came on acutely during an otherwise typical migraine 5 weeks previously. She had complained of blurred vision but had not noticed diplopia because she had developed a compensatory head tilt. She gave a 20-year history of migraine, but commented that the recent headaches were more sudden and paroxysmal in type without associated nausea or vomiting. Apart from the left fourth nerve lesion there were no other neurological findings. She was reviewed a month later. She had noticed a new symptom within the preceding month: when she leant her head backwards and to the right she developed a sudden surge of headache which cleared the moment she resumed a normal position. This symptom and the fourth nerve palsy raised the possibility of a lesion in the posterior midbrain or superior medullary velum blocking the fourth ventricle. A CT scan was performed. This revealed an enormous tumour extending from just behind the pineal, enveloping the back of the brain stem and up through the tentorial hiatus into both lateral ventricles, with a modest degree of hydrocephalus. Four-vessel angiography was normal. At operation the tumour

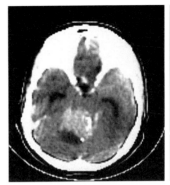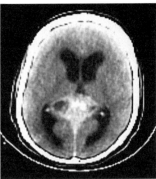

CRII. *Extensive tumour originating in the pineal region.*

was found to be arising in the vermis and had spread into both cerebellar and cerebral hemispheres and completely occluded the fourth ventricle. It was extremely vascular and contained multiple areas of haemorrhage. Post operatively the patient was in an akinetic mute state and a scan revealed massive haemorrhage into the extensions of the tumour in the lateral ventricles and upper brain stem. Histologically, the tumour was a malignant oligodendrocytic grade III glioma. Surprisingly she made a steady recovery and radiotherapy was given. Six weeks later retractory nystagmus was the only residual finding in the CNS. The patient survived for 3 years requiring subsequent shunting, although she was never able to return to work. Two years after the insertion of the shunt it became blocked by recurrent tumour. More extensive surgery and further radiotherapy were felt to be unjustified.

There are several lessons to be learnt from this case. Subtle changes in a patient's migraine should always be carefully reconsidered. Paroxysmal headache on altered head posture may be a very significant symptom and several other similar case reports are included in other chapters. The paucity of physical findings in a patient with an enormous tumour in a strategic area must be emphasized. Once again, it was historical features rather than physical findings that led to the early detection of the tumour.

Tolosa–Hunt syndrome is a recurrent unilateral orbital pain accompanied by transient extraocular nerve palsies and a very high ESR. CT scanning reveals evidence of thickening of the retro-ocular tissues. The dramatic response to steroids is diagnostic.

Wegener's granulomatosis is an extremely rare collagen vascular disease of which a midline ulcerating lesion affecting the nasopharynx is one variety. Haemorrhagic nasal discharge, an extraocular nerve palsy and a high ESR is a classic presentation of the condition.

CASE REPORT III

A 68-year-old man was referred to an ENT surgeon with a 4-month history of a blocked airway, marked reduction in his sense of smell and 3 weeks' severe headache worsened by straining or sneezing. He reported transient diplopia with lateral separation of the images lasting only 2 days. In view of a clinical suspicion of Wegener's granulomatosis the ENT surgeon was asked to arrange an ESR before the patient was seen. It was elevated at 66mm/hr. Further evaluation of the history suggested that the patient had had a transient sixth nerve palsy, and direct questioning revealed that he had felt generally unwell and had lost a stone in weight in the previous 3 months. With the exception of slightly protuberant bloodshot eyes, physical examination was normal. An examination of the nasopharynx under general anaesthesia and biopsy revealed granulomatous changes consistent with Wegener's granulomatosis. Further investigation excluded disease elsewhere, although tests for rheumatoid arthritis and smooth muscle antibodies were positive. He was treated with steroids and azathioprine and remained well until 5 years later, when he had a myocardial infarct. Yearly examinations of the postnasal space and biopsies had been negative. However, after his myocardial infarct the ESR had continued to rise and 2 months later he perforated a previously asymptomatic carcinoma of the transverse colon. He died 2 years later of a recurrent myocardial infarct, with no evidence of active granulomatous disease.

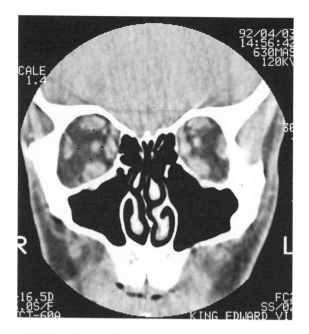

CRIV. *Extraocular muscle swelling in malignant exophthalmos.*

Other Conditions Simulating Nerve Lesions

Extraocular nerve palsies are usually all-or-nothing. Partial palsies are relatively rare, and usually all the muscles supplied by the nerve show some degree of weakness. In the case of a fourth or sixth nerve palsy only one muscle can be affected. Therefore, if two muscles supplied by **different** extraocular nerves are affected the following conditions should be considered.

Thyrotoxicosis

Weakness of the superior rectus muscle and the lateral rectus muscle commonly causes diplopia in thyrotoxicosis, irrespective of the presence of exophthalmos. The pathological changes in the muscles suggest that an inflammatory myopathic process is responsible. Thyrotoxic exophthalmos can also cause diplopia, purely by mechanical displacement of the globe.

Myasthenia gravis

Diplopia and ptosis of the eyelid are the common presenting symptoms of myasthenia gravis, and variable eye signs or fatiguability of the eyelid or eye movements should always raise this diagnostic possibility. In some patients more permanent or even apparently progressive signs occur and cause diagnostic confusion. In some instances even a Tensilon test may be negative (see Chapter 18). Patients have been known to have ophthalmological operations for squints which were later proved to be due to myasthenia gravis! Thyrotoxicosis can be associated with myasthenia gravis, further complicating the clinical picture.

CASE REPORT IV

A 62-year-old man was referred by an ophthalmologist with a 4 week history of vertical diplopia. A few months previously he had been diagnosed as myxoedematous and was on treatment with thyroxine. He had an extraordinary family history in that his father, grandfather and sister had all had pernicious anaemia, his mother had died of thyrotoxicosis in 1931, and both daughters were in renal failure, one due to Prader–Willi syndrome and the other due to autoimmune nephritis. On examination he had marked bilateral ptosis, impairment of up gaze in both eyes, bilateral weakness of abduction and almost no adduction of the left eye. All these signs cleared completely within 1 minute of 4 mg of edrophonium (Tensilon). Full autoimmune screening revealed no abnormality, and even thyroid and acetylcholine receptor antibodies were negative. He was treated with pyridostigmine and prednisolone, with variable control of his severe ocular symptoms. Azathioprine was therefore added to the regimen. Over the next few months his weight fell and he developed lid retraction and exophthalmos. Blood tests revealed that he was now thyrotoxic. Thyroid hormone was stopped, carbimazole was given and his antimyasthenia treatment continued. Over the next 3 months severe progressive malignant exophthalmos developed, with an admixture of diplopia due to globe displacement and variable weakness of different extraocular muscles. Very high doses of steroids were given, with near complete resolution of the exophthalmos and much better control of the myasthenic symptoms. Three years after the onset he remains euthyroid, with slight vertical diplopia when fatigued and slight exophthalmos. No other features of myasthenia have developed.

Over 3 years this patient has demonstrated ocular motility problems due to myasthenia gravis, mechanical displacement of the globe, and possibly thyrotoxic extraocular myopathy. The severity of extraocular muscle swelling related to the thyrotoxicosis can be seen on the CT orbital scans.

Latent Strabismus

Diplopia under conditions of fatigue, drowsiness or following impairment of vision in either eye is often due to the breaking down of a lifelong squint. A history of a childhood squint or previous orthoptic exercises often establishes the cause. If there is no previous history another form of cover test may be useful.

The examiner covers one of the patient's eyes and asks them to fix their gaze on a finger held about 18 inches away. When the other eye is uncovered it will be seen deviated inwards or outwards and will quickly pull back to line up with the other eye. This has unmasked a latent deviation requiring positive muscle action to keep it compensated. Fatigue allows the eye to drift, resulting in diplopia usually in the evenings while watching TV. The development of uncorrected impaired vision in one eye will also make it difficult for the patient to maintain binocular vision, and will unmask a latent squint.

Progressive Ocular Myopathy

This is a relatively rare form of muscular dystrophy in which the main progressive muscle weakness occurs in the extraocular muscles and eyelids causing ptosis and diplopia. Careful examination usually discloses that there is also weakness of the facial and limb girdle muscles (see also Chapter 18). Familial ptosis is probably a mild variant of this condition which usually starts in adulthood and may be associated with impaired upward gaze. Ptosis props fitted to the spectacle frames may be required to push the lid up off the pupil and may be useful in some patients.

Kearns–Sayre Syndrome

This is a very rare but important syndrome, an example of inherited mitochondrial DNA disease. It usually starts before 20 years of age, as a progressive external ophthalmoplegia associated with pigmentary retinal degeneration. Mental retardation and cerebellar ataxia are associated features. Cardiac conduction defects are usually present and often the cause of death.

Internuclear Ophthalmoplegia

Multiple sclerosis may present as an extraocular nerve palsy, usually a sixth nerve lesion. More often diplopia occurs without weakness of any individual eye movement due to disruption of the conjugate eye movement mechanism, and this is discussed fully in Chapter 7.

General Approach to Diplopia

Whenever a patient presents with the symptom of diplopia the following sequence of questions will usually establish the site of the lesion and provide a strong clue to the cause.

1. Was the onset acute or gradual? Clearly, one either has or has not got diplopia, but a relentless worsening suggests infiltration of the nerves or a mechanical displacement of the globe.

2. Is there any variability or remission? Extraocular nerve lesions of any cause are usually 'all or nothing'. If the symptom varies from time to time a latent strabismus or myasthenia gravis must be considered.

3. Is there any associated ptosis of the eyelid? An acute third nerve palsy usually includes complete ptosis of the eyelid. Lesser degrees of ptosis or variable ptosis should suggest myasthenia gravis or a progressive ocular myopathy. Occasionally, patients with allergic swelling of the eyelid are incorrectly diagnosed as suffering from a recurrent partial third nerve lesion: obvious oedema of the eyelid during an attack should establish the diagnosis.

4. Was there any pain? A painful onset usually indicates aneurysmal dilatation of a blood vessel, either a berry aneurysm causing a third nerve palsy or an aneurysmal dilatation of the intracavernous part of the carotid artery causing a third or sixth nerve palsy. Incomplete loss of eye movements and severe congestion of the eye should also raise the possibility of a granulomatous lesion in the orbit, either pseudotumour of the orbit or Tolosa–Hunt syndrome.

Herpes zoster opthalmicus with an extraocular nerve palsy should also be considered as the vesicular rash may take several days to appear, during which time there is severe pain in the distribution of the first division of the fifth nerve.

Migraine headache may be complicated by a transient extraocular nerve palsy. If there is a history of previous migraine or a positive family history this diagnosis may be readily suspected. In a first attack this can be a challenging diagnosis, particularly considering the vicious nature of migraine headaches that readily mimic more serious intracranial conditions. In the elderly, severe headache and extraocular nerve palsy should raise the possibility of cranial arteritis.

5. Is there any exophthalmos or proptosis? Protrusion of the globe, especially if associated with swelling and suffusion of the bulbar conjunctiva, suggests the presence of either an aneurysm in the cavernous sinus, thrombosis of the cavernous sinus with vascular congestion, or a tumour in the orbit. The rapidity of onset and the presence of pain usually enables the distinction to be made, but the inflammatory conditions of the orbit which respond to steroids should also be considered.

The fact that thyrotoxicosis is the commonest cause of exophthalmos should always be remembered, even if unilateral. The term 'exophthalmos' is most accurately applied to the bulging eye associated with thyrotoxicosis. A bulging eye due to all other causes is correctly referred to as proptosis.

Proptosis and Orbital Tumours (Figs. 5.17 and 5.18)

There are several interesting aspects of these lesions that allow firm clinical conclusions to be reached.

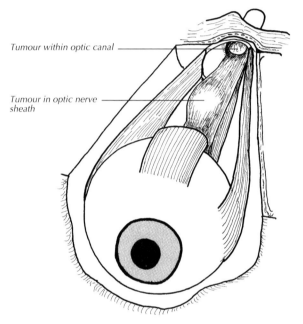

Tumour within optic canal

Tumour in optic nerve sheath

5.17   Lesion within the optic nerve sheath. (Early optic nerve compression with blindness)

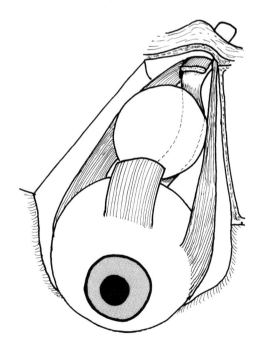

5.18   Lesion within the musclecone. (Proptosis but no visual impairment)

Visual Impairment

Tumours within the nerve sheath cause marked visual loss. Tumours within the muscle cone cause marked proptosis, but vision is often surprisingly unaffected. Tumours in the optic nerve canal cause very early visual loss, which is usually the presenting symptom.

Pain

Pain is not a feature in slow-growing tumours, even when proptosis is severe. Infective and metastatic lesions may cause severe pain before proptosis is apparent. If the eye is painful and red, thyroid disease, pseudotumour, caroticocavernous fistula and herpes zoster are the major conditions to be considered.

Eye Movements

If the eye movement abnormality seems to be purely due to displacement of the globe, the lesion is likely to be benign. If there is clear evidence of an extraocular nerve palsy, then infection, metastatic carcinoma or primary carcinomas in the orbit become more likely.

Some clue to the possible lesion can be found from the direction of displacement. (Fig. 5.19).

1. Lesions in the muscle cone displace the eye along the line of the nerve, laterally and slightly downwards, with marked proptosis. If an attempt is made to reduce the eye into the orbit a sensation as if the eye were being pushed against a marble will be noted.
2. Lesions in the lacrimal fossa displace the eye medially and slightly upwards.
3. Lesions of the ethmoid displace the eye laterally and slightly downwards.
4. Lesions of the maxillary antrum displace the eye upwards and laterally.

The Pupil

The pupil may be affected by direct damage to the ciliary nerve or secondarily affected by damage to the optic nerve itself, producing a Marcus Gunn pupillary response.

Age of Onset

In children, teratomas, dermoid tumours, haemangiomas, rhabdomyosarcomas, Burkitt's lymphoma, metastases from neuroblastoma and optic nerve tumours complicating neurofibromatosis are the likely causes. In adults, tumours of the lacrimal gland, carcinoma of the antrum, metastases, especially from the prostate, or malignant lymphoma may occur in the orbit.

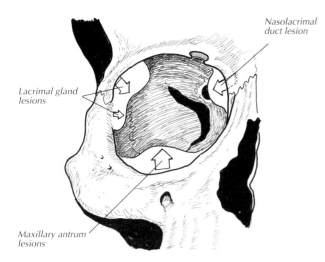

*Nasolacrimal
duct lesion*

*Lacrimal gland
lesions*

*Maxillary antrum
lesions*

5.19   Lesions invading the orbital margins.

Duration of Symptoms

Symptoms of gradual onset usually indicate benign lesions such as meningioma or neurofibroma. A rapid onset, particularly if painful, usually indicates infective or metastatic disease. A rapid bilateral onset without pain may indicate dysthyroid disease and, if painful, orbital myositis (pseudotumour of the orbit).

Clinical Examination of the Patient With Proptosis

An examination of the conjunctiva, iris and pupil should be routinely performed. The eyeball should be palpated for tenderness and attempts to reduce it into the socket should be made. The eyeball should be auscultated with the bell of a stethoscope for bruits. The retina and optic discs should be inspected. Primary optic atrophy would indicate a chronic lesion. Venous distension might indicate a sheath tumour compressing the ophthalmic vein, or an arteriovenous malformation. Occasionally the back of the globe can be seen to be indented from behind by the lesion causing the proptosis. Examination of the visual fields may provide evidence of an intracranial extension of the lesion, especially if an upper temporal defect is found in the other eye (see Chapter 3).

A general examination looking for evidence of systemic disease should always be performed in patients with proptosis or exophthalmos.

6. The Cerebellopontine Angle and Jugular Foramen

The Cerebellopontine Angle

The second major grouping of cranial nerves is found in the region known as the cerebellopontine angle. This consists of a shallow triangle lying between the cerebellum, the lateral pons and the inner third of the petrous ridge (Fig. 6.1). The vertical extent of the angle

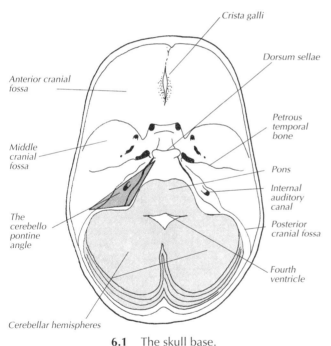

6.1 The skull base.

Crista galli

Dorsum sellae

Anterior cranial fossa

Petrous temporal bone

Middle cranial fossa

Pons

Internal auditory canal

The cerebello pontine angle

Posterior cranial fossa

Fourth ventricle

Cerebellar hemispheres

is from the fifth nerve above, on its course from the pons to the petrous apex, and the ninth nerve below, passing from the lateral medulla to the jugular foramen. The abducent nerve runs upwards and forwards on the medial edge of the area and the seventh and eighth cranial nerves traverse the angle to enter the internal auditory canal (see Fig. 6.7).

The hallmark of a lesion in this region is clinical evidence of damage to the seventh and eighth cranial nerves, so that a wide range of vestibular, auditory and

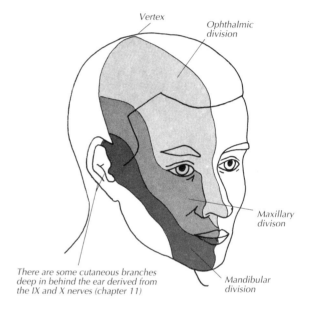

Vertex

Ophthalmic division

Maxillary divison

Mandibular division

There are some cutaneous branches deep in behind the ear derived from the IX and X nerves (chapter 11)

6.2 Cutaneous distribution of the fifth nerve.

motor abnormalities may occur. Several simple and benign conditions, such as Bell's palsy, enter into the differential diagnosis of more serious conditions such as acoustic nerve tumours. It is essential to be able to evaluate the nerves in the area at the bedside, and have at least an understanding of the methods and aims of eighth nerve tests, such as auditory function tests, the caloric test and brainstem evoked potentials. These are described and discussed in this chapter.

Clinical Evaluation of the Vulnerable Cranial Nerves

The trigeminal nerve conveys sensation from the face and provides the motor supply to the muscles of mastication. The cutaneous distribution is of great clinical importance. The sensory supply of the face is shown in Fig. 6.2. Notice that the area supplied by the first (ophthalmic) division extends back to the vertex, not to the hairline, and includes the nose and part of the upper lip. Embryologically this is the nerve supply of the frontonasal process. The third (mandibular) division has a relatively small area of supply and it is important to remember that there is a large area over the angle of the jaw supplied by nerve roots C2 and C3. Patients with non-organic sensory loss over the face usually claim anaesthesia extending to the line of the jaw and the hairline. The very complex anatomy of the trigeminal nerve is described below and illustrated in an exploded diagram which includes all the main branches in one illustration (Fig. 6.3a,b,c).

The Trigeminal Nerve (Fifth Nerve)

The trigeminal nerve is the largest cranial nerve. It arises from the middle of the pons and passes forwards and laterally across the subarachnoid space. Its large ganglion lies over the tip of the petrous bone, where the nerve divides into its three divisions.

The Ophthalmic Nerve (First Division of the Fifth Nerve)

The first division of the fifth nerve lies below the sixth nerve in the lateral wall of the cavernous sinus and is liable to damage by similar pathology. Because of its extensive sensory distribution severe pain in the forehead, nose and scalp, back as far as the vertex, may result from such damage.

The nerve divides into three branches as it enters the superior orbital fissure.

1. The lacrimal nerve runs along the lateral rectus muscle to the lacrimal gland and supplies the skin over the lateral eyelid and brow. It picks up secretomotor fibres from the zygomaticotemporal nerve which it conveys to the lacrimal gland. In the skin it receives proprioceptive filaments from the facial nerve.
2. The frontal nerve divides into two branches, the supratrochlear and supraorbital nerves, which supply the skin of the forehead and scalp to the vertex. They are liable to damage by minor injuries over the brow, and a causalgic syndrome may follow local trauma.
3. The nasociliary nerve has important autonomic and cutaneous functions:

   (a) The main trunk traverses the orbit and enters the anterior ethmoidal foramen into the intracranial cavity, runs across the cribriform plate and then exits from the through a slit in the crista galli to enter the nose. It supplies the mucosa of the nasal cavity and emerges at the lower end of the nasal bone to supply the skin over the tip of the nose, alar and vestibule.

   (b) In the orbit the nasociliary nerve gives off branches to the ciliary ganglion and two or three long ciliary nerves, which carry the pupillodilator sympathetic fibres and convey sensation from the cornea. These are of major importance for the protection of the very delicate cornea.

   (c) The infratrochlear branch arises just behind the anterior ethmoidal foramen and lies on the medial wall of the orbit. It supplies the skin of the upper medial eyelid and the upper side of the nose.

The Maxillary Nerve (Second Division of the Fifth Nerve)

The middle branch of the fifth nerve ganglion lies in the extreme lower lateral wall of the cavernous sinus and exits the skull through the foramen rotundum. It traverses the pterygopalatine fossa and enters the floor of the orbit through the inferior orbital fissure. At first it lies in a groove in the orbital floor and then enters the short canal and then onto the face through the infraorbital foramen. It supplies the skin of the cheek, midlateral nose and lateral part of the alar, lower eyelid and the mucous membranes of the cheek and upper lip. In its course, it gives off the following branches:

1. Meningeal branches to the floor of the middle cranial fossa
2. Two branches to the sphenopalatine ganglion conveying the secretomotor fibres destined for the lacrimal gland
3. The zygomatic nerve, which lies in the floor of the orbit and divides into the zygomaticotemporal nerve (secretomotor of the lacrimal gland and cutaneous sensation to the temporal area) and the zygomaticofacial nerve which, after penetrating the zygomatic bone, supplies cutaneous sensation to the prominence of the cheek.
4. The three alveolar nerves which supply the teeth, gums and adjacent palate, via the superior dental plexus. The anterior superior branch is the largest and supplies not only the incisor and canine teeth but also the lateral nasal wall, nasal septum, the lower eyelid and the skin of the upper lip.

The Pterygopalatine (Sphenopalatine) Ganglion

This very large ganglion is suspended from the maxillary division, deep in the pterygopalatine fossa. It receives its main connection from the nerve of the pterygoid canal. This carries preganglionic parasympathetic fibres from the nervus intermedius (seventh nerve) and sympathetic fibres from the middle meningeal artery. Both groups of fibres are then relayed by way of their complex course to the lacrimal gland. The main outflow

6.3 The Trigeminal nerve.

(a) Ophthalmic nerve.

(b) Maxillary nerve.

(c) Mandibular nerve.

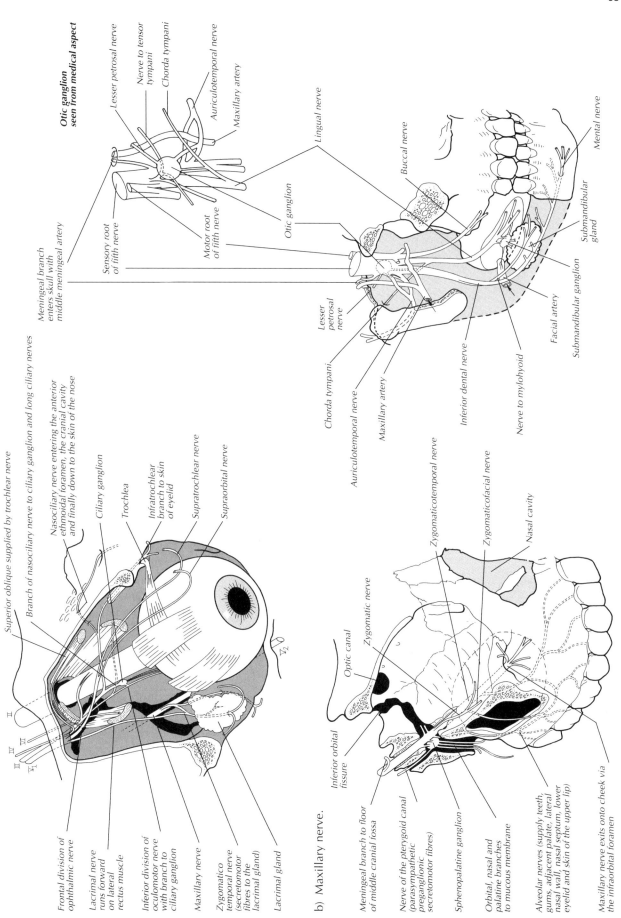

Otic ganglion seen from medical aspect

Lesser petrosal nerve

Nerve to tensor tympani

Chorda tympani

Auriculotemporal nerve

Maxillary artery

Lingual nerve

Maxillary artery

Meningeal branch enters skull with middle meningeal artery

Sensory root of fifth nerve

Motor root of fifth nerve

Otic ganglion

Buccal nerve

Mental nerve

Submandibular gland

Submandibular ganglion

Facial artery

Nerve to mylohyoid

Inferior dental nerve

Maxillary artery

Auriculotemporal nerve

Chorda tympani

Lesser petrosal nerve

Superior oblique supplied by trochlear nerve

Branch of nasociliary nerve to ciliary ganglion and long ciliary nerves

Nasociliary nerve entering the anterior ethmoidal foramen, the cranial cavity and finally down to the skin of the nose

Ciliary ganglion

Trochlea

Infratrochlear branch to skin of eyelid

Supratrochlear nerve

Supraorbital nerve

Frontal division of ophthalmic nerve

Lacrimal nerve runs forward on lateral rectus muscle

Inferior division of oculomotor nerve with branch to ciliary ganglion

Maxillary nerve

Zygomatico temporal nerve (secretomotor fibres to the lacrimal gland)

Lacrimal gland

Zygomaticotemporal nerve

Zygomaticofacial nerve

Nasal cavity

Zygomatic nerve

Optic canal

Inferior orbital fissure

Meningeal branch to floor of middle cranial fossa

Nerve of the pterygoid canal (parasympathetic preganglionic secretomotor fibres)

Sphenopalatine ganglion

Orbital, nasal and palatine branches to mucous membrane

Alveolar nerves (supply teeth, gums, adjacent palate, lateral nasal wall, nasal septum, lower eyelid and skin of the upper lip)

Maxillary nerve exits onto cheek via the infraorbital foramen is through the orbital, palatine, nasal and pharyngeal nerves to the mucous membranes of the orbit, nasal passages, pharynx, palate and upper gums.

The Mandibular Nerve (Third Division of the Fifth Nerve)

This is the largest branch of the fifth nerve and includes the motor component of the nerve. It leaves the skull through the foramen ovale. The main sensory trunk is joined by the much smaller motor root, in Meckel's cave, just outside the skull. A meningeal branch re-enters the skull with the middle meningeal artery through the foramen spinosum and supplies the lateral, middle and anterior cranial fossae. A small branch, the nerve to the medial pterygoid, supplies the medial pterygoid, tensor tympani and tensor veli palatini. The main nerve then divides into anterior and posterior trunks. The anterior trunk conveys the bulk of the motor root to supply the masseter, temporalis and the lateral pterygoid. The main branch of the anterior trunk is the buccal nerve, which merges with the buccal branches of the facial nerve to supply the skin over the buccinator, the mucous membranes of the cheek and the posterior part of the buccal surface of the gum.

The posterior trunk is mainly sensory and divides into three main nerves.

1. The auriculotemporal nerve passes behind the temporomandibular joint to join the facial nerve, with which it is distributed to the skin over the tragus, helix, auditory meatus and tympanic membrane and, by way of superficial temporal branches, to the skin over the temporalis. It also conveys secretomotor fibres to the parotid gland and fibres derived from the tympanic branch of the glossopharyngeal nerve from the otic ganglion.

2. The lingual nerve supplies sensation to the pre-sulcal tongue, the floor of the mouth and the lower gums. It conveys the taste fibres of the chorda tympani to the mucous membranes of the tongue. It also conveys secretomotor fibres from the submandibular ganglion to the sublingual and anterior lingual glands. It communicates with the hypoglossal nerve.

3. The inferior alveolar (dental) nerve enters the mandibular canal, running forwards within the mandible to emerge on the chin at the mental foramen, dividing into the incisive and mental branches and supplying the skin and mucous membrane of the lower lip, jaw, incisor and canine teeth.

The motor component of the posterior trunk leaves the inferior alveolar nerve, just before it enters the mandibular canal, as the mylohyoid nerve, supplying mylohyoid and the anterior belly of the digastric muscle.

Clinical Evaluation of the Fifth Nerve

The symptoms of fifth nerve damage may include spontaneous pain in the face, which may be indistinguishable at times from true tic douloureux, but this is very unusual (see Chapter 21). More often, patients present with an area of painless numbness over the face, usually in the distribution of one of the divisions. This is an extremely ominous sign, often indicating malignant infiltration of the nerve.

Although well recognised in adults, and a specific complication of secondary breast carcinoma in the jaw, this observation is true in all age groups. An eleven year boy presented with a ten day history of numbness of the right lower lip and chin, in the distribution of the mental nerve. This was shown by CT scanning to be due to marked enlargement of the medial pterygoid muscle. Biopsy confirmed a malignant rhabdomyosarcoma. In spite of intensive radiotherapy and chemotherapy, the tumour extended to involve all other cranial nerves at the base of the skull in the three months before death.

Damage to the motor supply causes weakness of the muscles of mastication, and yet if the damage is unilateral this rarely produces significant disability and it is unusual for the patient to be aware of the deficit.

The most sensitive component of the fifth nerve to compression or distortion appears to be those fibres subserving the corneal reflex. The earliest sign of fifth nerve damage is often an impaired or absent corneal response. If numbness of the entire face is found with an intact corneal response there are considerable grounds for doubting the organicity of the claimed loss. Patients with non-organic sensory loss claim that the numbness extends from the hairline to the angle of the jaw. This is an important point, as anaesthesia of the face is a fairly common manifestation in non-organic disease. In the case of organic damage subsequent blunting of sensation to pinprick and finally anaesthesia may occur, but loss of the corneal reflex is an important early sign.

The masseter is the most powerful muscle in the body, and even in the presence of obvious wasting of both the temporalis and masseter muscles on one side it is difficult to detect unilateral weakness of jaw closure. Jaw closure should not be tested with a finger in the patient's mouth – a human bite can be very unpleasant! Downward pressure with the thumb on the bony prominence of the patient's chin is usually sufficient.

Jaw opening is a much weaker movement (a fact well known to alligator and crocodile handlers) and although wasting in the pterygoids is not detectable, weakness is readily discernible. This is tested by putting a finger or fist under the patient's chin in the midline and asking them to open their mouth against moderate resistance and permitting the mouth to open slowly. If the muscle on the right is weak the jaw will be pushed across to the right side. This is because the action of the two obliquely arranged pterygoid muscles is to tip the jaw open and simultaneously pull it forward. It is the failure to move forward on the weak side that causes the jaw to deviate towards the affected muscles.

The fifth nerve does not supply any of the muscles of facial expression.

The Corneal Reflex (Fig. 6.4)

A wisp of cotton wool, twisted to a point, should be prepared. The examiner should hold the patient's lower lid down and ask them to look up and to the side. The area shown is stroked gently. The cotton wool should not be allowed to cross in front of the pupil or the patient will see it and blink. The less sensitive bulbar conjunctiva around the edge of the iris should not be stroked, as the poor response may be misinterpreted as a depressed corneal reflex. Both eyes should shut simultaneously if the corneal reflex is present. If the patient does not blink, always ask whether they felt the stimulus: some patients are very stoical and resist

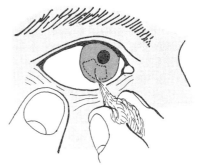

6.4   Correct way to elicit the corneal reflex

blinking and, when asked, readily confirm that it did indeed hurt.

The Abducent Nerve (Sixth Nerve)

The anatomy and clinical evaluation of the sixth nerve is fully detailed in Chapters 5 and 7.

The Facial Nerve (Seventh Nerve) (Fig. 6.5)

The seventh nerve is primarily motor to the muscles of facial expression. It also conveys the important taste

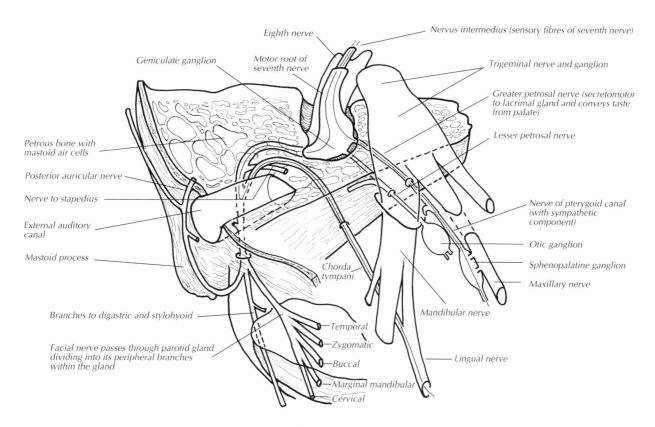

6.5   Course and connections of the facial nerve.
The angle of view is from the right side of the head looking downwards towards the midline.
The top of the petrous bone has been removed

fibres from the anterior two thirds of tongue in the chorda tympani and taste from the palate through the nerve of the pterygoid canal. A small but clinically important cutaneous supply to the skin of the external ear is carried via the vagus. These sensory fibres are contained in a separate trunk, the nervus intermedius, which runs with the eighth nerve rather than the seventh nerve in the subarachnoid space. The cell bodies of the sensory root lie in the geniculate ganglion. The nervus intermedius also carries preganglionic parasympathetic secretomotor fibres to the submandibular and sublingual salivary glands. These fibres originate in the superior salivatory nucleus in the brain stem.

Several important branches arise from the intrapetrous part of the nerve.

1. The greater petrosal nerve arises from the geniculate ganglion. It carries taste fibres from the palate and it conveys preganglionic parasympathetic fibres to the pterygopalatine ganglion, and thence via the zygomaticotemporal and lacrimal nerves to the lacrimal gland. It is joined by the deep petrosal nerve (derived from the sympathetic plexus on the carotid artery) to form the nerve of the pterygoid canal.

2. A branch from the ganglion joins the lesser petrosal nerve and is then carried to the otic ganglion. This conveys secretomotor fibres in the auriculotemporal nerve to the parotid gland. It also carries sympathetic fibres derived from the carotid artery to the blood vessels of the gland.

3. The nerve to stapedius arises 6 mm above the stylomastoid foramen.

4. The chorda tympani arises at the same level and runs forward across the middle ear to enter the canal in the petrotympanic fissure, grooves the spine of the sphenoid and joins the lingual branch of the fifth nerve, with which it is distributed to the presulcal part of the tongue.

5. At the stylomastoid foramen twigs join both the vagus and the glossopharyngeal nerve.

6. The posterior auricular nerve supplies the muscles of the ear and the occipital belly of occipitofrontalis.

7. The branches to the muscles of facial expression pass through the parotid gland, and from above downwards are the temporal, zygomatic, buccal, marginal, mandibular and cervical branches.

8. Cutaneous fibres are distributed with the auricular branch of the vagus, supplying the skin on both sides of the auricle and part of the external auditory canal and the tympanic membrane.

The Submandibular Ganglion

The submandibular ganglion lies on the lingual nerve. Its preganglionic fibres are derived from the superior salivatory nucleus in the brain stem and reach it via the facial nerve, chorda tympani and lingual nerve.

These fibres are secretomotor to the submandibular and sublingual glands. The sympathetic components are derived from the plexus on the facial artery and pass uninterrupted through the ganglion to the blood vessels of the same glands.

Clinically Important Features of the Seventh Nerve

It is often incorrectly thought that the fifth nerve has a motor supply to the muscles of facial expression and that the seventh nerve conveys sensory fibres to the face. For practical purpose the seventh nerve is almost purely motor, apart from the clinically important sensory component to the external auditory canal carried in the auricular branch of the vagus. It also carries the chorda tympani, conveying taste sensation from the anterior two-thirds of the tongue. As this nerve joins the seventh nerve in the middle ear, theoretically the presence or absence of impaired taste sensation ought to be of great localizing value, but in practice it is not particularly useful as these taste fibres are often spared in lesions proximal to the middle ear.

The nerve supplies the frontalis muscle and all the muscles of facial expression, including platysma. It also supplies stapedius, and this muscle, with tensor tympani (which is supplied by the maxillary division of the fifth nerve), contracts simultaneously to damp down the oscillation of the tympanic membrane and the stapes when the ear is subjected to high-intensity sound. A complete seventh nerve lesion will therefore alter auditory acuity on the affected side.

The seventh nerve does not contribute to normal eye opening but is certainly contributory to forced eye opening, and ptosis is not a feature of a seventh nerve palsy. However, there will be weakness of eye closure as the orbicularis in both the upper and lower lids is paralysed and the patient becomes unable to oppose and clench the eyelids shut to bury the eyelashes. The upper lid can only passively cover the cornea, providing incomplete protection in patients with a seventh nerve palsy. Ptosis is sometimes incorrectly included amongst the manifestations of a seventh nerve lesion. The posterior auricular branch supplies the auricular muscles, which are sometimes surprisingly well developed and under voluntary control in those patients who can 'wiggle their ears'.

It is often forgotten that the facial nerve supplies the platysma, which is a major muscle lying over the front of the neck. In some people the voluntary control of this muscle is highly developed and they are able to 'web' their neck by forced contraction of the muscle. This is best demonstrated when the patient tries to evert the lower lip.

Clinical Evaluation of the Seventh Nerve

One of the problems most often discussed and yet frequently misunderstood is the difference between an upper motor neuron lesion and a lower motor neuron lesion of the seventh nerve (Fig. 6.6). The difference is based on the supranuclear innervation of the seventh cranial nerve nucleus. This is discussed in detail in Chapter 8. In simple terms, the cerebral hemisphere is most concerned with facial expression and therefore exerts major control over the opposite lower facial muscles. The forehead and eye closure mechanisms are mainly concerned with reflex eye closure and therefore have a dual consensual innervation. Both eyes will shut simultaneously if either eye is threatened without hemisphere intervention.

The result is that a unilateral lesion of the upper motor neuron fibres from the hemisphere, as might occur in a typical cerebrovascular accident, will result in readily detectable weakness in the opposite lower face, whereas eye closure and forehead movement will remain relatively intact because the intact hemisphere pathways provide adequate cross-innervation. Very careful evaluation often reveals that there **is** slight weakness of voluntary forehead wrinkling and eye closure on the affected side.

In a lower motor neuron lesion of either the nucleus, the fascicle or the main seventh nerve trunk, **all** the muscles innervated by the seventh nerve will be affected, leading to complete loss of control of the facial muscles on the affected side.

The difficulty that beginners have seems to stem from the terminology: an upper motor neuron lesion affects only the lower face, whereas a lower motor neuron lesion affects the entire face.

Testing Seventh Nerve Function

When evaluating a patient with suspected facial weakness a systematic examination should be made.

1. The patient's ability to wrinkle the forehead is tested (occipitofrontalis muscle). This will be obviously impaired in a lower motor neuron lesion.

2. The patient's ability to shut the eyes and hold them tightly shut is tested. In the presence of a lower motor neuron lesion the eye can be seen rolling up as an ineffectual attempt to shut the eyelids is made (Bell's phenomenon). In an upper motor neuron lesion very slight weakness of eye closure is usually detectable as an inability to bury the eyelashes completely on the affected side.

3. The patient's ability to flare the nostrils, smile and forcibly show the teeth is tested. In a lower motor neuron lesion profound asymmetry is obvious. In an upper motor neuron lesion, slow and incomplete movement of the mouth on the side opposite the causal lesion may be noted. The weakness in an upper motor neuron lesion is rarely complete. A further variation results when the weakness is more apparent on emotional movement, such as a spontaneous smile, than on volitional movement such as forcibly showing the teeth. This is discussed further in Chapter 8.

4. The platysma muscle is tested. The best way to do this is to ask the patient to try and evert the lower lip while the examiner observes the neck muscles.

Upper motor neuron facial weakness – left side

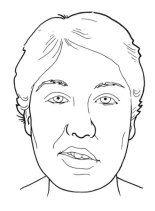

*Slight droop of mouth, palpebral fissure
slightly wider but upper face unaffected*

Lower motor neuron facial weakness – left side

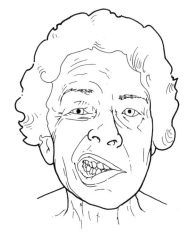

*Marked weakness of forehead, eye closure and
mouth, with gross facial asymmetry*

*Lower motor neuron facial weakness affects all the face
Upper motor neuron affects mainly lower face*

6.6   Upper and lower motor neuron facial weakness. (Patient is obeying command to show the teeth.)

Contraction of mentalis, which wrinkles the skin of the chin, will be seen and the neck will web, sometimes quite dramatically.

If it were as simple as this, there would be little problem, but there are three other considerations.

1. Almost all patients have some degree of facial asymmetry. It is often easy to speculate that the patient has facial weakness and clinical notes often contain the comment 'facial asymmetry, ? weakness'. If there is any doubt it is best to assume that the face is normal. The very slight but definite weakness of eye closure that is typical of an upper motor neuron lesion is the best check. If eye closure is quite normal and symmetrical, there is no facial weakness.

2. A patient with an incomplete lower motor neuron seventh nerve lesion often demonstrates relative preservation or early recovery of the muscles of the forehead and around the eye. This with the residual weakness of the lower face may mimic a rather severe upper motor neuron lesion.

3. Some patients have a greater degree of upper motor neuron control of the opposite seventh nerve than is usual. In such patients an upper motor neuron lesion can produce profound weakness of the mouth and moderately severe weakness of eye closure and even the forehead muscles, and mimic a recovering or incomplete lower motor neuron lesion.

In both the above situations other symptoms and signs may have to be used to establish the type of seventh nerve lesion with certainty. If there is any remaining doubt it is always worth obtaining old photographs of the patient and asking relatives' advice. If a close relative can see no change in the patient's facial expression then there is almost certainly nothing wrong.

Taste Sensation

Taste sensation should be tested in any patient who has a lower motor neuron lesion of the seventh nerve. The patient should be asked to protrude the tongue and the surface is dried. A drop of sweet, salt or sour flavour is placed on a cottonwool stick and stroked along each side of the tip of the tongue. The patient should then put his tongue back in his mouth but should not swallow until he has established whether the taste was appreciated on both sides. Taste may be completely lost or may be delayed, often with a slightly metallic flavour in incomplete lesions of the chorda tympani. Unimpaired taste sensation is unfortunately not a reliable indicator that the nerve lesion is distal to the middle ear, as these fibres are often spared, but if taste **is** affected it certainly confirms that the lesion is proximal to or in the petrous bone itself.

Testing the Corneal Response when there is Paralysis of Eyelid Closure

When a patient has a lower motor neuron lesion of the seventh nerve eyelid closure is affected so that the normal corneal response is impaired. It is essential to be certain that corneal sensation is intact in this situation. If it is impaired the patient clearly has more than a simple Bell's palsy, and from a management point of view the eye is at considerable risk from foreign bodies, if it is both **anaesthetic** and **unprotected**. In this situation testing should be performed as follows:

1. The patient is asked to compare the sensation on both sides when the cornea is lightly stroked with a cottonwool wisp, as described earlier.

2. The examiner should observe whether the eyeball rolls upwards and away from the stimulus. It should do so if the cornea is sensitive.

3. Also observe whether the other eye shuts simultaneously. The corneal response is a consensual reflex, like the pupillary response to light, and the unaffected eye should instantly shut tightly, as the cornea on the side of the paralysed eyelid is stimulated if corneal sensation is normal.

If the corneal reflex is impaired suitable protection for the cornea should be arranged immediately, either by a simple eye-patch as a short-term measure or a tarsorrhaphy as a longer-term measure, but also requiring protective glasses or by deliberate paralysis of the eyelid by botulinum toxin if there is already evidence of corneal ulceration.

The Auditory and Vestibular Nerve (Eighth Nerve)

The clinical physiology of the eighth nerve is a major subject and is more appropriately dealt with in greater detail at the end of this chapter.

Cerebellopontine Angle Lesions

The terms cerebellopontine angle tumour and acoustic neuroma are not interchangeable. There are several other less common lesions that may occur at this location (Figs. 6.7, 6.8)

Acoustic Nerve Tumours

When an acoustic nerve tumour develops in the cerebellopontine angle a typical sequence of events occurs. The tumour arises on the vestibular division of the nerve, but the earliest symptoms are usually auditory. Slowly progressive and often unrecognized loss of hearing develops, sometimes preceded by tinnitus.

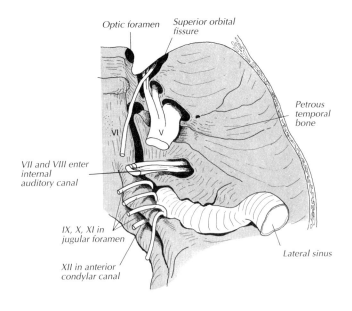

6.7 Normal cerebellopontine angle.

Optic foramen

Superior orbital fissure

Petrous temporal bone

VII and VIII enter internal auditory canal

IX, X, XI in jugular foramen

XII in anterior condylar canal

Lateral sinus

VI

V

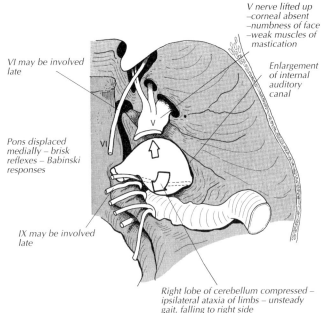

6.8 Acoustic nerve tumour.

V nerve lifted up
–corneal absent
–numbness of face
–weak muscles of mastication

Enlargement of internal auditory canal

VI may be involved late

Pons displaced medially – brisk reflexes – Babinski responses

IX may be involved late

Right lobe of cerebellum compressed – ipsilateral ataxia of limbs – unsteady gait, falling to right side

VI

V

Episodic vertigo is an unusual feature in the early stages of an acoustic nerve tumour, although such tumours are usually accorded an unwarranted high position in the differential diagnosis of vertigo.

CASE REPORT I

A 19-year-old man was referred for the investigation of deafness in one ear. This had been discovered when his local audio retailer had refused to replace a pair of earphones for the third time, particularly as everyone but the patient could hear perfectly normally through both speakers. He had not realized that he had become completely deaf in the left ear. He had some mild headaches and had recently felt slightly dizzy on sudden movement, but there were no other signs. CT scanning revealed a 1" diameter acoustic neuroma which was successfully removed. Unfortunately his life ever since has been seriously disrupted by constant unpleasant auditory hallucinations in the deaf ear. This is a very rare complication.

CASE REPORT II

A 38-year-old aircraft mechanic was referred because of attacks of giddiness on changing position and obscuration of vision on standing suddenly. An optician had detected gross papilloedema even though the patient somewhat reluctantly admitted to recent occasional mild headaches. When the history was taken he denied any other problems, but during routine assessment of the cranial nerves he was discovered to be completely deaf in the left ear. He apologized for not mentioning it before but related that this had been first discovered when he entered the RAF at the age of 18, and had been dismissed as 'one of those things'. He had gross papilloedema with visual impairment, nystagmus to the right and

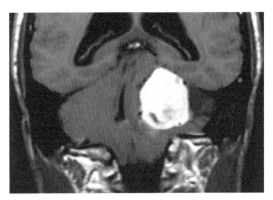

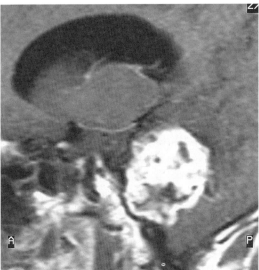

CRII. *Acoustic neuroma with 18-year history of deafness presenting as acute visual failure due to papilloedema.*

mild left-sided cerebellar signs. An enormous 2" diameter acoustic nerve tumour was successfully removed, but the facial nerve unfortunately could not be preserved.

CASE REPORT III

*A 57-year-old woman was referred with facial pain. For some 7 months she had been subject to intermittent attacks of sudden, vicious, paroxysmal pain, purely in the left nostril and left side of the nose. The pain had all the features of trigeminal neuralgia but the distribution was extremely unusual and the response to carbamezepine, given by her GP, disappointing. It transpired that 10 years previously she had been referred following the discovery of complete deafness in her left ear after a long period of tinnitus. She had been reassured at the time that it was 'one of those things'. Physical examination revealed loss of the left corneal response, which is **never** seen in trigeminal neuralgia. An MRI scan revealed an acoustic neuroma, which was successfully resected with full preservation of the facial nerve.*

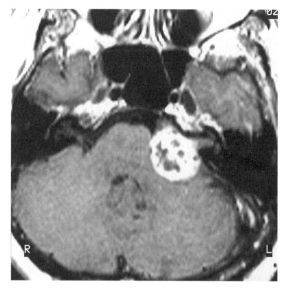

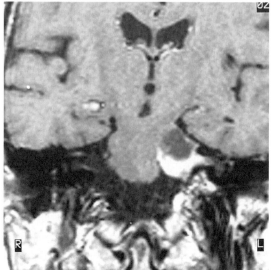

CRIII. *Acoustic neuroma presenting as trigeminal neuralgia.*

There are several important lessons to be drawn from these cases: it is obvious that unilateral deafness, discovered by accident, should never be dismissed without full investigation; the natural history of acoustic neuromas may be disarmingly long – 10–20 years in two of the above cases – without other dramatic events; an enormous tumour causing papilloedema does not necessarily cause dramatic headache, even when occupying a major part of the posterior fossa; and finally, it is dangerous to dismiss any physical finding as 'one of those things'. When the 'thing' is eventually shown to be a large benign tumour, this is a very embarrassing comment to have committed to the clinical record.

Although on anatomical grounds early damage to the seventh nerve would be anticipated, facial nerve palsy is in fact a very late and extremely unusual manifestation of an acoustic nerve lesion. However, some twitching of the facial musculature – a condition known as hemifacial spasm – may be a presenting symptom. If the seventh nerve is involved in this way the chance of finding a lesion other than an acoustic nerve tumour is greatly increased, and a meningioma or cholesteatoma (epidermoid tumour) become important differential diagnostic considerations.

The most consistent early physical sign is depression or absence of the corneal reflex. The fifth nerve is lifted up by the tumour and the afferent fibres for the corneal reflex seem to be very sensitive to such distortion. Numbness over the face may appear later, but a complete fifth nerve lesion with motor and sensory loss is very unusual indeed.

The ease with which the other cranial nerves in the vicinity can be stretched and distorted without clinical evidence of damage, is a striking feature of the natural history and accounts for the paucity of clinical findings in many patients with extremely large acoustic nerve tumours.

If undetected, the tumour eventually extends medially and starts to distort the brainstem and cerebellum and then produces more dramatic symptoms. Attacks of vertigo, which may be positional in type, ataxia of gait and a mild spastic tetraparesis may develop. The ataxia is usually most marked in the upper limbs on the side of the tumour. At this stage brisk reflexes and extensor plantar responses may be found, but there may be few local signs except for deafness and a depressed corneal response. If the patient is left untreated further distortion of the brain stem may block the cerebral aqueduct, leading to hydrocephalus, headache, papilloedema and even dementia.

The natural history of an acoustic nerve tumour can be as long as 30 years. Bilateral acoustic neuromas occur in patients with neurofibromatosis whose specific gene defect has now been identified. They are classified as having neurofibromatosis type II.

CASE REPORT IV

A 37-year-old man presented in 1977 with radicular pain in a T8 distribution on the left-hand side, at first only on exercise but constant at the time of referral. The only physical finding was an absent left upper abdominal reflex. Myelography revealed a neurofibroma on the left T8 nerve root, which was successfully removed. When told the nature of the tumour, he revealed that his mother had had bilateral acoustic neuromas. Re-examination revealed a few rather modest café-au-lait patches but no other evidence of neurofibromatosis. Five years later he developed a whistling noise in the left ear and noticed slight impairment of hearing. Otoneurological testing revealed bilateral loss of the caloric responses and high-tone deafness in the left ear. CT scanning repeated over 3 consecutive years failed to reveal any abnormality, in spite of deteriorating audiovestibular function. By that stage his elder brother had been found to have bilateral acoustic neuromas. In 1985 an MRI scan showed a 4 cm lesion on the left and a 1 cm lesion on the right acoustic nerves. The larger lesion was successfully removed, with preservation of the facial nerve. He was followed with 2-yearly MRI scans until early 1994, when the lesion on the right, which had increased markedly in size in the last 2 years, was starting to distort the brain stem and produce a mild degree of hydrocephalus. Removal became obligatory. The seventh nerve was preserved but the patient became totally deaf following this procedure. His eldest son, who was by then 24, who had had cutaneous evidence of neurofibromatosis when examined at the age of 14, now has bilateral acoustic nerve tumours, small and fusiform in shape, demonstrated on MRI scanning. His female cousin, who is 26, has needed an operation on one side. Genetic testing has revealed that his two youngest sons are not carrying the gene.

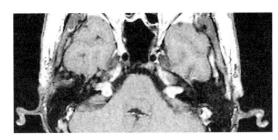

CRV. *Bilateral acoustic neuromas at age 24 in the son of above patient.*

CASE REPORT V

*A 46-year-old woman was referred by the biochemical investigation unit where she had been referred for investigation of diabetes insipidus. The biochemical diagnosis was confirmed and, as part of the routine assessment, an MRI scan was performed to demonstrate the hypothalamus and pituitary regions. Following this investigation she was referred for a neurological opinion because of the rather dramatic findings on MRI scanning. Her only other symptoms on detailed questioning were slight impairment of hearing on both sides and occasional giddiness if she moved suddenly. Physical examination revealed widespread café-au-lait patches and subcutaneous neurofibromata. There were **no** neurological signs. The MRI scans revealed multiple meningiomata, a pituitary lesion, a pineal lesion, bilateral cerebellopontine lesions, two neurofibromas in the cervical canal and a syrinx in the cervical spinal cord. She has been reviewed 6-monthly since these findings, with no significant change in her clinical condition over 2 years, and the diabetes insipidus is controlled by DDAVP. There are no known affected family members. (MRI scans on p. 72)*

This particular case again emphasizes something that has only emerged since the advent of scanning, which is how modest or non-existent the clinical signs can be in the presence of major pathology. In the past it was always assumed that failure to detect such lesions represented lack of clinical skill, but it is now perhaps more appropriate to marvel at how often lesions were detected when the clinical findings detailed throughout this volume were the only diagnostic tools available and the special investigations imprecise and often hazardous.

Other Cerebellopontine Angle Lesions

Meningiomas, cholesteatomas, haemangioblastomas, ectasia of the basilar artery and metastatic deposits of carcinoma or lymphoma may all occur in the cerebellopontine angle. Neuromas on the fifth, seventh, and ninth nerves are rare but can produce similar clinical pictures. In all these cases the exact sequence of clinical events may provide the clue to an alternative pathology. An early seventh nerve palsy is always an important clue, being very rare in acoustic neuromas. On occasions it is not until the lesion is exposed at surgery that its nature is revealed.

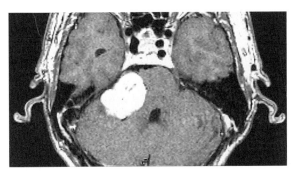

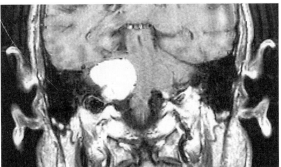

CRIV. *Acoustic neuroma in familial case. Tumour on opposite side removed previously.*

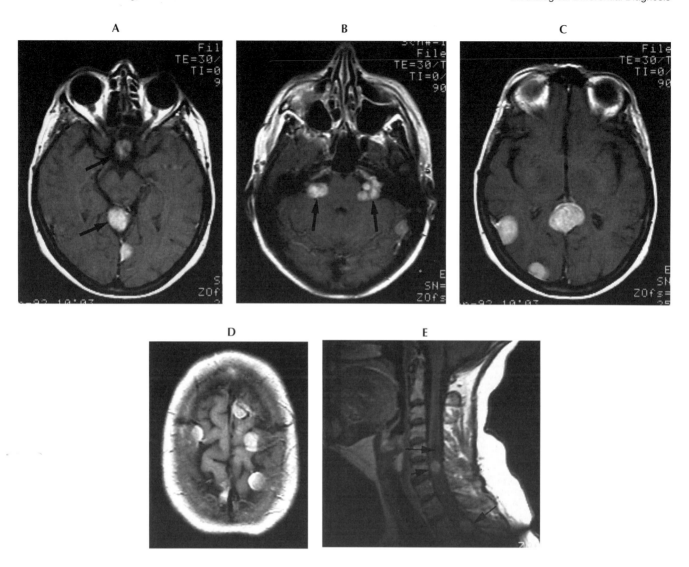

CRV.   ***A*** *Pituitary and pineal region tumours*   ***B*** *Bilateral cerebellopontine tumours*   ***C*** *Surface meningiomata and pineal lesion*
D *Multiple surface meningiomata*   ***E*** *Syringomyelic cavity and two neurofibromas in cervical canal*

A pontine glioma, a rare tumour of the brain stem, usually occurs in young boys and older patients with neurofibromatosis. They typically expand the pons and produce a series of projecting knobs of tumour on the surface of the brain stem. One of these knobs may project into the cerebellopontine angle and produce the clinical picture of an extrinsic tumour in that area. The fact that the patient is a child or has neurofibromatosis should always raise the possibility of this diagnosis. A coexistent sixth nerve lesion is a strong clue to this diagnosis, as pontine gliomas often originate in the region of the sixth nerve nucleus.

Medulloblastomas and astrocytomas of the cerebellum may push forward into the angle but the inevitable ataxia and the early development of the headache, papilloedema and vomiting, usually with a total history of a few weeks at the most, should point to this diagnosis. These tumours are usually found in children, but can present throughout adulthood.

Carcinoma of the nasopharynx may invade the skull base between the clivus and the petrous bone, where the sixth nerve is especially vulnerable. Malignant infiltration of the fifth nerve usually causes patches of painless numbness. This never occurs as an early feature of an acoustic nerve tumour. Carcinoma from distant sites may reach this area. Two patients with acute cerebellopontine angle lesions caused by metastatic Hodgkin's disease have been seen by the author. Local meningeal involvement by syphilis or tuberculosis were important causes of the syndrome in the past.

In general, whenever the possibility of a lesion in the cerebellopontine angle is raised the clinical history and the evaluation of the physical signs should be very carefully documented and compared with the typical clinical picture of an acoustic nerve tumour. Any unusual feature should indicate the possibility of another cause.

Investigation of Patients with Suspected Cerebellopontine Angle Lesions

Careful history-taking and examination may provide all the necessary information for a reasoned guess at the pathology of the lesion. The investigation of choice has become an MRI scan with gadolinium enhancement. There is little indication these days for plain skull films or the special views to demonstrate the internal auditory canals that used to take so much time and often gave such limited information.

The mortality rate of operations on these tumours used to be as high as 15–20%, owing to the difficulty caused by the vessels supplying the tumour also supplying the brain stem. Modern scanning and the use of the dissecting microscope have greatly reduced the mortality, although even in the best hands a fatal outcome following surgery is far from rare. If the tumour is very large, considerable morbidity from damage to adjacent cranial nerves and the brain stem is not uncommon. Preservation of the seventh nerve is a major aim of surgery, as the nerve is always intimately involved in the tumour. This can be very difficult to achieve.

Other Causes of Damage to Cranial Nerves in the Region

Fifth Nerve Lesions

There are four conditions to be discussed.

Trigeminal Sensory Neuropathy

This is a rare condition in which progressive numbness of the face occurs in the distribution of the fifth nerve. It may have its onset at any age and the differential diagnosis must include a continued search for a neoplasm in the nasopharynx. A period of up to 2 years may elapse before a neoplasm can be demonstrated, so that the diagnosis of trigeminal sensory neuropathy should not be made too readily and should be kept under regular review.

Tic Douloureux (Trigeminal Neuralgia)

This condition is discussed in detail in Chapter 21. The features of interest in this chapter are that the pain is not exclusively confined to one division of the nerve, but usually runs along the line between the third and second, and the second and first divisions respectively. If sensation is tested immediately after a burst of pain, some transitory impairment may be demonstrated. The general rule that there should be no sensory loss other than under this circumstance is valid, and a permanent area of numbness or loss of the corneal reflex excludes the diagnosis unless previous nerve section has been performed. The diagnosis is only tenable if there are no physical signs of fifth nerve damage. It is rare for trigeminal neuralgia to be due to an underlying lesion, in striking contrast to the much less common glossopharyngeal neuralgia, which is frequently associated with underlying pathology.

Herpes Zoster Ophthalmicus

This condition is also considered in Chapter 5 and Chapter 21. Although herpes zoster can affect any nerve root in the body, the thoracic roots are usually affected in the younger age groups. In the elderly the virus has a predilection for the first division of the fifth nerve.

The typical history is 2–3 days of excruciating pain in the forehead on one or other side. Between the third and fifth days small vesicles first appear in the eyebrow, and over the next 48 hours marked oedema of the whole face and neck on the same side may rapidly appear. At its height the rash may cover the entire cutaneous distribution of the nerve. Extraocular nerve palsies may occur, but usually recover completely over 6–8 weeks. The severe pain lessens with the onset of the rash in most cases, but if it does not, urgent treatment in an attempt to prevent the development of 'postherpetic neuralgia' is necessary. The use of narcotic analgesics to control the immediate pain and a combination of phenytoin and imiprimine may be helpful. There is no evidence that zivouridine prevents the development of postherpetic neuralgia, although it hastens healing and does reduce scarring.

Multiple Sclerosis

An episode of numbness of one side of the face in a young person, sometimes following local anaesthesia for dental work, is a surprisingly frequent symptom of multiple sclerosis. This typically recovers over 6–12 weeks but may later be complicated by trigeminal neuralgia. An attack of facial numbness as an initial symptom of MS seems to carry a poor prognosis, with a high likelihood of further episodes.

Sixth Nerve Lesions

The possible causes of a sixth nerve lesion have been fully documented in Chapter 5, and central lesions of the nucleus and fascicle are covered in Chapter 8.

Seventh Nerve Lesions

There are three important clinical conditions to consider.

Bell's Palsy

Bell's palsy is one of the most common neurological disorders. It consists of an acute lower motor neuron facial paralysis, often preceded by a history of aching pain in and around the ear in the 24 hours before the onset, which may be severe. The face is often described as feeling stiff or 'numb'. It is essential to be certain that there is no actual sensory loss, as this is quite incompatible with the diagnosis. The palsy is usually complete within hours of the onset, but recovery may occur so rapidly that the palsy may appear incomplete by the time the patient is first examined.

The prognosis is excellent, some 80% of patients making an uncomplicated recovery in 2–6 weeks. Where recovery is delayed, and begins after 12 weeks, the ultimate degree of recovery is usually incomplete and often further complicated by the development of facial synkinesis. This is due to the development of giant motor units when intact nerve fibres have taken over adjacent muscle fibres whose own nerve supply has not recovered. This can ultimately result in grimacing of the over-recovered side, sometimes giving the impression that the normal side is paralysed. This problem can be very effectively treated with botulinum toxin injections. There is considerable doubt that the prognosis of Bell's palsy is altered by the use of steroids, in spite of their enthusiastic and continued use for over 30 years.

The condition is thought to be related to a viral infection, the swollen nerve being damaged by entrapment in the facial canal. The most important underlying diseases that may predispose to Bell's palsy are diabetes and hypertension. Rare causes include Lyme disease, sarcoidosis and Melkersson's syndrome, the latter associated with oedema of the face and a fissured tongue. Recurrent and bilateral attacks may occur in all these conditions. The most frequent and frightening mistake is for the patient to be told that Bell's palsy represents a 'small stroke'. It does not! This term, with all its implications for the future of the patient, should never be used in discussing this benign condition.

Ramsay Hunt Syndrome (Herpes Zoster of the Seventh Nerve, or Geniculate Herpes)

In this condition the seventh nerve is damaged by the herpes zoster virus. This causes certain distinct differences in the clinical picture. Excruciating pain in the ear precedes the facial weakness by 24–72 hours, with the later eruption of vesicles in or around the external auditory meatus and over the mastoid process. At this stage massive oedema, redness and tenderness of the ear may occur. Examination of the external meatus will then become impossible. Other cranial nerves may be involved, notably the fifth nerve, with sensory loss over the face or numbness of the palate due to a ninth nerve

lesion. If the vesicles are not prominent or not detected the condition may be mistaken for a very severe bacterial infection of the ear. Sometimes a single vesicle in the external auditory canal or behind the ear may be the only superficial evidence of herpes zoster. This type of Bell's palsy is a surprisingly common complication of pregnancy, possibly due to altered immune status. The majority of patients recover but the possibility of incomplete recovery is slightly greater than with non-herpetic Bell's palsy.

Benign Hemifacial Spasm

This condition has many pathological similarities to trigeminal neuralgia, and in fact the conditions may co-exist. Both are now thought to be caused by minor anatomical variations of the blood vessels running along the nerves and presumably causing irritation of the nerve. Hemifacial spasm consists of continual twitching movements, usually maximal around the eye and mouth. The condition is annoying and embarrassing rather than painful or ominous. Consideration should always be given to the possibility of an underlying lesion, although as with tic douloureux the number of cases in which a lesion is found is small. The commonest demonstrable cause is a cholesteatoma (epidermoid tumour) in the cerebellopontine angle. These tumours are totally unrelated to the type of cholesteatoma that may occur in the external auditory canal related to chronic ear infection.

CASE REPORT VI

A 67-year-old man presented with rapidly increasing ataxia, nausea and vomiting, with 30-year history of left-sided hemifacial spasm. CT scanning revealed a massive hypodense lesion occupying the left half of the posterior fossa. The appearances were typical of an epidermoid tumour. The lesion was successfully removed but the patient was left with multiple lower cranial nerve palsies and died of aspiration pneumonia 6 weeks postoperatively.

Hemifacial spasm may occur in either sex at any age, but is usually found in older age groups, especially hypertensive females. Tumours in the cerebellopontine angle, basilar artery aneurysm or ectasia and lateral recess meningiomas may be responsible for this condition but in the majority of cases no definite cause is found. It can now be treated very effectively by botulinum toxin injections, which can achieve partial paralysis of the muscles in spasm without the complete weakness produced by previous treatments using alcohol injection or nerve avulsion techniques. When the condition has been present for many years, a mild weakness of the affected side of the face gradually develops which lessens the need for botulinum injections. In younger patients neurovascular decompression should be considered.

The Cochlear–vestibular Nerve (Eighth Nerve)

The eighth cranial nerve carries information from two highly specialized end organs, the vestibular apparatus and the organ of Corti. Both lie deep in the temporal bone. They are suspended in the bone in perilymph, which is basically CSF and is in continuity with the sub-arachnoid space. A highly specialized fluid with a high protein content, known as endolymph, fills the semicircular canals and the scala media of the cochlear.

The Vestibular Apparatus

The Semicircular Canals (Figs 6.9 and 6.10)

The semicircular canals are three fine tubes arranged as shown in Figure 6.9. Note that the lateral canal is tilted up 30° at the front; it is not horizontal. The six canals work as three matched pairs in three planes, as indicated in the figure. At the end of each canal as it joins the utricle is a swelling called the ampulla. This

Figure to show the Position of the Semicircular Canals in the normal position

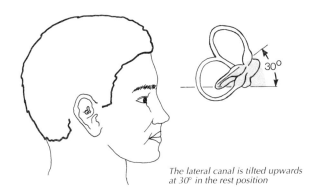

The lateral canal is tilted upwards at 30° in the rest position

Figure to show the Position of the Semicircular Canals during The Caloric Test

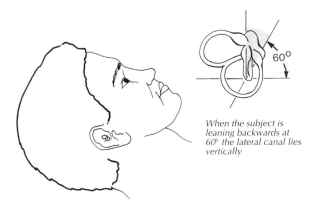

When the subject is leaning backwards at 60° the lateral canal lies vertically

6.9   Position of the semicircular canals in the normal position.

contains the cupola and the hair cells. The cells are polarized to respond to movement in one direction only by the position of the single kinocilium on each cell. In the lateral canal movement towards the utricle stimulates the cupola. The vertical canals are stimulated by movement away from the utricle (Fig. 6.10). Neural activity generated by the canals is transmitted to the vestibular nucleus on the same side of the brain stem and then to the eye muscle nuclei, as discussed in Chapter 7. The desired end result is that whatever the position of the head the eyes continue to look straight ahead.

The Otolith Organs (Fig. 6.10)

The Utricular Mechanism

The otolith organ in the utricle senses tilting of the head. It is shaped like a flat plate tilted up at the anterior end and is covered with hairs polarized towards the bend. Head tilt is sensed by the variation in pressure of the calcium carbonate crystals on the hairs produced by gravity.

The Saccular Mechanism

The organ in the saccule senses angular acceleration of the head. It is shaped like a shield, with a central ridge facing forwards. Forward movement forces the crystals to attempt to slide down the slope on either side proportional to the speed and angle of the movement.

Vestibular Function Tests

Gait

A patient who has a unilateral vestibular or cerebellar disorder will veer or fall to that side and tend to hold on to the wall on the affected side. The gait becomes wide-based as the patient attempts to improve their stability. These difficulties may be exaggerated by asking the patient to walk heel to toe. In patients who have diffuse cerebellar disease or central vestibular lesions generalized instability will be apparent. The patient will walk on a wide base and lurch in all directions, desperately holding on to anything that offers stability or support. Patients with gait ataxia due to posture sense loss walk unsteadily but with a high-stepping gait, which is an additional and virtually diagnostic feature. They will also fall over if they close their eyes.

The Romberg test   Postural instability can be best evaluated by the Romberg test. This is not a specific test of vestibular function and is often used to demonstrate loss of joint position sense, the patient falling

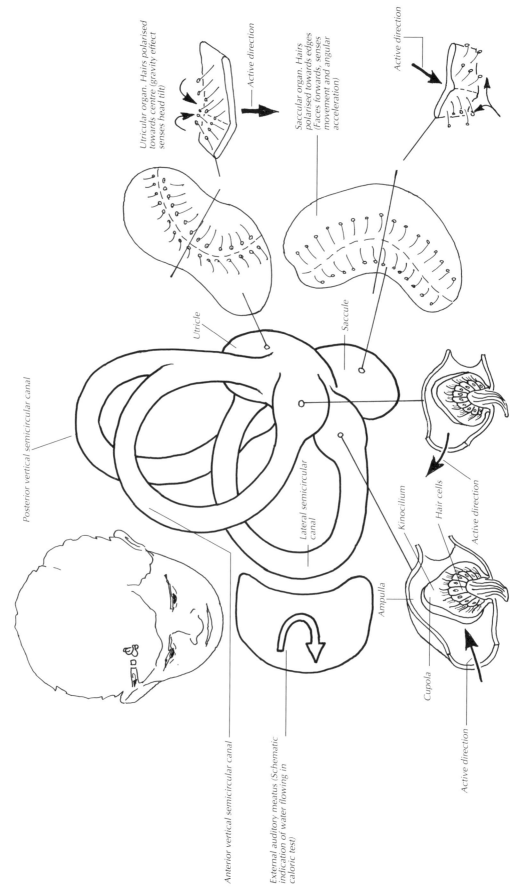

The angle of view is as indicated in the top left of the picture and water is shown schematically flowing through the auditory meatus to stimulate the lateral semicircular canal as in a caloric test (note that the polarization of the cupola in the lateral and anterior semicircular canal is in different directions as shown by the arrows and the polarization of the utricle and saccule are indicated by large arrows showing the direction of movement, and small arrows indicating the displacement of the kinocilia)

Utricular organ. Hairs polarised towards centre (gravity effect senses head tilt)

Active direction

Saccular organ. Hairs polarised towards edges (Faces forwards, senses movement and angular acceleration)

Active direction

Utricle

Saccule

Posterior vertical semicircular canal

Lateral semicircular canal

Kinocilium

Hair cells

Active direction

Anterior vertical semicircular canal

Ampulla

External auditory meatus (Schematic indication of water flowing in caloric test)

Cupola

Active direction

6.10   Right vestibular apparatus and its components.

when they close their eyes. The test was dramatically abnormal in patients with tabes dorsalis who had complete loss of posture sense.

The standard Romberg test consists of the patient standing, with feet together and eyes open and then closed. On eye closure the normal swaying may increase slightly but the patient should not fall or stagger. In unilateral vestibular or cerebellar disease the patient sways towards the damaged side. The enhanced Romberg test is similar except that the patient stands with one foot in front of the other with the arms folded against the chest. The same observations are made with the eyes open and then closed.

A further modification of this type of test is to ask the patient to march on the spot with their eyes closed. If the patient rotates round more than 30° or moves sideways more then 36 inches, the test is abnormal. The abnormal movement is towards the affected side.

Tests of Co-ordination

Past Pointing Tests   There are two ways of performing these tests which depend on normal strength and normal posture sense being established before deficits can be safely attributed to cerebellar or vestibular disease.

The patient is asked to place the tips of their index fingers together in front of them at eye level and hold them together. Then, with their eyes closed, spread the arms and then attempt to touch the finger tips together again. The hand on the affected side will miss the target finger repeatedly, with defect of range and direction.

An even more difficult modification is for the examiner to offer a target finger which the patient touches with the eyes open and then attempts to touch again with the eyes closed. Inaccuracy of the suspect arm should be readily detected.

Finger-nose and Heel-knee-shin Testing   These tests are mainly used to detect incoordination in cerebellar disease where the incoordination is as bad with the eyes open as when they are closed. They can also be used to indicate vestibular disorders and provided it has been established that joint position sense is normal, the patient will perform the tests accurately while looking but badly with the limb on the affected side when the eyes are closed. These tests are discussed in detail in Chapter 12.

It must be appreciated that these tests require multiple skills in the motor, sensory, vestibular and cerebellar components of posture and movement and correct interpretation requires **all** these factors to be considered before deciding which component is at fault. The most frequent error is to identify difficulties in a **weak** limb as due to abnormal vestibular or cerebellar function (see Chapter 12).

Nystagmus
Nystagmus is discussed in detail in Chapter 7.

The Caloric Test   This remains the most useful test of vestibular function in spite of the development of modern evoked potential testing. Ideally, a standardized test using thermostatically controlled water temperature should be used. The test is based on the fact that the cupola can be deflected by convection currents set up in the semicircular canals if they are heated or cooled. The lateral canals can be easily stimulated by hot or cold fluid running through the external auditory canal. A further advantage is that the patient's head can be held still, so that the resulting nystagmus is easily observed.

1. The patient sits on a couch with his head back at 60° to bring the lateral canals to the vertical position. This is because it is easier to produce convection currents in a vertical column of fluid. The test should not be performed if the eardrum is perforated.
2. Water at 30°C and 44°C is run into each ear in turn. A thermostat is used to keep the temperature steady and 250 ml of water are allowed to flow over 40 seconds in the standardized test.
3. While the water is running the patient looks at a point straight ahead. This produces vertigo and easily observed nystagmus as the canals are stimulated or inhibited and the eyes are pushed or pulled to either side. The duration of the nystagmus is timed. The normal duration is 2 minutes ± 15 seconds. The resulting nystagmus is now often documented by electronystagmography with the eyes closed.

The interpretation of the results of caloric testing are based on the following features (Fig. 6.11):

1. Cold water cools the apex of the canal and fluid flows towards the cool area away from the utricle. The cupola is inhibited.
2. Hot water heats the apex of the canal, setting up a convection current towards the utricle. This stimulates the cupola.
3. With the knowledge that an active semicircular canal moves the eyes to the opposite side, it follows that cold water upsets the balance and the normal canal pushes the eyes towards the cold stimulus. Conversely, the hot water activates the canal and pushes the eyes away from the stimulated ear. Thus two abnormalities may be detected: canal paresis and directional preponderance.

Canal Paresis   If the semicircular canals or the eighth nerve on one side are damaged an incomplete or defective response to both hot or cold water in the

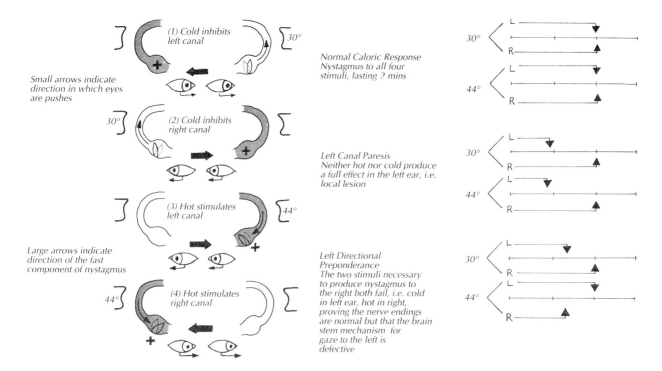

6.11 Mechanism of the caloric test.

affected ear will be found. Normal responses will be obtained from the other ear.

Directional Preponderance   The central connections of the vestibular nerve are such that cold water in one ear has the same effect as hot water in the other. If it is found that nystagmus cannot be induced to one particular side, it indicates that the vestibular nucleus on that side is defective. This is known as directional preponderance and indicates a lesion in the brain stem.

There are some situations in which both canal paresis and directional preponderance may coexist, for example when an acoustic nerve tumour or other posterior fossa lesion is damaging the nerve itself and also displacing the brain stem. This can produce confusing results which require expert interpretation.

The test can be further enhanced by recording the nystagmus with the eyes closed to remove optic fixation. The resultant nystagmus is suppressed with the eyes open and enhanced with the eyes closed. If there is a central lesion this enhancement cannot occur, producing further evidence of a central rather than a peripheral lesion, which is ultimately the main value of the test.

Positional Nystagmus

When a patient's main symptom is vertigo occurring only when the head is in a certain position, positional

testing may be helpful. The patient's head is held by the examiner with the patient sitting with his back towards the end of a couch. The patient is then quickly lowered, with his head turned to the right or left side, until the head is off the end of the couch and below the horizontal position. Acute vertigo with brisk nystagmus occurs when the affected vestibular apparatus is in the underneath position. There are two types of response:

1. Nystagmus starts after a 10–15 second delay, lasts some 30 seconds and is directed towards the underneath ear. If the test is repeated the response is less dramatic or even absent. This is the benign type and is a positioning response.

2. If the nystagmus comes on immediately, persists as long as the position is maintained or is in the opposite direction, it is of the central type. Repeated testing will produce repeated responses. There is a high likelihood that the patient will have a tumour in the posterior fossa. This a positional response.

More complex vestibular tests, including electronystagmography, will not be discussed in detail. Their main advantage lies in the fact that, using electrical recording with the eyes closed, the optic fixation reflexes are abolished. These reflexes are strong enough to suppress peripheral vestibular nystagmus but will have no effect on nystagmus due to central pathway or cerebellar disease. Another way of achieving this in the outpatient clinic is the use of Frenzel lenses, which defocus the patient's eyes and with the marked magnification of the patient's eyes enable the examiner to observe minimal nystagmus and abnormalities of saccadic movement more readily. Both techniques allow a distinction to be made that may be difficult on naked eye clinical examination. Other newly developed tests include pressure plate analysis of posture and sway, but these are so far of uncertain significance. These electronic and computerized tests are time-consuming and somewhat difficult to interpret, and the diagnostic precision of MRI scanning is such that an MRI scan rather than extensive otoneurological investigation is possibly quicker and less expensive when an acoustic nerve tumour, brainstem or cerebellar lesion is strongly suspected.

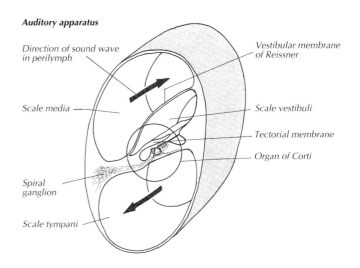

Auditory apparatus

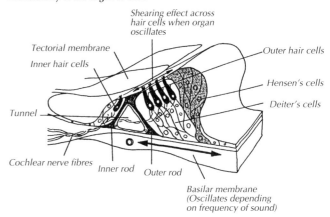

The Anatomy of the Organ of Corti

6.12   Section of part of the Cochlear Spiral and the organ of Corti.

The Auditory Apparatus (Fig. 6.12)

The organ of Corti has a similar basic structure to the vestibular apparatus and consists of receptor hair cells arranged in a fluid-filled spiral tube. The cavity of the tube is divided into three compartments by two membranes stretched across its centre, a roof membrane (of Reissner) and a tightly stretched basilar membrane. The closed cavity between them is filled with endolymph and the cavities on either side with perilymph. The receptor cells lie on supporting tissue arising from the basilar membrane. The hair processes are embedded in a thin membrane that bridges across the organ of Corti, known as the tectorial membrane. When the basilar membrane vibrates in response to a sound wave the tectorial membrane has a shearing effect on the hairs. At the apex of the cochlea the membrane has a diameter of 0.5 mm and at the base 0.04 mm, responding to low tones and high tones respectively. The pressure wave is transmitted through the perilymph by the pump-like effect of the stapes in the oval window, and the shock wave passes to the round window where the energy is dissipated.

Hearing can be tested at the bedside in the following ways:

1. A simple test can be performed with a wind-up watch and quantified by measuring the distance from the ear at which the watch can still just be heard. Unfortunately, modern electronic watches cannot be used!

2. If a watch cannot be heard at all a whispered voice at about 18 inches should be tried, gradually raising the voice until it becomes audible. It is essential to occlude the opposite ear with a finger while performing this test.

3. The tuning fork tests help distinguish between hearing loss due to middle ear disease (conductive deafness) and that due to eighth nerve damage (perceptive deafness).

The Rinne Test

A 256, 512 or 1024 tuning fork is held on the mastoid while the opposite ear is masked. It is then held half an inch from the external auditory canal and alternately on the mastoid until it is not longer heard in one of these positions. A Rinne positive test is documented when the tuning fork can still be heard in front of the ear but no longer heard on the mastoid. This is the normal situation and is documented as AC>BC. A Rinne negative test is recorded when the tuning fork is heard longer when placed on the mastoid than when placed in front of the ear canal, and is documented as BC>AC and indicates conductive deafness, as air-conducted sound depends for its transmission on intact auditory ossicles.

The Weber Test

If the tuning fork (256 or 512) is placed on the vertex it should be heard equally in both ears if hearing is normal. In perceptive deafness the fork will not be heard in the affected ear. In conductive deafness the fork will be heard louder in the affected ear as the auditory ossicles are circumvented.

The Noise Box

Some patients may claim total deafness in one or both ears that is suspected to be non-organic in type. A very simple test makes use of the same phenomenon that causes the noise level of conversation at parties get louder and louder. The loudness of the voice automatically rises if the background noise level is high.

The patient is asked to read aloud with the normal ear occluded and a wound up noise box is held next to the affected ear. When the catch is released and the noise begins, the patient will immediately raise their voice as they continue reading if the hearing is intact. This very simple and effective test can then be confirmed using electrophysiological tests of hearing and conduction in the auditory pathways.

Electrophysiological Tests of Hearing

Classic audiometric testing includes pure tone audiometry, speech audiometry and the measurement of tone decay. These tests require considerable expertise and patient cooperation, and are not easily used in young children. This is a subject in itself and can only really be appreciated by seeing the tests performed. Basically, pure sounds of known frequency and intensity or a series of words are presented to the patient via earphones. The positive or correct response is plotted on standard graphs and the distinction between conductive and perceptive deafness can be made.

Recent advances in electrophysiological testing not only allow hearing to be tested but also demonstrate neural activity in the cochlea, auditory nerve and brainstem pathways.

Acoustic or stapedius reflex testing is performed using an airtight probe in the external auditory meatus. The probe injects the sound, permits the pressure in the canal to be controlled and detects movement of the tympanic membrane. The stiffening of the membrane when a noise is presented to the ear is detected, requiring no cooperation from the patient.

Electrocochleography (ECog) is performed by inserting a long needle electrode through the tympanic membrane. Small potentials generated in the cochlea itself and in the auditory nerve and brain stem can be detected and studied using averaging techniques.

Brainstem Auditory Evoked Potentials (BAERs)

Of special interest to neurologists is the recording of a stream of potentials in the brain stem set up by an auditory stimulus. These are known as BAERs (brainstem auditory evoked responses). This consists of a series of five potentials detected by an electrode placed over the mastoid process and information about brainstem function can be obtained. The five potentials occur at different latencies, as indicated in Figure 6.13. The latency between potentials I and II represents activity in the cochlea and auditory nerve. The latency between II and III represents the first relay in the brain stem and between III and IV the further relays in the brain stem before the impulse reaches the inferior colliculus. Abnormal latencies between I and II indicate an acoustic nerve lesion. Abnormal delays in I–V or III–V indicate a lesion in the brain stem itself. These can be of value in detecting subclinical brainstem lesions in MS, although in those cases where there are no clinical correlates of BAER abnormality it is not unusual for subsequent MRI scanning to be unhelpful. BAERs have not achieved the diagnostic precision of VERs.

Clinical Disorders of the Eighth Nerve and its Connections

The insidious early development of deafness and the surprisingly late symptom of vertigo in cerebellopontine angle lesions has been repeatedly stressed. Only acute disorders of the eighth nerve and its connections produce dramatic symptoms such as tinnitus, acute deafness or vertigo. The most frequent manifestation of tinnitus is probably the pulsatile rushing noise, synchronous with the pulse, that occurs in elderly arteriopathic patients and which may cause severe depression. Most tinnitus remains unexplained and there is no effective treatment. Few patients find that a masker, a hearing aid-like device that emits a 'different' noise, of much value.

Vertigo is a common and distressing symptom. It is most important to establish that what the patient is describing really is vertigo. Patients frequently use the expressions 'dizzy' or 'giddy', and too often these terms are uncritically accepted as being synonymous with vertigo. Closer questioning may reveal that the patient actually means 'light-headed', 'woozy' or 'faint', but does not experience the characteristic spinning sensation of vertigo. Vertigo is best defined as an illusion of movement of either the patient or their surroundings.

Once 'non-vertiginous' patients have been excluded, relatively few disorders need be considered. In most instances the history alone is very characteristic and a fairly confident clinical diagnosis can be made. The

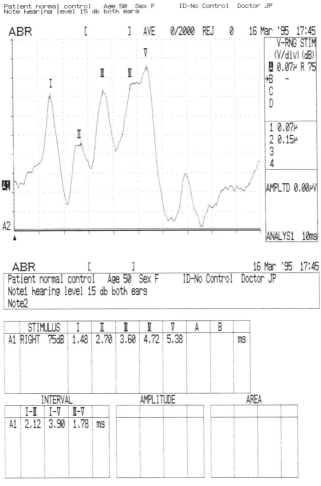

6.13 Brainstem auditory evoked responses (BAER's)

majority of patients in the 'non-vertigo' group are suffering from an anxiety state or hyperventilation syndrome. These conditions are fully discussed in Chapter 22. Very extensive, expensive and often unnecessary investigations may be performed on these patients unless strict clinical criteria for diagnosing vertigo are applied.

The history is all important in patients with vertigo and the type of sensation, the circumstances under which it occurs, the associated symptoms, duration and frequency of attacks must all be established.

The major causes of vertigo are:

Benign positional vertigo
Non-benign positional vertigo
Vestibular neuronitis
Menière's disease
Migraine
Multiple sclerosis
Drugs, including alcohol
Brainstem ischaemic attacks
Complex partial seizures
Perilymph fistula.

Benign Positional Vertigo

This condition occurs mainly in middle age but can present at any age. The history is very striking. The onset is always abrupt and the first attack often occurs after a few seconds delay, as the patient first gets out of bed. As they become upright they develop acute rotatory or somersaulting vertigo and they may stagger or fall, damaging themselves and bedroom furniture in the process. Within 15 seconds the attack is over, by which time the patient has usually managed to sit down on the bed. They may then move more cautiously and it will not happen again until they get back into bed and attempt to lie down. They then quickly discover that sitting up or lying down or looking up or looking down, particularly with the head rotated to one particular side, will provoke further attacks. They will also realize that there is a brief latent period, with a delay of perhaps 5 seconds, before the onset of the vertigo after they have made the provocative movement. The intense vertigo typically lasts only 10–15 seconds, usually too brief to cause nausea or vomiting.

A few courageous patients may also discover that just after an attack has occurred they can move with some impunity for 1–2 minutes before a further attack can be provoked, but very few dare to experiment! Some patients may be wakened by vertigo set off by turning over in their sleep. Others find that hanging washing on a line is particularly provocative, because of the tilting up of the head to the side while pegging up the clothing or towels.

The condition usually persists for between 2 and 20 weeks and may recur on two or three occasions over the next 1–2 years. It is particularly common in migraine sufferers, and in some instances seems to occur as a migraine variant showing the same cyclical pattern as the patient's conventional headaches. In children it is nearly always associated with migraine. About 30% of attacks are preceded by an upper respiratory viral infection and 30% follow head trauma, which may have been quite mild. In some 40% of cases no clear cause can be established.

Non-Benign Positional Vertigo

A more ominous variant of positional vertigo can occur which is associated with disease in the posterior fossa. It differs from benign positional vertigo in several critical ways.

CASE REPORT VII

A 58-year-old woman was referred with a 10-day history of occipital headache, nausea and impairment of balance. When summoned form the waiting room she stood up and fell forwards, and was caught by the attendant nurse. She had noted that any change of position, from lying to sitting in bed, or from sitting to standing, provoked the same response, and on some occasions the resulting giddiness had persisted long enough to cause vomiting. Physical examination revealed nystagmus to the left-hand side and minimal incoordination of the left arm. She had previously had a carcinoma of the breast treated by local excision 6 years before. Yearly follow-up had revealed no evidence of recurrence. A CT scan confirmed a midline cyst and an adjacent contrast-enhancing lesion in the left cerebellar hemisphere. Unfortunately the chest X-ray revealed six deposits in the lung fields.

This case demonstrates all the following features which are typical of the condition. The vertigo is of instantaneous onset, there is no latent period. It may be triggered by **any** sudden movement of the head in **any** direction rather than in one specific direction, and is of longer duration, often sufficient to cause vomiting, which may be sudden and projectile in type. It can also be immediately provoked by further movement as there is no refractory period after an attack. If the underlying cause is not established and treated the attacks will continue until other evidence of brainstem or cerebellar disease appears. The usual cause in the adult, where

primary posterior fossa tumours are rare, is a cerebellar metastasis. Personal experience suggests that metastases from large bowel tumours are particularly likely to spread to the posterior fossa and present in this way.

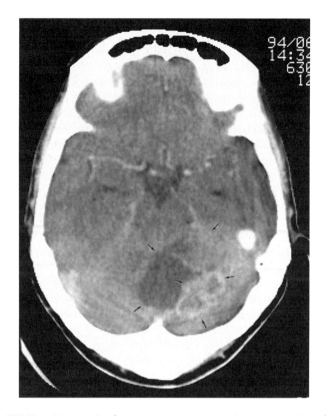

CRVII. *Metastatic breast cancer presenting as positional vertigo. Midline cyst and metastatic tumour.*

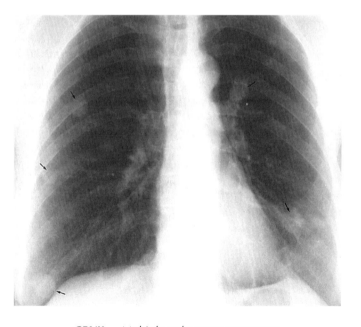

CRVII. *Multiple pulmonary metastases.*

Vestibular Neuronitis

This is a common benign disorder that occasionally occurs in epidemic form and is thought to be due to a viral infection of the vestibular ganglion, or of the brainstem vestibular system. The onset is abrupt, with very severe vertigo and ataxia, often accompanied by severe vomiting. There are no auditory components, which should exclude an attack of Menière's disease. The acute phase lasts 5–7 days and is often followed by a prolonged recovery period, during which benign positional vertigo occurs and progressively subsides. During the acute phase no position is completely comfortable and the patient preferentially lies quite still on their back. Vomiting may be so severe that the patient requires admission and intravenous fluids. It does not show any tendency to recur and is a benign but distressing condition.

Menière's Disease

Although this diagnosis is often suspected it is actually quite a rare condition, usually starting in middle age. The attacks are of very sudden onset, preceded by a full or bursting sensation in the head and followed by a roaring or hissing noise in the ear, which disappears as the ear becomes deaf later in the attack. Intense vertigo is present from the onset. The disturbance of otolith function is often the main problem, and patients may feel as though they are somersaulting over backwards and fling themselves in the opposite direction, ending up on the ground. The patient prefers to lie with the affected ear uppermost and perfectly still, any movement making the vertigo worse. Attacks may last up to 24 hours and leave the patient exhausted.

The associated auditory symptoms are the key factor in the history. The mechanism of the condition is still not understood, but is thought to be due to ischaemic damage altering the fluid balance in the various compartments in the inner ear. Some benefit may be achieved by a salt-free diet, diuretics and vestibular sedatives. Drugs that may improve the circulation to the inner ear, such as betahistine or calcium channel antaqonists, may be of some benefit. In some 80% of patients the condition remits over 5 years, so that destructive surgical procedures on the ear are only justified in chronic cases that are unresponsive to simple measures. Although it is a benign condition it is probably one of the most unpleasant disorders known. In some patients a close relationship to migraine is seen and migraine prophylactic drugs may confer some benefit. After repeated attacks progressive deafness occurs in the affected ear. It is at this stage that the diagnosis is often made.

Migraine

Nausea and vertigo are common components of the migraine syndrome and in some patients these symptoms are worse than the headache. The onset of a characteristic headache (see Chapter 20) should leave little doubt as to the diagnosis. Problems may arise when the headaches are completely replaced by the vestibular symptoms. It is essential to explore fully the previous headache history of any patient with unexplained attacks of vertigo and vomiting. Benign positional vertigo in childhood is very commonly a migraine variant. In adolescence basilar migraine with severe vertigo and other brainstem phenomena such as diplopia, dysarthria, tetraparesis and even cortical blindness may occur, attacks typically lasting 30–60 minutes and followed by headaches, which may be surprisingly modest in intensity. Some cases of Menière's disease may be related to migraine. Adult migraineurs may also experience short-lived benign positional vertigo-like attacks as a migraine variant.

Multiple Sclerosis

Although multiple sclerosis may cause episodes of acute vertigo, the majority of such patients will also have symptoms such as diplopia, numbness of the face, weakness or ataxia of a limb, or dysarthria to indicate a more widespread brainstem lesion. None of these additional symptoms occurs with simple disorders of the vestibular apparatus. Furthermore, in multiple sclerosis the cochlear fibres entering the brain stem may also be damaged, leading to deafness in one ear. This combination of signs could lead to diagnostic errors and Menière's disease may be suspected. The persistence of an attack over a 2–6-week period, the patient's age and other physical signs should exclude Menière's disease and indicate the possibility of multiple sclerosis. A surprising number of previous brainstem episodes in patients who subsequently develop other evidence of MS seem to have been incorrectly identified as Menière's disease at their initial presentation.

Drug-Induced Vertigo

Many drugs and alcohol can cause vertigo as a side-effect. The drugs include virtually all anticonvulsants, most sedatives, many antibiotics and antituberculous drugs, particularly streptomycin. Chloroquine, methysergide maleate and aspirin, may also cause tinnitus. A careful history of drug ingestion and dosage should be regarded as part of the routine questioning in any patient who complains of vertigo.

Brainstem Vascular Disease

Although vertigo is the single most common symptom of brainstem vascular disease, it does not follow that vertigo in an elderly patient is always due to vertebro basilar ischaemia. As in suspected multiple sclerosis, a careful enquiry for other symptoms of brainstem disease should be made. It is unwise to accept this diagnosis uncritically and other evidence of brainstem dysfunction should be present in order to make the diagnosis.

Brainstem vascular disease is very over-diagnosed in elderly patients who have experienced brief attacks of dizziness or vertigo on hot days, in bathrooms or when standing up suddenly. It is not unusual to encounter elderly patients with drug-induced Parkinson's disease who have been taking prochlorperazine unnecessarily for years after such an attack has been misdiagnosed as a brainstem ischaemic episode.

Complex Partial Seizures

Some patients with complex partial seizures experience vertigo as a prodromal symptom of an attack. Subsequent events should leave little doubt that the vertigo was part of an epileptic event. It is likely that epileptic discharges originating in the posterior temporal lobe are responsible (see also Chapters 10 and 22).

Perilymph Fistula

This distressing condition is very similar symptomatically to benign positional vertigo, but the individual episodes last longer and are accompanied by hearing impairment. It usually follows trauma to the ear or comes on during sudden exertion, and is due to rupture of the oval window. The condition tends to settle after 2–3 weeks if the patient avoids sudden exertion. One characteristic feature of a perilymph fistula is a remarkable sign known as the Tullio phenomenon. When the patient is subjected to a loud noise, acute vertigo, nystagmus, oscillopsia and postural imbalance is provoked. The mechanism of this phenomena remains uncertain but the condition subsides as the fistula heals.

The Jugular Foramen (Figs. 6.14 and 6.15)

The jugular foramen is an extremely difficult area both to illustrate and to understand. The ninth, tenth and eleventh cranial nerves enter the internal part of the foramen lying on the medial side of the sigmoid sinus. The foramen itself angles forwards and laterally under the petrous bone, which is excavated by the slight ballooning of the sigmoid sinus as it exits through the skull to become the jugular bulb. The three cranial nerves emerge in front of the jugular bulb, lying between it and the carotid artery, which enters the carotid canal just anterior to the emerging jugular vein. There are two other structures in the area of differential diagnostic importance to be considered:

1. The twelfth (hypoglossal) nerve, which exits through the anterior condylar canal posteromedial to the jugular foramen and comes into close relationship with the three other nerves **outside** the skull
2. The cervical sympathetic which **ascends** into the area on the carotid artery. It does not exit from the skull via the jugular foramen. It follows that if the cervical sympathetic is involved in a jugular foramen syndrome the lesion is certain to be outside the skull.

The Anatomy of the Last Four Cranial Nerves

The Glossopharyngeal Nerve (Ninth Cranial Nerve)

The glossopharyngeal nerve has sensory, motor and autonomic components. The sensory ganglion cells lie in the superior and inferior ganglia of the nerve, and the central processes pass to the nucleus of the tractus solitarius, conveying taste sensation, and to the nucleus of the spinal tract of the fifth nerve, conveying somatic sensation. The motor nucleus is the upper part of the nucleus ambiguus, which receives bilateral supranuclear innervation from corticobulbar fibres. This nucleus supplies the stylopharyngeus. The autonomic parasympathetic fibres arise in the inferior salivatory nucleus. These preganglionic fibres reach the lesser petrosal nerve by way of the tympanic branch and relay in the otic ganglion. The postganglionic fibres are distributed to the parotid gland by way of the auriculotemporal nerve.

The glossopharyngeal nerve emerges from the brain stem in line with the vagus and accessory nerves, and exits through the jugular foramen. It descends between the jugular vein and the carotid artery, picking up sympathetic fibres from the carotid plexus as it loops forwards and medially to reach the soft tissues of the oropharynx, posterior tongue and palate. In its course it gives off the tympanic (Jacobson's) nerve, conveying the secretomotor fibres for the parotid gland to the otic ganglion via the tympanic plexus and lesser petrosal nerve.

An important branch, the carotid nerve, innervates the carotid body and carotid sinus conveying, respectively, chemoceptor and stretch reflex information centrally for respiratory and circulatory reflex function. The final branches are the pharyngeal, tonsillar and lingual branches, carrying general sensation and taste from the appropriate areas.

The Otic Ganglion

The otic ganglion lies just below the foramen ovale, attached to the mandibular nerve but functionally con-

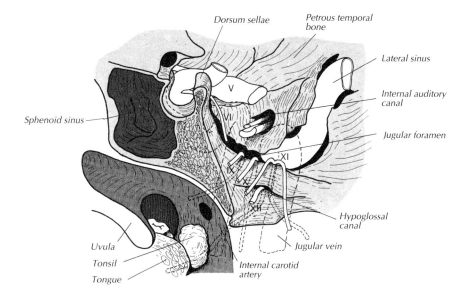

6.14 Jugular foramen sagittal section of skull base, right side shown.

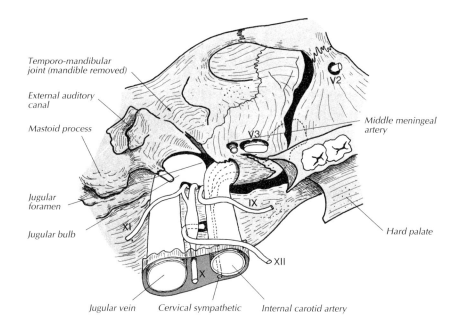

6.15 Jugular foramen seen from below and laterally on the right side.

veying information from the glossopharyngeal nerve. The parasympthetic fibres relay in it and supply the parotid gland by way of the auriculotemporal nerves. Sympathetic fibres picked up from the middle meningeal artery pass through the ganglion without synapse and are distributed to the blood vessels of the parotid gland in the same nerve.

The Vagus Nerve (Tenth Cranial Nerve)

The vagus nerve (the wanderer) is the most widely distributed cranial nerve. The central connections are similar to those of the ninth nerve.

1. The dorsal nucleus of the vagus contains motor and sensory components. The motor fibres are general visceral efferent to the smooth muscle of the bronchi, heart, oesophagus, stomach and intestine. The sensory fibres are general visceral afferent originating in the oesophagus and upper bowel, with cell bodies in the superior and inferior vagal gangila.

2. The nucleus ambiguus gives origin to fibres controlling the striated muscle of the pharynx and intrinsic muscles of the larynx. It has a bilateral supranuclear innervation.

3. The nucleus of the tractus solitarius is shared with the glossopharyngeal nerve and receives fibres from the taste buds of the epiglottis and vallecula.

4. The spinal nucleus of the fifth nerve receives general somatic afferent fibres from the pharynx and larynx.

Because of these extensive nuclear connections, multiple rootlets emerge from the anterolateral brain stem and form a flat cord which enters the jugular foramen. The superior and inferior ganglia lie both in the foramen and just below it, in an identical pattern to the glossopharyngeal nerve. Both ganglia make connections with the accessory and hypoglossal nerves and pick up fibres from the sympathetic plexus on the carotid artery. Below the inferior ganglion, the cranial root of the accessory nerve merges into the vagus nerve, which then distributes its fibres to the pharynx and larynx. The vagal branches of practical importance are as follows:

1. A meningeal branch supplying the dura of the posterior fossa is given off in the jugular foramen.

2. The auricular branch arises from the superior ganglion. It is joined by a branch from the glossopharyngeal and is distributed to the skin of the external ear with the branch of the facial nerve. These fibres all ultimately enter the nucleus of the descending tract of the fifth nerve.

3. The pharyngeal branch arises just above the inferior ganglion and distributes the accessory components to the pharyngeal plexus supplying the pharynx and palate.

4. The superior laryngeal nerve comes off the inferior ganglion and divides into two branches. The internal laryngeal nerve supplies sensation to the mucous membrane of the larynx and conveys proprioceptive information from the neuromuscular spindles and stretch receptors of the larynx. The external laryngeal nerve supplies the cricothyroid and contributes to the pharyngeal plexus, which is of considerable importance in speech mechanisms.

5. The recurrent laryngeal nerve has differing courses on each side. On the right it loops under the subclavian artery and on the left under the aortic arch. On both sides it then ascends on the side of the trachea to reach the larynx. It supplies all the muscles of the larynx, except the cricothyroid, and carries sensory fibres from the mucous membranes and stretch receptors of the larynx.

The Spinal Accessory Nerve (Eleventh Cranial Nerve)

The cranial part of this nerve is a detached portion of the vagus and the spinal part is motor to the sternocleidomastoid and trapezius. The cranial portion arises from the lower part of the nucleus ambiguus and a small component from the dorsal efferent nucleus of the vagus. The nerve rootlets emerge in line with the vagus, are joined by the ascending spinal component, and then run laterally to enter the jugular foramen. The cranial portion merges with the vagus at the level of the inferior vagal ganglion and is then distributed in the pharyngeal

and recurrent laryngeal branches of the vagus. These fibres probably supply the muscles of the soft palate.

The spinal root arises from the ventral horn cells from C1 to C5. The fibres emerge from the cord laterally between the anterior and posterior spinal nerve roots to form a separate nerve trunk, ascending into the skull through the foramen magnum. It then exits from the skull by way of the jugular foramen in the same dural sheath as the vagus. It runs posteriorly as soon as it emerges, to supply the sternocleidomastoid and the upper part of trapezius, and it receives a major contribution from branches of the anterior roots of C3 and C4 to form a plexus which supplies the cervical musculature. Surgical evidence suggests that these root components make important contributions, as upper cervical root section is required to completely denervate the sternocleidomastoid and trapezius. The peripheral portion of the nerve is easily damaged in lymph node biopsy and other operations in the posterior triangle of the neck.

The accessory nerve is unusual in that clinical evidence indicates that its supranuclear innervation is ipsilateral. In hemiparetic vascular lesions the weakness in the sternocleidomastoid is on the **same** side as the lesion. In epileptic fits originating in the frontal pole the head turns **away** from the side of the lesion, which indicates the the ipsilateral sternocleidomastoid is contracting. If this distribution is not recognized, the signs may seem to indicate that a patient with a left hemiparesis has a right accessory nerve lesion, and therefore a lower brainstem lesion, rather than a simple capsular cerebrovascular accident. This is a commonly made mistake.

The Hypoglossal Nerve (Twelfth Cranial Nerve)

The hypoglossal nerve arises from a nuclear column in the floor of the fourth ventricle derived from the same embryological cell groups as the nuclei of nerves III, IV and VI. Like nerves III and VI, the fascicular fibres have to traverse the full sagittal diameter of the medulla to exit from the ventral surface between the pyramid and the olive. The numerous rootlets combine and become two main fasciculi with their own dural sleeves, and exit by way of the hypoglossal canal just below the jugular foramen. The nerve therefore emerges deep to the other structures and has to course downwards and anteriorly to emerge between the jugular vein and the carotid artery, cross the inferior vagal ganglion and then course upwards and anteriorly on the hyoglossus, distributing branches to all the muscles of the tongue. It receives sympathetic fibres from the superior cervical ganglion, some fibres from the vagus and from the motor roots of C1 and C2 via the ansa cervicalis. Numerous filaments connect to and are distributed with the lingual nerve.

Fibres derived from the hypoglossal nucleus supply the styloglossus, hyoglossus, geniohyoid and genioglossus. The fibres derived from the C1 components are distributed to the sternohyoid, sternothyroid, omohyoid, thyrohyoid and geniohyoid. Although a twelfth nerve lesion paralyses one side of the tongue as its most obvious feature, the larynx is also pulled across to the opposite side on swallowing, as a consequence of the failure of the hyoid to elevate on the paralysed side.

The supranuclear innervation of the hypoglossal nucleus is usually bilateral but can be mainly contralateral. The nerve is particularly vulnerable to surgical trauma in operations on the neck for malignant disease and during endarterectomy. Paralysis during central venous catheterization has also been reported.

Clinical Evaluation of the Last Four Cranial Nerves

The Glossopharyngeal Nerve (Ninth Cranial Nerve)

There is no such thing as a 'ninth nerve palsy'. From a practical point of view the nerve is purely sensory and the sensory fibres terminate in the spinal tract of the trigeminal nerve when they enter the brain stem. The peripheral distribution is via the pharyngeal branches to the mucous membrane of the pharynx. The only muscle supplied by the nerve is the stylopharyngeus, which cannot be tested clinically. The error noted above is made because of the almost universal misconception of students that the ninth nerve is motor to the palate. When the gag reflex is tested the sensory stimulus is relayed via the ninth nerve, but the resulting visible palatal movement is mediated by the tenth nerve. This reflex is too gross for accurate clinical diagnosis of a glossopharyngeal nerve lesion.

Sensation should be carefully tested by touching the palate gently with an orange stick on each side and then, with the patient saying 'Aah', touching the posterior pharyngeal wall on each side. The patient should be asked to compare these gentle stimuli. If there is any doubt, pain sensation can be tested in the same areas, using a long sterile hatpin. It is vital to test for such sensory loss in all the clinical situations discussed below. Evaluation of taste sensation over the posterior third of the tongue has no proven value in clinical diagnosis.

The Vagus Nerve (Tenth Cranial Nerve)

The motor distribution of the vagus comprises the nerve supply to the palate and the vocal cords. Weakness of the palate may cause nasal regurgitation of food, and nasal speech. The paralysed side of the palate does not move and is pulled across to the intact side when the patient says 'Aah'. Paralysis of one vocal cord will allow that cord to lie permanently and limply abducted to the midline. This leads to hoarseness, loss of volume of the voice and an inability to cough explosively, the so-called 'bovine cough'.

Examination of the tenth nerve should include examination of palatal movements, the patient's voice, and the patient's ability to cough. The sensory fibres conveyed in the vagus are distributed in the auricular branch, which supplies the skin over the cranial part of the auricle and the posterior wall and floor of the external auditory meatus. This accounts for the referral of pain from malignant disease in the throat to the ear and auditory canal. These fibres terminate in the spinal nucleus of the trigeminal nerve when they enter the brain stem.

Spinal Accessory Nerve (Eleventh Cranial Nerve)

The spinal accessory nerve is motor to the sternocleidomastoid and the upper part of the trapezius muscle. The complex central control of this nerve is also discussed in Chapter 11. From a practical point of view, damage to the nerve results in wasting and weakness of the sternocleidomastoid and upper trapezius. Like so many things in neurology, these signs are very easily overlooked unless one is specifically alerted to the possibility of an abnormality.

The Hypoglossal Nerve (Twelfth Cranial Nerve)

The hypoglossal nerve is the motor nerve to the tongue. The tongue muscle, in addition to moving the tongue from side to side, also moves it up and down and in and out. In fact, the tongue is a piece of muscle pulling against itself. Unilateral damage to the nerve supply leads to wasting, weakness and fasciculation of that side of the tongue. The wasting and fasciculation are best seen with the tongue lying in the floor of the mouth. Normal tongues show slight flickering movements when held out for more than a few seconds, a source of considerable anxiety to generations of medical students! On attempted tongue protrusion the muscle on the weak side cannot balance the forward push of the muscle on the intact side, and as a result the tongue deviates **towards** the weak side. Patients do not notice unilateral involvement of the tongue. It is usually found by accident by the patient or their dentist and causes little or no disability. The commonest cause of this rare condition is a neurofibroma of the twelfth nerve. For some reason these are almost exclusively found in females. Bilateral involvement causes dramatic impairment of chewing, swallowing and speaking, and is responsible for the presenting symptoms in elderly patients with the bulbar form of motor neuron disease (see Chapter 11).

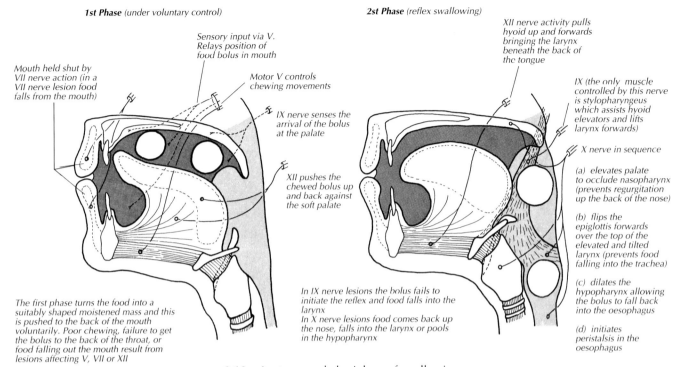

1st Phase (under voluntary control)

Mouth held shut by
VII nerve action (in a
VII nerve lesion food
falls from the mouth)

Sensory input via V.
Relays position of
food bolus in mouth

Motor V controls
chewing movements

IX nerve senses the
arrival of the bolus
at the palate

XII pushes the
chewed bolus up
and back against
the soft palate

The first phase turns the food into a
suitably shaped moistened mass and this
is pushed to the back of the mouth
voluntarily. Poor chewing, failure to get
the bolus to the back of the throat, or
food falling out the mouth result from
lesions affecting V, VII or XII

2st Phase (reflex swallowing)

XII nerve activity pulls
hyoid up and forwards
bringing the larynx
beneath the back of
the tongue

IX (the only muscle
controlled by this nerve
is stylopharyngeus
which assists hyoid
elevators and lifts
larynx forwards)

X nerve in sequence

(a) elevates palate
to occlude nasopharynx
(prevents regurgitation
up the back of the nose)

(b) flips the
epiglottis forwards
over the top of the
elevated and tilted
larynx (prevents food
falling into the trachea)

(c) dilates the
hypopharynx allowing
the bolus to fall back
into the oesophagus

(d) initiates
peristalsis in the
oesophagus

In IX nerve lesions the bolus fails to
initiate the reflex and food falls into the
larynx
In X nerve lesions food comes back up
the nose, falls into the larynx or pools
in the hypopharynx

6.16 Anatomy and physiology of swallowing.

The Cervical Sympathetic

Horner's syndrome has been discussed in detail in Chapter 2.

The Anatomy of Swallowing

Several cranial nerves are involved simultaneously in chewing, bolus formation and swallowing. The whole sequence of events is fully detailed and annotated in Figure 6.16.

Clinical Presentations

Owing to the proximity of the last four cranial nerves several combinations of nerve lesions are possible, depending on the exact site of the causative lesion. The presenting symptoms are similar whatever the diagnosis. They include loss of strength or hoarseness of the voice, nasal speech, difficulty in swallowing, with nasal regurgitation of fluids, or aspiration of food particles with attacks of choking.

Weakness of the sternomastoids and trapezii may be noticed by the patient, or tongue wasting noted by chance by a dentist, and lead to referral. Both the ninth and tenth nerves convey some sensation from the region of the external auditory canal and the area behind the ear. Deep aching pain in and around the ear may indicate damage to these nerves in the region of the jugular foramen. Headache may also occur as

these nerves convey pain fibres from the dura of the posterior fossa. Irritation of these fibres may cause referred pain in the occipital region.

As noted in Chapter 2, a Horner's syndrome can be easily overlooked but may occasionally be the presenting symptom. It is usually the droopy eyelid, rather than the small pupil, that is noticed.

The Syndromes

Vernet's Syndrome (of the Jugular Foramen)

This consists of evidence of damage to the three nerves that traverse the jugular foramen itself, i.e. cranial nerves IX, X and XI. A lesion inside the skull is more likely to cause this restricted syndrome because a lesion outside the skull is likely to also affect both the twelfth cranial nerve and the cervical sympathetic.

Collet–Sicard Syndrome (of the Posterior Lacerocondylar Area)

The Collet–Sicard syndrome consists of damage to the last four cranial nerves. From Figure 6.14 it will be seen that as the foramen opens from the skull it is adjacent to the foramen lacerum, just above the condyle of the occipital bone. The last four cranial nerves lie in close proximity in this area. This syndrome could also occur with a lesion inside the skull, but an intracranial lesion extensive enough to affect all four nerves (see Fig. 6.13) would be very likely to distort the brain stem or cerebellum, and produce signs of long tract damage or cerebellar disturbance.

Villaret's Syndrome (of the Posterior Retropharyngeal Space)

Referring to Figure 6.14, it will be seen that in the anterior part of the area lying immediately behind the nasopharynx, the cervical sympathetic, is extremely vulnerable. Villaret's syndrome consists of damage to the ninth, tenth, eleventh and twelfth nerves **and** a Horner's syndrome. The association with Horner's syndrome always indicates a lesion outside the skull.

Cause of Jugular Foramen Syndromes

Lesions Inside the Skull

Any of the lesions that can cause the cerebellopontine angle syndrome can also extend down towards the foramen magnum and involve the last four cranial nerves in numerical sequence. The diagnosis is easy if the fifth and seventh nerves are also affected, as there is no lesion that could occur outside the skull and produce such a combination. Tumours that specifically occur inside the skull in this region are neurinomas of the ninth, tenth or twelfth nerves. They occur most often on the twelfth nerve, with a marked predilection for young females, and occur on the left side in a ratio of 9:1. The reason for this is unknown. Meningiomas and epidermoid tumours (cholesteatomas) may also occur in this area and tend to cause distortion of the brain stem. This eventually produces long tract signs and symptoms such as a mild or intermittent tetraparesis. As noted previously, cholesteatomas in the posterior fossa are particularly prone to cause hemifacial spasm.

Lateral brainstem lesions are unusual except in vascular accidents. Although these syndromes may include a Horner's syndrome, they rarely cause diagnostic confusion because of the abrupt onset and the associated spinothalamic sensory loss over the opposite side of the body, which leaves do doubt that the cranial nerve damage is due to intrinsic brainstem disease. The classic vascular syndrome in this area is that of Wallenberg (see also Chapter 11).

Lesions in the Jugular Foramen or Outside the Skull

Of the lesions discussed above, both meningiomas and neurofibromas may extend out through the foramina, in a dumb-bell fashion, sometimes presenting as a mass

at the angle of the jaw. A Horner's syndrome is certain evidence that the lesion is outside the skull, as the cervical sympathetic ascends into the area and does not pass through the foramen. Attempts should also be made to see if a palpable mass is present at the angle of the jaw, or if there is any cervical lymphadenopathy. It is important to realize that a bony hard mass is normally palpable in this area: it is the tip of the transverse process of the atlas!

Other Causes

Polyneuritis Cranialis

This is a somewhat dubious entity which basically consists of multiple cranial nerve palsies for which no cause can be established and which may well recover. Several examples have been seen in elderly patients, in whom intensive investigations, including multiple nasopharyngeal biopsies, failed to demonstrate a cause and who recovered completely under observation. Some of the reported cases have also suffered from diabetes or syphilis, and the nerve lesions may represent a variety of transient nerve palsies similar to those that may involve the extraocular nerves.

An important practical point is that although the suspicion of metastatic carcinoma must be high, irradiation without tissue diagnosis is not justified unless relentless progression of the syndrome can be established. Isolated twelfth nerve palsies with recovery after a few weeks may occur, and may be due to a similar pathology to Bell's palsy. In all cases follow-up should be continued until full recovery has occurred.

Perhaps the most clearly identifiable condition of this type is the Fisher syndrome. a variant of Guillain–Barre syndrome, which specifically affects the cranial nerves. The picture consists of the rapid evolution of multiple cranial nerve lesions, particularly affecting the extraocular nerves, accompanied by marked loss of posture sense with resultant ataxia. In two of the author's cases almost complete deafness, without vertigo, accompanied the condition. The prognosis is excellent, with full recovery over several weeks. There are as yet no case reports of treatment with immunoglobulin infusion, although it seems likely that the condition would respond to this treatment.

Glomus or Carotid Body Tumours

These tumours arise in the chemoectodermal tissue that is normally present in the carotid body, and may be found ectopically in the inner ear and around the ninth and tenth nerves. Neoplastic changes in this tissue produce highly vascular erosive tumours which may destroy the petrous temporal bone and present as a vascular nodule in the external auditory canal.

Depending on the exact site of the glomus tumour, a cerebellopontine angle syndrome associated with an internal and/or an external jugular foramen syndrome may result. These tumours occur in either sex, with a peak incidence in the third and fourth decades.

Glossopharyngeal Neuralgia

This very rare form of neuralgia consists of attacks of severe pain in the throat when fluid or food is swallowed. The pain is excruciating and similar to that of tic douloureux. Exploration to cut the nerve often reveals aberrant vessels coursing across the nerve, or unsuspected neurofibromas or cholesteatomas adjacent to the nerve. Vascular decompression is now the treatment of choice if no other lesion is demonstrable. It is always wise to regard the syndrome as potentially symptomatic, indicating an underlying lesion, until proved otherwise by MRI scanning or surgical exploration.

Investigation of the Jugular Foramen Syndrome

Having established the combination of nerve palsies, the two most important additional clinical signs to be sought are a Horner's syndrome or evidence of brainstem compression. The former indicates an extracranial lesion and the latter an intracranial lesion. If the lesion is outside the skull routine haematological studies and chest and paranasal sinus X-rays assume significance, and direct examination of the nasopharynx and larynx should be part of the routine evaluation. Skull X-rays are rarely of value, although a careful skull base film should be taken. MRI scanning is now established as the investigation of choice in this region. The ability to see through bone permits the demonstration of lesions such as a neurofibroma on the vagus nerve, actually within the jugular foramen. Hitherto this was technically impossible, as in all other imaging techniques the bone prevented visualization.

CASE REPORT VIII

A 76-year-old man presented with a history of weight loss, a mass at the angle of his jaw, dysphagia and a hoarse voice. On examination the following signs were present:
There was a hard tender mass at the angle of his jaw
The left palate was insensitive to touch and pinprick
The left palate was weak and he had a bovine cough
There was wasting and weakness of the left sternomastoid and trapezius muscles

The left side of the tongue was slightly wasted, fasciculating and deviated to the left on protrusion
He had a left Horner's syndrome.

In this case the mass and the Horner's syndrome indicated that the lesion was extracranial. Biopsy revealed a squamous carcinoma, probably metastatic from the lung.

CASE REPORT IX

A very anxious 63-year-old woman was seen in 1976 with symptoms of presyncope following the initiation of treatment for significant hypertension (BP 180/120). There were elements of both postural hypotension and anxiety-based panic in her symptoms, but no physical signs. In April 1971 she had complained of a tightness in the throat and a shooting pain in the right ear. A barium swallow was normal and she was reassured by the ENT surgeons. She was re-referred to the ENT surgeons in 1986, with a 1-year history of hoarseness of the voice due to a paralysed left vocal cord. Laryngoscopy and bronchoscopy were otherwise normal, but a year later she was complaining of dysphagia for solids. She was first referred for a neurological opinion in October 1988. Her family thought that the speech disturbance had started in 1983, when her voice had become slightly 'croaky'. She had noticed difficulty with chewing and swallowing for the past 18 months and, in retrospect, at about the same time she had noticed wasting of the muscles of the left side of the neck and shoulder, which had been attributed by her GP to 'arthritis'. On physical examination at that time she had complete involvement of the left ninth, tenth, eleventh and twelfth nerves and an extensor plantar response on the left-hand side. There was no Horner's syndrome. It was felt that this combination had to indicate a lesion inside the skull or in the jugular foramen itself. An MRI scan revealed a neurofibroma almost certainly originating on the tenth cranial nerve, within and just below the jugular foramen. In view of her age (then 75) it was felt that any surgical approach to this lesion was unjustified, but that in view of the long history and presumed benign nature of the tumour significant further progression was unlikely. The extensor plantar remains unexplained.

A certain amount of easily acquired skill is necessary to detect multiple lower cranial nerve palsies. The provisional diagnosis and investigative approach depend on the accurate detection of associated signs. Jugular foramen syndromes are good examples of conditions where clinical findings alone provide nearly all the information necessary to identify the likely diagnosis. With MRI scanning now available to actually confirm the diagnosis, either surgery or radiotherapy can be accurately planned.

7. Conjugate Eye Movements and Nystagmus

The eyes have central connections that function like the steering linkage on a car, allowing them to move together, i.e. the movements are 'conjugate'. In the absence of these controlling mechanisms the eyes rove in an aimless way. If these mechanisms fail to develop, as in someone who is blind from birth, wild roving eye movements are a very obvious feature.

Three basic control mechanisms are established in the first few months of life, provided that the child has normal vision.

1. The ability to look in any desired direction until an object of interest is found. These movements occur as little flicks of the eyes, called 'saccadic movements'. They essentially supply the brain with a series of still pictures until the desired object is located. They are under voluntary control and are initiated in the frontal lobes.

2. The ability to hold the object on the same point of the retina in spite of any movement it may make. These pursuit movements of the eyes are smooth, to avoid jerky vision. They are controlled by the parieto-occipital area in close liaison with the visual cortex.

3. Ideally the eyes are held in the straight-ahead position most of the time. This is achieved by the continual adjustment of the eye position in relation to the position of the head in space, and is maintained by vestibular activity and proprioceptive information from the neck muscles integrated at brainstem and cerebellar level.

Eye movements require very rapid but small and absolutely synchronous contractions of the active muscles and, by reciprocal innervation, relaxation of those muscles resisting that movement. The muscles must then hold the new position. The rapid movement is called a saccade and the static holding phase is a tonic contraction of the same muscles.

The sudden movement is controlled by 'burst neurons' in the pons that fire at 600 cycles per second in brief bursts. The tonic or hold phase is maintained by a neural network that holds the eye in the predetermined position. The 'pause neurons' in the pons fire continuously and are inhibited during the saccade and come back into action the moment the saccade ends.

The sequence, when the eyes change position, is as follows: the pause cells are inhibited; the burst neurons discharge; a saccade occurs; and then the tonic and disinhibited pause cells hold the new position.

The various frontal, parietal, voluntary and involuntary pursuit mechanisms impinge onto these basic brainstem control mechanisms, with cerebellar and vestibular influences continually modifying the eye position, appropriate to the head position and body movement.

Pathways of Conjugate Gaze-Controlling Mechanisms

It must be stressed that many of the pathways to be discussed are only presumed to exist. None of the descending pathways can be followed beyond the general area of the pretectal region and the lateral pontine reticular formation. The approximate position of the pathways has been deduced from clinical evidence provided by lesions in the brain stem and their effects on eye movements.

Voluntary Gaze Mechanism (Fig. 7.1)

The cortical areas controlling voluntary gaze lie in the premotor strip of the fontal lobe (area 8). This area has an intimate connection with the parietal control area, which it can override at any time to change the direction of gaze. The descending pathways pass in the corona radiata through the anterior limb and genu of the internal capsule, closely associated with the corticobulbar fibres to the brainstem nuclei. From the internal capsule the fibres rotate to lie medially and dorsally in the cerebral peduncle (follow the arrows on the figure) and decussate in the upper pons and descend to the level of the sixth nerve nucleus into the paramedian pontine reticular formation.

Central mechanisms for eye movements seen from above and anteriorly

Start at circle to follow complete pathway   *Start at circle to follow complete pathway*

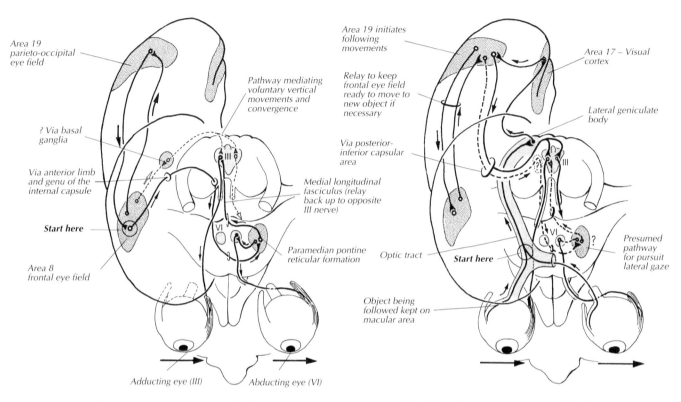

Area 19
parieto-occipital
eye field

Pathway mediating
voluntary vertical
movements and
convergence

? Via basal
ganglia

III

Via anterior limb
and genu of the
internal capsule

Start here

VI

Area 8
frontal eye field

Medial longitudinal
fasciculus (relay
back up to opposite
III nerve)

Paramedian pontine
reticular formation

Adducting eye (III)   Abducting eye (VI)

Area 19 initiates
following
movements

Area 17 – Visual
cortex

Relay to keep
frontal eye field
ready to move to
new object if
necessary

Via posterior-
inferior capsular
area

Lateral geniculate
body

III

Optic tract

VI

Start here

?

Presumed
pathway
for pursuit
lateral gaze

Object being
followed kept on
macular area

7.1   Voluntary eye movement mechanisms.   **7.2**   Pursuit eye movement mechanisms.

The adjacent sixth nerve nucleus is activated from this area and so is the opposite paired medial rectus muscle, by a very important relay, back across the midline and up to the opposite third nerve nucleus. Thus both eyes look to the left or fight simultaneously. The relay pathway is the medial longitudinal fasciculus. The fundamental importance of this tract is shown by its presence in all vertebrates. It is also the first tract to myelinate in man.

Pursuit Eye Movement Mechanism (Fig. 7.2)

The object to be followed is located by voluntary effort. The eyes 'lock in' on the object and then only move in response to movement of the object, which is kept focused on the macular part of the retina. Thus a direct relay from the visual cortex, forward to area 19, controls the movement. This area projects via corticotectal and corticotegmental fibres into the midbrain and pons, with a considerable ipsilateral component. There is also a considerable input from the vestibular nuclei and cerebellum modifying pursuit movements. This is dis-

cussed further in the next section. There is also a large forward projection that gives the frontal eye fields information as to where to direct voluntary gaze, although it is unlikely that the parietal area actively controls frontal eye field activity.

Paralysis of both voluntary saccadic gaze and pursuit gaze usually indicates damage at the subthalamic level, where both pathways come together, and is called the Roth–Bielschowsky syndrome.

Vestibular Influences on Eye Movements

These influences are best understood if we examine what happens when one lateral semicircular canal is stimulated. The lateral canal is only stimulated by forward movement of the endolymph within it (follow arrows on Figure 7.3, from the left labyrinth and see also Chapter 6). If the head is rotated sharply to the left, the fluid in the left labyrinth moves forward and stimulates the cupola. For the eyes to keep looking straight ahead – the ultimate aim of the whole process – the eyes must deviate to the right. This is controlled

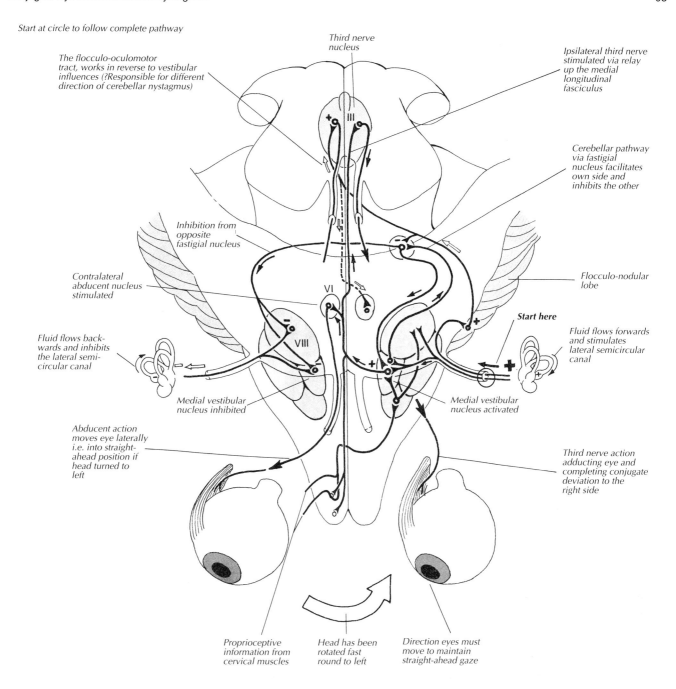

Start at circle to follow complete pathway

The flocculo-oculomotor tract, works in reverse to vestibular influences (?Responsible for different direction of cerebellar nystagmus)

Third nerve nucleus

Ipsilateral third nerve stimulated via relay up the medial longitudinal fasciculus

Cerebellar pathway via fastigial nucleus facilitates own side and inhibits the other

Inhibition from opposite fastigial nucleus

Contralateral abducent nucleus stimulated

Flocculo-nodular lobe

Fluid flows back-wards and inhibits the lateral semi-circular canal

Start here

Fluid flows forwards and stimulates lateral semicircular canal

Medial vestibular nucleus inhibited

Medial vestibular nucleus activated

Abducent action moves eye laterally i.e. into straight-ahead position if head turned to left

Third nerve action adducting eye and completing conjugate deviation to the right side

Proprioceptive information from cervical muscles

Head has been rotated fast round to left

Direction eyes must move to maintain straight-ahead gaze

7.3 Vestibular and cerebellar control.

by activity in the medial vestibular, nucleus, activated by the canal stimulation relaying across to the opposite sixth nerve, and back up the medial longitudinal fasciculus to the third nerve nucleus on the same side. Thus both eyes simultaneously move to the right.

The cerebellum plays some role through a facilitatory mechanism for the movement relayed through the fastigial nucleus of the cerebellar roof nuclei. Contributory information also comes from the proprioceptive organs of the neck via the spinovestibular tract.

Cerebellar Influence on Eye Movements

The role of the cerebellum is far from clear. In addition to the above, essentially vestibular, reflex pathway that is facilitated by cerebellar activity, there is a prominent flocculo-oculomotor tract, the only direct cerebellar connection with the eye muscle nuclei. This pathway, by its connection with the opposite third nerve, and presumably by a relay down to the sixth nerve on its own side, would tend to move the eyes in the opposite direction. Lesions in this area prevent smooth tracking and cause horizontal nystagmus with a downwards component. Experimental studies on the role of the cerebellum in eye movements have produced complex results and clinical lesions and stimulation experiments may even result in divergence of the eyes.

Whenever nystagmus is discussed cerebellar disease is always prominent in the discussion, although the mechanism of nystagmus caused by cerebellar disease is, clinically, the least understood. These pathways will be referred to in later discussion of the clinical features of nystagmus.

Horizontal Eye Movements

The main nucleus involved is the abducent nucleus. This includes those neurons that control the ipsilateral lateral rectus and those that project via the medial longitudinal fasciculus to the opposite third nerve nucleus controlling the contralateral medial rectus and activated by burst cells in the paramedian pontine reticular formation adjacent to the abducent nucleus, previously called the pontine lateral gaze centre. Vestibular influences possibly act directly on the abducent nucleus and not via the reticular formation. However, the basic neural control mechanisms for all integrated movements lie in the brainstem reticular formation and cerebellum.

Vertical Eye Movements

Vertical eye movements do not require the participation of the sixth nerve, and the controlling mechanisms lie mainly in the dorsal rostral midbrain beneath the superior and inferior colliculi.

There appears to be no actual centre for vertical gaze. The burst cells lie in the rostral interstitial nucleus of the medial longitudinal fasciculus just ventral to the aqueduct. These cells seem to be controlled by ascending influences from the pons and not by direct pathways from above.

Upward movement pathways pass through the superior colliculus, dorsal to the aqueduct to the nuclear components supplying the superior rectus and the inferior oblique. Downward movement pathways to the inferior rectus and the superior oblique pass ventrally to the appropriate nuclei. Lesions in the ventral brain stem affect down gaze. Lesions in the dorsal brain stem affect up gaze (Parinaud's syndrome). The importance of basal ganglia pathways to these movements can be deduced from some clinical observations to be discussed later.

Convergence Mechanism

The ability to converge the eyes is critical to maintaining close binocular vision. This movement utilizes both medial rectus muscles simultaneously. To do this it was theorized that a midline 'centre for convergence' existed, and this was long held to be in the nucleus of Perlia, which lies between the two third nerve nuclei. Experimental work has failed to confirm the validity of this view, and divergent squints may result from damage anywhere from the thalamus to the lateral pons or cerebellar peduncles. It is unlikely that a specific midline mechanism for convergence exists.

Clinical Disorders of Conjugate Gaze Mechanisms

In each of the controlling areas lesions that damage the pathways may cause imbalance between the two sides, by either overactivity or underactivity of the damaged area.

Lesions in the Frontal Cortex and Anterior Internal Capsule

Overactivity of the Frontal Eye Field (Fig. 7.4)

Epileptic seizures arising in the appropriate area of the frontal cortex cause what are called 'frontal adversive attacks'. In these episodes the attack commences with the head and eyes being forcibly deviated away from the side of the discharging frontal cortex. The side of the body to which the deviation has occurred may then be involved by focal motor activity, and ultimately the attack may progress to a generalized seizure.

Underactivity of the Frontal Eye Field

Damage to the frontal eye field due to vascular occlusion or following surgical removal of the frontal pole may result in the inability to look to the opposite side. This actual deficit is rarely seen, as rapid compensation occurs, and the eye movements appear to be normal within hours of the event. However, residual evidence may be found when the patient is shown to have difficulty in maintaining gaze in that direction, or with the development of nystagmus caused by this weakness when attempting to do so. If the patient is subsequently anaesthetized or becomes comatose, the eyes will deviate towards the damaged side of the cortex as the unopposed activity of the intact frontal lobe is unmasked. The unconscious patient with a frontal lesion therefore looks away from his hemiplegic side and towards the side of the lesion (Fig. 7.5).

Bilateral damage to the frontal cortex or the descending pathways in the internal capsule may lead to total loss of voluntary control over eye movements. There are several relatively rare causes of this condition.

A congenital variety exists called congenital oculomotor apraxia. The affected child has to move the whole head around to view the desired object.

**Diagrams to illustrate eye movement disorders
associated with seizures and hemiplegia**

Discharging focus in right frontal area (if area 8 included eyes look to opposite side)

Area shown would be damaged by a distal middle cerebral artery occlusion – the frontal eye field on this side is inactive

Damage to the right pons prevents the pontine centre for lateral gaze to the right from moving the eyes to the right

Right lateral pons is infarcted

Head turns to left, by action of right sternomastoid (see discussion in Chapters 6 and 11)

The intact frontal eye field on the left pushes the eye to the right

The eyes look AWAY FROM the paralysed limbs if the patient has a frontal lesion

The eyes look TO-WARDS the paralysed limbs in a patient who has a lateral pontine lesion

The intact left pontine centre moves the eye to the left

Left side progressively involved in seizure which may be of Jacksonian type

The right hemisphere damage causes a left hemiparesis (P)

The pyramidal fibres are damaged in the pons ABOVE the medullary decussation causing a left hemiparesis

extensor plantar

extensor plantar

7.4 Eye movement in frontal adversive seizures.

7.5 Eye movement with right frontal damage.

7.6 Eye movement with right pontine damage.

An acquired form of oculomotor apraxia may occur in arteriosclerotic patients who have suffered bilateral cerebral vascular accidents. If the lesions responsible are in the anterior internal capsule the loss of control of eye movements is often accompanied by other evidence of pseudobulbar palsy (see Chapter 9).

The insidious development of damage in both pathways is seen in progressive supranuclear degeneration, multisystem atrophy and Steele–Richardson–Olzewski syndrome. It may also occur as a component of Creutzfeld–Jakob disease (see Chapter 10). All these conditions are complicated by dementia.

Lesions in the Parieto-Occipital Cortex

Overactivity of the Parieto-Occipital Cortex

Seizures originating in the parieto-occipital area cause deviation of the eyes to the opposite side, but in this situation the eye movements will often be accompanied by visual hallucinations. These usually consist of flashing lights and coloured blobs. A generalized convulsion may ensue but focal motor activity, other than the eye movement, is not a feature of a focal seizure arising in the occipital lobe.

Underactivity of the Parieto-Occipital Cortex

Damage to the parieto-occipital cortex is often associated with other parietal lobe difficulties, which may make testing difficult. If a homonymous hemianopia coexists, as it often does if the lesion is a vascular one, the patient may be unable to follow the target because it keeps vanishing into their hemianopic field. In these cases it is essential to keep the object to be followed just inside the midline, in the intact half of the patient's vision, and to move it slowly. In a patient who has a dominant hemisphere lesion coexistent dysphasic difficulty may prevent them understanding the instruction to follow an object, and formal testing may prove impossible.

Optokinetic Nystagmus

The nystagmus that occurs while watching passing telegraph poles from a moving train is dependent on the integrity of the parietal fixation mechanism. Loss of this so-called optokinetic nystagmus to one side is important clinical evidence of a lesion in the opposite parietal lobe. It is tested by spinning a drum marked with vertical lines, in front of the patient, and asking them to watch the lines. The drum is then spun in the opposite direction to provoke nystagmus to both right and left. This can be voluntarily suppressed by the patient fixing their gaze beyond the drum. This can be prevented by the used of suitable lenses to prevent the patient looking beyond the drum. It is a good test for non-organic blindness. The drum is spun in front of the suspect patient's eyes; if nystagmus occurs, in the direction of rotation, vision is intact.

Optokinetic nystagmus is of major value in diagnosing vestibular disease as it remains intact in peripheral eighth nerve or vestibular end-organ disease and is impaired in central vestibular disorders and lesions of the opposite parietal cortex.

Lesions Affecting Basal Ganglia

Although the anatomical pathways that link the basal ganglia with eye movements are unknown, there is adequate clinical evidence of their importance. The posteromedial thalamus and rostral pretectum are the major areas concerned in the generation of saccadic movements for both horizontal and vertical eye movements.

Overactivity of Basal Ganglia

Uncontrolled overactivity of the basal ganglia is the cause of oculogyric crises. These attacks usually consist of a fixed deviation of the eyes in an upward direction. Lateral deviation or downward deviation occurs less frequently. Such attacks were a major feature of postencephalitic parkinsonism. In this condition compulsive thoughts or actions and a frank confusional state often coexisted with the attack. Currently the main causes are phenothiazine hypersensitivity and post head injury states. The phenothiazine drugs that have powerful antiemetic effects are the worst cuplrits and severe sustained oculogyric crisis can occur after a single postoperative dose for postanaesthetic vomiting. Young females are particularly vulnerable to this complication, and hysteria may be suspected unless this very dramatic and rare complication is recognised.

Underactivity of Basal Ganglia

Impairment of vertical gaze is quite a frequent normal finding in elderly persons. Impaired upward gaze with square-wave jerky movements is an early and frequent physical sign found in both parkinsonism and Huntington's chorea. In both diseases attempted upward gaze may cause jerky vertical nystagmus, owing to weakness of the conjugate movement.

Lesions Affecting the Collicular Area

The collicular area receives input direct from the retina via the lateral geniculate body, which clearly plays a role in visually guided pursuit eye movements. This area lies superficially in the colliculus. The deeper region is purely motor and receives input from both frontal and parietal cortical centres and feedback from the occipital cortex, and is involved in object localization and following movements.

There are several manifestations of lesions in this area. The signs are thought to be caused by pressure and distortion of underlying structures in the midbrain, and not by damage to specific pathways that traverse the colliculi. The general name for the clinical picture produced is Parinaud's syndrome. Any combination of impaired upward or downward gaze, pupillary dilatation, loss of the accommodation reflex and retraction of the eyelids may occur.

Loss of upward gaze associated with dilated pupils that are fixed to light but constrict on convergence, suggests a lesion at the level of the superior colliculus. A more dramatic sign of a lesion at this level is seen when attempts to look upwards provoke convergence–retraction nystagmus, the eyes literally appearing to be pulled back into the orbit and to jerk in and out.

Loss of downward gaze, normal pupil reactions to light and loss of convergence and therefore loss of the pupillary accommodation reaction, suggest that the lesion is slightly lower, in the area of the inferior colliculus. Progressive distortion at either level may lead to skew deviation, in which the eyes may be divergent and one elevated and one depressed. Lesions originating in the pineal gland, ranging from pinealomas, teratomas, gliomas and undifferentiated pineal tumours, may produce this clinical picture. Thalamic tumours may extend down into the area and produce similar clinical findings. Other causes are rare, but include aqueduct stenosis, encephalitis, multiple sclerosis, Wernicke's encephalopathy, neurosyphilis and tuberculoma. A similar constellation of signs may occur in children with Nieman–Pick disease, Tay–Sachs disease and maple syrup urine disease.

Lesions Affecting the Pontine Area

Pontine Gaze Palsy

Damage to the paramedian pontine reticular formation results in an inability to look to the side of the lesion. There is often a coexistent sixth nerve palsy on the same side, but the failure of the other eye to move on attempted lateral gaze clearly indicates a gaze palsy. If there is an associated hemiplegia it will be on the opposite side, as the lesion is above the pyramidal decussation. Therefore, in a patient who is unconscious owing to a unilateral brainstem lesion the eyes will deviate towards the hemiplegic side (Fig. 7.6). This situation may also be seen with basilar artery thrombosis, multiple sclerosis, pontine gliomas and Wernicke's encephalopathy. The detailed clinical picture of a lateral pontine lesion is discussed in Chapter 11.

Internuclear Opthalmoplegias (Fig. 7.7)

There are two main varieties of internuclear opthalmoplegia due to damage to the medial longitudinal fasciculus which links the eyes together, resulting in disconjugate gaze in which the eyes move independently on attempted lateral gaze.

Anterior Internuclear Opthalmoplegia (Fig. 7.7a)

Patients are seen in whom, far from there just being weakness of convergence, the eyes are actually diverged. Essentially, there is paralysis of both medial recti. This condition occurs in hypertensive haemorrhagic brainstem lesions and multiple sclerosis. The divergence may be complicated by skew deviation of the eyes, in which one eye looks up and out and the other looks down and out. This may be further dramatized by the presence of see-saw nystagmus, in which the eyes jerk up and down alternately.

Posterior Internuclear Opthalmoplegia (Fig. 7.7b)

In this classic variety the medial longitudinal fasciculus is damaged between the sixth nerve nucleus below and the opposite third nerve nucleus above, the medial rectus failing to move synchronously with the contralateral lateral rectus on attempted lateral gaze to either side. Yet when each eye is tested separately medial rectus function is evident but may be incomplete. This is tested by covering the abducting eye and watching the adducting eye continue to follow the finger, having arrested in mid-position when the abducting eye has reached it outer limit. In a typical example the abducting eye demonstrates course jerky nystagmus with little

or no nystagmus in the adducting eye. The situation reverses when the patient looks to the opposite side, a condition which used to be called 'internuclear ophthalmoplegia with ataxic nystagmus'. The mechanism of nystagmus in these cases is much disputed and no widely accepted explanation exists. The further the intact eye moves from the rest position, the more marked the nystagmus in it, suggesting that the degree of deviation alone may be critical. The majority of bilateral examples of this condition occur in multiple sclerosis, and the condition is almost pathognomonic of this disease.

In a child with neurofibromatosis a pontine glioma may be responsible for this clinical picture, because tumours do not respect the midline. Unilateral internuclear opthalmoplegia is usually caused by an occlusive vascular lesion of the paramedian area of the brain stem because the vessels are strictly unilateral and supply up to the midline (see Chapter 11). Asymmetrical internuclear opthalmoplegia can also occur in multiple sclerosis.

An important benign cause of transitory bilateral internuclear opthalmoplegia with nystagmus is a toxic level of anticonvulsant drugs, particularly diphenylhydantoin or carbamazepine.

CASE REPORT I

A 23-year-old woman presented during her third episode of multiple sclerosis with a left lower motor neuron seventh nerve palsy and complete divergence of the eyes. Three days after starting a course of ACTH the facial weakness had cleared and the eyes improved to the extent that she then had a classic internuclear ophthalmoplegia. Within a week her eye movements returned to normal. She thus demonstrated consecutively the two main varieties of internuclear ophthalmoplegia.

CASE REPORT II

A 56-year-old man had been treated with insulin shock therapy in the Middle East, during a toxic confusional state. On recovery he had diplopia on looking to the left side. When seen a year later he had a unilateral internuclear ophthalmoplegia. This presumably resulted from a vascular lesion during a variety of metabolic insults caused by fever, dehydration and hypoglycaemia.

Another eye movement disorder also seen quite frequently in multiple sclerosis is the reverse of a posterior internuclear ophthalmoplegia. On attempted lateral gaze to either side the abducting eye shows incomplete movement while the adducting eye achieves a full range. At first sight this appears to be a bilateral sixth nerve palsy, but if each eye is tested independently a near complete range of abduction can be obtained in both eyes. The mechanism of this is uncertain but a postulated site is shown in Figure 7.7c.

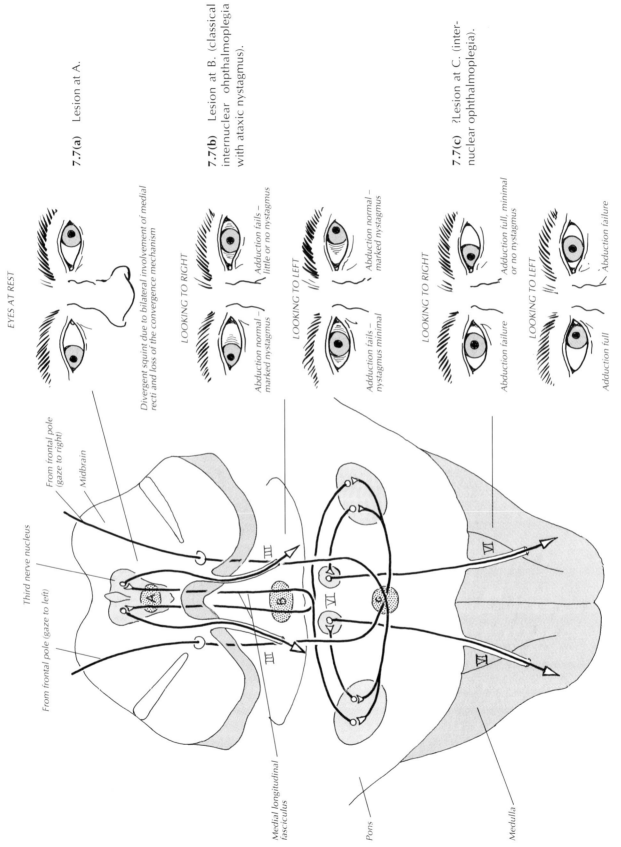

EYES AT REST

7.7(a) Lesion at A.

Divergent squint due to bilateral involvement of medial recti and loss of the convergence mechanism

7.7(b) Lesion at B. (classical internuclear ohphthalmoplegia with ataxic nystagmus).

LOOKING TO RIGHT

Adduction fails – little or no nystagmus

Abduction normal – marked nystagmus

LOOKING TO LEFT

Abduction normal – marked nystagmus

Adduction fails – nystagmus minimal

7.7(c) ?Lesion at C. (inter-nuclear ophthalmoplegia).

LOOKING TO RIGHT

Adduction full, minimal or no nystagmus

Abduction failure

LOOKING TO LEFT

Abduction failure

Adduction full

From frontal pole (gaze to right)

Midbrain

Third nerve nucleus

From frontal pole (gaze to left)

III

III

Medial longitudinal fasciculus

VI

VI

Pons

Medulla

7.7 Internuclear ophthalmoplegias.

Nystagmus

The basic pathological features common to all causes of nystagmus is that there is either weakness in maintaining the conjugate deviation of the eyes or an imbalance in the postural control of the eye movements. In either case there is a tendency for the laterally deviated eyes to drift slowly back to the central position – this is the pathological component – and to regain the original position by a fast flick. The latter is the movement that is traditionally recorded as the direction of the nystagmus.

One of the major problems for the student arises from the fact that nystagmus is defined in the direction of the fast movement, which is not the abnormal part of the process. Minor degrees of nystagmus may only be manifest on full lateral gaze to the weak side. If more severe, it may appear on the slightest deviation to the weak side. If very marked, it may also be apparent at rest as fine jerky movements of the eye from side to side. Qualitatively, it may be defined as fine or coarse, based on the amplitude of movement and horizontal, vertical or rotatory, depending on the direction of movement. The other quality, usually described as pendular, is a specific feature of ocular nystagmus and is discussed separately below.

Although at first sight the quick movement of nystagmus would appear to be a deliberate attempt by the occipitoparietal motor area to restore fixation, the movement persists even following transcollicular section of the brain stem. The activity is clearly generated in the pons. However, the occipitoparietal motor area does have significance in the physiological phenomenon of optokinetic nystagmus discussed earlier. It is the absence of optokinetic nystagmus that is pathological, and this finding points to a lesion in the pursuit gaze pathway of the opposite parieto-occipitotemporal cortex or the pathways, down to pontine level.

In vestibular and cerebellar nystagmus the optic fixation reflexes may be strong enough to inhibit the slow drift and prevent nystagmus from occurring. This can be demonstrated by electronystagmography, performed in the dark with the eyes closed and the eye movements recorded electrically from electrodes placed over the eyelids.

Since the original edition of this text was completed in 1975, there has been an explosion of knowledge of the physiology of eye movements and nystagmus, making an already complex subject even more difficult. Sadly, the clinical application of this knowledge has made little impact on diagnosis or management. Even the advent of MRI scanning has not always confirmed the presence of central lesions which have been suspected as a result of neuro-otological electro physiological abnormalities. Because of this discussion will be confined to those situations producing demonstrable abnormalities detectable at the bedside in patients who clearly have conditions causing vertigo, nystagmus, diplopia and incoordination.

Examining for Nystagmus

1. Make sure that the ambient lighting is adequate to observe the patient's eyes clearly.

2. Often the movement of a spot of light reflected in the patient's eye from an adjacent lamp or window clarifies the range and direction of any movement observed, and is sometimes more easily seen than the iris itself.

3. If the patient has ptosis or a narrow palpebral fissure, use the left hand to hold the eyes open to facilitate observation (as shown in Fig. 7.8).

4. Ask the patient to fix their gaze on your index finger, a pencil or the handle of a tendon hammer about 18 inches (0.45 m) in front of the eyes to avoid convergence.

5. Observe the patient's eyes for abnormal movements at rest. Any nystagmus in this position is called first degree nystagmus.

6. Move the object alternately to the right and left. Do not move it too quickly or even normal patients may appear to have jerky eye movements. Do not move it too far (take the iris of the inward-looking eye just to the caruncle) and then hold the position and continue to observe the eye. Jerky oscillations called nystagmoid jerks will occur if the eye is taken too fast or too far. The latter can be a particular problem in patients who have a wide palpebral fissure, where the outward-looking eye is taken further than usual. Continue to observe any movement of the eye at the correct end point (Fig. 7.9).

7. Take the eyes back to the neutral position, watching carefully for any overshoot or oscillation before the eye stabilizes at the primary position.

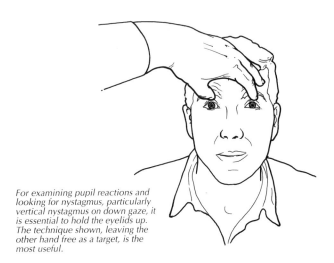

For examining pupil reactions and looking for nystagmus, particularly vertical nystagmus on down gaze, it is essential to hold the eyelids up. The technique shown, leaving the other hand free as a target, is the most useful.

7.8 Position for examining holding eyelids up.

8. Take the eyes upwards (elderly patients often have limited up gaze) and in addition to watching for lateral and vertical movement of the eyes at the end point, also for any tendency of the eyes to converge or retract, especially if the range of movement is abnormal for the age.

9. Take the eyes downwards, which is easier if the patient extends the head slightly and the examiner holds both eyelids up with the finger and thumb of left hand (Fig. 7.8). There is always a slight tendency for the eyes to converge as the examiner almost always inadvertently moves the target object slightly closer to the patient in this position.

10. Finally, once it is established that there are no abnormal eye movements, the object can be deliberately moved closer to check that convergence is

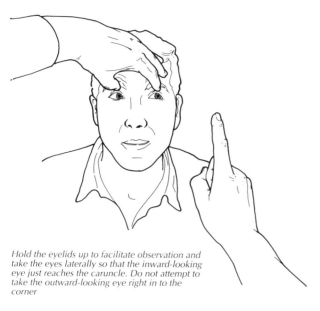

Hold the eyelids up to facilitate observation and take the eyes laterally so that the inward-looking eye just reaches the caruncle. Do not attempt to take the outward-looking eye right in to the corner

7.9   Looking for nystagmus.

normal and that the accommodation reflex is intact. This is a considerable economy of time and effort, provided that the examiner remembers to make all the appropriate observations.

11. Record the findings simply as 'EOM full without nystagmus' if entirely normal or, if abnormal, make a simple chart on a grid indicating the position, extent, direction and, if necessary, any rotatory components of the nystagmus observed. It is also worth documenting whether the patient was examined lying, half reclining or sitting upright, as this can sometimes influence the nature and severity of the nystagmus.

Rather than attempt a classification based on experimental knowledge of nystagmus, we will consider nystagmus merely in a clinical diagnostic context at the bedside.

Clinical Evaluation of Nystagmus

Diagnostic Pitfalls in Evaluating Nystagmus

Nystagmoid Jerks

These are jerky movements subsiding after two to three beats at the extremes of gaze when the examiner moves the target too far and too fast. It is not a physical sign of pathological significance.

Congenital Nystagmus

This has usually been noted since birth or in the neonatal period and is often familial with dominant inheritance. It is present in the primary position and exaggerated when the eyes move in any direction, including vertical gaze. In all positions it is side to side and of equal rate and amplitude. It is also called pendular nystagmus for this reason. Perhaps the most important feature is that the patient is usually unaware of the movement and in many cases a compensatory head movement synchronous in the opposite direction stabilizes the image. In some families the nystagmus may only appear on movement and is not present in the primary position.

CASE REPORT III

A neurological consultation was requested on an 18-year-old girl with nystagmus who had already had a full negative neurosurgical work-up (bilateral carotid angiograms and air encephalography). She demonstrated all the clinical features of congenital nystagmus. Arrangements were made to discuss this with her parents and siblings. When the neurological team were summoned to meet them, the whole family was sitting by the bed, heads and eyes wobbling in unison!

Spasmus Nutans

This rare condition of childhood includes three features in the classic form, although the picture may be incomplete in some cases. It starts between 6 months and 3 years of age and usually lasts a few weeks. The cause is unknown. The triad consists of torticollis, head nodding which is not compensatory, and pendular nystagmus in one eye. If the apparently unaffected eye is observed with a +15 or +20 diopter lens in the ophthalmoscope a shimmering movement can be detected. There are rare examples of the condition occurring in association with developmental disease of the CNS and with lesions in or around the optic chiasm. Further investigation is clearly indicated if the signs fail to subside over a few weeks as anticipated.

Monocular Nystagmus

Monocular vertical nystagmus may be seen with acquired blindness in one eye. As noted in Chapter 5, incomplete or recovering extraocular nerve lesions affecting eye movement may cause sufficient weakness to allow drift from the direction of gaze of the affected muscle, and the saccadic jerks to restore the position may mimic monocular nystagmus.

In myasthenia gravis weakness of a single eye muscle may produce nystagmus but in these cases it is often the **unaffected** paired muscle that demonstrates nystagmus. This can occasionally happen with an extraocular nerve palsy, but nystagmus in the **contralateral** eye is very typical of ocular myasthenia.

Superior oblique myokymia is another very rare condition in which for a few seconds at a time the superior oblique muscle on one side contracts rhythmically, producing a most distressing jerky diplopia with oblique separation of the images. The condition may respond to carbamazepine and may be generated in the brain stem. The condition remits and relapses and appears to be benign.

Nystagmus due to Serious Visual Abnormality

This is also known as acquired sensory nystagmus. Children with serious visual difficulty but not complete blindness develop nystagmoid movements of pendular type. This will occur with aniridia, achromatopsia, albinism, optic nerve agenesis, congenital cataracts or macular disease due to Leber's congenital amaurosis. Any child with apparent congenital nystagmus but no family history should be carefully assessed for other ocular developmental anomalies.

Adults who become blind develop nystagmoid movements, but these are not as dramatic as the random oscilations of the congenitally blind patient, in whom wild constant roving eye movements are the rule.

Nystagmus due to Vestibular Disease

Nystagmus due to disease of the vestibular apparatus or the vestibular nerve has several characteristics. It can, however, become very complicated when a lesion such as an acoustic neuroma may, in addition, to the pure nerve lesion, distort the brain stem and produce components more typical of a brain stem vestibular pathway lesion.

Peripheral Vestibular Nystagmus

- Will always be associated with vertigo, usually rotational, although somersaulting or rocking vertigo may occur in the acute phase
- A vestibular lesion usually inhibits vestibular function on that side (i.e. has the same effect as cold water in the ear)

- The sense of rotation is therefore away from the side of the lesion
- The fast phase of the resulting nystagmus will always be away from the side of the lesion whatever the direction of gaze
- The patient will past-point, stagger or fall, away from the side of the lesion
- The nystagmus and resulting giddiness can be reduced by fixing gaze and lying quite still in a neutral position
- Nausea and vomiting are prominent features of the acute phase
- Deafness or tinnitus may be associated (typical of Menière's disease or a vascular lesion of the middle ear)
- The nystagmus and vertigo settle quickly because of central adaptation to the altered vestibular input

Nystagmus due to Central Vestibular Disease

- It is usually due to distortion, tumour, infarction or inflammatory disease of the brainstem
- Onset may be acute but difficulties due to other brainstem dysfunction may dominate the symptoms, the vertigo being a milder but persistent component as central adaptation cannot occur
- The nystagmus will rarely be associated with auditory phenomena
- The nystagmus may be multidirectional and include vertical and rotary components. True vertical nystagmus is always indicative of brainstem dysfunction.
- Visual fixation has no effect on the nystagmus or vertigo, and lying still with eyes closed or open confers little benefit
- There may be accompanying fixed deviation of the eyes towards the side of the lesion, the eyes pushed in that direction by the unopposed activity of the contralateral intact vestibular nucleus

Positional Vertigo and Nystagmus

It is appropriate here to review the relationship between positional vertigo and nystagmus (see also Chapter 6). Positional vertigo is a very common and important condition. In the present context it is worth reiterating the following points to enable a clear distinction to be made between central positional vertigo, which often has a serious cause and peripheral positional vertigo, which is usually due to a benign condition.

Central Vertigo
- Occurs instantly on position change, without a latent period
- Is provoked by movement in any direction

- Does not fatigue and further movement causes another episode
- May be mild but often associated with vomiting on position change

Peripheral Vertigo

- Always has a 5–10 second latent period
- Is only provoked by movement in one direction
- Rapidly fatigues and will not recur on repeated movement
- Is very severe but brief, usually less than 20 seconds duration
- Vomiting is so unusual that the diagnosis should be reconsidered
- Is usually self-limited and settles in 6–12 weeks

Nystagmus due to Other Brainstem Causes

Nystagmus associated with internuclear opthalmoplegia has been discussed earlier in this chapter. Whether or not there is associated nystagmus and vertigo is dependent on simultaneous involvement of the vestibular nuclei or connections. The striking feature is that the nystagmus is more marked in the abducting eye.

Vertical nystagmus, the eyes moving up and down, always implies a brainstem lesion. Up-beating vertical nystagmus shows a high correlation with lesions of the cerebellar vermis, and is often seen in children with medulloblastoma. Down-beating vertical nystagmus has a very high association with lesions of the cervicomedullary region and may occur in patients with platybasia, basilar invagination and Arnold–Chiari malformation. It can also be seen with vascular, demyelinating and neoplastic lesions in the same area.

CASE REPORT IV

A 17-year-old boy presented with brief attacks of vertigo that had occurred while indulging in a peculiar modern style of dancing at a Christmas party. There were no other symptoms but down-beating vertical nystagmus was found on gaze to the left-hand side. MRI scanning revealed a tumour involving the cerebellar tonsil extending into the cisterna magna and cervicomedullary junction. This was successfully excised.

Nystagmus due to brainstem dysfunction can be caused by alcohol intoxication, abnormal metabolic states, and toxic levels of most anticonvulsants, sedatives and phenothiazine tranquilizers. These are the commonest situations in which vertical nystagmus will be encountered. Symmetrical nystagmus in all directions of gaze should always raise the suspicion of drug intoxication.

Nystagmus due to Cerebellar Disease

Whenever students are asked about their knowledge of nystagmus they always mention cerebellar disease as

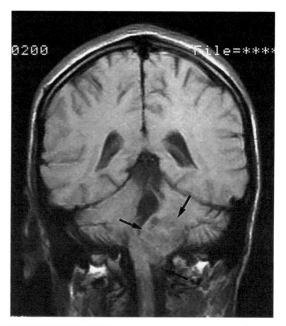

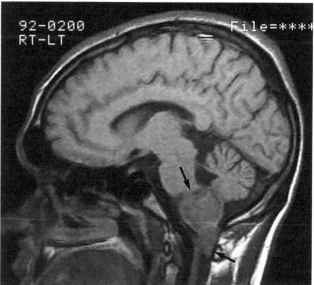

CRIV. Low-grade glioma originating in cerebellar tonsil.

an important cause. In relative terms cerebellar causes of nystagmus are uncommon. Even patients with cerebellar tumours, which classically produce nystagmus with its fast phase **towards** the side of the lesion, often have much more complex nystagmus, due to coincidental distortion of the brain stem, and pure cerebellar nystagmus is extremely rare. In the majority of patients there is no detectable nystagmus. In cerebellar degeneration and demyelinating disorders affecting the cerebellum, coexistent lesions in brainstem pathways make the extent of the cerebellar contribution difficult to evaluate.

There are a few conditions where cerebellar components are important:

1. Lesions of the cerebellar vermis cause vertical nystagmus with up-beat components.

2. Lesions of the flocculus impair smooth visual tracking and cause horizontal gaze nystagmus with a down-beat component.

3. Lesions of the nodulus may cause both down-beat and positional nystagmus.

4. Fastigial nucleus lesions cause saccadic dysmetria and may cause the square-wave jerks typical of neurodegenerative disorders of the cerebellum and the extrapyramidal system.

5. Dorsal medullary lesions and cerebellar lesions may cause periodic alternating nystagmus, which is a horizontal nystagmus that changes direction every few minutes.

With progressive cerebellar lesions three very discrete eye movement abnormalities develop in sequence:

1. Ocular dysmetria is a side-to-side oscillation of the eyes seen as they return to the primary position from lateral gaze, for a few moments before they stabilize.

2. Ocular flutter occurs when, without any attempt to move the eyes, brief bursts of oscillation of the eyes in the neutral position are observed. This is always associated with ocular dysmetria.

3. Opsoclonus (also called saccadomania) is the description given when the eyes conjugately, spontaneously and continuously oscillate in a variety of directions. This is beyond the patient's control and continues in sleep. In children this condition occurs specially in association with neuroblastoma. In adults an occult carcinoma should be excluded. It can occur as a postinfectious condition, when it is often accompanied by ataxia and myoclonus. It may be modified by steroids and if the patient recovers it proceeds to recovery through stages 2 and 1.

Voluntary Nystagmus

Voluntary nystagmus is an ability that some people have to produce brief bursts of rapid jerks of the eyes, lasting seconds only. They usually initiate the jerking with the eyes closed. It is blocked when the eyes are open, which is the reason it subsides so quickly. It is a 'party trick' without pathological significance.

The importance of testing for nystagmus correctly, and recording in detail the quality, direction and other features, is not sufficiently appreciated. The almost universal finding recorded in the neurological examination of patients – 'few nystagmoid jerks' – does not indicate great clinical acumen. On the contrary, it demonstrates poor clinical technique and a failure to distinguish this from a true physical sign.

8. The Cerebral Hemispheres: The Lobes of the Brain

Although the brain functions as an integrated unit certain areas have a major influence on specific functions, hence the search for features in the history or on clinical examination that may have localizing significance. Such evidence remains the 'gold standard' for differential diagnosis, otherwise only a somewhat unsatisfactory diagnosis that there is 'something wrong with the brain' can be advanced.

Intellectual and Behavioural Disorders

For the highest levels of intellectual functioning the entire brain must be intact. Yet quite extensive lesions in some areas may produce little or no identifiable deficit, whereas a small lesion in the dominant hemisphere may have a devastating effect on speech function and comprehension. In the presence of a cerebral neoplasm additional features such as raised intracranial pressure, cerebral oedema and brain displacement may add non-specific generalized intellectual or behavioural changes to the focal signs of the underlying lesion. For this reason, any statement by a patient's relative to the effect that a recent intellectual decline or change in personality has occurred, should be taken very seriously, even if no definite abnormality is detectable on simple testing or clinical examination. So often the patient himself is unaware of or actually denies such a change, and it is always vital to obtain reports from employers and work-mates to supplement the history given by the patient and his family.

It can be very difficult when the family contacts the doctor revealing important evidence of such problems while stating that under no circumstances must the patient ever find out that they had given such details. Short of pretending to be clairvoyant, this can be an extremely tricky situation to handle (see first case below). Memory impairment, loss of concentration, irritability, loss of motor skills or inappropriate behaviour may all mark the onset of symptoms of a cerebral lesion.

CASE REPORT I

A 58-year-old man was referred following a generalized convulsion. No focal features were observed. He had had a single-vessel bypass operation 8 months previously without complication. On examination, with the exception of slightly increased reflexes in the right arm and leg, there were no abnormal physical signs. His sense of smell was not tested. His family, unknown to the patient, had described him as having become a rather withdrawn, solitary man in recent years, who in addition to his daytime work as a personnel manager spent several hours a night editing a bridge magazine, even though they conceded that his behaviour had always been somewhat peculiar. On this basis it was decided to investigate him fully in spite of the clinical suspicion that the fit might have been related to a vascular event during cardiac surgery. An EEG revealed a few sharpened wave forms in the left frontal region. A CT scan revealed a large left frontal lesion, which at surgery was shown to arise from the olfactory groove. He subsequently revealed that he had lost his sense of smell several years previously. His postoperative course was complicated by CSF leakage through the cribriform plate, requiring surgical repair. Unfortunately his already difficult behaviour was if anything worse following surgery, and he did not manage to resume employment, although he continued his obsessional interest in the game of bridge.

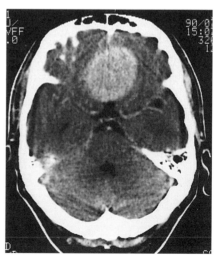

CRI. *Olfactory groove meningioma arising from floor of anterior cranial fossa.*

CASE REPORT II

A middle-aged industrial chemist, always an extrovert, became more expansive in his behaviour and one day while driving with his wife suggested that she should drive for a while. As soon as she stepped from the car to go round to the driving seat, he drove off and left her stranded. He had no explanation for this behaviour. The only physical sign was a right Babinski response. Investigation demonstrated a large meningioma overlying the left parietal area. No satisfactory explanation can be advanced for the behavioural upset but his behaviour returned to normal following the removal of the meningioma.

CASE REPORT III

The doorman at a large London hotel started greeting eminent guests at the door in a familiar manner. By lunchtime numerous complaints had been received by the manager, who found the doorman entertaining the occupants of the entrance hall to a selection of army songs. On examination he had bilateral extensor plantar responses and mild papilloedema. His behaviour until that day had been exemplary. A chest X-ray revealed a large carcinoma of the lung and subsequently multiple cerebral metastases were demonstrated by a radioisotope scan.

More specific disabilities may provide clues as to the localization of the underlying lesions.

1. Frontal lobe lesions cause striking memory impairment to the point of dementia, often coupled with marked physical inertia (see later explanation). A frequently associated feature is a deterioration in social behaviour, especially in respect of micturition. This is probably related to the location of the cortical centre for micturition in the second frontal gyrus. Urinary incontinence occurring in the early stages of the history in a patient with intellectual decline should always be regarded as indicating a frontal lesion until proven otherwise. The unusual use of bad language in inappropriate circumstances is another feature often encountered.

2. Temporal lobe disorders may also cause personality changes with memory impairment. The slow deterioration may be punctuated by episodic bizarre personality change, with sudden onset and cessation. These often turn out to be complex psychomotor seizures and may last for days at a time, with residual confusion between the more obvious attacks. The possibility of a temporal lobe disorder should be considered in any patient with sudden attacks of altered behaviour.

3. Parietal lobe lesions produce manifestations that vary depending on the patient's cerebral dominance. The majority of patients (including the majority of left-handed patients) are left hemisphere dominant.

Dominant hemisphere parietal lesions produce dysphasia, with either inability to understand commands, inability to speak or a combination of both. The evaluation of patients who are unable to communicate requires some degree of skill and time. A very common error and dangerous assumption is that poor communication is synonymous with confusion.

CASE REPORT IV

A middle-aged alcoholic woman became irrational and 'confused'. This was attributed to an amnesic syndrome and she was transferred to a mental hospital, where it was discovered that she was dysphasic. Subsequent investigation and operation disclosed a glioma in the left temporal lobe, her dominant hemisphere.

CASE REPORT V

An elderly man was taken to hospital and left by his relatives, who departed before giving any history. His was 'confused' and could give no account of himself. The neurological service was asked to see him at their leisure, with a diagnosis of 'chronic brain syndrome'. Examination revealed both receptive and motor dysphasia, a mild right hemiparesis and a slightly dilated left pupil in an extremely drowsy man. Immediate investigation revealed a massive subdural haematoma, which was successfully evacuated.

The methods available for screening patients for dysphasia will be detailed later, but the main point must be reiterated: speech difficulties can easily be mistaken for confusion by the unwary examiner.

Lesions affecting the non-dominant parietal lobe do not affect speech function but cause unusual deficits in acquired skills, such as cutting up food, dressing, getting out of the bath and geographic orientation. The complete preservation of speech function, which enables the patient to discuss the nature of his problems while being unable to explain them, is a feature of the condition, which is known as dyspraxia.

CASE REPORT VI

A man came home to find his 70-year-old wife sitting in an empty bath making repeated but ineffectual efforts to get out. She could not understand why she was having such difficulty and may have been stuck in the bath for 4 hours. After her husband had helped her from the bath she needed help to dress. There was evidence of a right hemisphere lesion on physical examination, which proved to be due to a cerebrovascular accident.

CASE REPORT VII

A 56-year-old carpenter suffered a series of attacks of paraesthesiae in the left arm during an influenzal illness. There were no definite sequelae. On the day he returned to work he took 2 1/2 hours to travel the half mile to work and was seen wandering in the wrong direction by neighbours. When he arrived at work he was unable to find his way to his bench and was unable to use his tools. He was sent home and his wife found that he had great difficulty putting on his pyjamas. No abnormality was found on angiography but a vascular lesion of the non-dominant parietal lobe was suspected (this was in 1970, before CT scanning).

Combinations of peculiar behaviour, wearing clothes back to front, inability to dress, getting lost around the house or in the street, or sudden inability to perform skilled tasks such as carpentry are all suggestive of a lesion in the non-dominant parietal lobe.

Sometimes the apparent localization based on clinical features can be misleading, as in the following case.

CASE REPORT VIII

A 55-year-old man was admitted to hospital following the acute onset of a severe headache while playing hockey. His wife reported that he had been behaving strangely for some weeks: he had arrived back from a business trip to Ireland with 20 pairs of shoes, and she found a drawer full of unopened packets of underpants that he had purchased. The final straw was when she realized that he had remortgaged the house to buy an enormous caravan, which she discovered when it was delivered to their home. There were no clear-cut physical findings and no evidence of raised intracranial pressure. A frontal lesion was suspected. He was polycythaemic but there were no other haematological or biochemical abnormalities. CT scanning revealed a large cerebellar lesion but no other lesions, and there was no evidence of hydrocephalus. Following surgery the lesion was found to be a metastatic carcinoma of the lung. There is no obvious explanation for his extraordinary behaviour, which the patient remained unable to explain before his death a year later.

Bedside Evaluation of Intellectual Function

An assessment of the patient's mental state, intelligence and specific evaluation for dysphasia should be made. Considerable information in all these spheres can be obtained while passing the time of day with the patient and during the actual history-taking. Their mood, attitude towards the disability and attitudes towards the examiner and third parties are readily detectable without specific testing.

Mental State

Formal testing of the mental state is often confined to establishing the patient's orientation for time and place. If there seems to be any uncertainty this can be taken further by asking the patient the date and day of the week, the season or details of recent weather. Anyone who has spent more than a few days in a hospital bed will know how difficult this becomes! The monotony of routine, the irrelevance of the date and the isolation from the outside world readily produces some degree of confusion about time and date in the most alert patient. More immediate questions, such as the name of the ward, the ward sister or the consultant in charge

may be more appropriate. General questions on the content of the day's newspaper, or the news on the radio, are usually much more useful, although they are at first sight less specific than the date. Nursing reports of the patient's behaviour and manner are also extremely useful in making this general evaluation. An assessment of the patient's memory for remote, recent and immediate events should be made and, wherever possible, checked with a relative. Due allowances for the patient's special interests should also be taken into consideration.

Screening Tests for Intellectual Function

Although some testing can be performed at the bedside, subtle alterations are unlikely to be detected by the occasional examiner. A series of traditional bedside tests have been formalized into a composite group called the 'mini-mental state' and this serves to make sure that several different intellectual functions have been assessed, but formal psychometric testing is essential, especially where no immediately obvious abnormalities are detected in a patient who is thought to be demonstrating altered behaviour or loss of intellectual skills.

One of the traditional tests is the 100 minus 7 test, where the patient is asked to subtract 7 from 100, and then 7 from the product and so on. For full interpretation both the accuracy and the time taken are important. This test is badly affected by anxiety and to base the whole assessment on it would be entirely inappropriate. A less demanding but similar test is to ask the patient to count forwards and backwards to and from 20.

Another traditional test is the ability to learn a lengthy sentence. Both perseveration of errors and the time taken to learn the complete the sentence give useful information. The traditional test sentence (which anyone who has trained at the National Hospital for Nervous Diseases should definitely know by heart!) is:

'There is one thing that a nation must have to be rich and great, and that is a large, secure supply of wood.'

Most patients can learn this sentence accurately in three to five attempts. However, the test is subject to all the problems of anxiety, speech difficulty and memory disturbance. The results are not specific for any condition.

Other tests of memory and concentration consist of asking the patient to learn a sequence of numbers forwards and backwards. Normally patients can learn seven numbers forwards and five backwards. As an ongoing test of both short- and long-term memory, the patient can be asked to memorize a six-figure telephone number or an address immediately and again 10 minutes later, and finally after completing all the other tests.

Explaining the meaning of proverbs and general knowledge tests, the names of public figures, names of countries and their capitals can be very difficult, as the general interests of the patient will influence their performance.

A dysphasic patient unable to name any simple objects or describe the meaning of simple words such as brunette was asked the meaning of 'piscatorial'; his face lit up and he answered in a flash 'appertaining to a fish'. Needless to say, he was a keen fisherman.

Screening Tests for Dysphasia

Formal dysphasia testing is best left until one has a clear idea as to how confused or disorientated a patient is, yet it is important to be certain that the patient has full comprehension of the spoken word and is capable of making a well-informed, appropriate answer to a question **before** taking the case history. It is essential that the patient is not distressed by testing and it is best not to pursue any difficulty for too long, and certainly not in front of an audience.

First establish that the patient can understand the spoken word by testing his ability to close his eyes, stick out his tongue and show either his right or his left hand to command. A severely confused demented or dysphasic patient may stick out his tongue at the first command and may continue to stick it out on every subsequent command. This may represent perseveration or may be the only motor act that the patient can understand or be persuaded to perform.

If the patient cannot understand spoken commands he may be able to read them. The same simple responses should be requested in writing, i.e. 'put out your tongue' etc., showing the command to the patient on a card.

The patient's spoken answers, if any, should be recorded. Patients with nominal aphasia (difficulty in naming objects) have a remarkably good command of language but the sentences lack nouns. To avoid this problem they will use alternatives. A patient who was asked to name his wedding ring, pointed to his wife and said, 'I've been with her a long time'; another, when asked to name his glasses, called them 'looks'.

A very interesting and common observation in this situation is that the patient who is quite unable to name his glasses when they are handed to him, a few moments later when asked to put his glasses on, will reach out without hesitation and pick them up! Similarly, many patients, when asked the time, will look at their watch but are quite unable to name it, or indeed tell the time.

The patient may be able to express himself better in writing and should be asked to write his name and address and a simple sentence to dictation.

Object-naming is a very simple test and is perhaps the most useful at the bedside. Usually the patient's ability to name their watch and its various components, identify a pen and its clip, or objects such as fruit on the bedside locker or the buttons on their pyjamas, is tested. If they fail, it can be most distressing for the patient, and bystanders should not be allowed to listen to or show amusement at their difficulties.

The patient should attempt to read and paraphrase a passage from a book or newspaper to test their ability to both read and understand what they are reading. Some patients may sit all day holding a book upside down, conveying the incorrect impression of thoughtful reading, only formal testing reveals the severity of the problem.

Abnormalities in the performance of these tests indicates impairment of understanding the written or spoken word, and implies dysphasia and therefore damage to their dominant parietal lobe. In almost all instances this will be the left hemisphere. Only one left-handed patient in 10 is actually right hemisphere dominant. Once dysphasic difficulty has been detected the site of damage is localized to the dominant hemisphere, and it is unlikely that further useful localizing information can be obtained by more exhaustive testing.

Screening Tests for Dyspraxia

Dyspraxia is the difficulty produced by damage in the non-dominant parietal lobe, usually the right hemisphere. The presenting history may include examples of loss of acquired skills, such as difficulty in simple household tasks or in the workplace. Everyday activities normally performed without thought, such as removing clothes, opening a book, closing a newspaper, lighting a cigarette or putting a cup back on to a saucer, may suddenly present great difficulty. A clue to this difficulty is often seen in the total disorganization of the patient's bedside locker and objects scattered around their bed.

Allowances for any motor deficits or ataxia should obviously be made but in many cases these functions are normal, making the considerable difficulty that the patient has with apparently simple actions even more dramatic.

Constructional tests using either matchsticks to copy simple figures, or drawing a clock face, a man or a bicycle from memory, all fall into the same category. Drawing a clock face, in particular, may demonstrate left-sided neglect, which is a common feature of non-dominant parietal lesions, with the numbers 1–12, all crammed into the right half of the circle.

At a higher level of testing the patient's ability to draw a plan of the ward or of an area of his home can be tested. A taxi driver performed well on all tests until asked to sketch a plan of Trafalgar Square – this explained his main complaint of difficulty in doing his job!

One of the most striking dyspraxic difficulties is dressing apraxia, where the patient may be quite unable to sort out and put on their clothing. One patient even demonstrated left-sided neglect in association with this problem. He appeared from behind his screens wearing only the right trouser leg tied round the top of his right thigh, the left trouser leg dangling free, and his right arm inserted into the left sleeve of his jacket, which was worn back to front! Even in the days before scanning, an accurate localizing diagnosis was possible faced with this amazing picture. The patient had a right parietal tumour.

As with dysphasia, the demonstration of dyspraxia in one sphere of activity provides accurate localizing information and always indicates a lesion in the non-dominant parietal lobe.

In summary, patients may appear to be confused owing to general depression of intellectual function, which may vary with the conscious level. This may be because of dysphasic problems, producing difficulty in both understanding and communicating verbally. Alternatively they may have problems in the performance of simple tasks due to dyspraxia. Distinction between these various possibilities is vital. Dysphasia or dyspraxia indicates a focal abnormality in the dominant and non-dominant hemispheres respectively, whereas confusion may indicate an altered level of consciousness, an infective disorder, multiple lesions, or metabolic disorder affecting the whole brain. The latter requires an entirely different approach to further investigation and management. Currently, in such cases, the relative ease with which CT scans can be obtained has tended to lead to scanning first and thinking later when no focal lesion has been demonstrated.

Motor and Sensory Evaluation in Hemisphere Disease

Because physical examination for motor and sensory abnormalities in patients with cerebral disorders can be so critical and difficult, the correct method of examination will be discussed in detail in the following sections and will be presumed to have been understood in all the following chapters.

Motor Disorders in Hemisphere Disease

For normal motor function the patient must have intact sensory feedback and cerebellar input to control his limbs. Patients often say that they are 'unsteady' or 'numb' when they actually mean 'weak'. If these descriptive terms are taken at face value an entirely incorrect view of their disability will be obtained. It is essential to ask the patient to elaborate on these terms

in the same way as they should be asked to elaborate on the term 'blackout'.

Preliminary testing is best performed by asking the patient to hold the arms outstretched. This is a very useful test for screening and should be evaluated systematically.

1. Observe the outstretched hands. Are there any abnormalities of the hands themselves, such as finger clubbing; do the hands shake? does one arm have difficulty in maintaining its position? If one arm drifts down, that arm is likely to be found to be weak on further testing.

2. Can the patient play the piano in mid air quickly and rhythmically? If not, the less efficient hand may be affected by a mild pyramidal lesion. In a right-handed patient these movements are always slightly better performed with the right hand.

3. The patient is then asked to close their eyes. When the eyes are closed do the hands remain level; does one arm rise up or oscillate, which may indicate cerebellar disease; does one arm fall away, which may indicate defective sensory feedback or frank weakness? The latter should already have been excluded, when the arms were outstretched with the eyes **open**.

If the patient is drowsy or will not move his limbs to command because of dysphasic difficulty, spontaneous movements of the limbs should be observed. If the examiner pinches the skin on the patient's anterior chest wall, the patient will invariably use his best arm to pull the examiner's hand away. If the good arm is then held down while the test is repeated the affected limb will move if it is able to do so. The legs may be tested by painful stimuli to each leg in turn, which may be achieved by pinching the skin or pricking the foot. While performing these tests, the gross sensory function of the two sides can also be assessed.

Evaluation of Motor Function in the Presence of a Hemisphere Lesion

Gross defects of motor function in the semiconscious patient have been considered above. In most instances one is looking for a very subtle deficit and the secret of evaluation lies in knowing how and where to look for minor motor disability.

The Face

The problem of the asymmetrical face and the frequent assertion that this represents a mild upper motor neuron lesion was discussed in Chapter 6. Upper motor neuron facial weakness as encountered in patients with hemisphere lesions presents further difficulty.

There are two types of facial movement, voluntary facial grimacing and smiling, and involuntary grimacing and smiling as a true emotional response. The former function is probably mediated through classic motor pathways from the motor strip and the emotional responses through supplementary motor areas lying deep in the insula and temporal lobes. The facial movements should be carefully observed during history-taking and spontaneous smiles provoked and carefully observed. Then a forced smile should be tested and the patient's ability to show the teeth, with the almost inevitable patient response 'they are false'.

Quite obvious facial weakness on one test may be coupled with normality of the other. The type of weakness noted may have localizing significance. If weakness is only apparent during emotional changes of facial expression it is likely to be due to a lesion in the temporal lobe. It should be recalled that the weakness will be maximal around the mouth. Eye closure may be very mildly affected and forehead wrinkling is usually spared (see Chapter 6).

The Limbs

When testing limb function we are looking for evidence of tone change and "pyramidal weakness". This concept is vital for accurate diagnosis, and yet is surprisingly neglected in most textbooks and teaching, as indicated by the number of doctors who test limb power by assessing the hand grips and the strength of the quadriceps muscles. These are the two movements least likely to be affected by pyramidal pathway disease!

Tone

Tone is best tested in the arms by holding the patient's hand as if shaking hands and gently rotating the forearm and flexing and extending the wrist, and then the elbow. If tone is increased the limb will be felt to suddenly stiffen and resist further movement. This will be most marked when pulling against the biceps, the wrist flexors and the finger flexors. If the examiner suddenly pulls and maintains firm pressure against any of the stiff muscles, clonus may be elicited. Clonus is the rhythmic contraction and relaxation of a stretched muscle. In the arm this is most easily detected on attempts to externally rotate the forearm or extend the wrist.

In the leg tone is tested by holding the patient's knee between both hands and gently rotating the hip. When the limb is rolling freely, suddenly lift the knee off the bed. In the normal situation, the knee will bend and the heel will never leave the bed. If the leg is even slightly spastic, the whole leg will fly up. Minor abnormalities can be confirmed by comparing with the opposite limb.

If the upper leg is thought to be spastic, patella clonus may be present. This is tested by holding the patella at its upper margin with the thumb and index finger and, with the leg lying flat on the bed, pushing down sharply on the patella towards the foot and **maintaining** the downward pressure. If there is patella clonus the patella will jerk up and down rhythmically as long as pressure is maintained.

At the ankle, the classic test for clonus can be applied. With the knee slightly bent the foot is sharply dorsiflexed, pressing against the ball of the foot. The oscillations will continue as long as this pressure is maintained.

Reflex Responses

In the presence of cerebral disease we are looking for enhanced reflexes. It is important that the reflexes are elicited with the limbs in exactly the same position if side-to-side comparisons are to be made. The upper limbs are best tested by flexing the arm at the elbow and laying the forearm across the patient's chest. Each limb will have to be tested separately, but this position makes it particularly easy to see the responses and to strike the triceps tendon accurately.

The supinator, biceps and triceps jerk should be elicited routinely. All these reflexes will be enhanced on the affected side. The pectoralis jerk should be included (elicited by placing the hand on the pectoralis towards its insertion on the arm and striking the back of the fingers firmly with the patella hammer). The muscle will be felt to contract and the shoulder will jerk forwards.

The finger jerk should also be enhanced in this situation (elicit by the examiner holding the patient's half-flexed fingers with his own, which are then tapped with the tendon hammer). The patient's fingers will be felt to jerk, and if the free thumb is observed this will be seen to flex at the same time. If the finger jerk is pathologically enhanced it may be possible to elicit the Hoffman reflex. With the patient's hand in a relaxed semiflexed position, the terminal phalanx of the patient's middle finger should be flexed with the examiner's thumb and then suddenly released. This allows the phalanx to suddenly extend. As it does so, the terminal phalanx of the thumb will be seen to flex.

It should be stressed that all the reflexes discussed above are normally present: it is only asymmetrical enhancement (or absence) that constitutes an abnormal finding. In a very anxious patient generalized enhancement of the reflexes is not necessarily pathological. The reflexes are arbitrarily documented as '+', '++' or '+++', the latter indicating marked enhancement and '+' the normal state. Where the reflexes are rated '+++', tone should be increased and clonus easily elicited. The legs are discussed in chapter 13.

Weakness

The distribution of weakness is best remembered by recalling the typical posture and gait of a patient recovering from a stroke. The arm is flexed (the flexor group of muscles being strong) and the leg extended (the extensors being strong). Functionally this is ideal; if the situation were reversed few patients would ever regain the ability to walk after a stroke. From this posture it can easily be deduced that in the arm the weak groups will be those controlling shoulder abduction, elbow extension, wrist extension and finger abduction. The intact but spastic groups will adduct the arm to the side of the body and flex the arm at the elbow and wrist.

In the leg, the weak groups will be the hip flexors, the hamstrings and the dorsiflexors of the foot. The strong spastic muscles are the glutei and quadriceps, which hold the hip and knee stiff, and the plantar flexors which keep the foot slightly flexed, causing it to scrape along the ground as the patient walks. This pattern of weakness indicates damage to pyramidal pathways. This may be in the main motor pathways at capsular level, the corticospinal tracts in the brain stem or the spinal cord pathways. This residual pattern of muscle strength is maintained by non-pyramidal pathways and is **entirely** dependent on normal cortical function in the appropriate area.

If the whole area of **cortex** supplying a limb is damaged the extrapyramidal pathways are unable to take over and an acute global flaccid weakness of the limb occurs, which at first may be associated with depressed or absent reflexes and no clear plantar response. Later, the reflexes return and the plantar response becomes extensor but flaccid paralysis remains. This explains why a patient with a small infarction in the left internal capsule has a good prognosis for recovery, because non-pyramidal mechanisms are able to take over, whereas if the left middle cerebral artery is occluded with infarction of the overlying cortex, the prognosis for recovery is poor and the patient has the added problem of dysphasia due to the damage to the speech cortex. This is amplified further in the next chapter.

Motor evaluation should answer the following questions:

1. Is there any facial weakness, either voluntary or emotional?
2. Is there any fall away of the outstretched hands?
3. Is there any disparity between piano-playing movements of the hands or toe wiggling, the equivalent test in the feet?
4. Is there any tone increase on the affected side?
5. Is there any reflex asymmetry (brisker on the affected side) or an extensor plantar response?

6. Is there weakness in a pyramidal distribution, bearing in mind that more powerful proximal movements such as shoulder abduction or hip flexion may be demonstrably weak when the only peripheral signs are impaired fine movements?

Sensory Disorders in Hemisphere Disease

Damage to the sensory cortex may cause rather modest sensory symptoms on the opposite side of the body, the most dramatic of which is sensory epilepsy. This usually consists of episodes of tingling, progressing to post-ictal numbness. It is very unusual for focal pain to be produced although it can happen. Owing to a considerable motor representation in the sensory cortical area the sensory symptoms are often associated with some twitching of the same limb or limbs. Surprisingly often focal motor epilepsy is found to have its origin in the sensory strip, with minimal sensory phenomena. Any sensory symptoms should be strictly unilateral.

Even with full knowledge of these peculiarities, some clinical situations can present impossible diagnostic problems.

CASE REPORT IX

A 45-year-old woman was referred with a 2-year history of sensory disturbance affecting the right leg. This had started while using a proprietary slimming machine, which massaged the back via an electrically driven belt. During the procedure she had had a sudden sensation as if someone had snapped two cheese-cutting wires up the back of both legs. The symptoms then became more marked on the right, with a mixture of numbness, tingling, clumsiness and weakness of the right leg, which slowly progressed over 2 years. At night she suffered attacks of tingling and spasm in the right leg, which in a letter written at that time were noted as 'almost convulsive in type'. Physical examination then revealed bilateral brisk reflexes and unsustained clonus in both legs, a left extensor plantar but no response on the right because of a profound spinothalamic deficit extending to T9. The picture was highly suggestive of multiple sclerosis, but over the next few months all the then available investigations (VERs, myelogram and CSF IgG) were negative, although there was a slight response to course of steroids. Six months later, while pushing a supermarket trolley, she suffered five attacks of what sounded like uncontrolled clonus down the right side and two similar episodes while lying in bed, which ceased the moment she straightened her back. The motor signs were still bilateral but the sensory loss was confined to the right side below T9. Six months later there was no change but she had noticed that she would occasionally develop a tingling sensation in the right leg, which could be immediately relieved by extending her neck, seeming to add further support to the diagnosis of demyelinating disease. Matters came to a head 3 months later when, following a 1 hour shuttle flight during which she had been forced to sit with her head angled forwards, she tried to stand up and both legs had become paralysed.

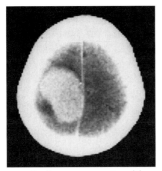

CRIX. *Surface meningioma presenting like remitting multiple sclerosis. (note: in this old scan the lesion is on the left side. Early scans were viewed from above).*

It was 90 minutes before she could stand and walk without assistance. At the same time she noticed that her face had become tingly and numb, placing the lesion, if there were one, above cervical level, A CT scan was performed and revealed an enormous left-sided parasagittal meningioma, which was successfully removed with complete resolution of her symptoms.

This extraordinary case demonstrates a completely misleading spinothalamic sensory deficit with an apparent spinal level which was ultimately shown to be due to a cortical lesion. This, when coupled with bilateral pyramidal signs in the legs, and in the total absence of any symptoms suggesting intracranial pathology, explains the diagnostic delay, but a great many of the features of this case remain inexplicable.

A similar case with rather more immediate clarification of the true situation follows.

CASE REPORT X

A 70-year-old man complained of severe low back pain and pain radiating down the entire right leg. He had already had a normal myelogram. When re-examined by his orthopaedic surgeon brisk reflexes and an extensor plantar response were found in the right leg. He was referred urgently and when seen the next day he had become densely hemiplegic and semiconscious overnight. A large metastatic deposit in the leg area of the sensory strip was found. It seems likely that his early symptoms can be regarded as a form of sensory epilepsy.

An example of longstanding sensory epilepsy which escaped identification for 23 years until a major epileptic fit occurred, represents the other end of the spectrum of possible presentations of sensory cortical lesions.

CASE REPORT XI

A 42-year-old engineer had suffered from attacks of tingling and numbness of the left hand, extending to the left side of the chest and head, since the age of 19. As these episodes often occurred at mealtimes they had long been ascribed to 'indigestion'! Three weeks before admission he suffered two major epileptic fits, each beginning with these sensory symp-

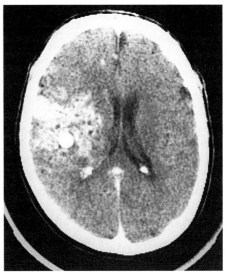

CRXI. *Right-sided arteriovenous malformation presenting as epilepsy with lifelong bruit.*

toms but progressing to focal jerking of the arm and face and then loss of consciousness. A loud bruit was heard over the entire right side of the head, and angiography revealed an angioma occupying the bulk of the right hemisphere. The patient had been aware of the bruit all his life and had therefore assumed that it was normal. Twelve years later he developed a progressive left hemiparesis, and a CT scan and angiography suggested severe intracranial steal syndrome. An attempt to ablate the massive angioma was made surgically, but the patient unfortunately suffered severe damage to the hemisphere during surgery and has required full-time nursing care ever since.

The sensory loss caused by a superficial lesion is rarely complete. In fact, total loss of all sensory modalities down one side of the body is extremely unusual, and should raise doubts as to the organicity of the findings. Due to bilateral cortical projections and some sensory appreciation of poorly localized touch, pain and vibration at thalamic level, these sensations may be relatively spared. The modalities that are specifically affected by a cortical lesion are accurate localization of touch, two-point discrimination, joint position sense and temperature appreciation. Other popular modalities, such as the recognition of numbers scratched on the skin and stereognosis (recognition of an object placed in the hand), are really composite sensory functions requiring all modalities to be intact, and are not specific forms of sensation, but because they depend especially on those sensations appreciated at cortical level they will be very severely impaired by a cortical lesion. A useful screening test is to ask the patient to compare the textures of bed covering, but this is subject to the same objection of relative non-specificity. If unilateral, abnormalities of these tests suggest diffuse damage to the sensory cortex. If the findings are bilateral, spinal cord or peripheral nerve disease must be suspected.

To detect very minimal dysfunction the test for sensory extinction is used. The theoretical basis of the test is probably the same as that for extinction hemianopia, illustrated in Figure 3.3. The patient is lightly touched on either limb and occasionally simultaneously on both limbs with the eyes closed. The ability to recognize a light touch on one limb, but failure to detect the same touch when both limbs are touched at the same moment and in the same location, is called sensory extinction and has the same significance as cortical sensory loss.

If the lesion lies deep in the hemisphere at thalamic level or in the subthalamic area, more dramatic sensory loss will be found. In the early stages of a progressive lesion, or in the recovering stages of a vascular lesion that has damaged the sensory pathways at thalamic level, extremely unpleasant, deep, poorly localized pain with a scalding or burning quality down the opposite side of the body may occur. These sensations may occur spontaneously or be provoked by any stimulus to the affected side of the body. This is called the Dejerine–Roussy syndrome and is discussed further in the next chapter.

CASE REPORT XII

A 52-year-old woman presented with a 2-month history of difficulties affecting the right side. This had started as a tingling in the right hand and simultaneous numbness of the right big toe. At the same time she became aware that the right leg was clumsy. Over the following 6 weeks the entire right side became numb, and yet hypersensitive to touch. For 4 weeks she had noticed increasing weakness of the right arm and right leg. She had had a slight left-sided headache throughout. She had had a left mastectomy 7 years previously for carcinoma of the breast. Examination revealed a hemiplegic gait, with minimal weakness on formal testing and flexor plantar responses. There was severe impairment of all sensory modalities on the entire right side of the body. Investigation and craniotomy revealed a large necrotic metastasis in the posterior part of the left thalamus.

This is a typical example of the history of a thalamic lesion and a good example of the type of sensory deficit to be found in such cases. Another case report is included at this point to emphasize the quality of sensory pathway damage in the brain. The patient had a lesion in the brainstem but presented with such typical symptoms they are worth documenting here for emphasis.

CASE REPORT XIII

A 70-year-old woman presented with a 3-week history. On an extremely cold day she developed a sensation over the left side of the head as if she were being tickled by hairs. Later the same day she noticed that the left hand felt tingly and numb, although there was no motor dysfunction. On several occasions the left leg had felt transiently numb, during which time it had dragged. Physical examination revealed no motor

signs but she was totally unable to detect the difference between a sharp and a blunt object, or cold sensation down the entire left side, and even a 3 inch separation of two points in the left hand was not detected in spite of normal touch sensation and her ability to detect two points at 5 mm on the unaffected side. These symptoms had progressed over 3 weeks and an MRI scan revealed a ring-enhanced lesion in the dorsal aspect of the right cerebral peduncle. Two similar lesions were visible in the right hemisphere at the vertex. There was no known primary lesion and the patient elected not to undergo further investigation or treatment. Her symptoms rapidly progressed until she died 10 weeks later.

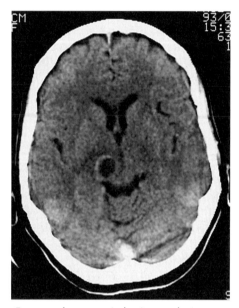

CRXIII.   *Presumed metastatic brainstem lesion presenting as pure sensory syndrome.*

Evaluation of Sensory Function in the Presence of a Hemisphere Lesion

Light Touch Sensation

Traditionally a wisp of cotton wool is used to test light touch sensation. A mere touch with a fingertip is just as effective and can be very accurately repeated from side to side, and this is the ideal method when testing for sensory extinction as described above. It would be very unusual for light touch to be affected with a hemisphere lesion.

Pain Sensation

Pain sensation used to be tested with a pin or needle carried in the examiner's lapel. This practice was to be deprecated, even before the advent of AIDS. It is now standard practice to use either disposable pins in plastic mounts or any of the highly effective disposable, sharpened, plastic instruments now available. It is essential to be sure that it is the painful sensation that is appreciated and not just the touch. This particular point will be enlarged on later when discussing spinal cord disease, but it should be mentioned here that one of the classic errors in sensory diagnosis is to regard the patient's answer that they can feel the pin, as indicating that pain sensation is intact. They **must** be aware that the sensation is painful.

Pain sensation is unlikely to be significantly affected in cerebral disease, but altered perception where pain assumes an increasingly unpleasant or bizarre quality may well be found. In this situation a single prick may feel like a bunch of needles and a dragged pin may produce a sensation as if the skin were being slashed with a scalpel. It is important to ask the patient to identify qualitative differences in the sensation by comparing the two sides when pain sensation is being tested.

Two-Point Discrimination

Two-point discrimination can only be tested when the patient has already been shown to appreciate and localize a single light touch accurately. Clearly there is no point in performing the test otherwise. The test is only reliable at the fingertips. The average female should be able to detect 3–5 mm separation and males (especially manual workers) 5–8 mm separation. Although it is stated that appreciation of greater than 4 cm separation on the legs is abnormal the figure varies so widely that the test must be regarded as unreliable in the lower limbs.

Joint Position Sense

Joint position sense can be accurately tested in both the hands and the feet. The distal interphalangeal joint should be steadied by holding each side of the joint, and the distal phalanx moved up and down by holding the

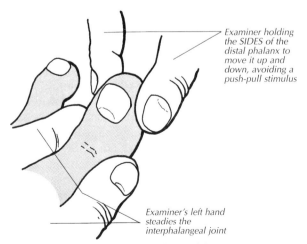

Examiner holding the SIDES of the distal phalanx to move it up and down, avoiding a push-pull stimulus

Examiner's left hand steadies the interphalangeal joint

8.1   Correct way to test joint position sense.

sides of the finger or toe (Fig. 8.1). If the pulp and nail are held the 'push–pull' stimulus will modify the results.

Always start with the patient watching the toe or finger so that they understand what is required. They may then close their eyes for formal testing once they understand what they must do.

In the fingers, deflections of 2–3 mm should be easily detectable and become easier the further from the mid-position the phalanx is moved. Patients also sense extension movements more than flexion movements, as there is more resistance to extension and the pull on the tendons adds to the sensation. The same is true in the toes, where movements of 3–5 mm should normally be detected. In both the upper and lower limbs, the ability of the patient to detect the neutral position with the eyes closed is a very striking confirmation of normal function.

Patients with marked spasticity in the arm or leg may demonstrate the effect of pulling on the tendons very dramatically, sensing only upward movements in the finger and toe as the phalanx is moved against the spastic muscle. Flexion movements of the fingers and toes may not be detected at all.

Joint position sense is very dramatically affected by a lesion in the sensory cortex and the patient may be unable to sense even movements at the wrist and ankle. Joint position sense should be specifically and carefully tested in all patients with suspected cerebral disease.

Vibration Sense

Vibration sense is tested with a 128 Hz tuning fork applied to various bony prominences on the limbs and trunk. It is a test of dubious clinical value as vibration is not a specific modality carried in a specific pathway. The sensation probably travels in both dorsal columns and spinothalamic pathways and is appreciated bilaterally at thalamic level. In hemisphere lesions vibration sense will only be lost in association with dense loss of other modalities due to a lesion in the region of the thalamus. The value of vibration sense in the diagnosis of peripheral nerve and spinal cord lesions will be discussed in a later chapter.

Temperature Sensation

Temperature sensation need rarely be tested routinely. With cortical lesions the loss is usually identical to the pain sensation loss. Temperature sense loss is never found in isolation. The correct method of testing is fully detailed in Chapter 13 in situations where it has greater clinical significance.

Routine sensory testing when screening a patient with a suspected hemisphere lesion should include the following:

1. Light touch is tested on both sides and extinction testing performed as described.

2. Joint position sense is tested on both sides.

3. Pain appreciation is evaluated on both sides. Remember that a qualitative difference in pain appreciation can be as important as actual loss of pain sensation.

4. Two point discrimination is tested in both hands.

If these simple tests are normal further testing is unlikely to add further diagnostic information.

Clinical Disorders of the Lobes of the Brain

The Frontal Lobes (Fig. 8.2)

The frontal lobes include all the hemisphere anterior to the Rolandic fissure. They extend much further posteriorly than is generally appreciated. The surface marking of their posterior extent is at the vertex. The two lobes are interconnected in the midline by the corpus callosum, which unfortunately provides a route for easy spread of frontal lobe tumours across the midline in a 'butterfly' distribution.

The areas of major clinical importance are the motor strip (area 4), the supplementary motor area (area 6), the frontal eye fields (area 8), the cortical centre for micturition (the medial surface of the frontal lobe) and the important connections with the temporal lobe, parietal lobe, basal ganglia, hypothalamus and cerebellum. In addition, in the dominant hemisphere the frontal lobe includes Broca's speech area. This area controls the motor mechanisms concerned with articulation. The olfactory bulb and tract and the optic nerve lie immediately under the lobe.

Clinical Features of Frontal Lobe Damage

Personality Change

The frontal lobes play a major role in personality, particularly in respect of acquired social behaviour. Patients with frontal lobe lesions will often present with personality disorders. Loss of drive, apathy, decreasing concern about personal appearance, personal hygiene, family affairs or business all occur and what is best described as an apathetic dementia results. In some cases

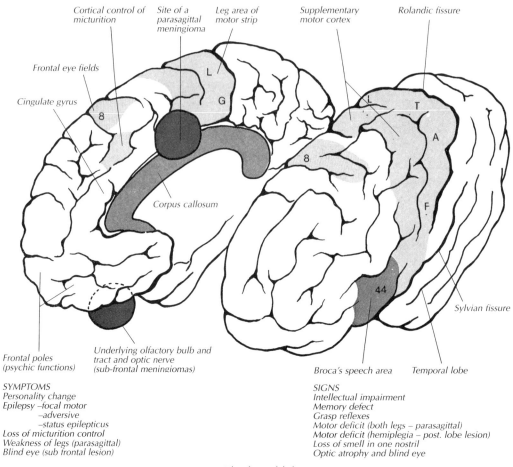

SYMPTOMS
Personality change
Epilepsy –focal motor
             –adversive
             –status epilepticus
Loss of micturition control
Weakness of legs (parasagittal)
Blind eye (sub frontal lesion)

SIGNS
Intellectual impairment
Memory defect
Grasp reflexes
Motor deficit (both legs – parasagittal)
Motor deficit (hemiplegia – post. lobe lesion)
Loss of smell in one nostril
Optic atrophy and blind eye

8.2   The frontal lobes.

increasing disinhibition causes trouble. This may well include urinating in public, inappropriate bad language and antisocial behaviour without concern for the effect on others. The frontal lobes also play a major role in information processing and a severe decline in intellect is often coupled with memory impairment until obvious dementia occurs. In any demented patient where there is a history of personality change or micturition problems before the dementia becomes established, urgent consideration should be given to the possibility of a frontal lobe tumour. Patients with parasagittal lesions are particularly likely to present in this way.

CASE REPORT XIV

A 60-year-old woman had been behaving somewhat peculiarly for nearly 5 years. The earliest symptom was apparent while driving, when passengers noticed that she always drove in and out of bus stop bays, to the alarm of the people waiting at the bus stop. Her business acumen declined and she was unable to cope with the introduction of the new value added tax. On one occasion, while driving in the country she apparently got out of her car to pass water behind a tree, and afterwards could not find her car, which was later returned to her by the police, having been found parked in the middle of the road astride a double white line. Surprisingly, no action was taken in spite of her lack of explanation for this extraordinary event. Her son in Canada complained that her air-letters were difficult to read because when he tore off the edges part of the letter went with it. The next letter arrived apparently empty, until he steamed it open and found that she had only written on the glued sections! At that point he came to England to see what was going on. He found her extremely peculiar in affect and slightly hypomanic, but there were no definite neurological signs. Investigation demonstrated a large right subfrontal meningioma. Following operation, it was clear that she had no memory for events of the previous 5 years. She remained a somewhat eccentric woman.

The particular type of micturition disturbance associated with a frontal lobe lesion is an abrupt awareness that the bladder is full coupled with the inability to prevent it from emptying immediately i.e. the patient loses the ability to inhibit the micturition reflex. As personality changes ensue this causes less and less concern to the patient.

CASE REPORT XV

A 56-year-old woman became increasingly uninterested in her household duties and incontinent of urine. However, it was not until she voided on her husband's prize roses that he sought advice on her account. When she was originally seen in the outpatients clinic, the registrar placed her on the inpatient waiting list, to come in for investigation of Parkinson's disease. On admission, the picture was that of an apathetic dementia with generalized rigidity and bradykinesia, but there was no tremor or cogwheel rigidity. A frontal lesion was suspected and an enormous parasagittal meningioma was demonstrated on angiography and removed. Full recovery ensued.

CASE REPORT XVI

A 47-year-old woman with a lifelong history of severe migraine, associated with vomiting and visual disturbances, presented with a sudden change in the severity and location of the headache and four episodes of apparent transient global amnesia with headache. The feature that had to make this diagnosis questionable was that she was incontinent of urine during one of the attacks and incontinent of faeces during another. She said that she actually felt as if she were dreaming that she was passing urine, and then to her horror realized that she was. On another occasion, at a self-service restaurant, she walked past her sons as if she did not recognize them, sat down at a different table and kept asking whether she had paid for her meal. She was personal secretary for her husband in a very important business and the whole family felt that her intellectual skills and memory had deteriorated dramatically in recent weeks. Physical examination revealed absolutely no abnormality in the CNS. She was started on treatment for migraine and an MRI scan was arranged for 2 days later. This revealed an enormous parasagittal meningioma arising from the free edge of the falx, and re-examination, even armed with this information, still revealed no abnormality. It seemed more likely that these peculiar amnesic episodes represented prolonged complex partial seizures, rather than transient global amnesic attacks,

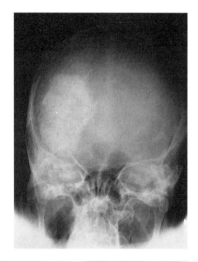
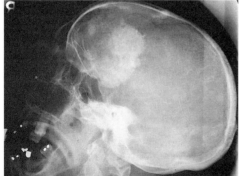

CRXIV. Right subfrontal meningioma presenting as dementia with behavioural disorder. Capillary phase of angiogram (1976)

and the incontinence of urine has to be regarded as a major diagnostic clue. The tumour was completely resected without sequelae. Her migraine continues.

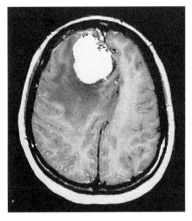

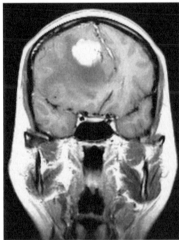

CRXVI. *Parasagittal meningioma.*

Epileptic Events in Frontal Lobe Lesions

Epileptiform attacks are a frequent feature of frontal lobe lesions. There are four types of seizure that point to a frontal lobe disturbance.

Adversive Fits

Due to the presence of the frontal eye fields in area 8, a discharge in this region often causes the head and eyes to turn away from the discharging cortex. These are called 'adversive seizures' and are typical of a frontal lesion.

Focal Motor Epilepsy

Focal Jacksonian fits and unilateral motor convulsions ought to be due to a lesion in or near the main motor cortex, which lies in the precentral gyrus of the frontal lobe. Surprisingly frequently the lesion is actually found

in the parietal area. The discharge in these cases probably arises in the motor cells in the sensory strip. The simultaneous onset of tingling paraesthesiae with the focal fit should indicate this possibility.

Status Epilepticus

As many as 50% of patients who suffer an attack of status epilepticus as a presenting symptom or early in the course of their illness are eventually shown to have a frontal tumour. Status epilepticus in patients with long-established epilepsy does **not** have the same sinister significance.

Temporal Lobe Attacks

The intimate connections of the orbital surface of the frontal pole to the temporal lobe can lead to epileptic events, with all the features of temporal lobe epilepsy, and the causal lesion may lie in or under the frontal pole.

CASE REPORT XVII

In 1987 a 15-year-old girl was referred with a history of two events. On the first occasion her classmates saw her look up in the air to the right-hand side and she fell face first on to her desk, convulsed and bit her tongue. Three weeks later, while talking to her mother, she suddenly answered in a series of unrelated words and as her mother looked towards her she turned to the right-hand side and her right arm flew up into the air. She did not fall and was taken out into the garden, where she quickly came to and asked what she was doing. There was a history of a single febrile convulsion at the age of 11 months. An EEG showed a persistent asymmetry in the right frontotemporal region and treatment with carbamazepine was begun. Over the next year there was no hint of further episodes, but a year later there was a short flurry of four or five attacks which were controlled by an increase in medication. The benign nature of her condition seemed certain when her 13-year-old sister had two epileptic events while in hospital for a dental procedure. Over the next 4 years occasional attacks continued to occur, with episodes increasingly typical of complex partial seizures, with very frequent déjà vu attacks, particularly at mealtimes. No focal motor features had occurred since the onset. A repeat EEG was performed which still showed persistent right frontal slowing. CT and MRI scans revealed a lesion either within or below the right frontal lobe. This proved to be a hamartoma, which was resected with relative ease, since which time she has been seizure free.

This somewhat embarrassing case is important for several reasons. The very early febrile convulsion under 1 year of age should have been viewed with greater suspicion. The slight abnormalities on the EEG might have prompted earlier CT scanning but tumours presenting as epilepsy in childhood are so uncommon that routine scanning is hard to justify, and the advent of

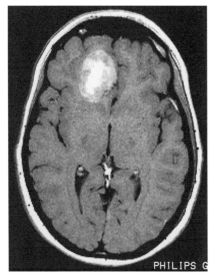

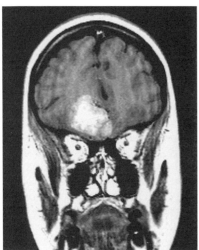

CRXVII. Hamartoma presenting as complex partial seizures.

epilepsy in a sibling added further misleading reassurance. It was only the persistence of attacks in spite of all measures, and the far from dramatic but similar second EEG, that prompted scanning. There were no physical signs. It should be emphasized that she has recovered from surgery without sequelae and is unlikely to have been disadvantaged by the delay in diagnosis of this congenital anomaly. This remains a superb example of a frontal lesion producing attacks indistinguishable from complex partial seizures, even the motor events of the first two episodes were false lateralizing.

Extracerebral Manifestations of Frontal Lobe Damage

Patients with lesions in the orbital part of the frontal lobe, or subfrontal lesions such as olfactory groove or sphenoidal ridge meningiomas, are particularly prone to develop intellectual deficits due to frontal lobe damage. These lesions may also cause blindness in one eye or loss of sense of smell in one or other nostril, and these problems may not be noticed by the dementing patient. For this reason it is essential to examine vision and sense of smell extremely carefully in demented patients. Because the motor strip is so far back, compared with the size of the frontal lobe, intellectual deterioration, micturition disturbance or focal epileptic attacks are often the earliest symptoms of a frontal lobe tumour, long before definite physical signs appear. The possibility of a frontal tumour should always be pursued as far as possible on suspicion alone, even if there are no physical signs. Motor signs tend to come on dramatically suddenly when the tumour becomes oedematous and patients are often seen with a tumour occupying most of the frontal lobe, who have only had dramatic symptoms for a few days.

CASE REPORT XVIII

A 64-year-old bus driver complained of a variety of unexplained symptoms and was eventually dismissed on medical grounds. About a year later he began to become morose and uncommunicative and complained of headaches. He rapidly deteriorated and memory difficulties were noted. The picture was thought to be due to a severe retarded depression and he was admitted to a mental hospital for electroconvulsive therapy. After three treatments he became drowsy and developed a mild left hemiparesis. Neurological examination revealed gross papilloedema and a mild left hemiparesis. A very large oedematous grade 3 astrocytoma was resected from the right frontal lobe. Following surgery the patient had no motor deficit and no recollection of events for several weeks prior to his admission. Once again, amnesia was, in retrospect, a surprisingly severe part of the syndrome.

Physical Signs of Frontal Lobe Lesions

As discussed above, physical signs may be a late feature of a frontal lobe lesion. The need to look for optic atrophy and check for normal vision in both eyes, and careful testing of the sense of smell, has already been emphasized in patients with altered personality, behaviour or amnesic syndromes.

The Grasp Reflex

One of the most useful tests is the grasp reflex. It is also difficult to elicit correctly. In the fully conscious patient stroking the palm of the hand is liable to serious misinterpretation! It is easier if the examiner holds the patient's hand with two or three fingers in the palm, while gently rotating and flexing the arm as tone is assessed. Then, as the examiner releases his grip, gentle pressure is exerted against the base of the patient's fingers. An involuntary increase in the patient's grip, which traps the examiner's fingers, is a positive response. The harder the examiner pulls, the harder the patient will grip, even if the pull threatens to pull the patient off the bed or couch. A unilateral grasp reflex provides strong evidence of a disturbance in the opposite frontal lobe. A bilateral grasp reflex is a less significant finding which has no localizing value but may indicate bilateral frontal damage, and is quite a significant finding in a demented patient and may well indicate a structural lesion.

If the lesion is situated posteriorly in the lobe, damage to the motor strip may cause increased reflexes and an extensor plantar response on the opposite side of the body. If the dominant hemisphere is affected the patient may also have motor aphasia – the inability to speak but with full understanding of instructions. This is also known as Broca's aphasia. This will almost always be coupled with obvious weakness of the right face and arm.

Parasagittal lesions are particularly likely to cause micturition disturbances and intellectual upset as they affect both hemispheres. As the area of cortex supplying the leg lies either side of the midline at this point, increased reflexes in both legs and bilateral extensor plantar responses may be found. This can lead to a very rare but classic trap into which even experienced neurologists may fall.

CASE REPORT XIX

A 66-year-old woman developed a mild spastic paraparesis over 9 months. There was some modest mid-thoracic backache. She was otherwise well. Myelography revealed a mid-dorsal disc lesion with cord compression. This was decompressed using a lateral approach, and for some 6 weeks the patient showed significant improvement and was discharged for further rehabilitation. She then suddenly deteriorated and became slightly confused. She was re-admitted and CT scanning revealed a parasaggital meningioma. This was removed and she again started to improve. She unfortunately succumbed to a pulmonary embolus 6 weeks after the second operation. It is impossible to say which of these two lesions was the main cause of her clinical picture. Both were an equally acceptable cause of her symptoms.

Direct disruption of frontal lobe influences over the basal ganglia and cerebellum may cause 'pseudoparkinsonism' or 'pseudocerebellar' signs in addition to the apathy due to dementia. It is easy in such a case to make the mistaken diagnosis of arteriosclerotic dementia and parkinsonism. For this reason the majority of neurologists insist on full investigation before a patient is allowed to be labelled as demented, with the hopeless prognosis that this diagnosis carries. As an example of pseudocerebellar signs, the following case report is instructive.

CASE REPORT XX

A 50-year-old woman with known carcinoma of the breast presented with a 10-day history of headache, difficulty in walking and clumsiness of the left side. She had vomited several times. Physical examination revealed left-sided cerebellar signs and a left-sided extensor plantar response. There were no reflex changes and no nystagmus or dysarthria. A left-sided cerebellar metastasis was confidently diagnosed and a solitary right frontal metastasis demonstrated on the

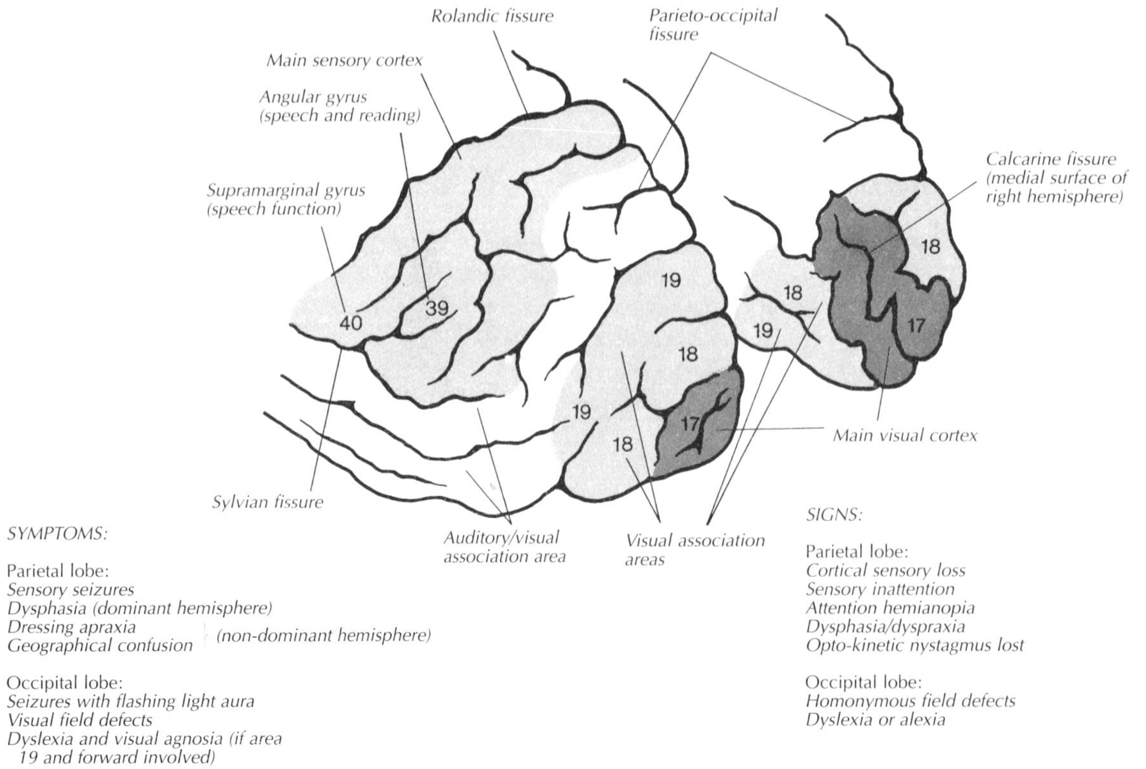
Rolandic fissure
Parieto-occipital fissure
Main sensory cortex
Angular gyrus (speech and reading)
Supramarginal gyrus (speech function)
Calcarine fissure (medial surface of right hemisphere)
40
39
19
18
17
18
19
18
17
19
18
18
17
Main visual cortex
Sylvian fissure
Auditory/visual association area
Visual association areas
SYMPTOMS:
Parietal lobe:
Sensory seizures
Dysphasia (dominant hemisphere)
Dressing apraxia
Geographical confusion
(non-dominant hemisphere)
Occipital lobe:
Seizures with flashing light aura
Visual field defects
Dyslexia and visual agnosia (if area 19 and forward involved)
SIGNS:
Parietal lobe:
Cortical sensory loss
Sensory inattention
Attention hemianopia
Dysphasia/dyspraxia
Opto-kinetic nystagmus lost
Occipital lobe:
Homonymous field defects
Dyslexia or alexia

8.3 The parietal and occipital lobes.

CT scan! Evidence of metastases elsewhere precluded surgery.

The Parietal Lobes (Fig. 8.3)

The parietal lobes are quite small, extending from the Rolandic fissure anteriorly to the parieto-occipital fissure posteriorly and the temporal lobe below. The functional overlap between parietal, occipital and temporal lobe function in this area, and the physical continuity of the lobes, makes anatomical boundaries of little practical significance. The sulci that delineate the lobe are quite shallow, unlike the deep Rolandic and Sylvian fissures that delineate the frontal lobe.

The sensory cortex is organized in the same way as the motor strip, with a large representation for information from the face and arm on the lateral surface and that of the trunk, leg and genital areas at the vertex and into the parasaggital area. Speech function is concentrated in the supramarginal and angular gyri, and in the upper part of the adjacent temporal lobe. The visual association area (area 19) is adjacent to the occipital lobe (see extinction hemianopia, Chapter 3). The same region is also the control centre responsible for the phenomenon of optokinetic nystagmus discussed in Chapter 7.

Clinical Features of Parietal Lobe Damage

The clinical features of dominant and non-dominant parietal lobe dysfunction have been discussed earlier in this chapter. To summarize, the following physical signs should be sought in patients with a suspected parietal lobe disorder:

1. Evidence of cortical sensory loss or sensory inattention
2. Evidence of dysphasia if a dominant hemisphere lesion is suspected
3. Evidence of dyspraxia if a non-dominant hemisphere lesion is suspected
4. Evidence of an attention hemianopia or a frank hemianopia if a parietotemporal lesion is present
5. Loss of optokinetic nystagmus (see Chapter 7)
6. 'Soft' motor signs, such as slightly increased reflexes, mild facial weakness and an extensor plantar response on the side opposite the suspected lesion.

The Occipital Lobes (Fig. 8.3)

The occipital cortex has already been described in Chapter 3. Tumours in the occipital pole have considerable epileptic potential but are relatively rare. Seizures, preceded by visual hallucinations consisting of unformed flashes of light and colours, should be regarded as arising in the occipital lobe. Any field defect that is produced by a tumour in the lobe will not spare the macular cortex (a feature of vascular lesions, see Chapters 9 and 3). Damage to areas 18, 19 and 37 in the adjacent parietal lobe responsible for visual association may cause varying degrees of psychic blindness, such as visual agnosia (inability to recognize objects) or alexia (inability to read).

CASE REPORT XXI

A middle-aged architect suffered from attacks of flashing lights in the right field of vision for 10 years. Following one attack he also had great difficulty in reading, writing and spelling, indicating damage to the adjacent parietal area. This was not consistent with a simple vascular lesion as it involved two arterial territories, and further investigation and operation revealed an occipitoparietal astrocytoma.

CASE REPORT XXII

A 54-year-old woman was referred via her optician whom she had consulted because of difficulty in reading over the previous 3 months. She had had some low-grade morning headaches and occasional difficulty in remembering names and words. On examination she had a right upper quadrantic homonymous hemianopia and mild nominal aphasia, but no other abnormalities. A CT scan revealed a left occipital pole tumour which proved to be an anaplastic oligodendroglioma. Her visual fields recovered to normal postoperatively. Repeat scans 3 months later showed no residual tumour, but 3 months after that her headaches and hemianopia recurred. Repeat surgery revealed a glioblastomatous change in the tumour. This was followed by radiotherapy. On this occasion the hemianopia did not clear and sadly she died 6 months later, with increasing dysphasic difficulty as the recurrent tumour extended forwards into the parietal lobe.

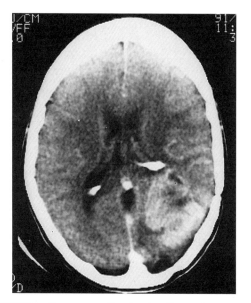

CRXXII. *Recurrent oligodendroglioma in occipito parietal region.*

The Temporal Lobes (Figs 8.4, 8.5)

The anatomy of the temporal lobe is extremely difficult to grasp owing to the way the lobe is folded in on itself under the overhanging frontal and parietal lobes and the extensive and important areas that are rolled in under the medial hemisphere. Furthermore, the connections of the lobe to the hippocampal area, the cingulate gyrus and the insula make the 'functional' temporal lobe much more extensive than its physical boundaries. The 'limbic system', which includes many of these areas, is discussed in Chapter 12.

One can only summarize some of the many functions of the temporal lobe that find expression in clinical disorders. These include:

1. The central representation of auditory and vestibular information in the superior and marginal gyrus
2. Memory function in the hippocampal gyrus
3. Visual association areas posteriorly
4. Central representation of taste and smell in the uncus
5. The upper homonymous visual field pathways (see Chapter 3)
6. The entire visual radiation at the parieto-occipital–temporal junction
7. Supplementary motor areas concerned with facial expression, eating, emotional responses to pain and pleasure
8. Many aspects of behaviour via frontal lobe connections
9. Central control of visceral motility, sexual and respiratory function.

Clinical Features of Temporal Lobe Damage

The clinical symptoms of temporal lobe disease can be of bewildering complexity. Fortunately the great frequency with which the disordered function is 'epileptic' in nature makes recognition of the lesion possible. The important clinical pointer is that however bizarre and whatever the nature of the upset, the sudden onset and offset of the disturbance points to a paroxysmal disturbance in the temporal lobe, previously known as a 'psychomotor' or temporal lobe seizure but now generally called a complex partial seizure. These terms all emphasize the prolonged and often bizarre behavioural upset that can be a feature of such attacks, quite unlike any other form of epilepsy. Consciousness is not necessarily lost and motor dexterity is often maintained, allowing complex automatisms to occur. These disorders are discussed in greater detail in Chapters 12 and 22.

Patients may relate a variety of typical prodromal events closely related to temporal lobe functions. They may describe vertigo, auditory or visual hallucinations, hallucinations of smell and taste respectively called olfactory and gustatory hallucinations, unpleasant visceral symptoms, déjà-vu (already seen) or jamais-vu (never seen) sensations, uncontrollable deep breathing,

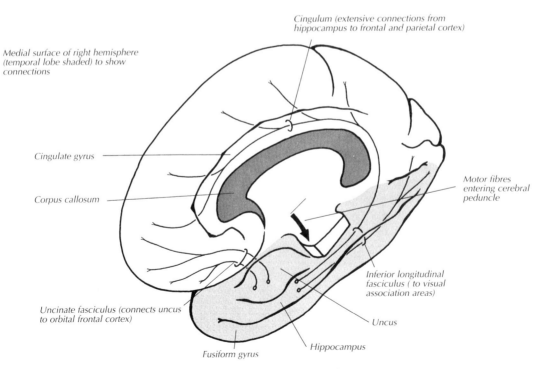

8.4   The right temporal lobe medial aspect.

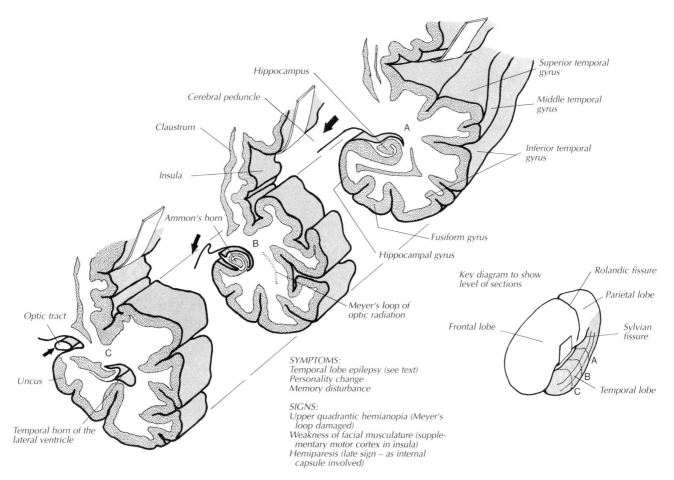

8.5   Lateral surface of left temporal lobe (anterior part shown cut off, Sylvian fissure pulled open).

sexual fantasies or just a peculiar feeling 'as if something awful is going to happen'. Déjà vu and jamais vu are usually very brief in nature, but sometimes patients have a more prolonged experience where they feel that everything that is going on around them has happened previously and they can predict what is going to happen next, or a more terrifying sensation when they are suddenly unable to recognize their own room or home or even the people they are with.

Motor accompaniments vary considerably, and peculiar grimacing, chewing, lip-smacking, sucking or kissing mouth movements, repeated fiddling with clothing and sometimes even removal of clothing may occur.

Patients may continue to drive many miles during an attack and become lost. Patients on foot may find that they have walked half a mile in the wrong direction.

Focal motor seizures affecting the face and arm in particular (by activation of supplementary motor areas in the insula) may occur and the seizure may progress to loss of consciousness and a major convulsion. When attacks originate in the temporal lobe association areas, bilateral changes of facial expression such as

smiling or snarling or grimacing may belie the focal onset of the attack. If a focal episode is confined to just half the face, it is more likely to have originated in the motor cortex of the frontal lobe.

Following a complex partial seizure the patient remains very confused and in this state may even to assault over-helpful bystanders. Contrary to popular opinion, aggressive behaviour during the attack is very unusual, and attempts to demonstrate that criminal behaviour is commonly due to or associated with epilepsy are unconvincing.

Physical Signs of Temporal Lobe Lesions

Lesions in the temporal lobe frequently cause temporal lobe epilepsy unless they are extremely acute, such as haematomas, highly malignant gliomas or herpes simplex encephalitis, which usually starts unilaterally and often mimics an acute cerebral abscess. In all these situations the clinical picture consists of a confused drowsy patient who is rapidly becoming hemiplegic. In all cases it is quite clear that the situation is a neurological emergency.

CASE REPORT XXIII

A 57-year-old man on anticoagulants following a prosthetic heart valve replacement was brought to the accident centre 1 hour after being struck in the left temple by a golf ball, hit at full power from 30 yards. He had not lost consciousness and was not drowsy, but had a headache and felt slightly nauseous. No signs were found by a non-neurological resident. He returned to the accident centre the next morning as the headache had worsened, but he was again examined and allowed home as there were no signs. He was brought back 12 hours later, having become progressively drowsy and confused during the previous 8 hours. On examination, he was so drowsy that he fell asleep between questions. His speech included completely irrelevant and inappropriate sentences and he was convinced that the prime minister was the Queen. His speech was slightly slurred. There were no other abnormalities. Power tone and coordination were equal, the reflexes were normal and both plantars were flexor. Immediate CT scanning revealed a 2-inch diameter intracerebral haematoma in the temporal lobe with marked midline shift. This was evacuated 4 hours later, following reversal of his anticoagulation, prompted by a sudden dramatic deterioration in his clinical state. He survived without significant sequelae.

Only 10% of patients who present with temporal lobe seizures are harbouring a tumour. Previously, careful follow-up was the main method of excluding the possibility, unless an EEG provided strong evidence of an underlying neoplasm. It was always wise to do a repeat EEG 6 months to a year after the first to see if any progressive change could be detected.

CASE REPORT XXIV

A 45-year-old carpenter presented with a single epileptic fit. There were no focal features at the onset and an EEG was entirely within normal limits. As a self-employed person he was extremely unhappy about the driving restriction. A routine follow-up EEG was booked for 6 months ahead. Four weeks before this was due, his workmates noticed a slight change in personality and his wife noticed that he had become very irritable. On the Saturday morning prior to his clinic attendance, following a very minor family altercation, he went into the garden and totally demolished his garden shed and a greenhouse with an axe. This behaviour was totally out of character. A repeat EEG was performed and revealed a gross disturbance in the right temporal region. Subsequent investigation disclosed a right middle cranial fossa meningioma, which was successfully removed.

With the advent of CT scanning most patients are scanned at their first attendance, although the pick-up rate is as low as 1%. In some instances the initial scan has failed to detect a tumour that was found subsequently. It would seem that the old-fashioned technique of following the patient still has some merit, even if modern investigations suggest that there is no reason to do so.

The main reasons for reopening investigation in such patients would be the advent of further symptoms or

physical signs. Subtle personality changes may occur. These are less dramatic than in frontal lobe lesions and may mimic depressive or psychotic disorders more often than dementia. There is a high incidence of impotence in males with temporal lobe tumours, so that this symptom combined with personality change should arouse suspicion. Unilateral lesions rarely cause significant memory impairment.

A careful search for an upper quadrantic homonymous hemianopia is very important. This would provide evidence of damage to Meyer's loop in the anterior temporal lobe (see Chapter 3). If a complete hemianopia is present the lesion has spread back into the adjacent parietal lobe and appropriate parietal lobe problems may be found, including dysphasia or dyspraxia, depending on the lateralization.

The face area of the motor cortex is the part most likely to be affected by a temporal lobe mass, therefore a mild facial weakness of the emotional type should be sought. Otherwise physical signs occur extremely late in the course of the disease and the picture then becomes one of a rapidly developing hemiparesis with confusion, headache, dysphasia (if on the dominant side) and personality change, indicating a rapidly expanding lesion. Prior to scanning some patients would be followed up for 10 years or more before this acute change unmasked the underlying lesion.

Diagnosis and Investigation of Cerebral Tumours

The cardinal symptoms and signs of a cerebral tumour are said to be headache, vomiting and papilloedema. In fact, these are very rarely the presenting symptoms unless the tumour is in the posterior fossa or has blocked the flow of CSF. In children, who are more likely to have posterior fossa tumours, these clinical features apply but in the adult the majority of tumours produce more subtle symptoms and signs, or even no signs at all, as already clearly indicated in the case histories in this chapter.

Headaches

Headaches are discussed in detail in Chapter 20. In relation to cerebral tumours the following features are worth considering:

1. Contrary to popular belief, headache is not an inevitable symptom of a cerebral tumour and is often so mild that the patient only mentions it in response to a direct question. The majority of patients with cerebral tumours do not have a significant headache.

2. Less than 0.1% of patients referred to hospital with headaches have a cerebral tumour.

3. If headache does occur it is not necessarily particularly severe. It is more likely to have a dull relentless quality. An association with vomiting markedly increases the chances of finding a serious cause, but as a broad generalization the more severe the headache the less likely it is to be due to a tumour. Such headaches are usually due to migraine.

Recent-onset headache associated with vomiting, particularly if both the headache and the vomiting are provoked by position change, is the only situation in which exclusion of a tumour becomes the first consideration. The differentiation of such headaches from migraine is discussed in more detail in Chapter 20. As examples of remarkably pure headache of pathological significance, the following case reports are important; again, the lack of physical findings, in particular the absence of papilloedema, must be emphasized.

CASE REPORT XXV

A 42-year-old accountant was due to return to his position in the Middle East the day after seeking advice for the following symptom, which had been present over the past 6 months. Exclusively while having his bowels open, if he strained while leaning forwards he developed a sensation as if he had been struck over the back right-hand side of the head with a mallet. The pain then pulsed in that area for five to ten paroxysms, each of lessening severity until it subsided. It did not make him feel giddy or sick. Physical examination was entirely normal but it was thought prudent to perform a CT scan, as he would not be returning to G.B. for 2 years. The scan revealed marked hydrocephalus due to a meningioma of the tentorial edge completely blocking the tentorial hiatus.

CASE REPORT XXVI

A 35-year-old man complained of severe headache in only one position. He was otherwise asymptomatic. For the previous 18 months, every evening as he bent over to reach the handle of his up-and-over garage door, he was struck by a sudden vicious headache, so severe that it made him stumble and fall on several occasions and always caused nausea, although he had never vomited. After standing for a few seconds, holding on to his car, the symptoms would clear. Physical examination revealed no abnormality. CT scanning demonstrated massive dilatation of the right lateral ventricle, which proved to be due to a papilloma entirely occupying and expanding the ventricle. The papilloma was successfully removed but unfortunately he was left with postoperative epilepsy.

Epileptic Seizures

Epileptic seizures in relation to tumours at different sites have already been discussed. As with headache, it is essential to have a sense of proportion about epilepsy and cerebral tumours.

1. In patients under 20 years of age the incidence of cerebral tumours causing epilepsy is 0.02%. The author has only seen four patients in this age range with a cerebral tumour causing epilepsy in 35 years.

2. Even patients in the age group 45–55 years, the decade with the highest incidence of cerebral tumours, only some 10% of patients with recent-onset epilepsy ultimately prove to have a cerebral tumour.

3. Epileptic seizures are more likely to occur when the underlying tumour is an infiltrating glioma rather than a surface lesion such as a meningioma. As gliomas occur twice as frequently as meningiomas, the patient who has a fit due to a tumour will usually prove to have a malignant glioma or astrocytoma. As an exception to this generalization chronic benign surface lesions that indent the cerebral hemisphere sometimes behave more like an intrinsic tumour.

From this it follows that a first seizure occurring in a patient aged 21 or more does not automatically mean that they have a tumour. Modern investigational techniques have allowed fairly confident exclusion of cerebral tumours as a cause of epilepsy following the first fit. It is still instructive to perform an EEG, as this will sometimes indicate that the patient is merely manifesting a lifelong tendency to epilepsy for the first time. Where minor focal features are seen on the EEG, particularly in one or other temporal lobe, it is almost the rule that subsequent scanning will **not** detect a lesion. Surprisingly often, it is the patient with a normal EEG at the first attendance who is later found to have an underlying lesion. Sometimes the EEG may provide evidence of underlying disease when even an MRI scan appears to be normal.

CASE REPORT XXVII

A 51-year-old woman was referred following an epileptic fit. In the previous 3 weeks she had stumbled over the occasional word in conversation. Her husband thought that during the attack the right side of her face was distorted. Another fit occurred in the casualty department without focal features. She was transferred to a neurosurgical unit, and following a normal CT scan was returned to the referring hospital, where a normal spinal fluid sample was obtained. She was transferred for a further neurological opinion. The only finding on examination was a major degree of receptive aphasia, which recovered over the next 24 hours. An EEG showed a marked slow-wave abnormality in the left temporal region. An MRI scan was reported as normal, although a dissenting view thought that there was slight oedema in the left posterior temporal region. She was put on phenytoin and remained perfectly well until she collapsed with a further fit while playing golf in Florida 9 weeks later. A second MRI scan revealed a temporal lobe glioma with marked oedema, although remarkably little shift, and again the only physical finding was receptive aphasia. The tumour was a malignant astrocytoma showing considerable pleomorphism and she was treated

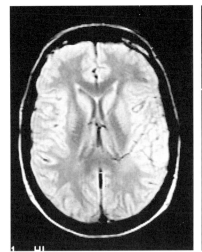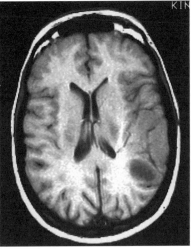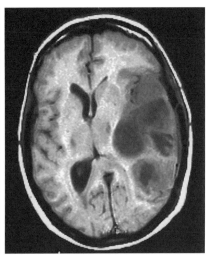

CRXXVII.   Rapid evolution of scan appearances over 6 months in malignant glioma.

with radiotherapy. Following a partial improvement, her clinical situation deteriorated markedly 5 months later and she died 9 months after the first fit.

It is therefore wise to continue to follow up patients with late-onset epilepsy and to repeat the investigations if any new features or physical findings appear.

A complete set of negative investigations early in the course of the illness does not exclude a neoplasm. Occasionally 5–10 years may elapse before other evidence of a slow-growing tumour becomes apparent. These need not necessarily be regarded as wasted years if the patient has remained in good clinical condition and has controlled epilepsy. Sadly, the patient's problems usually start when the tumour is finally diagnosed.

Epilepsy due to a tumour is not particularly difficult to control and difficulty in controlling epilepsy is not evidence of an underlying tumour. However, if the epilepsy starts as an episode of status epilepticus there is a 50% risk that the patient has a frontal tumour, and full investigation is indicated in this instance.

In childhood the majority of cerebral tumours occur in the cerebellum (medulloblastomas or cystic astrocytomas), the pons and the optic nerve or chiasm. Supratentorial tumours are rare. Therefore early headache, vomiting, ataxia or visual disturbance are common features of a tumour in the child, and conversely epilepsy is very unusual. (Clinical details of posterior fossa tumours in childhood are to be found in Chapters 3, 6, 11 and 12.)

In the adult supratentorial tumours account for 90% of cerebral neoplasms, increasing the likelihood of an epileptic presentation and decreasing the incidence of headache as there is more space available for tumour expansion. Only cerebellar tumours (in the adult hae-mangioblastomas and metastases) and tumours that block CSF flow (pinealomas, ependymomas of the fourth ventricle and intraventricular tumours) cause headache and vomiting as early features. The differential diagnosis of this presentation in the adult must include the possibility of the late presentation of congenital aqueduct stenosis or benign intracranial hypertension. Both conditions may present like cerebral tumours, causing raised intracranial pressure.

CASE REPORT XXVIII

A 24-year-old man was referred by an ophthalmologist to whom he had presented with vertical diplopia. This had been present since childhood and he had adopted a headtilt to the right to compensate for it. This was confirmed from old photographs. He had a left superior oblique palsy. While giving the history he suddenly mentioned that he had neurofibromatosis, and displayed café au lait patches and numerous subcutaneous neurofibromas. He confirmed that he had always had a large head and poor concentration. For the past 7 months he had had sudden explosive headaches associated with vomiting, and his mother thought that his head tilt had worsened. He had become extremely drowsy and had been found asleep in front of his computer at work on more than one occasion. On examination he had a very large head (circumference 62 cm) and walked with his head tilted to the right and back. He had unequivocal papilloedema in the left eye. He had a left superior oblique palsy with considerable overaction of the opposite inferior rectus, producing complex diplopia in all directions of gaze. His reflexes were slightly depressed but the right plantar response was extensor. Compensated aqueduct stenosis was suspected, but MRI scanning revealed a 3 cm diameter pineal tumour with severe hydrocephalus. This was treated by bilateral shunting and partial resection. The tumour was a low-grade glioma of subependymal origin. Apart from shunt revision he has remained well since surgery.

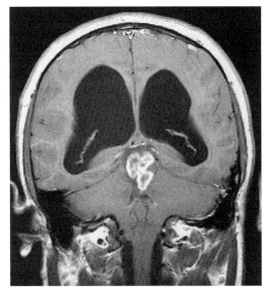

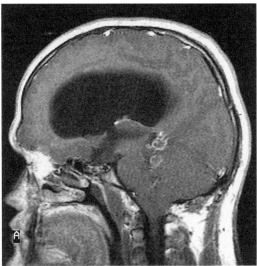

CRXXVIII.   Pineal tumour with hydrocephalus.

Pathological Features and Clinical Management

Childhood

In childhood, tumours usually occur in the cerebellum and preoperative pathological diagnosis is difficult. Half the tumours consist of a small-cell astrocytoma associated with a large cystic cavity. Complete removal with a low risk of recurrence is usually possible. The others are highly malignant medulloblastomas, which are tumours of disputed tissue origin usually arising in the vermis and extending down the superior medullary velum or peduncles into the brain stem, with little possibility of complete resection. They also tend to seed via the CSF and secondary deposits are found throughout the CNS, including the lumbar theca. They are usually radiosensitive and combined surgery and radiotherapy (including the whole spinal canal) may achieve impressive cure rates. Unfortunately, the effect of the treatment on the child is fairly devastating and survival is often blighted by the impact of these complications. This is not always the case, but sadly there is a risk of late recurrence even after an apparently successful outcome.

CASE REPORT XXX

A girl of 13 developed unsteadiness of gait, nausea and vomiting. A diagnosis of hysteria was entertained elsewhere and treatment including hypnotherapy was started. Shortly afterwards she collapsed, became unconscious and was transferred to the neurological unit in a decerebrate state, with fixed dilated pupils. She was transferred to a neurosurgical unit on a mannitol drip and a medulloblastoma was excised. She was referred for further treatment out of the area and

CASE REPORT XXIX

A 26-year-old driver of heavy earth-moving equipment was seen with what appeared to be benign positional vertigo. When he looked back over his left shoulder – a necessarily frequent action in his job – he became extremely giddy and had fallen from his machine on several occasions before being put off work. Otoneurological testing was normal and recovery was anticipated. Six months later he developed a new symptom. While standing passing water if he looked down his legs would suddenly buckle under him and he would fall to the ground. If he looked straight ahead this did not happen. There were no physical signs and it was postulated that he had a tumour in the fourth ventricle acting like a ball-valve, which blocked the outlet of the fourth ventricle when he flexed his neck. This very speculative diagnosis was confirmed by ventriculography and an intraventricular arachnoid cyst of the fourth ventricle was successfully removed, with complete resolution of all his symptoms. There was no headache at any stage.

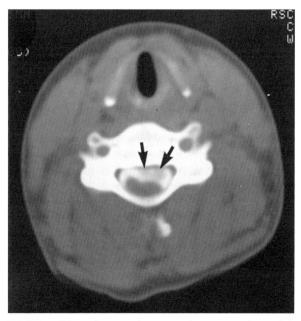

CRXXX.   CT myelogram demonstrating metastatic medulloblastoma in cervical canal 10 years after initial diagnosis.

was not seen again until she was 23 years of age. She was then referred with intractable C5 root pain in the left arm. Two years previously she had had a baby and 1 year previously had been investigated for epilepsy; a tumour which proved to be recurrent medulloblastoma had been removed from her right temporal lobe. MRI scanning of the whole spinal cord revealed tumour nodules throughout the spine, one in particular on the left C5 root, and the cauda equina had the appearance of a bunch of grapes. Apart from pain control no therapy could be entertained, and she died a few weeks later. It is likely that her tumour reactivated during the hormonal changes of her pregnancy.

Pontine gliomas are discussed in Chapter 11 and optic nerve gliomas in Chapter 3. Neither are really resectable but seem to be moderately radiosensitive, although it is thought that the natural history of these tumours is favourable. Whether radiotherapy should be used, particularly in the case of optic nerve gliomas, remains controversial.

In the adult, pontine gliomas occur with greatest frequency in patients with neurofibromatosis, and when they become symptomatic it is usual practice to treat the patient with radiotherapy, although the rarity of these tumours makes its value uncertain.

Adulthood

Primary posterior fossa tumours are extremely rare in the adult. Unlike childhood, 20%–30% of cerebral tumours prove to be metastases, particularly those in the posterior fossa. In the male metastatic carcinoma of the bronchus is the most frequent cause, and in the female metastatic carcinoma of the breast. Therefore a chest X-ray and careful breast examination are the first and most important investigations in any patient with a suspected cerebral tumour.

Any other tumour may metastasize to the brain but large bowel tumours, renal carcinoma and malignant melanoma are those most likely to do so. Large bowel tumours, particularly of the rectosigmoid, show a tendency to metastasize to the cerebellum, and in general metastases occur more frequently in both the parietal lobe and cerebellum than would be anticipated if spread were on a random basis.

Primary cerebral tumours occur in the lobes in a frequency roughly proportional to the size of the lobe, i.e. frontal/temporal/parietal and occipital. The only primary cerebellar tumour that is likely to occur in the adult is a haemangioblastoma. These consist of a small, highly vascular nodule of tumour, often in association with a large haemorrhagic cyst. Complete resection is often possible and the prognosis is probably the best for any cerebral tumour. Occasionally these tumours produce erythropoietin and cause polycythaemia. They may also be associated with vascular tumours in the retina (von Hippel–Lindau disease).

CASE REPORT XXXI

A 60-year-old man was admitted following acute collapse with severe headache. He had rapidly lapsed into a coma, with signs of an acute posterior fossa lesion. He was hypertensive and a diagnosis of primary intracerebral haemorrhage was made. He was transferred home direct from the neurosurgical unit following successful evacuation of the clot. He was not followed up but was readmitted 3 years later in a similar state, and quickly succumbed. A review of the investigations performed after the original surgery revealed a haemoglobin of 22:g/l. Unfortunately, the possible significance of this had not been realized. Post mortem revealed that he had re-bled into a haemangioblastoma.

In the cerebral hemispheres half the tumours are malignant gliomas or astrocytomas, with four grades of malignancy, I–IV, in order of increasing malignancy. An important subvariant is the oligodendroglioma, which occurs mainly in the frontal lobe and shows the greatest tendency to calcify. Many patients survive 15–25 years with this type of tumour, owing to its exceedingly slow growth. The following case was thought to be an oligodendroglioma until surgery revealed otherwise.

CASE REPORT XXXII

A 68-year-old woman was referred for further advice on the management of the epilepsy which she had had for 35 years. The attacks had always consisted of episodes of uncontrolled laughter or humming and singing, and were typical of complex partial seizures of temporal lobe origin. Several EEGs had been performed over the years which had shown idiopathic epileptic changes, as did the recording taken when she was first seen in 1989. The addition of clonazepam to carbamazepine and the withdrawal of barbiturate-based

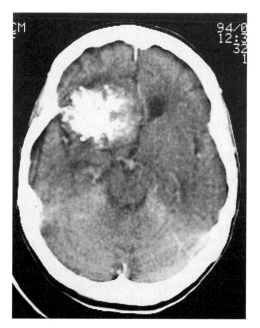

***CRXXXII.** Cavernous haemangioma discovered after a 35-year history of complex partial seizures.*

drugs produced a marked improvement in her mental state and virtual cessation of the attacks. At the age of 72, over a period of a few months, she became apathetic and physically slowed down, although no new findings appeared and the epilepsy remained controlled. It was suspected that she was developing dementia of Alzheimer's type, although the speed of onset was surprising. A CT scan revealed a heavily calcified left frontal lesion which, after 35 years, was clearly beginning to produce a mass effect. Pre-operatively this was thought to be an oligo-dendroglioma. At surgery this proved to be a cavernous haemangioma which shelled out quite easily. The postoperative course was complicated by frontal lobe oedema.

This case is full of lessons for the unwary. In spite of the rarity of epilepsy due to a tumour there is no stage at which one can regard a tumour as totally excluded. Headache is not the usual symptom of cerebral tumours, contrary to popular belief, and once again the 35 years of relatively normal life enjoyed by this patient can be regarded entirely as her good fortune, as it is possible that discovery and attempted resection of her lesion at her original presentation might have left her with unacceptable deficit and epilepsy. She did well to conceal it so successfully for so long.

The general prognosis of gliomas and astrocytomas is related to both the site and the histological grading: 75% of patients with grade IV tumours are dead within 9 months, and even with grade I and II tumours 75% of patients are dead within 3 years. Sadly, there is little to be gained by early diagnosis of these infiltrating malignant tumours. One of the disappointments of the advent of scanning is the discovery that there seems to be no such thing as a small cerebral tumour. Even when patients have only had symptoms for a few days, the scan nearly always reveals a massive tumour, surrounded by oedema, that is already inoperable or at least incurable. If one is fortunate enough to find a small tumour, it is often in a critical area of the brain. There is therefore considerable reluctance to tackle this surgically for fear of producing unacceptable deficit a few months ahead of the inevitable deficit that will be produced by the tumour itself.

It is therefore true to say that tumours arising in silent areas, in regions not associated with specific symptoms or signs, tend to remain asymptomatic until very large, and even then may carry a better prognosis because they are accessible and resectable by virtue of their site. Tumours arising in vital areas cause early symptoms and signs, but are often inoperable because the deficit produced by surgery would be unacceptable. The chance of useful operative intervention depends on the site of the tumour and the chances of prolonged survival on the histological grading. Paradoxically, it is probably better to have a highly malignant glioma in the frontal pole than a low-grade glioma in the parietotemporal region! However, the accuracy of localization per-

mitted by MRI scanning and improved surgical techniques, including operating in the dominant speech area, with the patient conscious, may improve the outlook in the future.

It is beyond the scope of this book to discuss the relative merits of radiotherapy or the possible benefits of chemotherapy, but it is reasonable to say that the prognosis for any patient with a malignant cerebral tumour remains grim, and there is still little sense of satisfaction in successfully diagnosing a cerebral tumour of this type, although the impression is often given that failure to diagnose a cerebral tumour within hours of first seeing the patient is the worst crime in neurology. The relative incidence of tumours in different sites is shown in Figure 8.6.

Tumours outside the substance of the brain include meningiomas, intraventricular lesions, pinealomas and neurofibromas. They produce either local signs if strategically sited, or non-specific signs and raised intracranial pressure if they interfere with the circulation of the CSF (Fig. 8.7).

(Figures show percentage frequency in hemisphere)

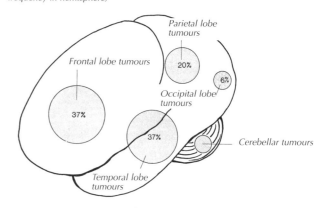

8.6 Tumour incidence in the different lobes.

Note. The shaded areas are intended to represent the site and not the relative frequency of occurrence

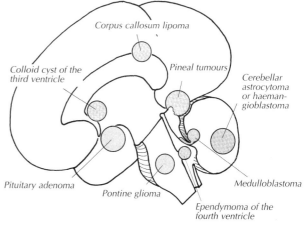

8.7 Other tumour sites.

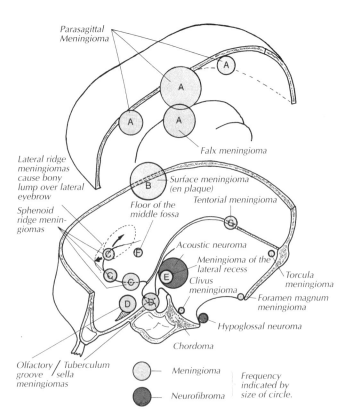

8.8 Common sites for meningiomas and neurofibromas.

Meningiomas

Meningiomas account for 20% of intracranial tumours and arise from the dura, particularly in areas where it is densely adherent to bone. The sites and relative frequencies are indicated in Figure 8.8. Lesions along the falx (A), are known as parasagittal tumours and typically produce frontal syndromes and cause technical complications by their tendency to invade the sagittal sinus. Surface meningiomas (B) are at first sight highly favourable, but often present formidable technical problems and successful removal may be marred by considerable neurological deficit. It is also a feature of these lesions that the clinical picture may be very atypical indeed, and there are several examples elsewhere in the text.

Tumours along the sphenoid ridge (C) tend to produce extraocular nerve palsies at the inner end and middle third, and marked hyperostosis if in the lateral third, producing a bony boss over the pterion. Complete surgical removal is usually technically impossible and relentless progression of signs and frequent recurrences are the rule.

Lesions at (C), the olfactory groove or tuberculum sellae, cause anosmia, visual failure and dementia. Meningiomas in the lateral recess (E) are a rare cause of the cerebellopontine angle syndrome (see Chapter

6). Those on the free edge of the tentorium (G) or at the confluence of the great veins (H) tend to obstruct CSF flow and produce the symptoms and signs of obstructive hydrocephalus (headache, vomiting and papilloedema). Rarely, meningiomas arise on the front of the brain stem and in the foramen magnum. Their clinical features will be found in Chapters 11 and 15 respectively.

Neuromas

Neuromas account for 7% of intracranial tumours and nearly all arise on the acoustic nerve (see Chapter 6). They may also occur on the fifth, ninth, tenth and twelfth cranial nerves (see also Chapter 7). This is one field where recent advances in imaging and surgical technique have produced dramatic improvements in the mortality and morbidity rates following surgery.

Pituitary Adenomas

Pituitary adenomas account for 10% of all primary intracranial tumours and are discussed in detail in Chapter 3.

Other Intracranial Tumours

Other extracerebral tumours are rare, and each account for 1% or less of cerebral tumours.

Intraventricular tumours include pedunculated meningiomas, ependymomas (particularly in the floor of the fourth ventricle), gliomas extending into the ventricle, and benign colloid cysts of the lining of the third ventricle or the septum pellucidum.

Lipomas of the corpus callosum are rare and may achieve considerable size before producing clinical features.

Pinealomas tend to infiltrate the midbrain (see Chapters 2 and 8) and usually cause early obstruction of the aqueduct. As an example of a very slow evolution of a pineal tumour, the following case report is remarkable.

CASE REPORT XXXIII

An 18-year-old man was referred in 1974 with loss of upward gaze and fixed dilated pupils. No pineal lesion was demonstrable by the then available technique of air encephalography. His symptoms progressed and a course of external beam irradiation was given on clinical grounds. Three years later he noticed further visual difficulties and developed a progressive bitemporal hemianopia and optic atrophy. This behaviour of pineal tumours was well recognized and tumour spreading round via the optic tract had been referred to in older literature as 'ectopic pinealomas'. Repeat air encephalography did not demonstrate a suprasellar lesion, but over the next 3 years he developed panhypopituitarism, requiring full replacement therapy. Throughout the 1980s his visual acuity progressively decreased to less than 6/60 and he was registered blind. He then developed progressive deafness. He became more and more uninterested in his surroundings and sat humming to himself all day and answered in monosyllables. A CT scan in 1989 revealed no definite abnormality. He eventually died in 1993, and at post mortem his upper brain stem was found to be encircled by a tumour of pineal origin which had infiltrated the medial and lateral geniculate bodies, the optic tracts the hypothalamus and the pituitary fossa.

Tumours in the ventricle can often be resected via the ventricle. Pinealomas can now be directly approached by a trans callosal route and treated by irradiation if appropriate, the obstructed aqueduct being bypassed if necessary by a shunt procedure.

Cerebral Abscess and Infective Granulomas

The most important differential diagnosis of cerebral tumour is cerebral abscess. The diagnosis may be extremely difficult to make. This is particularly true in those situations where a chronic low-grade abscess has developed in the absence of overt underlying disease. This used to be confusing to the extent that it was not until pus was encountered during needle aspiration of a cerebral mass that the diagnosis became apparent. CT scanning has made the preoperative diagnosis more certain.

In a classic case of cerebral abscess the presentation is acute, with a toxic 'meningitic' onset with fever quickly followed by confusion and focal neurological signs over a matter of days. This typical course usually occurs in patients in whom the risk is recognizable. This includes patients with pneumococcal pneumonia, patients with rheumatic heart disease and patients with cyanotic heart disease (venous blood bypasses the filtering effect of the lungs). In the pre-antibiotic era patients with chronic osteomyelitis, septic foci in the sinuses and chronic ear disease were also at great risk. Although this risk has been reduced, so has awareness of the possibility of cerebral abscess, and this is thought to account for the delay in diagnosis that is so often fatal. Finally, cerebral abscess may complicate head injuries, particularly those involving the paranasal sinuses and the middle ear. This is discussed further in Chapter 23.

A clue to the possible source of infection can sometimes be found in the site of the abscess. Bloodborne infections from the lungs or heart, like cerebral metastases and emboli, tend to lodge in the parietal lobes. Frontal abscesses are usually secondary to disease in the paranasal sinuses and temporal lobe and cerebellar abscesses from disease in the middle ear. The infecting organism, particularly from local lesions in the sinuses and ears, is usually the pneumococcus, although in some instances no definite organism can be cultured. For this reason, penicillin in adequate dosage (up to 24: Mu per 24 hours) is the most reliable treatment unless cultures and sensitivities suggest otherwise.

Too often, inadequate treatment with newer antibiotics in the mistaken belief that the abscess is due to an unusual or resistant organism, is responsible for therapeutic failure. Blood cultures, CSF cultures (if the fluid can be safely obtained – see below) and aspirated pus from the abscess should be obtained.

Suspected cerebral abscess is probably the most dangerous situation in which to perform a lumbar puncture. With the meningitis-like onset – a patient with headache, fever, confusion and perhaps a stiff neck – the immediate reaction is to arrange a lumbar puncture. It is now standard practice to perform a CT scan in all such patients **before** lumbar puncture, even when meningitis is suspected, to avoid this risk. In the days before scanning fine clinical judgement was called for in managing this difficult situation. Due to the rapid onset of the considerable oedema that usually occurs around an abscess, the risk of coning was high. Papilloedema rarely had time to develop and its absence could not be taken as evidence that there was no risk. This is another situation where management has been transformed by the availability of modern scanning techniques. In spite of this, sadly, the prognosis for patients with cerebral abscess has improved little in the last 30 years. The following cases may be cited as examples of the different types of presentation of cerebral abscess.

CASE REPORT XXXIV

A 60-year-old man with known compensated cyanotic heart disease presented with a 7-day history of headache, drowsiness and increasing dysphasia. He had been running an intermittent fever. A lumbar puncture at the referring hospital revealed a pressure of 260: mmHg and the fluid contained 56 cells, 50% polymorphs and 50% lymphocytes. The protein was 100: Mg% and the CSF sugar normal. Further investigation revealed an abscess in the left temporal lobe, which was successfully drained.

The history, presentation and underlying disease made the diagnosis obvious in this patient, but he was fortunate to survive the ill-advised lumbar puncture.

CASE REPORT XXXV

A 32-year-old woman who had had a normal pregnancy and delivery 2 years previously presented with a 2-month history of headache and focal epileptic seizures involving the left face and left arm. In retrospect, it was possible that an isolated focal fit had occurred a year previously. Prior to admission an attack left her with permanent weakness of the left face and arm and a peculiar affect. Right carotid angiography revealed an avascular mass in the right frontal lobe. At craniotomy for glioma pus was encountered and a ß-haemolytic streptococcus was cultured. She made a full recovery following surgery.

This history is typical of the subacute 'space-occupying' lesion type of presentation, in a clinical setting in which the original source of infection is not certain.

Other infective diseases causing cerebral masses are relatively rare in Great Britain. The syphilitic intracerebral gumma has become a museum disease and intracranial tuberculoma an extremely rare disease, although in India tuberculosis accounts for 20% of all intracranial masses. Hydatid cysts are rare in Europe but account for 30% of intracranial tumours in several South American countries. Clearly, these disorders must be considered in immigrants and those who have served overseas in endemic areas.

Unfortunately, the advent of AIDS has introduced a completely new range of previously extremely rare conditions in Britain. With the exception of cryptococcal meningitis in patients with malignant lymphoma, cerebral disease due to fungal infections was almost unknown. Now, when multiple cerebral lesions with scan appearances like a cerebral abscess are found, fungal infection of the brain has to be considered in the differential diagnosis in patients known to be at risk.

Two other conditions that need to be considered in the same group of patients presenting with evidence of diffuse cerebral dysfunction are progressive multifocal leukoencephalopathy due to an opportunistic infection by a polyoma virus, and multiple primary cerebral lymphoma. Both conditions were almost reportable 20 years ago but have now become relatively common. (Other infectious diseases of the nervous system are discussed in Chapter 24.)

Investigation of a Suspected Cerebral Mass

In the previous edition of this book several pages were devoted at this point to methods of investigation, and a whole chapter later in the book amplified these techniques further. Many of these investigations are now consigned to the history books in the developed world. The main constraint on modern investigations remains their availability and expense.

1. The history and physical examination remain the gold standard for the initial assessment of any patient suspected of suffering from a primary or secondary cerebral neoplasm. Examples in this chapter emphasize the paucity of physical signs in many instances.

Routine chest X-rays and a careful breast examination in females will exclude the majority of underlying neoplasms. All previous surgical procedures should be reviewed. Very often patients have not been told of or have forgotten the removal of a malignant tumour many years previously. Previous tumours of the thyroid gland and kidney are notorious for producing cerebral metastases many years later, and any patient who has had a malignant melanoma in the past should be regarded as at risk for the rest of their life.

2. Plain skull films are almost always normal. Erosion of the dorsum sella was usually found only in the presence of chronic raised intracranial pressure and pineal shift was thought to occur only in patients who would have very obvious clinical evidence of a large mass in one hemisphere. Since the advent of CT scanning one of the surprises has been the massive intracranial brain displacements that can be found in a patient who has walked into the clinic and given their history and who have little or nothing to find on physical examination. Clearly, sella erosion and pineal shift on straight X-rays were extremely crude and unreliable signs but they were all we had!

Abnormal intracranial calcification may still occasionally provide a diagnostic clue to the presence of a meningioma, craniopharyngioma or oligodendroglioma. These days intracranial calcification is usually a chance finding when the patient has skull X-ray following mild head trauma. At least it is now possible to evaluate this finding further without subjecting the patient to unpleasant and dangerous investigations.

Skull X-rays are usually abnormal in patients with a pituitary tumour, and plain skull films and a coned view of the sella are still an inexpensive and reliable way of confirming the suspicion of a pituitary lesion.

3. For 50 years an EEG has been regarded as a useful screening test for the presence of cerebral tumour. In general it is more likely to be abnormal in the presence of an intrinsic tumour, and it is well known that slow-growing surface lesions often produce little or no abnormality on the EEG. This means that the EEG is more likely to be confirmatory in those cases where there is little clinical doubt that there is a problem, and in those cases where it could be of most help there has to be considerable reservations about its value. At present electroencephalography is of most value in the assessment of patients who have presented with an epileptic fit, although it may be misleadingly normal. Some of these problems were discussed earlier in this chapter. Interpretation by the clinician in charge of the case is more likely to avoid unnecessary investigation of dubious abnormalities. It is always useful to personally review and discuss the EEG with the reporting neurophysiologist.

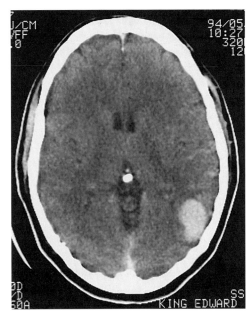

CRXXXVI. Surface lesion thought to be a meningioma presenting as possible transient ischaemic attacks over 5 years.

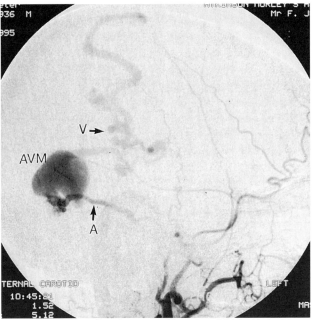

Note: (A) rapid filling of arteriovenous malformation, AVM the blush of the AVM itself and (V) large venous drainage vessel.

CRXXXVI. External carotid subtraction angiogram in same case shows an arteriovenous malformation.

CASE REPORT XXXVI

A 59-year-old man was seen on three occasions in the outpatients clinic over 5 years. On the first occasion the history suggested an epileptic event with a dysphasic component, but an EEG was entirely normal. On the second occasion the attack was longer lasting and accompanied by some facial asymmetry and clumsiness of the hand, and a transient ischaemic attack had to be considered. No risk factors were identified and an EEG was again normal. On the third

occasion, 4 years later, an attack readily diagnosable as a transient ischaemic episode occurred, with dysphasia, numbness and weakness of the right face and arm lasting 15 minutes. An EEG was again normal. On this occasion it was decided that a CT scan looking for evidence of previous vascular insults should be performed, and what appeared to be a meningioma the size of a plum, overlying the left parietal cortex, was demonstrated. Subsequent angiography revealed that this was in fact a dural arterio-venous malformation. This was successfully surgically resected.

4. Ultrasound investigation first found its place in clinical investigation in cerebral disease. The basic problem of detecting the midline echo through the thickness of the skull with reflection of the sound waves from the inside of the skull was never really solved, and convincing midline shift was only really demonstrable when the clinical situation was already obvious. It is no longer used for this purpose, but fortunately other applications in the field of cardiology and obstetrics have prevented its demise and ultrasound scanning of the neck vessels has become the most important non-invasive technique for investigating the cerebral circulation.

5. The advent of CT scanning in the 1970s and MRI scanning in the 1980s has transformed investigation. The original manuscript for the first edition of this book was completed in 1975, and it was only while revising this text that the full magnitude of this change became apparent. A great deal of the previous edition was written with the intention of guiding logical and, wherever possible, harmless investigation to exclude or confirm the presence of neurological disease. Our ability to harm the patient with inappropriate, inadvisable or dangerous investigations was such that a great deal of time was spent anguishing over the indications for the various investigations then available. Today's neophyte neurologist can have little concept as to how difficult this was, and there seems to be a danger that much important clinical knowledge will disappear as the requirement for sound clinical judgement is apparently replaced by scanning. If the same strict criteria for reaching diagnostic conclusions **before** investigation continue to be applied, then hopefully the best and most economical use of these valuable but expensive modern investigational techniques will be achieved.

Within a few years of the advent of CT scanning it was apparent that the distinction between cerebrovascular accidents and tumours was not always clearcut, and serial scans had to be performed to clarify the initial findings. Many conditions still remain undiagnosed and undiagnosable by CT scanning.

MRI has resolved some of these difficulties and has added conditions such as multiple sclerosis to those that can now be diagnosed by scanning techniques, but the pathological basis of the changes seen on MRI remain uncertain and there is still much to be learned.

6. Angiography retains a small role in the investigation of cerebral tumours, particularly in demonstrating the vascular supply of meningiomas. It is no longer a front-line investigational technique in the management of suspected cerebral tumour, and the amazingly detailed signal void of the flowing blood in the cerebral vasculature on MRI scans can give better visualization of the exact anatomy of the blood vessels than is achievable by angiography, and dynamic MRI scanning will improve this further.

As a final example of the application of all the clinical skills, history taking, examination, investigation and the outcome from surgery for even benign lesions, the following case is instructive.

CASE REPORT XXXVII

*A 61-year-old lady was referred with chronic depression. Seven years before her husband had died unexpectedly, and she became depressed and gave up her work. Her sons left home and she found even voluntary jobs impossible because of poor concentration. There were no other symptoms. On examination, she was very mentally and physically slowed with a parkinsonian gait. She had a palmar mental reflex on the **left** side, a **left** grasp reflex and possible bilateral extensor plantar responses. Smell sensation was normal. There were no other signs of extrapyramidal disease. A CT scan revealed a large **right** subfrontal meningioma with extensive oedema. During surgery she suffered massive intra-operative bleeding and post-operative scans revealed bilateral frontal oedema and infarction in the left anterior cerebral distribution. Six months later she remains apathetic, poorly motivated and incontinent of urine and faeces.*

The early history was reasonably regarded as depressive by her general practitioner. The clinical picture of mental and physical slowing was very strongly suggestive of frontal lobe damage. In spite of the diagnosis being confirmed by scanning within an hour of her being seen in the clinic, the ultimate

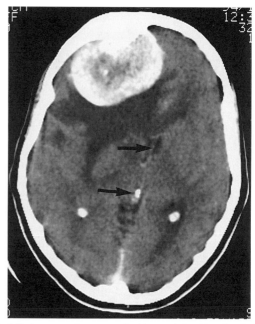

Marked displacement of septum pellucidum and pineal in spite of which patient had minimal physical signs

CRXXXVII. *Subfrontal meningioma presenting as an atypical depression*

outcome is a sad example of the unpredictable aspects of even 'benign' cerebal cerebral tumours. It is certainly proof that the expressions 'benign' or 'malignant' in the field of cerebral tumours are relative terms.

The diagnosis of cerebral tumours is based in the first instance on the history and physical signs. Subsequent management is based on investigations as seem appropriate to the clinical diagnosis. At all stages a continual review of the situation and the evidence provided by the tests already performed should be evaluated and the need to repeat the investigations considered. It is quite possible to fail to demonstrate a tumour at the first attempt, and it should always be remembered that there is still no absolutely exclusory test. Even CT and MRI are not infallible. Any patient in whom there was sufficient suspicion to investigate for a tumour should remain under clinical review until any uncertainty is resolved.

9. The Cerebral Hemispheres: Vascular Diseases

In the previous chapter the anatomy of the hemispheres was described and this knowledge applied to the detection of dysfunction in various areas, in particular the features of damage in the various lobes of the brain. This has special application in the detection of cerebral tumours.

When we consider the blood supply of the cerebral hemisphere the single most important point that emerges is that each lobe does not have an individual blood supply, so that vascular disease produces an entirely different group of clinical syndromes, although on occasions some overlap with disease affecting specific lobes can occur.

At the simplest level a 'hemiparesis' or 'hemiplegia' means no more and no less than that there is an abnormality in the opposite hemisphere. A very common error is to assume that 'hemiparesis' or 'hemiplegia' is synonymous with a 'stroke', an assumption that may lead to a serious diagnostic error and a treatable condition such as a subdural haematoma being missed.

To make the clinical differentiation between a neoplastic or other space-occupying lesion and a stroke one must rely very substantially on the temporal history, and yet the abruptness of onset that characterizes a vascular lesion may occur with a cerebral tumour, and conversely but much less frequently a stroke may have a subacute onset that mimics a tumour. Therefore, a very accurately plotted anatomical extent of the lesion can be critical in making the differential diagnosis.

The use of the term 'a small stroke' should be avoided. It is often used loosely in an attempt to suggest diagnostic precision, but in reality it cloaks clinical uncertainty. The smaller the postulated stroke, the more precisely the area of damage and its arterial supply should be identified. This label falls into the same category as the ubiquitous 'trapped nerve' so beloved of fringe medicine practitioners and the public. Unfortunately, neurologists are obliged to define precisely which nerve is involved; the 'nerve to the arm' will not suffice!

The advent of CT and MRI has made the detection of intracerebral haemorrhage more certain and has revealed that, in the past, many cases that would have been regarded as infarction were indeed haemorrhages, but the distinction between a cerebral infarct and a low-grade glioma can still be difficult and require serial scanning to be certain of the diagnosis.

The Arterial Blood Supply of the Cerebral Hemispheres

The hemispheres are supplied by the terminal branches of the carotid and basilar arteries. There are anastomoses between the various branches over the cortex, and the efficiency of these collateral supplies is often critical in determining the final extent of infarction following major vessel occlusions (Fig. 9.1).

The Anterior Cerebral Artery (Fig. 9.2)

The anterior cerebral artery arises from the internal carotid artery in the cavernous sinus and sweeps forward and over the genu of the corpus callosum and then backwards, dividing into two vessels, the pericallosal and callosomarginal arteries, supplying the parasaggital cortex, including the entire motor and sensory cortex controlling the leg. The supply of the vessel extends posteriorly to the Rolandic fissure. Shortly after its origin the anterior cerebral artery gives off an inconstant branch known as the recurrent artery of Huebner. If present, this vessel contributes to the blood supply of the descending motor fibres in the internal capsule destined to supply the cranial nerve nuclei and the arm on the opposite side.

The two anterior cerebral arteries are joined together by a short anterior communicating artery which allows collateral flow to the opposite hemisphere if the carotid artery is occluded on either side. Whenever carotid ligation or embolization is contemplated in the treatment of an aneurysm or arteriovenous fistula, the patency of this vessel should be demonstrated angiographically

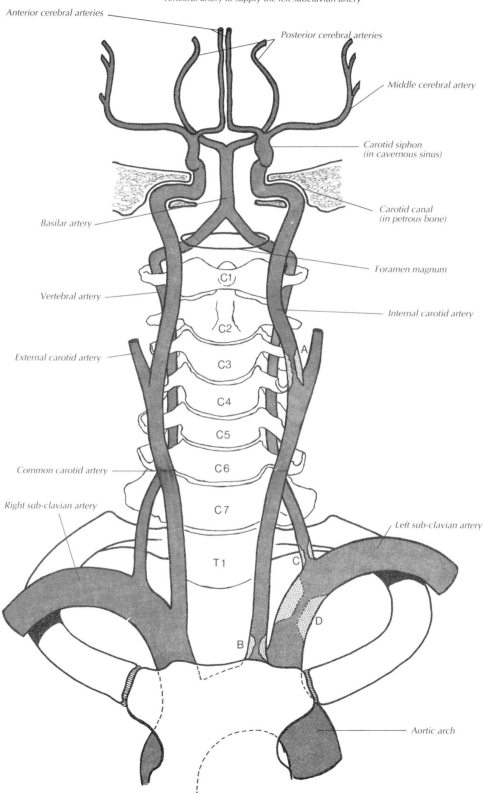

A, B, C are common atheroma sites
Lesions at A & B produce transient hemiparetic ischaemic attacks
Lesions at C produce brainstem ischaemic episodes
Lesions at D produce the "subclavian steal syndrome" – blood
passes up the left carotid artery and back down the left
vertebral artery to supply the left subclavian artery

Anterior cerebral arteries

Posterior cerebral arteries

Middle cerebral artery

Carotid siphon
(in cavernous sinus)

Basilar artery

Carotid canal
(in petrous bone)

Foramen magnum

Vertebral artery

Internal carotid artery

External carotid artery

Common carotid artery

Right sub-clavian artery

Left sub-clavian artery

Aortic arch

C1
C2
C3
C4
C5
C6
C7
T1

A
C
B
D

9.1   The extracranial circulation of the brain.

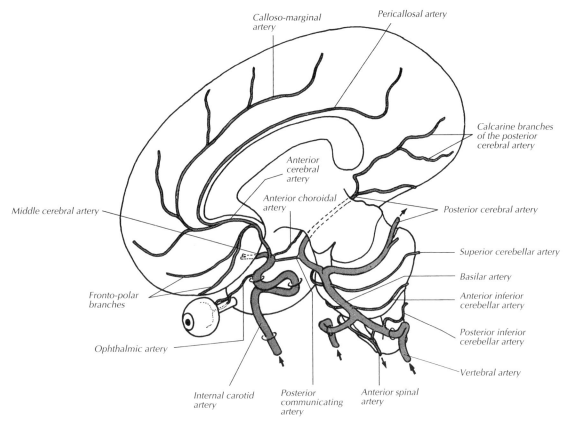

9.2   Intracranial circulation of the brain.

before treatment. Patency is also critical in patients who sustain complete occlusion of one carotid artery, and an adequate collateral circulation through this vessel may prevent the development of disability.

The Middle Cerebral Artery (Fig. 9.4)

This artery originates at the bifurcation of the internal carotid artery just above the cavernous sinus. The vessel then passes laterally between the upper surface of the temporal lobe and the inferior surface of the frontal lobe to reach a position deep in the Sylvian fissure. Here it divides into three main vessels, the trifurcation of the middle cerebral artery, where large emboli are prone to lodge as the arterial lumen suddenly narrows dramatically. These vessels pass upwards and backwards in the fissure, giving off branches that exit along the length of the fissure to supply the lateral surface of the hemisphere. These are the precentral, central, posterior parietal and posterior temporal arteries.

As the middle cerebral artery passes laterally it gives off a series of six to twelve long thin penetrating vessels that enter the anterior perforated substance to supply the basal ganglia and part of the internal capsule. These are the lenticulostriate arteries.

Terminal branches of the main vessel reach the occipital pole (see below) and possibly provide an additional blood supply to the macular cortex at the tip of the lobe.

The Posterior Cerebral Artery

The posterior cerebral arteries are formed by the bifurcation of the basilar artery in the interpeduncular space (Figs 9.2 and 9.4). Each vessel passes round the cerebral peduncles lying between the medial surface of the temporal lobe and the upper brain stem. Along its length each gives off vessels supplying the inferior medial surface and hippocampal area of the temporal lobe. A series of penetrating vessels supplies the dorsolateral brain stem, the thalamus, posterior internal capsule and sublenticular and retrolenticular visual radiations. These are the thalamogeniculate and thalamoperforating arteries.

The main vessel continues as the calcarine artery, supplying the visual cortex with the exception of the macular cortex at the tip of the pole. This has an additional blood supply from the middle cerebral artery (see macular-sparing hemianopia, Chapter 3).

Clinical Features Produced by Cerebral Blood Vessel Occlusions

The term occlusion is used reservedly. Following a cerebrovascular accident it is unusual to find a vessel actually occluded. This is because most occlusions are now known to be due to temporary embolic blockage,

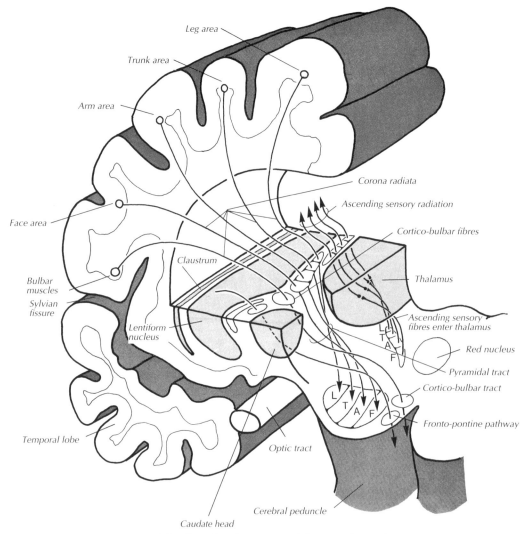

9.3 Functional anatomy of the capsular region.

with rapid subsequent recanalization. However, a few minutes' obstruction of flow in any vessel leads to irreversible damage to the territory supplied. There are three main patterns of damage that can occur:

Occlusion of the main trunk of the parent vessel
Occlusion of one of the important penetrating arteries
Occlusion of one of the terminal branches

These three possibilities will be considered for each vessel in turn.

Anterior Cerebral Artery Occlusion (Fig. 9.5)

Main Trunk Occlusions

Anterior cerebral artery occlusions are quite rare. The picture depends to some extent on whether or not the recurrent artery of Heubner is present.

1. If there is no recurrent artery the face and arm will not be affected, but the entire leg area of the cortex is destroyed. This causes flaccid paralysis of the leg, with cortical sensory loss.

2. If there is a recurrent artery and the block occurs proximal to its origin, the anterior internal capsule will also be infarcted giving rise to a typical upper motor neuron facial weakness and a spastic arm, with considerable potential for recovery (because the overlying arm cortex is intact) but a useless flaccid leg (because all cortical control, both motor and sensory, is lost, with poor potential for good recovery).

Because the paracentral lobules are also damaged, voluntary control of micturition is often impaired, with incontinence of urine a common consequence. In such instances the patient is unable to inhibit the desire to pass water the moment they are aware of the full bladder, with sudden uncontrolled bladder emptying (see Chapter 15). In some instances this

9.4 Blood supply to the capsular region.

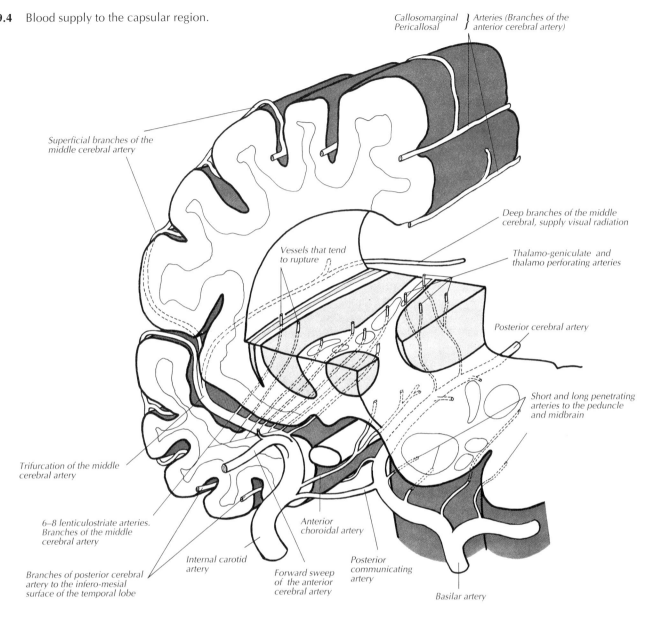

Callosomarginal ⎫ Arteries (Branches of the
Pericallosal ⎬ anterior cerebral artery)

Superficial branches of the
middle cerebral artery

Deep branches of the middle
cerebral, supply visual radiation

Vessels that tend
to rupture

Thalamo-geniculate and
thalamo perforating arteries

Posterior cerebral artery

Short and long penetrating
arteries to the peduncle
and midbrain

Trifurcation of the middle
cerebral artery

6–8 lenticulostriate arteries.
Branches of the middle
cerebral artery

Anterior
choroidal artery

Internal carotid
artery

Posterior
communicating
artery

Branches of posterior cerebral
artery to the infero-mesial
surface of the temporal lobe

Forward sweep
of the anterior
cerebral artery

Basilar artery

combination of incontinence and flaccid weakness of the leg may prompt an ineffectual search for a cauda equina lesion. The clinical evidence against this possibility would be that in spite of the flaccidity of the leg the reflexes rapidly return and become brisk, and the plantar response is extensor. These findings would be very unusual with a cauda equina lesion, which usually causes areflexia and absent plantar responses (see Chapter 15). Furthermore, considerable intellectual deficit and memory disturbance may occur owing to damage to frontoparietal and frontotemporal fibres in the cingulate gyrus. In all cases, if there is any evidence that the other leg is also affected (i.e. the lesion is not strictly unilateral) a parasaggital tumour must be excluded. Vascular occlusions affecting the hemisphere should not produce bilateral signs.

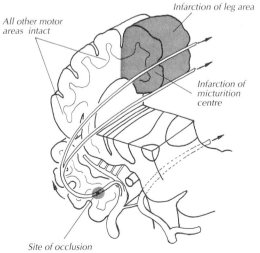

Infarction of leg area

All other motor
areas intact

Infarction of
micturition
centre

Site of occlusion

9.5 Anterior cerebral artery occlusion.

Perforating Artery Occlusion

If the recurrent artery of Heubner is present and is occluded, weakness of the face and arm will occur; this will be of pyramidal type. Even if the dominant hemisphere is involved dysphasia does not occur because the cortex is unaffected. This is a very rare syndrome.

Terminal Branch Occlusion

The terminal vessels primarily supply the cortex controlling the leg and infarction affects both motor and sensory function. Flaccid weakness of the leg with brisk reflexes and an extensor plantar response will be found. The sensory loss affects accurate touch perception and joint position sense. It is of the cortical type. This makes it almost impossible for the patient to mobilize, as even with splints to stiffen the leg they have no awareness of its position. With distal lesions intellectual disturbances and bladder dysfunction may be less severe than those caused by a main trunk occlusion.

Middle Cerebral Artery Occlusions

Main Trunk Occlusions (Fig. 9.6)

Middle cerebral artery occlusion causes massive infarction of the bulk of the hemisphere. There is often considerable cerebral oedema, which may cause coma and eventual death. There are also important differences between the hemispheres, with global dysphasia if the dominant hemisphere is affected and severe dyspraxia or even denial of the existence of the whole left side if the non-dominant hemisphere is affected.

From a motor point of view the lesion destroys both pyramidal and extrapyramidal mechanisms, hence a

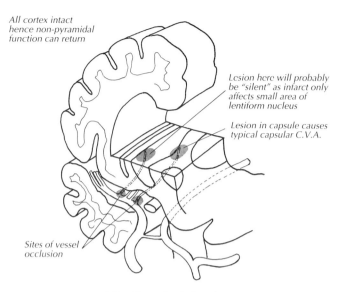

9.7   Capsular infarction.

flaccid type of weakness of the face and arm, with little or no potential for recovery, is found. The leg cortex is spared but is so extensively 'undercut' by the lesion that even the leg rarely improves significantly. This is quite the most devastating type of cerebrovascular accident, with very minimal improvement to be anticipated and a real chance that the patient may die from the acute swelling of the infarcted hemisphere, because the oedema due to a vascular lesion is unresponsive to treatment with high-dose steroids or osmotic agents. Hemianaesthesia and a complete hemianopia are usually associated with the hemiparesis.

The clinical picture can be identical with that produced by total occlusion of the carotid artery in the neck, with cross-circulation via the anterior communicating artery keeping the anterior cerebral area perfused and the posterior cerebral circulation functioning normally. These anastomoses may be so efficient that patients are sometimes seen who have developed complete carotid artery occlusion and have sustained no neurological deficit.

Perforating Artery Occlusions (Capsular Cerebrovascular Accident) (Fig. 9.7)

A cerebrovascular accident due to occlusion of one of the lenticulostriate vessels is both the most frequent type and the most favourable. Several of these vessels may be occluded without demonstrable effect. The evidence for this statement takes two forms. First, extrapyramidal syndromes are extremely rare in vascular disease of the brain and infarction in the basal ganglia may occur with little clinical deficit. Yet a substantial part of the basal ganglia is supplied by these vessels. Secondly, there is the evidence provided by a 'pseudobulbar palsy'. The explanation of this condition

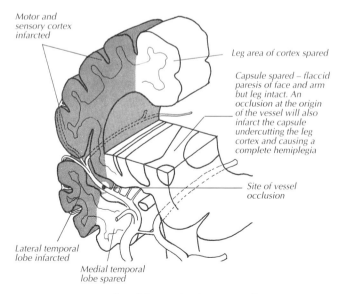

9.6   Distal middle cerebral artery occlusion.

is rarely understood by students. The mechanism is as follows: a vessel supplying the corticobulbar fibres to the brainstem nuclei on one side, is occluded. Because most of these nuclei have 50:50 innervation from each hemisphere, little or no deficit occurs and the episode may pass unnoticed. If some time later, the corticobulbar fibres on the other side are damaged the cranial nerve nuclei are abruptly deprived of all control. The result is the acute onset of serious difficulty with speaking, chewing and swallowing, with a grave risk of aspiration. Significant recovery is unusual: patients often need tube feeding or gastrostomy for the rest of their life, and recurrent aspiration pneumonia occurs. The syndrome is most often seen in diabetic or hypertensive patients, as both groups are prone to develop widespread small-vessel disease.

When one of the vessels supplying the main motor pathways of the capsule is occluded a typical 'capsular cerebrovascular accident' occurs. Usually the only evidence of corticobulbar fibre damage is a mild upper motor neuron facial weakness, but if the patient is seen very soon after the onset transitory weakness of palatal and tongue movements may be detectable for a few hours on the same side as the facial weakness. Initially a flaccid hemiplegia will be found. In this acute stage no reflexes or plantar responses can be elicited.

Within hours, tone starts to return, the reflexes become brisk and an extensor plantar response will appear. As tone increases power will return in a pyramidal distribution (see Chapter 8). The flexor groups in the arm and the extensor groups in the leg become stronger. The functional importance of this distribution of power results in the majority of patients leaving hospital with the typical hemiplegic gait, the arm flexed up in front of the chest and the leg stiff and circumducting to avoid scuffing the ground. Physiotherapy can capitalize on this functional distribution and help the patient learn to make the best use of the compromised limbs, but contrary to the patient's perception, physiotherapy is not responsible for the recovery which is to be anticipated.

There is rarely any sensory deficit or visual field defect, as both these pathways lie in the vascular territory of the posterior cerebral artery. A combination of hemiplegia, hemianaesthesia and hemianopia is not typical of capsular infarction, and the prognosis in such cases is poor. These patients have either had a complete middle cerebral artery occlusion (see above), an anterior choroidal artery occlusion (see later), or a haemorrhage into the internal capsule, which does not respect arterial territories.

A capsular lesion in the dominant hemisphere is not accompanied by dysphasia because the overlying parietal cortex is unaffected. A distinction must be made between dysphasia and dysarthria. Dysarthria means poor phonation. With a capsular lesion in the acute stages severe weakness of the face may lead to slurring of speech, but the patient understands the spoken word and uses words correctly. There is really no reason at all for there to be any confusion about the use of these terms. Dysphasia is defined as difficulty in understanding the written or spoken word and the inability to formulate an appropriate answer, even though the patient is capable of phonation.

Terminal Branch Occlusions

There are four major peripheral branches on each side, with different clinical manifestations depending on cerebral dominance.

Dominant Hemisphere. The precentral artery supplies the motor areas for the face and arm and Broca's speech area. Occlusion of this vessel causes flaccid paralysis of the face and arm and total inability to speak, but with full comprehension. As the patient is also unable to write his anguish and frustration are considerable. Recovery is minimal, although speech therapy may occasionally have a modest success in helping these patients to say a few key words, and word-finding boards or electronic communication devices may be helpful. If the central artery is occluded weakness of the face and arm occurs, with mild dysphasic difficulties.

Occlusion of the posterior parietal artery produces complete aphasia with loss of comprehension and loss of speech, even though the patient may well be able to phonate and even say single irrelevant words, or new words of his own making (neologisms), or incoherent sentences of otherwise normal words (word salads). There may be a mild hemiparesis and cortical sensory loss but the latter is usually impossible to ascertain owing to the lack of communication.

Occlusion of the superior temporal artery tends to cause receptive aphasia. The patient may be able to speak but the sentences are irrelevant and inappropriate to the examiner's question.

Non-Dominant Hemisphere. Superficial branch occlusions in the non-dominant hemisphere produce similar findings, although the dysphasic difficulties are replaced by dyspraxia. Precentral and central branch occlusions cause a flaccid monoplegia of the arm and face. Occlusions of the posterior parietal and superior temporal arteries may cause mild sensory difficulties in the left face and arm and more generalized difficulties such as dressing apraxia or geographical disorientation and difficulty with skilled tasks.

Posterior Cerebral Artery Occlusions (Fig. 9.8)

Main Vessel Occlusions

The effects of a complete posterior cerebral artery occlusion can be very variable as there are numerous anastomoses between the vessel and the middle cerebral arteries. Variable degrees of confusion and memory deficit can occur, but these are more suggestive of bilateral damage due to occlusion of the basilar artery than occlusion of a single posterior cerebral artery. There may be some memory deficit with unilateral lesions and it has been postulated that in some patients there is a dominant hemisphere for memory. There may also be some sensory deficit and a field defect due to thalamogeniculate artery occlusion, damaging the posterior limb of the capsule and the visual radiations.

Perforating Vessel Occlusion

Occlusion of one of the thalamogeniculate vessels produces a more readily recognizable clinical picture. The posterior limb of the internal capsule, part of the thalamus and the visual radiation are affected, resulting in hemianaesthesia with loss of all sensory modalities and complete hemianopia (the visual radiation is damaged in its entirety). Often a good recovery is achieved but the main risk is the subsequent development of the Dejerine–Roussy syndrome which may follow this type of cerebrovascular accident. When this happens the initial numbness is replaced by paraesthesia, or a painful sensation which becomes excruciating in severity when the affected limb is touched, or even continual pain without provocation. This is typically a scalded, burning sensation as if the side were on fire or conversely as if the side were covered in icy-cold slime. Both sensations are extremely unpleasant and may drive the patient to suicide. It is rarely responsive to drugs or surgical procedures. Occasionally control may be achieved with diphenylhydantoin or carbamazepine combined with imipramine or chlorpromazine.

If the branches to the upper brain stem are affected hemiballismus may occur. This is the only extrapyramidal syndrome typically produced by vascular disease. It consists of the abrupt onset of wild flinging movements of the limbs on one side of the body. It may subside spontaneously but can usually be arrested dramatically by 50 mg chlorpromazine intramuscularly. For longer-term control, if the movements continue tetrabenazine 12.5–25 mg t.d.s. may be helpful (see Chapter 12 for further discussion).

Terminal Branch Occlusion

Occlusion of the calcarine artery causes a macular-sparing hemianopia (see Chapter 3). This can occur in otherwise fit young persons during the course of a migraine attack. Incomplete lesions can cause a variety of incomplete hemianopias but in all cases the deficit will be absolutely congruous and will spare the macular, making identification easy. A CT or MRI scan will usually demonstrate the area of damage and is always worth performing. A surprisingly high yield of unanticipated intrinsic or extrinsic tumours, especially meningiomas, may be found in this area, presenting with a vascular-type onset.

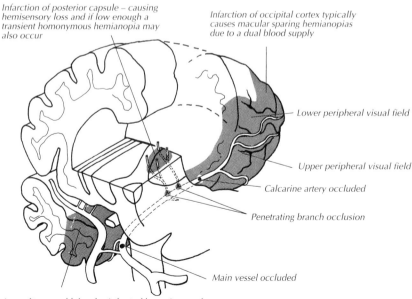

Infarction of posterior capsule – causing hemisensory loss and if low enough a transient homonymous hemianopia may also occur

Infarction of occipital cortex typically causes macular sparing hemianopias due to a dual blood supply

Lower peripheral visual field

Upper peripheral visual field

Calcarine artery occluded

Penetrating branch occlusion

Main vessel occluded

Area of temporal lobe also infarcted by main vessel occlusion but unless bilateral minimal memory deficit occurs

9.8   Posterior cerebral artery occlusions.

Anterior Choroidal Artery Occlusions

The anterior choroidal artery arises directly from the carotid artery and runs backwards along the optic tract to the area under the internal capsule, eventually supplying the choroid plexus of the lateral ventricle. It has a variable distribution that includes the optic tract and the basal ganglia. At one stage surgical ligation was attempted as a possible treatment for parkinsonism, but this occasionally produced devastating disabilities including hemiparesis, and was quickly abandoned. It seems likely that some patients who develop hemiparesis, hemisensory loss and hemianopia, and who clearly have not had a middle cerebral artery occlusion as there is no flaccidity, no drowsiness, no dysphasia or dyspraxia, may have suffered an occlusion of the anterior choroidal artery and have infarcted the subcapsular area and the optic tract.

Development of Symptoms and Signs of a Vascular Accident

The clinical pictures produced by infarction of various areas of the central nervous system have been outlined. If the damage is clearly in one of these territories, the chance that the lesion is a vascular one is high. However, the majority of diagnoses of 'stroke' are based on historical features. We will examine some of these features critically to show how valuable an accurate topographical diagnosis can be in substantiating a clinical impression.

Abrupt Onset of Symptoms

The term 'stroke' emphasizes the single characteristic feature of a vascular accident – its very abrupt onset. Yet so often the patient, often elderly and living alone, is found drowsy, confused and dysphasic and the mode of onset cannot be established. In such instances it is safest to pursue other diagnostic possibilities.

Drowsiness or increasing neurological deficit over a period of hours can occur following a middle cerebral occlusion, but if the onset was not very abrupt, metabolic disorders, subdural or extradural haematomas, meningeal infection or herpes simplex encephalitis must be excluded. In the elderly patient meningitis may present as a stroke-like illness, with confusion, minimal pyrexia and little or no neck stiffness.

A further cause of acute hemiparesis with or without confusion that should always be considered is hypoglycaemia. There is clinical and experimental evidence that poor perfusion of one hemisphere may lead to focal symptoms such as hemiparesis when the blood sugar reaches dangerously low levels.

CASE REPORT I

A 52-year old woman presented with a 1-week history of recurrent transient hemiparesis. An attack was seen during which a purely motor deficit of the left face and arm developed lasting less than 5 minutes. It was accompanied by a mild headache but the patient was otherwise normal. There was no pallor, sweating or confusion. She was normotensive and because of a bed crisis could not be admitted immediately for investigation. She was given aspirin and a booked admission was arranged. Two days later she was brought to the accident centre with a rather more dramatic episode, a dense left hemiparesis lasting 30 minutes. Again she was otherwise asymptomatic. She was admitted and the routine fasting blood sugar, part of the vascular work-up, was 1.8 m.mols. Further investigation revealed an islet-cell tumour in the head of the pancreas, which was successfully removed. Six weeks postoperatively the patient collapsed at home, was admitted as an emergency and died of complications related to the surgery.

Conversely, the extremely abrupt onset of disability can occur with a cerebral tumour. Previously this situation was always attributed to haemorrhage into the cerebral tumour, and yet such haemorrhage was a surprisingly rare finding at post mortem. Since the advent of scanning it is apparent that haemorrhage into tumours is extremely rare, with perhaps metastatic melanoma being the only exception. The cause of sudden deterioration appears to be acute oedema developing around a tumour, with sudden brain shifts. The patient below was seen in 1961, before sophisticated investigation was available, but is included as an extraordinary example of this type of presentation.

CASE REPORT II

A 28-year-old pregnant woman collapsed and became deeply unconscious while preparing a meal. She had a complete right hemiparesis and fixed dilated pupils. A skull X-ray revealed half an inch of pineal shift to the left side. She died while further investigations were being arranged. She was found to have an extensive infiltrating glioma of the left thalamus. She had been asymptomatic until she collapsed.

A Stuttering Onset of Symptoms

Whenever a neurological event has occurred it is always important to establish whether there were any premonitory symptoms. For example, however abrupt the onset of a hemiparesis, if there was a prior history of several weeks' headache, personality change or ill health, the diagnosis of a stroke would certainly be in doubt.

Repeated identical brief episodes of hemiparesis with full recovery quite often occur, and such episodes are called transient ischaemic attacks. These are widely regarded as a sign of an impending stroke, and carotid artery ultrasound and possibly angiography should be considered in an attempt to locate an operable atherosclerotic lesion in the appropriate carotid artery. Even this assumption is not always reliable.

CASE REPORT III

A 56-year-old man gave a history of several brief attacks of left-sided weakness over a 6-week period. There were no residual signs and he was extremely hypertensive. Hypotensive therapy was begun and angiography was not performed in view of the very high blood pressure. A few weeks later a similar episode occurred without recovery. An angiogram performed elsewhere revealed a glioblastoma in the right hemisphere.

This is a good example of the 'vascular' presentation of a neoplasm. Occasionally the reverse may occur and this is a particular feature of complete carotid artery occlusion.

CASE REPORT IV

A 38-year-old woman gave a 10-month history of intermittent sensory symptoms affecting the left side, headache, memory impairment and some personality change. Over a period of 5 days she developed a moderately severe left hemiparesis. Full investigation showed no sign of cerebral tumour but there was almost complete occlusion of the right carotid artery, confirmed by angiography.

CASE REPORT V

A 49-year-old military contracts manager for an aeroplane manufacturer gave a 3-week history of episodic tingling and numbness in the left limbs. This had been associated throughout with a dull right frontal headache. Examination revealed a left attention hemianopia, left-sided facial weakness and impairment of sensation over the entire left side, but no motor signs in the limbs. A tumour was suspected but a carotid angiogram revealed complete occlusion of the right internal carotid artery.

CASE REPORT VI

A 58-year-old company director complained of pins and needles in his left hand for 2 weeks, which had been treated by neck traction. This was followed by attacks of clumsiness of the left hand, weakness of the left side of his face and difficulty in articulating, each attack lasting seconds only. Over 3 weeks things worsened until progressive weakness of the left side was apparent and he became forgetful and drowsy, but denied headache. On admission he was extremely drowsy, with a left hemiparesis and a left extensor plantar response; sensory testing was impossible. A right carotid angiogram showed complete carotid occlusion. Despite attempts to control cerebral oedema he deteriorated and died several days later.

The similarities in the latter case histories are remarkable, and yet when the last patient was seen only 6 weeks after the second, the diagnosis of carotid artery occlusion did not seem likely on the clinical evid-

ence. Carotid artery occlusion may mimic a cerebral tumour so closely that a tumour is almost invariably the suspected diagnosis. CT and MRI have made the evaluation of such cases much easier. All the cases quoted above occurred in the pre-scanning era and serve to emphasize how difficult neurology was in the very recent past, and how dramatic the changes in diagnostic evaluation have been.

Steady Improvement of the Neurological Status

Any abrupt neurological event with rapid recovery certainly qualifies for the term 'a vascular event' and in the majority of instances it will prove to be due to a vascular accident. Unfortunately, in some instances, as already discussed, recovery is not the rule and in the case of a middle cerebral artery occlusion the subsequent oedema may lead to deterioration, coma and even death. An intracerebral haemorrhage may produce a similar picture. This is discussed later.

Immediate loss of consciousness or an epileptic fit are extremely unusual events in an uncomplicated cerebrovascular accident. A major embolus from a fibrillating heart, an intracerebral haemorrhage or a subarachnoid haemorrhage should be suspected if either of these events occurs. Loss of consciousness or an epileptic fit should never be dismissed as being due to a 'small stroke'. They are so unusual in major strokes that the likelihood of their occurring during an otherwise subclinical stroke seems remote.

Headache

Although severe headache of abrupt onset associated with neurological signs is most likely to occur during some form of cerebral haemorrhage, headache of moderate severity is by no means unusual in an uncomplicated occlusive cerebrovascular accident. Occasionally patients with migraine are unfortunate enough to suffer an occlusion during an attack of migraine. This is very often an occlusion of the posterior cerebral artery or its terminal branches. Headache should be regarded as a symptom of uncertain significance in suspected cerebrovascular accidents. It has been suggested in the past that headache in occlusive vascular disease is due to the opening of collateral blood vessels, but these vessels would be in arterial territories that are thought to be insensitive to pain and it is difficult to understand how headache could result. Only the first centimetre of the major blood vessels inside the skull is thought to be pain sensitive.

These problems and illustrative case histories have been included to highlight the fact that, however obvious the diagnosis of 'stroke' may appear to be, the subsequent physical examination should be performed to answer the question 'are these signs compatible with a cerebrovascular accident in a specific vascular territory?' This is essential to avoid compounding an error that may have started with a misleading history.

Other Types of Cerebrovascular Accident

Thrombotic Lesions

Whenever a non-haemorrhagic cerebrovascular accident has occurred some basic disease processes that may predispose to intravascular thrombosis must be excluded, especially in the young patient. Haematological disorders, including polycythaemia rubra vera, thrombotic thrombocytopaenic purpura, disseminated lupus erythematosus, polyarteritis nodosa, coagulopathies and the heavy protein diseases should be excluded.

Diabetes mellitus and syphilis should be considered at any age, and in the elderly a high erythrocyte sedimentation rate (ESR) should be regarded as being due to temporal (cranial) arteritis until proved otherwise. In the younger patient an elevated ESR in addition to collagen vascular disease may indicate an atrial myxoma, another rare cause of transient ischaemic attacks or vascular accidents. All the necessary exclusory tests can be performed quite easily, and should be a routine part of the investigation of any patient with a suspected stroke. Embolization from auricular fibrillation may be the first evidence of thyrotoxicosis, or indicate a recent myocardial infarction; and subacute bacterial endocarditis frequently presents as a cerebrovascular accident.

Haemorrhagic Cerebrovascular Accidents

There are three main types of haemorrhagic cerebrovascular accident. It is now known that many small vascular lesions previously thought to be thrombotic are small lacunar haemorrhages. Because the blood does not burst into the ventricles or subarachnoid space, this type of haemorrhage cannot be distinguished from a small occlusive lesion in the internal capsule or brain stem. CT scanning has indicated that these small intracerebral haemorrhages are both more frequent and have a better prognosis than was ever previously suspected. Unfortunately, it is also probable that many of these patients may have been inappropriately anticoagulated in the past, because there was no way of confirming such lesions with the investigations then available. It is now obvious that clear CSF was not an adequate exclusory investigation for cerebral haemorrhage of this type.

Intracerebral Haemorrhage

A classic intracerebral haemorrhage usually results from the rupture of one of the more peripheral lenticulostriate arteries in the region of the external capsule. The haemorrhage rapidly strips the soft tissue under the cortex and may rupture into the Sylvian fissure or into the lateral ventricle. In either event the typical clinical picture is of a sudden fulminating headache with rapidly deepening loss of consciousness and tentorial herniation. First the ipsilateral pupil and then both pupils dilate and become fixed to light. In a typical case death ensues within 15 minutes to a few hours of the onset (brainstem haemorrhage is discussed in Chapter 12).

Arteriovenous Malformations (Previously Called Angiomas)

A less dramatic form of cerebral haemorrhage is associated with cerebral arteriovenous malformations. Many such lesions remain asymptomatic throughout the patient's life. In many cases uncontrolled focal epilepsy is a major problem and in some instances the first epileptic event seems to occur following a small haemorrhage into the lesion. On CT or MRI scanning there is often evidence of recent haemorrhage, and this is frequently confirmed during subsequent surgery on the lesion. The following case reports exemplify the typical onset that leads to the discovery of arteriovenous malformation.

CASE REPORT VII

A 53-year-old man was admitted after awakening with a slight headache. Two hours later he had difficulty holding objects in his left hand and felt slightly unsteady. Two days after the onset he had a more severe headache, by which time the difficulty with the hand was improving. A CT scan revealed a right parietal intracerebral haemorrhage, and subsequent MRI scanning revealed an extremely large right frontoparietal arteriovenous malformation with evidence of several areas of previous haemorrhage. The lesion was completely resected surgically but unfortunately the patient has been left with focal epilepsy. The risk of a fatal haemorrhage has been completely obviated.

CASE REPORT VIII

A 19-year-old man was referred following a focal epileptic fit affecting the left arm while playing golf. There had been no headache. A CT scan on admission revealed a small parasagittal area of haemorrhage. Two further focal fits occurred over the next 24 hours. In view of his age, haemorrhage into a small arteriovenous malformation was suspected and MRI scanning confirmed the presence of a small vascular lesion, which at surgery proved to be a cavernous haemangioma which was totally excised. Following a postoperative transitory hemiparesis, he recovered fully with only slight clonus and an extensor plantar response in the left leg. No further epileptic events have occurred over a 5-year period, although he remains on prophylactic anticonvulsants.

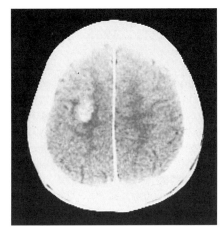

CRVIII.   Cavernous haemangioma presenting as focal epilepsy in a 19 year old.

CASE REPORT IX

A 42-year-old man was admitted after an epileptic fit. He had been on a 6-week business trip, had missed a lot of sleep and been awake for 36 hours prior to the event. He had also had six double whiskies on the evening of his return home. There were no physical findings and an EEG was slightly abnormal, with a suspicion of abnormal activity in both temporal lobes, more marked on the left. In view of the provocative circumstances no further investigations were performed at that time. He remained well for 3 years. A second 'attack' occurred, again associated with jet lag, alcohol and sleep deprivation. His wife had actually documented at least nine episodes prior to the arrival of the ambulance and six more before he reached hospital. This constituted an episode of status epilepticus, and in view of the possible association with frontal lesions a CT scan was performed. This revealed a small calcified lesion in the right frontal pole. An MRI scan suggested that this was a small vascular lesion, but subsequent angiography showed no feeder vessels and surgery was not recommended. He was treated with anticonvulsants and remained well until 1994 (3 years later) when, while on a business trip to Austria, he again went into status epilepticus. This was felt to provide ample justification for surgical excision of the lesion, which had the appearance of gliosis and old haemorrhage, although no definite vascular lesion could be identified histologically. It is thought that it was a small cavernous haemangioma which had self-destructed during one of the haemorrhages, and that the attacks of status were probably consequent upon acute haemorrhages.

In other patients recurrent subarachnoid haemorrhages may occur and as a rule there is a good recovery between attacks. This is because the haemorrhage is from sinusoidal vessels under low pressure, lacking the destructive power of a jet of arterial blood from a ruptured berry aneurysm or an artery. Unfortunately, progressive neurological disability may result from communicating hydrocephalus due to blood products damaging the arachnoid granulations, and in others progressive disability due to the shunting effect of a

large malformation may produce a similar picture. For all these reasons, in recent years a much more aggressive approach to the investigation and surgical removal of arteriovenous malformations has been implemented.

Finally, an acute intracerebral haemorrhage with the development of signs due to a stable intracerebral haematoma may be the first symptom of an arteriovenous malformation.

CASE REPORT X

A 52-year-old man had lunch and drinks with friends. A little later, while walking his dog, he was seen to stumble and fall down a bank. When helped to his feet he was noted to have clumsiness of the right leg. He insisted on going home and for several hours seemed to be well. However, the next morning he had a series of Jacksonian fits, starting in the right arm and becoming generalized. During one of these he fell and injured the occipital region and remained drowsy. He was admitted to hospital. On examination he was drowsy, with a flaccid weakness of the right arm and a spastic weakness of the right leg. He had bilateral extensor plantar responses. The differential diagnostic possibilities were legion but rapid deterioration in his conscious level required urgent surgical help. He was found to have an intracerebral haematoma in the posterior frontal pole associated with two separate arteriovenous malformations. Following evacuation of the haematoma he made a good recovery.

It has now been established that the risk of further haemorrhage is of the order of 1% p.a. and a variety of treatment options are now available. Small lesions may be treated by stereotactic radiosurgery, larger lesions by endovascular embolization, and very large lesions by open surgery with progressive ligation of feeder vessels and removal of the collapsed arteriovenous aneurysm. Because the brain in the area of a congenital malformation is non-functional, the deficit resulting from operating on very large lesions is surprisingly small. Recurrent subarachnoid haemorrhage may cause dementia due to hydrocephalus. This is thought to occur when the arachnoid villi become blocked by blood products and CSF resorption is impaired. A shunt procedure will often be of benefit to the patient in this situation.

Subarachnoid Haemorrhage

Subarachnoid haemorrhage due to aneurysms arising from the vessels traversing the subarachnoid space is a common and frequently lethal cause of intracranial haemorrhage. Although these aneurysms may arise at embryologically weak points on the vessel wall, they are no longer regarded as congenital.

Aneurysms are only found in children in association with coarctation of the aorta or hypertension due to renal disease. At all ages the presence of an aneurysm tends to parallel the height of the blood pressure. This is most dramatically demonstrated by the sudden change in sex ratio after the age of 50. Until then the ratio of females to males is 3:2. Over 50 it rises to 10:1. This is thought to be due to the better long-term survival of females with significant hypertension, leading to the development of aneurysms in the 50–70 age group.

Less than 15% of patients have symptoms prior to rupture and these usually consist of premonitory headaches over a few days. These headaches may be very non-specific indeed, and some confusion has been caused by articles originating in neurosurgical centres which claim that premonitory symptoms of subarachnoid haemorrhage are very common and frequently missed, with fatal results. Such statements rarely take account of the vast number of patients who appear at GP surgeries and in A and E departments 24 hours a day, with mild, modest or severe headaches, and if all such cases were immediately referred to neurosurgical departments as incipient subarachnoid haemorrhage they would be totally overwhelmed and perhaps would become slightly less critical of colleagues who fail to detect the one patient among thousands whose symptoms might be indicative of a pending subarachnoid haemorrhage!

Even when frank haemorrhage has occurred, the similarity of the headache to an ordinary migraine is striking. One clue may be the **simultaneous** onset of vertigo and vomiting with the onset of headache. In migraine the giddiness and vomiting may precede the headache by 30 minutes or more, or occur as a later feature in the course of the headache rather than simultaneously. To further compound the difficulty, photophobia and neck stiffness may occur in a severe migraine. Headache, acute nausea, vomiting and neck stiffness are the hallmarks of both subarachnoid haemorrhage and meningitis. These diagnostic dilemmas are further discussed in Chapter 20.

Transient cardiac arrhythmias or glycosuria often occur in a patient who has had a subarachnoid haemorrhage, for reasons that are not clear. Aneurysm sites and associated symptoms are fully illustrated in Figure 9.9. If there are no signs except those of subarachnoid blood (headache, photophobia, neck stiffness, vomiting, bilateral extensor plantar response) no prediction as to the site of the aneurysm can be made. With the dramatic improvements in techniques, including anaesthesia, the dissecting microscope and better clip design, a direct surgical attack on aneurysms has become the treatment of choice.

Conservative management of a subarachnoid haemorrhage is only applicable to those patients where immediate and follow-up angiograms 1 month later have failed to reveal an aneurysm as the cause. The immediate investigation of choice to confirm the diagnosis, to exclude a life-threatening intracerebral clot, and sometimes even demonstrate the causal aneurysm, is a CT scan. This will reveal blood in the subarachnoid space and, surprisingly often, blood in the ventricular system itself, even when the source of haemorrhage is

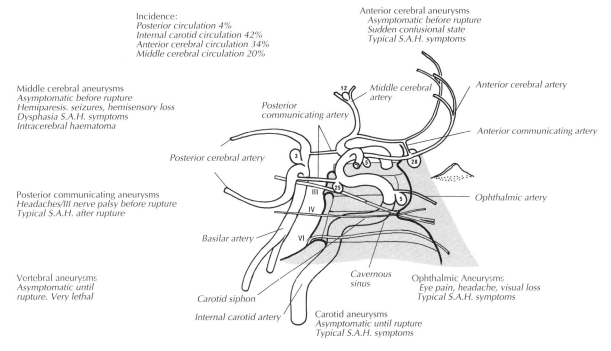

9.9   Aneurysm sites. (Figures indicate % occurence rates at that site – other sites 22% of the total)

not within the ventricle. This rather surprising finding has not been explained but is typified by a CSF/blood fluid level at the back end of the lateral ventricles, in the recumbent scanning position. Rarely will a lumbar puncture be required to confirm the diagnosis.

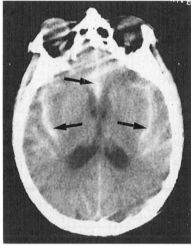

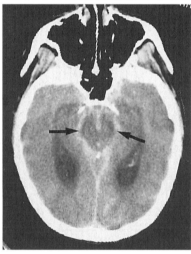

Severe subarachnoid haemorrhage (blood is seen in between the hemispheres, the Sylvian fissure and surrounding the brainstem. This was from an anterior communicating aneurysm

The ideal operative window is still controversial. In the first 7 days coexistent spasm may complicate surgery and lead to infarction, but with the most frequent rebleeds occurring between days 7 and 10, delay beyond 7 days may subject the patient to the compound risk of a fatal outcome from a second bleed. Following successful surgery a repeat CT scan is recommended at 6 weeks, especially if the patient is not making good progress postoperatively, as secondary communicating hydrocephalus may occur and require shunting.

Haemorrhage Into Tumours

When a patient who has a cerebral tumour develops symptoms very rapidly, it is often assumed that there has been a haemorrhage into the tumour. This is a very rare event: the sudden symptoms are usually produced by necrosis and oedema in the tumour as it outgrows its blood supply. Since CT scanning has been available the great rarity of haemorrhage into tumours has been more than adequately confirmed. The only tumour that characteristically becomes haemorrhagic is a metastatic deposit from a malignant melanoma: many patients with cerebral metastases from malignant melanomas present with what at first sight is a simple subarachnoid haemorrhage.

CASE REPORT XI

A 36-year-old man collapsed while cycling uphill into a head wind. He was found semiconscious and hemiplegic. On admission he had a stiff neck and a dense left hemiplegia with sensory loss. CSF examination revealed heavily bloodstained fluid. Twelve years previously he had had a malignant melanoma resected from his leg. Angiography revealed an avascular mass in the right parietal lobe. Craniotomy revealed a haematoma and the remains of a melanotic deposit into which the haemorrhage had occurred.

Investigation and Management of Suspected Cerebral Vascular Disease

The three considerations that should be applied to this clinical situation are:

1. Is the site and extent of the lesion typical of occlusion of an identifiable vessel?
2. Is there any underlying haematological or biochemical disorder that could have predisposed to or mimicked a cerebrovascular accident?
3. Are there any causative factors such as hypertension, auricular fibrillation, vessel stenosis or myocardinal infarction that can be identified and treated?

This entire chapter has been devoted to the recognition of symptoms and signs that are typical of a vascular accident. Anything that casts doubt on this diagnosis should prompt immediate further investigation. Underlying disorders that predispose to cerebrovascular accidents include anaemia, polycythaemia, diabetes mellitus, malignant or severe hypertension, inflammatory vascular disease and, in the elderly, temporal (cranial) arteritis. Heavy protein diseases such as myelomatosis should also be excluded.

Cardiac causes, including arrhythmia, valvular heart disease and subacute bacterial endocarditis should always be excluded by clinical examination, ECG and blood cultures. Thyrotoxicosis should be considered if the patient has auricular fibrillation, as in the elderly the clinical evidence of this disorder may be minimal or absent.

Two special conditions related to diabetes mellitus are of great importance.

1. Hypoglycaemia may cause focal signs such as a hemiparesis persisting for 24 hours or more with recovery. This possibility should always be considered with an intermittent clinical picture, and it important to realize that the patient may remain fully conscious throughout the episode. It may occur in patients on oral antidiabetic drugs or insulin, and occasionally as a presenting symptom of primary hypoglycaemia (see Case report I above).

2. The exact relationship of hyperosmolar non-ketotic coma to diabetes is uncertain. The biochemical syndrome consists of marked hyperglycaemia: a glucose level over 1000 mg% (50mmol/l) is not unusual, with marked dehydration and a gross increase in serum osmolarity. Many patients with this condition develop focal neurological signs before becoming comatose. The condition is fatal unless recognized. An important clue is marked dehydration in a patient who has only been ill for a few hours. There is no ketosis, which is the main distinguishing feature from diabetic coma. This condition is discussed in further detail in Chapter 24.

Once it has been established that the patient has had a cerebrovascular accident without evidence of underlying disease, the problem of further management arises. Management depends on the clinical situation.

The Patient who has a Completed Infarct

Angiography is unnecessary, as the surgical restoration of circulation to the damaged hemisphere may cause haemorrhage into the infarct. Anticoagulants may have the same effect. It is generally recommended that anticoagulants should not be started until 6 weeks after a major infarction to avoid this possibility. Unfortunately, if the infarct was a consequence of a major embolus from a fibrillating heart, there is a substantial risk of a further embolus within 6 weeks and the decision to start treatment has to be taken on a patient-by-patient basis.

Ultrasound examination of the unaffected carotid territory should be undertaken, and some would feel that angiographic demonstration of the rest of the cerebral vasculature is indicated to see if other surgically remediable lesions are present that could threaten other vascular territories. This consideration is still the subject or ongoing evaluation in a multicentre trial of carotid endarterectomy.

The Patient who has made a Complete Recovery

This situation constitutes a 'transient ischaemic attack'. The classification of such attacks depends on the duration of the deficit, and two main categories are now defined. A transient ischaemic attack (TIA) is defined as an episode with complete clearance of neurological findings within 24 hours, and an attack lasting longer than 24 hours but with complete clearance of signs within 7 days is now called a reversible ischaemic neurologic deficit (RIND). These specific definitions are important for research purposes and both indicate a warning vascular event. A search for the possible mechanism and attempts to avert further and more lasting deficits are the objective of modern management of cerebrovascular disease.

1. Any source of emboli should be identified. It should be remembered that in some series as many as 30% of emboli originated in the heart, often in an area of myocardial infarction or associated with valvular heart disease or atrial myxoma. If a cardiac source is confirmed, anticoagulants are indicated unless there are any specific contraindications; there is no age limit, provided that the patient is not significantly hypertensive. An INR level of between 2.5 and 3.0 is the preferred range for anticoagulation.

In recent years, soluble aspirin 75–150 mg daily has been used as an alternative to anticoagulants where a cardiac cause for the emboli has not been identified. The ideal dose and degree of protection provided has varied enormously in different studies and even at these low doses the risk of upper gastrointestinal haemorrhage should be considered as a relative contraindication in patients with a previous history of peptic ulceration. Aspirin has been shown to produce its protective effect by reducing platelet stickiness.

2. If the blood pressure is significantly elevated not only are anticoagulants contraindicated but the blood pressure should certainly be treated. In some patients recurrent TIAs may cease immediately when the blood pressure is controlled. Hypotensive therapy should be pursued aggressively in this situation, whatever the patient's age. There is no evidence to support the previous belief that lowering the blood pressure is harmful to these patients. Even if they develop symptoms of postural hypotension this does not cause further cerebrovascular accidents. The only proviso to this consideration is that immediately after a vascular accident the blood pressure is often elevated by altered autoregulatory reflexes, and the initial very high levels may be misleading. Hypotensive medication should be introduced cautiously and monitored carefully over the first few days, and may even prove unnecessary when the situation stabilizes.

3. If no source of emboli is identified and the patient is normotensive the question of cerebral vascular angiography must be considered. Even using the trans-femoral catheter approach the investigation is not totally without hazard, and should only be undertaken when serious consideration is being given to sub-sequent carotid endarterectomy. The presence of a bruit over one or other carotid artery, or narrowing demonstrated by ultrasound, provides the clearest indication for proceeding to angiography. Fortunately the use of modern ultrasound techniques is rapidly replacing angiography in many centres, offering non-invasive information that is sufficient to guide the neurosurgeon.

The value of carotid endarterectomy is still under multicentre trial evaluation. From results so far published, patients who have high-grade stenosis (greater than 70% stenosis) have been shown to benefit from endarterectomy, and where there is stenosis of less than 30% no advantage for surgery over conservative management has been demonstrated. Surgery will also depend on the patient's age and coexistent medical conditions. Whether carotid endarterectomy is of value in the critical 30%–70% group is still under active investigation. This trial was long overdue: original enthusiasm for a surgical approach arose when the narrowed artery was seen purely as an obstruction to blood flow. The recognition of the critical role of the narrowed area as a source of microemboli, which may be prevented by aspirin or anticoagulation, required that this procedure be thoroughly reappraised. In the past many patients were damaged by angiography in an attempt to demonstrate a lesion that might be amenable to surgery.

The Patient who is having a Series of Attacks with Increasing Disability

This situation is sometimes referred to as a 'stuttering hemiparesis' or a 'stroke in evolution'. In this very rare group of patients a progressive thrombosis of a major vessel is usually responsible and the risk of completing the thrombosis during angiography must be high. Immediate heparinization and the use of low molecular weight dextran may have some value in management, but even this may be unsuccessful in preventing completion of the stroke. Such cases are so uncommon that there is no consensus view on best management.

CASE REPORT XII

A domiciliary visit was requested for a 48-year-old man who had returned that morning from a business trip to Tokyo. He

was complaining of variable giddiness, variable slurred speech and variable intermittent diplopia. This had all started 5 days previously and was originally attributed by the patient to sitting in the direct draught of the air-conditioning in a taxicab. He was seen an hour later; at first there were no obvious abnormalities and the possibility of myasthenia gravis arose. However, his past history included a myocardial infarction at the age of 36 and he was known to be both hypertensive and a smoker. During the history-taking, at the end of a particularly long discussion he complained of double vision and the right eye was noted to deviate inwards, his speech became slurred and he developed lower motor neuron weakness of the right side of the face and giddiness with nystagmus. There was some tingling in the left limbs. He stopped speaking and within minutes everything returned to normal. The whole picture was repeated on two or three occasions in the following 15 minutes, as if there was 'claudication of the brain stem'. He was admitted to hospital urgently, given intravenous heparin and an infusion of low molecular weight dextran. In spite of this the attacks became more frequent, recovery less complete and within 8 hours he became drowsy, anarthric and tetraplegic. He died 2 hours later. At post mortem, he was shown to have complete occlusion of both the right vertebral and basilar arteries and a very small left vertebral artery. Presumably his brain stem had been perfused from above via the posterior cerebral arteries. The exact time at which these occlusions occurred is uncertain, but this is a typical example of this rare situation.

Each patient with cerebral vascular disease presents an entirely different set of problems and the statistics of cerebral disease and its outcome become meaningless when faced with an individual patient. There is still uncertain evidence of the advantages of carotid endarterectomy in the majority of cases, and because angiography is not totally risk-free there should be considerable discussion in each case before embarking on a surgical route. It is small consolation to the patient whose condition deteriorates as a result of investigation to be reassured that no surgically remediable abnormality was found. Decades of intensive investigation by retrospective and prospective studies of cerebral vascular disease and its treatment has still left many controversies in the ideal management of this common and potentially lethal problem. The patient's best chance of averting further problems lies in the discovery of an underlying condition that is amenable to specific treatment, and the recognition and early treatment of hypertension is probably the most important treatment that alters the short and long term prognosis.

10. The Cerebral Hemispheres: Disorders of the Limbic System and Hypothalamus

There is a borderline area between psychiatry and neurology that is concerned with acute and chronic disorders of personality, behaviour and intellect. Patients in these categories present considerable diagnostic problems as in many instances they are unable to give a coherent account of their illness. A third-party history from friends, relatives and workmates is vital if an accurate account of the course of the illness is to be obtained. It often transpires that an apparently acute illness has been preceded by several weeks' history of altered personality, headaches, speech disorder and loss of motor skills, which may provide important clues to the presence and site of an underlying lesion. A history of drug or alcohol abuse, previous malignant disease or recent head injury will completely alter the approach to the investigation and management of a patient with altered personality, behaviour or intellect.

There are four major types of disorder in which particular care must be exercised. If the incoherent, confused, aggressive or hallucinating patient is regarded as a diagnostic challenge rather than as a disposal problem, diagnostic errors will be avoided. It is essential that a complete neurological examination and any necessary investigations are performed before the patient is transferred to a mental hospital for psychiatric treatment or custodial care. The role of the neurologist in rescuing such patients from inappropriate detention in mental institutions is an important and difficult one.

CASE REPORT I

A 55-year-old man, previously in entirely normal health, was referred to a neurologist with a possible diagnosis of Parkinson's disease. The diagnosis was confirmed and treatment with dopamine suggested but no arrangements for follow-up were made. Five months later the patient was admitted to a mental hospital in an acute confusional state with marked mental and physical inertia. He was thought to be profoundly depressed. The admitting doctor was uneasy about the patient's clinical condition but was unable to obtain urgent advice from the original neurologist. The patient was therefore sent to the accident centre as an emergency. On examination the patient was lying rigidly on the trolley, mumbling incoherently. It was impossible to tell whether he was confused or just unable to speak. His mouth was dry, his lips excoriated and he was clinically profoundly dehydrated. There was severe cogwheel rigidity in all four limbs and little or no voluntary movement was possible. The plantar responses were flexor. His serum sodium was 192mmol/l. Other biochemistry was surprisingly normal. He was rehydrated overnight with considerable caution and, as soon as he could swallow, given 100mg amantadine hydrochloride. Within 24 hours he was able to talk normally and move all four limbs, and in 48 hours was walking almost normally. Dopamine was then added back into the regimen. It transpired that he had become increasingly slowed in all spheres – mental and physical – and his family had not realized that he was hardly eating or drinking over a period of nearly 3 weeks before the crisis. The patient undoubtedly owes his life to the admitting officer at the mental hospital. Two years later his Parkinson's disease was under good control on modest doses of medication.

Toxic Confusional States

Toxic confusional states may be due to drug overdose or idiosyncratic reactions to drugs such as antiparkinsonian agents. Pneumonia may cause a similar picture due to hypoxia, fever or general toxicity. In the elderly an afebrile course is possible and the physical signs of pneumonia are easily missed. Congestive cardiac failure, uraemia, liver failure, meningitis, subarachnoid haemorrhage, hypercalcaemia or hypoglycaemia may all present as a toxic confusional state. Patients with a history of alcoholism may develop a toxic confusional state with seizures when alcohol is withdrawn – the condition known as delirium tremens. This may happen when the patient is hospitalized for another condition. It is also important to remember that alcoholics do develop other forms of cerebral pathology and are particularly prone to sustain subdural haematomas from trauma occurring while drunk. Many patients have been seen who had been misdiagnosed as suffering from delirium tremens because of a history of alcoholism who in fact had subdural haematomas, and one even had a temporal lobe glioma.

CASE REPORT II

One Sunday afternoon in 1964, the neurological registrar who happened to be in the hospital was asked if he would like to see an example of delirium tremens on the professorial medical unit for his own interest. The patient was an elderly horse-racing correspondent and known to be a heavy drinker. He was confused and hallucinating, but was surprisingly drowsy and drifted into sleep during lulls in the examination. Examination revealed a slightly dilated right pupil, downward drift of the left outstretched hand, a left grasp reflex and bilateral extensor plantar responses. His relatives were telephoned and related that 3 weeks earlier he had been admitted to hospital for overnight observation after being struck by a car on a pedestrian crossing while inebriated. His condition was deteriorating so rapidly that burr holes were made by a general surgeon under local anaesthetic, and a massive right-sided subdural haematoma under very high pressure was evacuated, leading to a dramatically sudden and full recovery.

Patients with confusional states tend to be referred direct to psychiatrists if hallucinations or paranoid delusions dominate the clinical picture, and to a neurologist if they become stuporose or develop any sort of epileptic disturbance. It is important that psychiatrists have some neurological skills and it is incumbent on neurologists to be able to identify psychiatric conditions in their neurological patients.

Dysphasic Confusion

Patients who have disease in the dominant parietal lobe present an extremely difficult group of disorders, in which the communication problem is due to receptive or expressive dysphasia or combinations of these problems, and where there is a grave danger that the patient will be classified as 'confused' or 'demented'.

CASE REPORT III

A 60-year-old woman had been admitted direct to a mental hospital in a confusional state. She was referred for an urgent neurological opinion because the psychiatrists were unable to obtain any sort of history from her, although she seemed to be trying very hard to answer their questions. No neurological signs had been detected but the psychiatric team were unconvinced that the patient was psychiatrically unwell. Neurological evaluation quickly established that she had complete nominal aphasia and was unable to name any single object, or indeed complete any sentence. Subsequent investigation revealed a left parietal infarction.

Sadly, the recognition of dysphasia not only reveals the presence of a focal lesion in the dominant hemisphere but often indicates a poor prognosis, as extensive surgical procedures in the dominant parietal lobe are technically difficult and infarction rarely permits significant recovery. However, this should not preclude full investigation, as occasionally a subdural haematoma

or a small lesion with massive oedema may be found which may be amenable to a surgical attack, with minimal residual deficit of speech function.

Temporal Lobe Automatism

Prolonged disturbances of temporal lobe function can occur in complex partial seizures (formerly called psychomotor epilepsy) or temporal lobe ischaemia during migraine associated with transient global amnesia (see Chapter 22). In complex partial seizures bizarre and totally uncharacteristic behaviour may result, sometimes leading to difficult situations.

CASE REPORT IV

A 28-year-old man with complex partial seizures since his early teens experienced two extraordinary situations. On the first occasion he came to himself standing in a bus queue holding in his hand the remnants of his umbrella, which he had bent and broken across his knee during an attack. He was surrounded by alarmed passengers. On a second occasion he found himself in the window of a shop selling light fittings, striking the suspended display with an umbrella. Fortunately, on that occasion he was armed with a note from his neurologist which he was able to show to the shop owner and the policeman who had been summoned. Following this event, it was suggested that he discontinued carrying an umbrella! His attacks remained refractory to all anticonvulsants.

Any episodes of unusual behaviour should always be regarded as possibly due to complex partial seizures until proved otherwise, the main clue to this diagnostic possibility being the sudden onset and offset of the episode. Further problems may result in these situations if a bystander tries to interfere: the patient may react aggressively and end up in custody.

In contrast, transient global amnesia is characterized by the patient continuing to behave absolutely normally, with no recollection afterwards of events over a period that may extend to several hours. They tend not to get into difficulties because of the attack and colleagues or family may notice little untoward at the time. This fascinating subject is dealt with in much greater detail in Chapter 22.

The rare condition known as acute auditory hallucinosis, which complicates alcoholism, is possibly due to a metabolic disturbance in the temporal lobe. In this state non-stop auditory hallucinations are often coupled with paranoid behaviour, which may persist for several days in the presence of an otherwise intact sensorium.

CASE REPORT V

A naval rating was facing a serious charge as a result of an attack on a Chief Petty Officer. While crossing the Bay of Biscay in a severe storm, all the sailors had been seasick and had missed their rum ration, which was still provided at that time (1964). When the storm ended the sailor concerned suddenly started hearing music playing continuously. It was the same tune over and over and was very distressing. He became convinced that the CPO was deliberately playing a transistor radio to annoy him, and he started to jump round corners, look beneath lifeboat coverings and suddenly open doors to try to find the radio and its owner. He finally cracked and launched a savage attack on the CPO. He was detained, and while in custody suffered an epileptic fit. He was repatriated and underwent full neurosurgical investigation, including air encephalography, to exclude a tumour causing the epilepsy and behavioural disturbance. No neurological opinion was obtained. He was transferred to the hospital convalescent home and had a further series of epileptic fits following an alcohol 'binge' when he was allowed home for a weekend. Subsequent investigation revealed that he was an extremely heavy drinker and that the whole episode was the consequence of alcohol withdrawal during the storm.

Many of the psychiatric complications of alcohol follow alcohol withdrawal, so that in addition to the usual problem of the patient not admitting excessive intake, the relatives often conceal this information because they think that as the problems occurred when the patient had stopped drinking there is no connection, so the alcohol habit need not be mentioned. Sometimes the family are genuinely unaware of the problem.

CASE REPORT VI

A 32-year-old woman was referred following an episode that occurred while on holiday in Wales with her husband and two young children. Two days after arrival, she suddenly started to act in a frightened and strange way and asked her husband why a military band was practising in their back garden. As there was nothing, apart from a few sheep in a field a few hundred yards away, her husband was slightly concerned. This continued for 2 more days, during which time she also mentioned some strange animals around the house, but not the small creatures usually seen by patients with delirium tremens. On the third day she had an epileptic fit. On her return she was referred for consultation. At the consultation she was noted to be slightly unsteady on her feet but there was no smell of alcohol and she adamantly denied drinking. A blood alcohol level, taken at the consultation, contained 160:mg% of alcohol. Two weeks before the holiday she had been involved in a multiple car crash with her two small children in the back, and had not been breathalysed! Her husband had no idea of her addiction.

Any episodic, confusional or behavioural episode of this type should always raise the suspicion of alcohol or drug abuse, and the frequent association with epileptic events may cause diagnostic confusion if the epilepsy is regarded as more important than the preceding behavioural change. In the desire to exclude organic conditions the actual cause may be missed. It would be naive to expect that the patients willingly admit to this problem and make the diagnosis easy. In the elderly a clue to excessive alcohol intake may be found in their preference for disposing of their empty bottles in unmarked brown paper bags!

Many patients with migraine can recognize an impending attack by a change in behaviour or mood in the hours before the headache develops. This is probably due to impaired perfusion in the territory of one or both posterior cerebral arteries. A dramatic example of this type of transient temporal lobe dysfunction in migraine is detailed below.

CASE REPORT VII

A 46-year-old carpenter of previously exemplary character went swimming with his daughter early one Sunday morning. On his return he completed his income tax forms and started to mow his lawn. Shortly afterwards he went indoors and told his wife his vision was 'funny' and he thought he was developing a headache. He went to lie down, and a few minutes later when his wife took him a cup of tea he complained that he could not see or hear. He then became drowsy, and if disturbed became extremely violent. He remained in this state for 48 hours. CSF examination to exclude a subarachnoid haemorrhage and blood sugar determination to exclude hypoglycaemia were both normal. At this stage it was discovered that both his father and brother suffered from severe migraine. A tentative diagnosis of a somnolent state with a rage reaction due to medial temporal lobe ischaemia was made. On the third day the patient sat up in bed very bewildered and completely normal mentally. He had no recollection of events after his wife had come into the room. He was able to relate that the visual upset was loss of the right visual field, and that this had happened on previous occasions and had been followed by a headache. There seems little doubt that these were isolated migraine headaches. Several EEGs taken during the period of confusion were within normal limits.

This case indicates the extremely narrow area between 'normal' and 'abnormal' behaviour, not dependent on a gross disturbance of cerebral function but due to quite limited areas of dysfunction affecting the region known as the limbic system, or its cortical connections.

Dementia

Dementia is a problem common to neurology and psychiatry and is usually divided somewhat arbitrarily into presenile (onset before age of 65) and senile dementia. This classification places undue emphasis on the presenile group, because at any age dementia is a devastating problem for the patient and even more so for the distraught relatives. At any age full investigation to exclude any treatable cause is vital. This topic is of increasing importance due to the increasing prevalence of dementia in the ageing populations of developed countries, and has already become a major health problem, as most patients ultimately require institutional care and with good nursing may live for many years after their illness has destroyed their independence. A later section of this chapter is devoted to the causes and investigation of dementia.

The patient is to some extent protected from the full impact of their illness by loss of insight into their condition. There are many diagnostic and management problems in dementia, two of which are worth mentioning at this stage. A previously intelligent patient may react to the onset of dementia by developing obsessional behaviour patterns to avoid embarrassment, or by becoming severely depressed. In either case it is easy to overlook the underlying intellectual decline. In the later stages of dementia patients may react with paranoid suspicion, often directed at the closest relatives, whose concern is regarded with suspicion by the patient, who may alter his will in others' favour. Testamentary capacity in these patients is a difficult medicolegal problem, as favoured relatives often become involved in the patient's delusional system. It is most important to document in the notes at what stage it was felt that the patient's testamentary capacity became impaired. If a will is contested, an opinion may well be sought from the patient's medical advisers as to whether the patient was capable of making a valid will at **that** time. The basic requirement for valid testamentary capacity is that after discussion with the patient the medical examiner can confirm that

the patient is aware of his assets, including property, insurances and valuables, and aware of surviving family members to whom he ought to consider leaving these items. Sometimes this judgement has to be made in retrospect, based on the patient's general behaviour at the time, if it is subsequently discovered that they had altered their will once the illness had started.

Although dementia indicates diffuse loss of cerebral substance, occasionally exactly the same situation is produced by quite local lesions, particularly in the parasagittal or subfrontal regions. Typical case histories have been quoted in Chapter 8. Symptomatic dementia of this type is often due to interference with the activity of the cingulum or the orbital surface of the frontal lobe, both areas with important connections to the limbic system.

To understand the wide range of clinical features and disturbances of mood and affect that occur in diseases affecting these regions a broad grasp of the anatomy of the interconnections of the cerebral cortex and the limbic system and hypothalamus is necessary.

Limbic System (Fig. 10.1)

There are several definitions of the limbic lobe, depending on whether anatomical or physiological con-

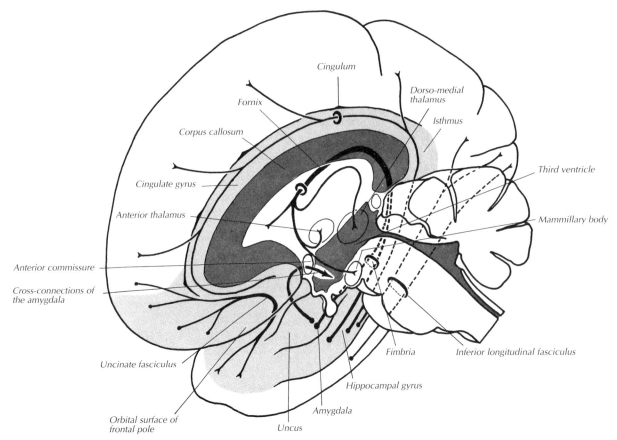

10.1   The limbic system.

siderations are paramount. Most current definitions exclude much of the olfactory apparatus and its central connections. The older terms – rhinencephalon, fornicate lobe or 'smell' brain – are not therefore synonymous with what is known clinically as the 'limbic system'.

The limbic system includes the hippocampus and hippocampal gyrus, the uncus, amygdala, cingulate gyrus, part of the insula, the septal area, the isthmus, Broca's olfactory area and the orbital surface of the frontal pole. Embryologically the inner surface of the temporal lobe rolls in on itself, forming the curved groups of cells known as Ammon's Horn, which lie in the floor of the lateral ventricle as the hippocampus. The hippocampal gyrus is the area overlying the hippocampus which is visible on the medial surface of the posterior end of the temporal lobe immediately behind the bulge overlying the amygdala.

The main fibre tract from the hippocampal area is the fimbria, which is joined by other fibres from adjacent areas to form a dense bundle called the fornix, which sweeps posteriorly at first and then up and over to pass anteriorly to distribute to all areas of the hypothalamus, but particularly to the mammillary body and parts of the thalamus. Some fibres from the fimbria decussate directly to the opposite hippocampus and there are also important cross-connections between the amygdala on each side through the anterior commissure.

Damage in the region of the amygdala is associated with rage reactions, hyperphagia (overeating) and increased sexual activity. Lesions in the region of the uncus are associated with olfactory and gustatory hallucinations, which have also been called 'uncinate fits'. In fact, seizures starting in any part of the temporal lobe have a unique opportunity to spread and involve other areas or both temporal lobes, resulting in the wide range of physical and emotional phenomena that may occur during a complex partial seizure.

The cingulate gyrus lies above the corpus callosum, its connecting pathways traversing the isthmus posteriorly and extending as far forward as Broca's olfactory area. Operations directed at these pathways and the connections from the cingulate gyrus to the thalamus (see also Fig. 10.2) form the basis of some psychosurgical procedures. These include frontal leukotomy and cingulotomy, which may be performed in patients with phobic anxiety states and chronic pain syndromes; in the latter case the emotional response to pain is blunted although the pain itself is not abolished. In recent years direct attacks on pain pathways have become more popular than psychosurgical procedures in the treatment of patients with intractable pain, but these are of limited value and are not in general use.

Hypothalamus (Fig. 10.2)

Although the hypothalamus is not included in the limbic system, from a functional point of view its exclusion is hard to understand as much of the expression of activity in the limbic system occurs via its important connections with the hypothalamus.

The main afferent connections of the hypothalamus are derived from the fornix, which is distributed to all the hypothalamic nuclei and then terminates in the mamillary body. Olfactory information reaches the hypothalamus via the medial forebrain bundle, which also receives information from other areas of the limbic system and forms the main longitudinal tract linking the various hypothalamic nuclei as it runs along the lateral border of the hypothalamic area. Cortical activity reaches the hypothalamus directly and via the thalamus.

From below, the hypothalamus receives visceral and gustatory sensation via both the dorsal longitudinal fasciculus and the reticular formation. Much of this visceral sensation is relayed to the cortex via the mammillothalamic tract and the thalamus.

The efferent connections of the hypothalamus include ascending projections into the limbic system, the cortex and thalamus, and descending projections to the tegmentum, the reticular formation and the cranial nerve nuclei over the pathways already described (note: in the illustration the medial forebrain bundle and both afferent and efferent components of the main tracts are not shown, to avoid overcomplicating the diagram).

Hypothalamic activity is mediated in three ways:

1. By control of the activity of sympathetic and parasympathetic nervous system, including the adrenal medulla
2. By extensive projections into the reticular formation
3. Through control of pituitary function by both direct neural connections (the supra optico hypophyseal and tubero hypophyseal tracts) and via the portal vascular system, which carries the various releasing factors to the gland which then secrete trophic hormones.

Functional Grouping of Hypothalamic Nuclei (Fig. 10.3)

A detailed knowledge of the names and positions of the various hypothalamic nuclei is not essential for clinical purposes, but there are some rough generalizations that can be made as to the functional grouping of the nuclei.

The anterior hypothalamus includes the supraoptic and paraventricular nuclei, which are particularly concerned with fluid balance via ADH (antidiuretic hormone) secretion and control of the thirst mecha-

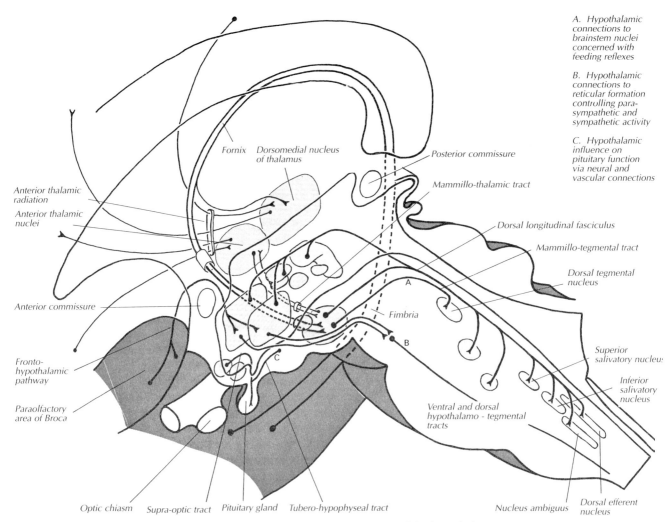

A. Hypothalamic connections to brainstem nuclei concerned with feeding reflexes

B. Hypothalamic connections to reticular formation controlling para-sympathetic and sympathetic activity

C. Hypothalamic influence on pituitary function via neural and vascular connections

Fornix   Dorsomedial nucleus of thalamus

Posterior commissure

Mammillo-thalamic tract

Anterior thalamic radiation

Anterior thalamic nuclei

Dorsal longitudinal fasciculus

Mammillo-tegmental tract

Dorsal tegmental nucleus

Anterior commissure

A

Fimbria

B

Fronto-hypothalamic pathway

Paraolfactory area of Broca

Superior salivatory nucleus

Inferior salivatory nucleus

C

Ventral and dorsal hypothalamo - tegmental tracts

Optic chiasm   Supra-optic tract   Pituitary gland   Tubero-hypophyseal tract   Nucleus ambiguus   Dorsal efferent nucleus

10.2   Main afferent and efferent connections of the hypothalamus.

These functions are based on animal experiments and the effects of clinical lesions in man. Because both pathways and nuclei are indiscriminately affected only rough area effect correlations can be made and in man the resulting combination may include features of damage to several areas

Lateral lesions cause hyper-somnolence, shivering, pilo-erection, small pupils. hypothermia and low blood pressure

Altered body temperature reg-ulation – hyper-pyrexia

Impairment of ADH secretion – produces dia-betes insipidus

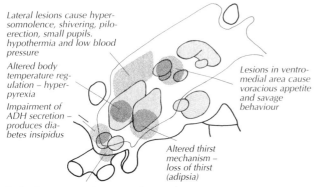

Lesions in ventro-medial area cause voracious appetite and savage behaviour

Altered thirst mechanism – loss of thirst (adipsia)

Lesion here causes pulmonary oedema and gastric erosion. Reason unknown. Also alters all circadian rhythms and may cause prolonged wakefulness.

10.3   Hypothalamic nuclei

nism. The central nuclei are concerned with body temperature regulation by control over skin blood vessels and sweating mechanisms. Damage to these areas may cause diabetes insipidus, complete adipsia, hyper-pyrexia, pulmonary oedema or acute gastric erosions. Damage to the suprachiasmatic nuclei alters circadian rhythms. This part of the hypothalamus is particularly likely to be damaged by pituitary tumours, cranio-pharyngiomas, head injuries and intracranial surgery directed at tumours in this region.

The posterior hypothalamus contains the dorsal nuclei, the posterior hypothalamic nucleus and the supramammillary and mammillary nuclei, and is mainly concerned with appetite, satiety, feeding reflexes, peri-stalsis and the control of the various secretions associated with eating and digestion. Lesions in this region are fortunately unusual and may be associated with total loss of appetite, leading to gross emaciation, or gross overeating with obesity and altered personality, often characterized by extremely bad temper and aggression.

Study of the lateral hypothalamic area is complicated by the fact that the interconnecting pathways run through the area, so that the clinical signs may indicate damage to either the nuclei or the tracts. Lesions in the lateral area are characterized by somnolence, disturbances of body temperature control and occasionally altered appetite. The following case histories give some idea of the problems presented by hypothalamic disorders.

CASE REPORT VIII

An 18-year-old boy became obese and somnolent and complained of visual failure. A suprasellar lesion was found which at surgery proved to be an extensive craniopharyngioma. Following surgery he was blind, and developed diabetes insipidus coupled with total loss of the thirst mechanism. Frequent episodes of drowsiness and epileptic seizures paralleled gross changes in hydration, which could not be controlled by hormone replacement therapy and careful fluid balance control. He died a few weeks later.

CASE REPORT IX

A 32-year-old Indian woman flew to England to join her husband, who had emigrated 2 years earlier. The husband had been informed prior to her arrival that she had been unwell with a personality disorder and had needed psychiatric treatment. He did not recognize her at the airport. Her weight had increased by 60 lb, she was apathetic and sleepy, and took little interest in her surroundings. It was suspected that she had a visual disturbance of some sort. The optic discs appeared normal but formal field testing was impossible as the patient kept falling asleep. Her body temperature was low, at 35°C, and she woke up only long enough to eat a meal. Investigation revealed a large suprasellar mass and she died during surgical exploration. Post mortem revealed an extensive craniopharyngioma.

Clinical Disorders of the Temporal Lobe and the Limbic–Hypothalamic System

Owing to the anatomical extent of the limbic system and its widespread cortical connections, lesions in many areas can give rise to an unusually complex range of symptoms. Because the area has considerable importance in special sense perception and visceral function these symptoms take unusual forms, often including hallucinations. The area also has considerable importance in memory function and consciousness, and several rare and unusual disorders of memory and sleep may have a basis in disordered limbic function.

Complex Partial Seizures (Temporal Lobe or Psychomotor Epilepsy)

The most varied range of abnormalities undoubtedly occur in temporal lobe epilepsy, and we can now consider some of these in an anatomical setting (see also Chapter 8).

The cortical representation of hearing and balance is found in the upper temporal gyri just below the Sylvian fissure, and discharges starting in this area typically produce auditory and vestibular symptoms.

CASE REPORT X

A 19-year-old shop assistant complained that for 6 months he had had brief attacks of a 'whirring noise' in the head followed by a sensation as if he was pitching forwards, which on several occasions had led to a fall. These attacks had occurred as often as six times a day and had never lasted more than 30 seconds. He had not lost consciousness. An EEG revealed seizure discharges originating in the right temporal lobe. The attacks ceased when he was treated with carbamazepine.

CASE REPORT XI

A 36-year-old police constable complained that he kept hearing voices on his communication set and that when he answered no-one was calling. There were absolutely no other symptoms and physical examination and an EEG were normal.

No definite diagnosis could be entertained. A year later, while in a police vehicle with two other officers, he heard voices on the car radio and asked why the others were not responding; they told him that there were no voices. He was noted to be a little pale and staring, and a few seconds later he went into a major convulsion. Investigation revealed an extensive right parieto temporal lesion which biopsy showed to be a grade I glioma. His fits were controlled with medication and 7 years later he was still working as a police constable.

Seizures originating in the visual association areas in the parieto temporal occipital region may give rise to complex visual hallucinations. However déjà-vu phenomena, in which the patient's surroundings suddenly seem frozen and familiar, may have their origin in memory function abnormalities and are more likely to be due to hippocampal dysfunction. Jamais vu is the reverse situation, where the patient suddenly finds familiar surrounding totally alien and may not recognize even their own house; it occurs less often than déjà vu.

Discharges arising in the region of the amygdala or uncus typically cause olfactory or gustatory hallucinations. These are very brief in duration and usually unpleasant in nature, often likened to 'rotting cabbage' or 'burning rubber'. The brevity of the attack causes difficulty in identifying the odour: patients often complain that before they can take a second sniff the smell has gone. Persistent unpleasant smells are unlikely to indicate temporal lobe dysfunction. Such symptoms are often psychogenically determined as part of a depressive illness or due to chronic suppurative sinus disease (sometimes known as ozema).

Altered awareness during the period of an attack, or sometimes half-recalled events, is characteristic of a temporal lobe attack and is probably related to hippocampal dysfunction, preventing complete sequential memory storage. Often bystanders cannot detect any change in the patient apart from rather deliberate movements, frequently described as 'zombie-like'. Sometimes overtly peculiar behaviour may occur, as described in the case report IV earlier in this chapter.

The insular cortex deep in the Sylvian fissure is concerned with the involuntary motor activity of visceral function. Common motor accompaniments of a temporal lobe attack are lip-smacking or chewing movements, which often provide an important diagnostic clue in episodes that might otherwise be mistaken for petit mal. Occasionally other visceral activity occurs and one patient frequently terminated her attacks by involuntary defecation, which she was quite unable to prevent although conscious.

Another characteristic feature of temporal lobe attacks are visceral sensations. These commonly include epigastric 'rising sensations', nausea, increased peristalsis and colicky pain, or peculiar tingling and numbness in the perineum. Several children have specifically commented on an icy-cold feeling in the perineum as the first symptom of an attack. This also tends to 'rise up' through the body, culminating in the full-blown episode. These are sensations that are normally relayed through the reticular formation to the thalamus and hypothalamus and ultimately discharged to the temporal and frontal cortices. Patients always describe these sensations as 'horrible' and 'frightening' in their own right, and not just because they know that they may end in a full-blown seizure.

A few patients have been reported whose attacks included heightened sexual activity, including masturbation to orgasm. The responsible discharges seem to arise in the medial temporal lobe. A central representation for sexual function in this region may be responsible for impotence in patients with temporal lobe neoplasms (see also Chapter 15).

It is important to remember that 'temporal lobe' phenomena may occur when cortical areas with close connections to the temporal lobe are damaged. These regions particularly include the orbital surface of the frontal lobe and the parasagittal region. Occasionally tumours quite remote from the temporal lobe may cause complex partial seizures. This is particularly true of subfrontal lesions (see Case report XVII in Chapter 8).

Disorders of Memory

Memory disorders usually follow damage to the medial temporal lobe and its connections to the mammillary body and upper brain stem. It follows that symmetrical lesions are usually responsible, and unilateral temporal

lobe lesions or surgical extirpation of one temporal lobe should have minimal effect on memory. Bilateral removal of the anterior temporal lobe produces the Kluver–Bucy syndrome, which is characterized by psychic blindness (inability to identify friends and relatives), pathological overeating, heightened sexual activity and altered emotional responses. Some of these features may reflect the short-term memory impairment, the continued eating and sexual activity perhaps reflecting incomplete recollection of previous indulgences.

Because bilateral damage is more likely to produce disorders of memory, metabolic or infective processes require exclusion. These include anoxia, hypoglycaemia, limbic encephalitis (sometimes associated with malignant disease) or herpes simplex encephalitis. Bilateral posterior cerebral artery occlusion due to an embolus lodged at the bifurcation of the basilar artery, or sometimes occurring during a migraine attack, may cause transient or permanent memory deficit. It is highly likely that prolonged vascular spasm causing ischaemia in this area is the pathological basis of transient global amnesia. This very important and surprisingly common form of amnesia is discussed in greater detail in Chapter 22, as the differential diagnosis includes epilepsy and other 'funny turns'.

Severe head injuries typically cause amnesia for the events of the injury and sometimes for the period immediately preceding it. This may be due to acute cell trauma, bilateral temporal lobe bruising, or dysfunction secondary to anoxia from other injuries or posttraumatic cerebral swelling. (see Chapter 23)

Two particularly interesting causes of amnesia are electroconvulsive therapy (ECT) and Korsakoff's psychosis. In ECT electric shocks sufficient to provoke an epileptic seizure are applied to one or both frontal lobes. Surprisingly, this not only produces amnesia for the ECT but also causes amnesia for events prior to it, and following a large series of treatments patients may suffer permanent memory deficits. The explanation of this is unknown. Korsakoff's psychosis occurs in alcoholics, usually as a permanent sequel to an attack of Wernicke's encephalopathy. The brainstem symptoms, nystagmus, extraocular nerve palsies and dysarthria usually respond to vitamin therapy, but a permanent memory deficit with a particular tendency to upset temporal relationships occurs. This may be the cause of confabulation, which is a striking feature of Korsakoff's psychosis but not unique to that condition. There is often defective recognition of events and defective sequencing, so that the patient inaccurately relates past events as if they had happened recently. The responsible lesions are found in the mammillary bodies and the dorsal median nucleus of the thalamus. Significant recovery is unusual.

Memory deficit is a constant feature of dementia and this problem is discussed in detail later in this chapter.

Disorders Affecting Sleep and Eating Habits

There are a few rare and peculiar disorders in which sleep and sometimes appetite are affected. Many have no known pathological basis, and yet the association of the clinical features strongly suggests an underlying disorder of hypothalamic/limbic function.

Various encephalitic conditions cause pathological disorders of sleep, including African trypanosomiasis and particularly Von Economo's encephalitis or encephalitis lethargica. In this disorder excessive sleeping and complete reversal of the diurnal sleep pattern were major features of the acute stage. Survivors later developed parkinsonian syndromes, but in acutely fatal cases the bulk of the pathological changes were found in the periaqueductal grey matter rather than in the basal ganglia.

A very rare peculiar disorder that has been described particularly in adolescents is the Kleine–Levin syndrome. This may follow an infective illness and is characterized by prolonged periods of sleeping coupled with peculiar behaviour and voracious appetite during the periods of activity. Attacks lasting days to weeks may occur over several years. No pathological basis has been demonstrated and some cases may be of psychogenic origin. A lesion affecting the hypothalamus should be excluded in all cases.

At the opposite extreme are the conditions known as anorexia nervosa and bulimia, which usually occur in young women and are now regarded as psychiatric disturbances associated with secondary endocrine dysfunction.

The 'Pickwickian' syndrome, named after the fat boy in Dickens's novel *The Pickwick Papers* is a combination of extreme obesity, alveolar hypoventilation and carbon dioxide retention, and is characterized by frequent brief attacks of sleep with sleep apnoea in a setting of continual drowsiness. The sleep component may be a combination of fatigue due to sheer bulk and metabolic factors, but the whole syndrome is a common feature of hypothalamic disorders. The patient quoted earlier who had a craniopharyngioma represents a minor degree of this syndrome. (Case Report VIII.)

Rarely, cerebral tumours, particularly pinealomas and midbrain tumours, may produce pathological drowsy states in which the patient may appear to be in a coma; however, the eyes remain open and the patient may be able to indicate alertness by eye movement. This state is known as 'akinetic mutism' and the alert but immobile condition as 'coma vigil'. The lesions responsible usually damage the midbrain reticular formation and include the tumours mentioned above and vascular lesions, particularly thrombosis of the upper segment of the basilar artery. However, recent pathological examination of the brain of the longest survivor of the persistent vegetative state after head trauma, has demonstrated that the main damage was in the thalamic nuclei, which suggests that thalamic projections may play a major role in maintaining the alert state.

Narcolepsy

Narcolepsy is a much under recognized condition. There are possibly 20 000 sufferers in the UK, only half of whom have been identified. There are several reasons for this. Some patients will present with **difficulty** sleeping at night because they tend to waken suddenly and dramatically, and the subsequent daytime drowsiness is incorrectly attributed to the lack of sleep at night. In contrast, the main differential diagnostic condition of hypersomnolence is characterized by prolonged deep nocturnal sleep and continuing daytime drowsiness in spite of this. The best basic definition of narcolepsy remains 'a sudden irresistible desire to go to sleep'. This may lead to inappropriate sleep, i.e. sleep in mid-sentence, while driving, or even falling into food at mealtimes. The resulting sleep may be relatively brief but is very refreshing and the patient will wake and feel fully alert. In contrast, hypersomnolence results in the patient drifting in and out of sleep which is not refreshing, the patient remaining drowsy in a state of sub-wakefulness with poor concentration and a high risk of accident or injury.

Narcolepsy can be most readily diagnosed if associated with the other classic features, or if there is a positive family history of the condition, which is present in some 30% of cases. The HLA antigen DR2 has been demonstrated in nearly all patients with narcolepsy and is present in only 20% of the population.

The narcolepsy component can occur in any situation that might result in drowsiness in a normal person: warmth, quiet, boredom, rhythmic noise and after heavy meals. The onset is sudden and irresistible, however hard the patient tries to stay alert.

Cataplexy is now regarded by some as being essential to the diagnosis of narcolepsy, but this seems unnecessarily restrictive. It consists of a tendency to buckle at the knees or fall when emotionally excited or suddenly surprised. Laughter, shock, anger, fear or sudden coughing may all be provocative. The patient can immediately pick themselves up again without difficulty, but is quite unable to prevent the fall when provoked. This component of the condition is remarkably well controlled by imipramine or trimipramine (10–25 mg t.d.s. of either drug).

Hypnagogic hallucinations consist of dramatic dreams occurring just as the patient is going to sleep or awakening, the transition being so fast that the patient is in effect dreaming while awake. As the dreams are often extremely vivid and sometimes frightening, this can be doubly disconcerting for the patient, especially if it is coincidental with sleep paralysis. This occurs when the patient wakes so fast that their motor pathways are not yet active, and for what may seem like several minutes–sometimes while dreaming vividly–the patient is unable to move or get away from the threatening components of their dream.

The main feature in the sleep pattern of patients with narcolepsy is the speed with which they enter REM (rapid eye movement) sleep. Normal subjects enter REM sleep after several hours of normal sleeping. Patients with narcolepsy are in REM sleep often within 10 minutes of going to sleep, and this is repeated following any awakenings.

The condition is best treated with dexamphetamine sulphate in a dose titrated to suit the patient, usually between 5 and 20 mg two to three times daily. The nocturnal sleep pattern usually improves when daytime sleepiness is controlled. Unfortunately, the alternative agent methylphenindate is only available to named patients in the UK.

Other Causes of Nocturnal Sleep Disorder

In recent years, the importance of nocturnal sleep apnoea due to upper airways obstruction as a cause of daytime somnolence has been increasingly recognized. It is characterized by disturbed sleep, restlessness, loud snoring and frequent prolonged periods of apnoea lasting 30–60 seconds and culminating in a loud grunting snort, which usually awakens the patient briefly. If surgical management of the upper airways obstruction is unsuccessful, positive airways pressure via the nose or mouth during the night will usually control the condition. The patient is often unaware of the sleep deprivation that results in their daytime drowsiness. They have often been relegated to the spare bedroom by their spouse many months or years before the potentially serious nature of their problem has been identified!

The rarer causes of sleep apnoea include Ondine's curse (an infant who is unable to maintain breathing mechanisms once asleep), brainstem lesions due to cerebral vascular accident or tumour, and paralysis of the respiratory muscles by motor neuron disease. In the past many poliomyelitis sufferers who were able to maintain adequate respiration during the day had to sleep in a cuirasse respirator because their breathing became inadequate while sleeping.

Dementia

In previous chapters dementia has been referred to as a presenting symptom. It is wise to regard dementia as a symptom and not as a diagnosis. The only exception is in the very elderly, in whom dementia is usually due to senile changes in the brain. Dementia should always be regarded as a symptom requiring urgent and complete investigation.

Dementia may be simply defined as failing intellectual function. There are three major components and various admixtures of the three may cause very variable clinical syndromes.

Cognitive Dysfunction

This includes memory deficit, failing judgement, difficulty in abstract thought and rumination on the past, progressing to total confusion of time and place and failure to identify very close relatives. In the very early stages perseveration of thoughts, losing the thread of conversations and even confabulation may occur, the latter not being a specific problem of alcoholism but occurring in any disorder in which recent memory is impaired.

Disorders of Mood and Affect

Patients' responses to developing dementia vary widely. Some patients become extremely anxious and seek reassurance. Others react in a short-tempered way with relatives who cannot keep up with their disordered thought processes. Patients of an obsessional nature may try to cope by keeping minute-by-minute diaries and checklists, and may successfully conceal failing intellect for months or years by this device. Some patients become extremely depressed, to the extent that the underlying dementia may be mistaken for gross psychomotor retardation. Visual hallucinations may be a problem, particularly when the situation is complicated by the use of drugs such as barbiturates, antiparkinsonian agents, alcohol, or during a fever. One severely demented patient who also took alcohol to excess had frequently attacked his wife during the night while suffering from hallucinations in which he thought he was being attacked by 'savage swans'.

Disorders of Behaviour

Disinhibition is a feature of confusional states due to organic disease, alcohol or drug abuse. Any change in a patient's behaviour, such as a previously sober man taking to alcohol, or minor criminal acts such as indecent exposure, should arouse the suspicion of early dementia. Clergymen may become profane and previously mild-mannered men may become subject to temper outbursts. All these features can occur in psychiatric disease but may also indicate the onset of dementia. Even though the disease is now relatively rare, neurosyphilis should be excluded in any patient in whom personality change is the main feature. At any age hypoglycaemia should also be considered, particularly if the attacks of abnormal behaviour are short-lived, although an epileptic attack arising in the temporal lobe should remain the main diagnostic consideration in such patients. The distinction may be very difficult.

CASE REPORT XII

A 58-year-old woman presented with a 2-year history of episodes lasting several minutes at a time where she became vague and remote. There had been no additional features such as lip-smacking or involuntary movements, but her husband had noted that the attacks usually occurred mid-morning and that she became pale and sweaty after the episode. Although she seemed perfectly normal at the time blood was taken, her serum glucose was only 1.5 mmol/l. Investigation revealed an islet-cell tumour in the tail of the pancreas, which was successfully removed.

Investigation of Dementia

The importance of detecting historical and physical evidence of a focal cerebral lesion has been repeatedly stressed. The fact that frontal tumours which typically cause dementia may not produce any physical signs, should be reiterated.

In addition to cerebral tumours other causes of dementia include drugs, chemicals (particularly bromides) and alcohol. A complete history of drug use is essential, including apparently innocuous 'over the counter' remedies. In the past many contained bromides. Patients taking high-dose steroids may also develop acute psychotic confusional states. Remember that alcohol intake may be denied or grossly underestimated by the patient and their relatives.

Specific infections, diseases such as AIDS, neurosyphilis, tuberculous meningitis or fungal meningitis should be considered, particularly in patients with an acute onset of confusion. Similarly, metabolic disorders such as renal or hepatic failure, hypercalcaemia, hypoglycaemia and the hyperosmolar non-ketotic coma typically cause confusional states of acute onset in a previously normal patient.

Patients may become demented followed head injuries, repeated subarachnoid haemorrhages, meningitis or recurrent epilepsy. In some cases the dementia may be due to communicating hydrocephalus secondary to the blockage of the subarachnoid CSF pathways, and a shunt procedure may be of benefit.

Normal pressure hydrocephalus

Closely related to these latter disorders is the condition known as normal pressure hydrocephalus, in which the ventricles become enormously enlarged and compress the thinned cortex against the inner table of the skull. The cause in many instances remains obscure, and although dramatic improvement may follow shunting there is a considerable risk of post operative subdural

haematoma, and subsequently the ever-present risk of bacterial colonization of the shunt with resultant meningitis or septicaemia. The typical syndrome produced by this condition consists of a triad of symptoms: memory disturbance and confusion, which may be episodic; progressive gait disability, with a tendency to walk in tottery little steps; and difficulty in urinary control, which may result in incontinence. The similarity of this picture to that resulting from multiple cerebrovascular accidents is immediately obvious. The clinical distinction should be the stepwise onset when the condition is due to multiple vascular accidents, and the insidious development when due to normal pressure hydrocephalus. Fortunately, modern scanning techniques usually enable the final distinction to be made.

Specific degenerative diseases which include dementia as part of the syndrome include the following:

Huntington's chorea (dementia coupled with choreiform movement disorders) (see Chapter 12)

Creutzfeld–Jakob disease (dementia which may be coupled with extrapyramidal, cerebellar and lower motor neuron dysfunction). A striking feature in most cases is the advent of myoclonic epilepsy, which is a major diagnostic clue. The relationship to a similar disorder in animals known as bovine spongiform encephalopathy remains uncertain

Steele–Richardson–Olzewski syndrome (dementia associated with specific impairment of conjugate eye movements and pseudobulbar palsy). This is now referred to as one of the multisystem atrophy disorders and is discussed further in Chapter 12.

The majority of patients with dementia fall into a non-specific group in which no cause can be established antemortem, and are now classified senile dementia, Alzheimer's type (SDAT). Postmortem examination in many cases reveals diffuse diagnostic changes in cerebral neurons, and only then may the condition be confirmed as Alzheimer's disease.

A more restricted form of degeneration affecting the frontal lobes particularly severely is known as Pick's disease. This is inherited as a dominant gene and is one of the more identifiable presenile dementias. The diagnosis can be confirmed by the distribution of atrophy on CT scanning.

Dementia often occurs in the later stages of parkinsonism and is a complication in 10% of patients who are suffering from motor neuron disease.

Patients with extensive multiple sclerosis, particularly those with lesions affecting frontal lobe connections, become demented. In fact, the majority of patients with multiple sclerosis who were previously described as 'euphoric' are actually demented and have little insight into their predicament. The pathological basis of this is only too obvious in the massive demyelination demonstrable in the cerebral white matter in these patients. This was previously only demonstrable at post mortem. With the advent of MRI the almost universal occurrence of cerebral white matter lesions has become a diagnostic feature, and the severity and extent of this in many patients a source of surprise.

In all patients with suspected dementia the most important test is formal psychometry to confirm the diagnosis. The typical findings are a fall in the performance IQ to 100 or less and a disparity between this and the premorbid (verbal) IQ, which may be 120 or higher. Sometimes in severe dementia the premorbid IQ can only be judged from the patient's educational, employment and social achievements. In some patients the performance IQ may be as low as 50. Psychometry will also identify patients who are severely retarded due to depression and detect the occasional case of 'pseudodementia' due to a functional nervous disorder.

Physical examination should always include a search for signs of neurosyphilis, alcoholism, involuntary movement disorders, parkinsonism, motor neuron disease and non-specific signs such as pout reflexes (tap the upper lip and watch the lips pout); the palmar mental reflexes (scratch the palm of the hand and observe wrinkling of the patient's chin on the same side); grasp reflexes and extensor plantar responses. A unilateral grasp reflex reliably indicates a lesion affecting the opposite frontal pole.

In the past arteriosclerosis was widely accepted as the basis of dementia. This diagnosis was always suspect, and current opinion is that the majority of patients with dementia do not have cerebral vascular disease as the cause. However there are two syndromes that are acceptable on a vascular basis. One is due to extensive small vessel disease producing multiple small areas of infarction in the region of the basal ganglia and internal capsule. This produces a combination of dementia, pseudobulbar palsy, emotional lability and the characteristic gait described as 'marche au petit pas', with short, shuffling steps, often mistakenly diagnosed as parkinsonism. This may occur in a setting of several unequivocal cerebral vascular events or may come on insidiously. It used to be claimed that such patients had tortuous hardened peripheral arteries or absent pedal pulses which indicated cerebral arteriosclerosis, but it is obviously unwise to draw any conclusions as to the state of the cerebral circulation from such findings. Many patients diagnosed as having 'arteriosclerotic dementia' are found to have other disorders when investigations are completed.

The second condition has only been identified since CT scanning became available. This is the syndrome of multi-infarct dementia, which consists of widespread areas of ischaemic damage to the cerebral hemispheres which may have occurred in the absence of any clear-cut previous history of identifiable cerebral vascular events. What is no longer acceptable is that dementia is a consequence of poor generalized cerebral perfusion.

CASE REPORT XIII

A 55-year-old senior aircraft maintenance engineer was referred because his family were concerned about his memory and concentration. Apparently no difficulty had been noted at his place of work. He was markedly confused and unable to give a coherent account of himself but, with the exception of brisk reflexes and dubious extensor plantar responses, there were no detectable abnormalities. His performance IQ was 80 and CT scanning revealed multiple areas of cortical infarction involving both hemispheres. Retrospective history-taking still failed to reveal any identifiable events related to any of these lesions. Presumably these lesions in relatively silent areas of the brain caused problems only when their sheer volume compromised cerebral function.

Special Investigations

1. The special importance of formal neuropsychiatric evaluation cannot be overstated. Simple screening tests such as the minimental state and the simple tests described in Chapter 9 may give some indication of the degree of difficulty the patient is experiencing, but they are no substitute for skilled psychometric studies by an experienced clinical neuropsychologist.

2. Routine haematological and biochemical studies, including ESR, urea, calcium, fasting sugar, liver function and thyroid tests (to exclude myxoedema in particular) should be carried out.

3. Serological tests for syphilis were of great importance in the past and tests for HIV infection have achieved importance in the last 10 years. Both tests remain appropriate in the setting of dementia investigation.

4. Serum B_{12} and folate levels can be of value, even if routine haematological studies are normal. Some 25% of patients with neurological complications of vitamin B_{12} deficiency have a normal blood film. Where appropriate, drug levels should be estimated, although elderly patients on high doses of sedatives or bromide-containing mixtures are now fairly rare.

5. CT or MRI scanning should be considered in most cases. Occasional surprises are the rule even in patients with no physical findings, with subfrontal meningiomas and bilateral subdural haematomas regularly detected, and the occasional recognition of a normal pressure hydrocephalus may result in dramatic improvement if correctly identified and treated by shunting. It is important to remember that the diagnosis of Alzheimer's disease cannot be made by scanning: it is other conditions that can be detected or excluded.

The necessity for careful physical examination and the exclusion of all possible metabolic and toxic causes of dementia will remain the responsibility of the neurologist. The demented patient is demanding of both time and effort, but some 10% of such patients may be found to have a remediable cause and unless all patients are carefully screened, further avoidable deterioration may occur before an alternative diagnosis is identified. It seems likely that in the future this will become an increasing part of the neurologist's workload.

11. The Brain Stem

The anatomy of the brain stem is very complicated but the structures that cause most of the complexity – the extrapyramidal, cerebellar and vestibular pathways – produce clinical signs of relatively limited localizing value. The functional importance of these pathways is undeniable and and they are detailed in other chapters, but for localizing brainstem lesions they are of limited help.

A brainstem lesion can be localized in the transverse plane by using the evidence provided by signs of damage to the long motor and sensory tracts. The level and vertical extent of the damage can then be established by the demonstration of associated cranial nerve lesions. The findings are then used like a grid reference on a map. To do this effectively it is necessary to be able to visualize the brain stem in three dimensions. Two series of diagrams that can be used to localize a lesion in two planes have been prepared for this chapter. These illustrations run in parallel with two figures showing the same information from a different angle of view in each illustration. The first series is drawn from a more conventional angle looking at the brain stem from in front and from the left-hand side (Fig. 11.1). This permits a better demonstration of the emergence of the individual cranial nerves and the basilar artery itself. The second series is drawn from an unusual angle, viewing the brain stem from behind and above, an angle which allows the relative positions of all the important structures to be seen in a single view (Fig. 11.2). It is hoped that these composite views will make brainstem anatomy less daunting and permit even the novice neurologist to attempt an accurate localizing diagnosis, which is critically important in the differential diagnosis of brainstem lesions.

Anatomy of the Brain Stem

The internal brainstem structures are arranged in layers (Fig. 11.3). The ventral layer mainly contains the motor pathways, the intermediate layer carries the sensory pathways and the dorsal layer in the floor of

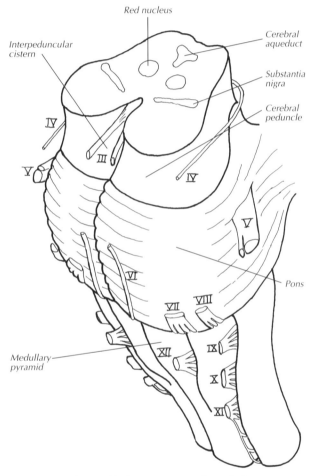

11.1 Brain stem: anterolateral view.

the aqueduct and fourth ventricle contains the cranial nerve nuclei. The extrapyramidal, cerebellar and vestibular connections run across all layers and cannot be considered in detail without adding confusion to this basic arrangement, and this additional knowledge does not greatly help clinical localization. The anatomy of these pathways will be found in greater detail in Chapters 5, 7 and 12.

11.2 Key Diagrams to show angle of view.

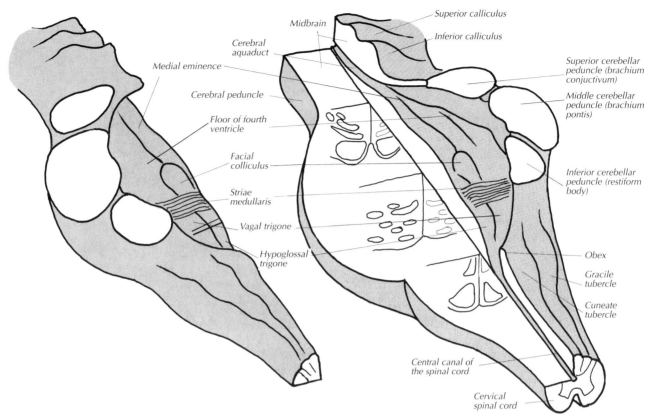

Superior calliculus

Inferior calliculus

Midbrain

Cerebral
aquaduct

Medial eminence

Cerebral peduncle

Floor of fourth
ventricle

Facial
colliculus

Striae
medullaris

Vagal trigone

Hypoglossal
trigone

Superior cerebellar
peduncle (brachium
conjuctivum)

Middle cerebellar
peduncle (brachium
pontis)

Inferior cerebellar
peduncle (restiform
body)

Obex

Gracile
tubercle

Cuneate
tubercle

Central canal of
the spinal cord

Cervical
spinal cord

Note. *The brain stem is viewed from behind with the cerebellum removed. The left dorsal quarter of the brain stem is shown cut away to enable us to imagine we are looking inside the left half of the entire brain stem. The pathways on the left side of the brain stem are shown in all the subsequent diagrams.*

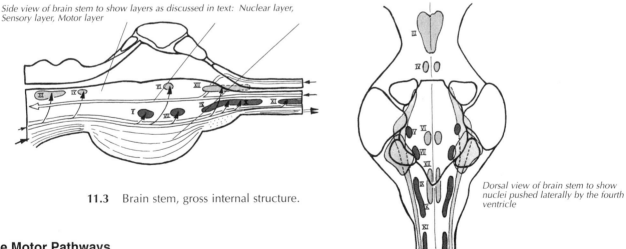

Side view of brain stem to show layers as discussed in text: Nuclear layer, Sensory layer, Motor layer

11.3 Brain stem, gross internal structure.

Dorsal view of brain stem to show nuclei pushed laterally by the fourth ventricle

The Motor Pathways

Corticospinal Pathways (Fig. 11.4)

As the corticospinal fibres descend into the midbrain they rotate into the medial part of the cerebral peduncle, the fibres carrying information to the leg lie laterally and the fibres to the arm lie medially. At pontine levels the pathways are broken up into a series of bundles by the transverse pontine fibres, which sweep across to the opposite cerebellar hemispheres. In the lower third of the pons the fibres come together again as a preliminary to their decussation in the medullary pyramid.

The anatomy of the decussation is of some importance. The arm fibres lie medially and cross the midline above the leg fibres to assume a medial position in the corticospinal tract on the opposite side of the cord. They are then in the ideal position to supply the ventral

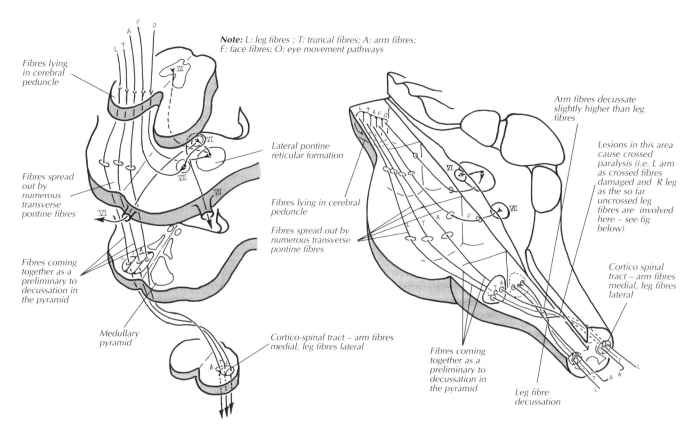

Note: L: leg fibres ; T: truncal fibres; A: arm fibres;
F: face fibres; O: eye movement pathways

11.4 Corticospinal pathways.

horn cells which control the muscles of the arm, which now lie adjacent to the medial aspect of the tract.

As the decussation of the leg fibres occurs slightly lower down than that of the arm fibres it is possible for a discrete lesion to cause weakness of one arm and the opposite leg, a clinical condition that might easily be dismissed as hysterical unless this anatomical possibility is appreciated. Similarly, it is anatomically possible for weakness of both arms to occur with little or no detectable weakness in the legs. The anatomy of these different lesions is shown in Fig. 11.5.

The majority of the corticospinal fibres cross in the medullary pyramid; those that do not do so decussate in the anterior commissure of the cord at cervical level. Ultimately, all pyramidal fibres reach the opposite side of the cord.

Corticobulbar Pathways (Fig. 11.6)

These extremely important pathways are usually given scant attention in anatomical and neurological textbooks. A knowledge of their functional anatomy is essential to an understanding of the physical signs in patients with brainstem lesions.

The corticobulbar fibres pass via the genu of the internal capsule to the most medial part of the cerebral peduncle with the rotation of the motor tract. This places them in the ideal position to cross the midline to

innervate the cranial nerve nuclei on the opposite side of the brain stem. (The pathways to the nuclei innervating the extraocular muscles have already been

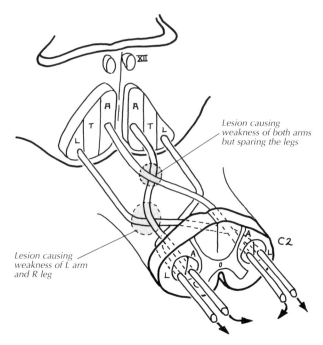

11.5 Corticospinal pathways. Detailed view of decussation in the medullary pyramid.

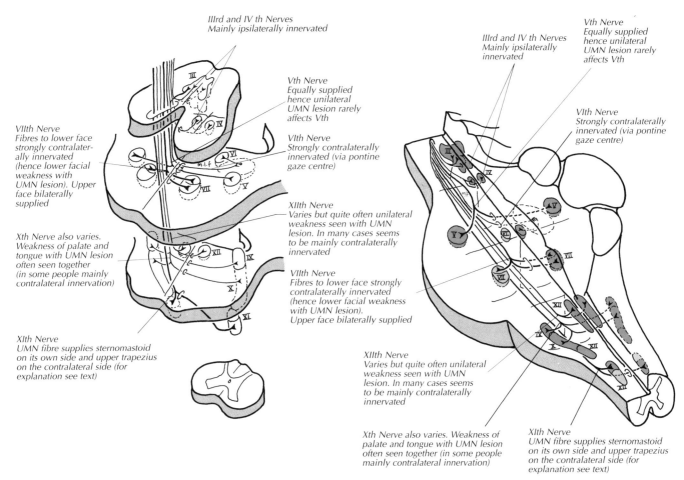

IIIrd and IV th Nerves
Mainly ipsilaterally innervated

VIIth Nerve
Fibres to lower face strongly contralaterally innervated (hence lower facial weakness with UMN lesion). Upper face bilaterally supplied

Vth Nerve
Equally supplied hence unilateral UMN lesion rarely affects Vth

VIth Nerve
Strongly contralaterally innervated (via pontine gaze centre)

Xth Nerve also varies. Weakness of palate and tongue with UMN lesion often seen together (in some people mainly contralateral innervation)

XIIth Nerve
Varies but quite often unilateral weakness seen with UMN lesion. In many cases seems to be mainly contralaterally innervated

VIIth Nerve
Fibres to lower face strongly contralaterally innervated (hence lower facial weakness with UMN lesion). Upper face bilaterally supplied

XIth Nerve
UMN fibre supplies sternomastoid on its own side and upper trapezius on the contralateral side (for explanation see text)

IIIrd and IV th Nerves
Mainly ipsilaterally innervated

Vth Nerve
Equally supplied hence unilateral UMN lesion rarely affects Vth

VIth Nerve
Strongly contralaterally innervated (via pontine gaze centre)

XIIth Nerve
Varies but quite often unilateral weakness seen with UMN lesion. In many cases seems to be mainly contralaterally innervated

Xth Nerve also varies. Weakness of palate and tongue with UMN lesion often seen together (in some people mainly contralateral innervation)

XIth Nerve
UMN fibre supplies sternomastoid on its own side and upper trapezius on the contralateral side (for explanation see text)

11.6   Corticospinal pathways (nuclei receiving main supply from descending left corticobulbar tract are heavily stippled).

discussed in Chapter 7, including their important internuclear connections.)

The motor nucleus of the fifth nerve, which controls the muscles of mastication, derives only half of its innervation from the opposite hemisphere, which means that it is equally innervated from its own hemisphere. This 50:50 innervation ratio means that a unilateral lesion of the supranuclear pathway rarely leads to detectable deficit in these muscles. For example, in a patient who has a cerebrovascular accident (CVA) affecting the internal capsule, motor power of the jaw is rarely impaired.

The supranuclear innervation of the seventh nerve, which controls the muscles of the facial expression, is more complicated (Fig. 11.7). The supply ratio to the forehead muscles is 50:50, so that a unilateral supranuclear lesion will not affect the forehead muscles (see upper motor neuron lesion in Fig. 6.6). The part of the nucleus supplying the lower face is almost exclusively innervated by decussating fibres with little ipsilateral control, similar to the pyramidal fibre distribution to the limbs. Therefore a unilateral supranuclear lesion produces marked weakness of the lower face.

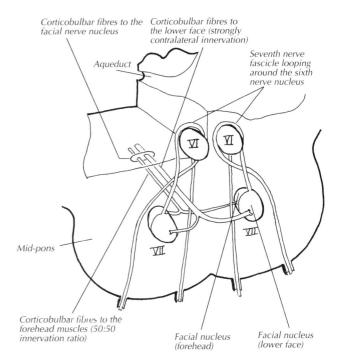

Corticobulbar fibres to the facial nerve nucleus   *Corticobulbar fibres to the lower face (strongly contralateral innervation)*

Aqueduct

Seventh nerve fascicle looping around the sixth nerve nucleus

Mid-pons

Corticobulbar fibres to the forehead muscles (50:50 innervation ratio)

Facial nucleus (forehead)   *Facial nucleus (lower face)*

11.7   Dual supranuclear innervation of the facial nerve nuclei.

The supranuclear control of the nucleus ambiguus (the motor nucleus of cranial nerves IX, X and XI) is clearly more variable. In the majority of patients with a capsular lesion there is no detectable weakness of the palate or vocal cords, suggesting that a 50:50 innervation ratio is the rule. In some patients a transient weakness may be found, suggesting that a greater degree of contralateral supranuclear innervation can occur. The same is true of the twelfth nerve nucleus (motor to the tongue). Usually there is no detectable weakness of tongue movement in a typical unilateral capsular CVA. When unilateral weakness of the tongue is found it is usually combined with weakness of the palate on the same side, suggesting that these lower cranial nerves are innervated in a 50:50 ratio but are contralaterally innervated in some patients.

This anatomical variation is of clinical importance for two reasons. At first sight the demonstration of tenth and twelfth nerve lesions on the same side as a hemiparesis might be thought to indicate two brainstem lesions, affecting the cranial nerve nuclei on one side and the pyramidal pathway above the pyramidal decussation on the other. This would be extremely unusual anyway, and knowing that an upper motor neuron 'hemiparesis' of these lower cranial nerves can occur

will avoid this diagnostic error. Furthermore, the prognosis for eventual recovery of a lower motor neuron cranial nerve lesion due to a brainstem CVA is extremely poor, but if it is due to a 'pseudobulbar' cranial nerve palsy from a lesion higher up, the signs will usually recede over several days in parallel with the improvement of the hemiparesis as intact ipsilateral innervation takes over. Thus diagnostically and prognostically the distinction is important. The sooner the patient is seen and examined after a CVA, the more likely it is that these transient pseudobulbar palsies will be detected and cause diagnostic confusion.

The supranuclear control of the spinal part of the eleventh nerve nucleus is also unusual. The hemisphere exerts control over the sternomastoid muscle on the same side and the upper fibres of the trapezius on the opposite side. At first sight this might appear to be an unnecessarily complex arrangement, but the functional importance is obvious when it is realized that the right sternomastoid turns the head to the left. Were the left sternomastoid active simultaneously with the left limbs, the head would turn in the wrong direction!

Thus a patient with a right capsular CVA and a left hemiparesis will be found to have weakness of the right sternomastoid. This is another finding that may lead the

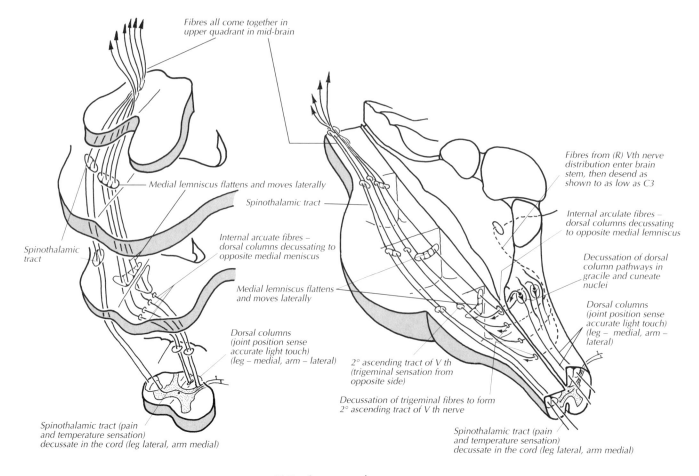

Fibres all come together in upper quadrant in mid-brain

Medial lemniscus flattens and moves laterally

Spinothalamic tract

Spinothalamic tract

Internal arcuate fibres – dorsal columns decussating to opposite medial meniscus

Medial lemniscus flattens and moves laterally

Dorsal columns (joint position sense accurate light touch) (leg – medial, arm – lateral)

Spinothalamic tract (pain and temperature sensation) decussate in the cord (leg lateral, arm medial)

Fibres from (R) Vth nerve distribution enter brain stem, then desend as shown to as low as C3

Internal arculate fibres – dorsal columns decussating to opposite medial lemniscus

Decussation of dorsal column pathways in gracile and cuneate nuclei

Dorsal columns (joint position sense accurate light touch) (leg – medial, arm – lateral)

2° ascending tract of V th (trigeminal sensation from opposite side)

Decussation of trigeminal fibres to form 2° ascending tract of V th nerve

Spinothalamic tract (pain and temperature sensation) decussate in the cord (leg lateral, arm medial)

11.8   Sensory pathways.

unwary examiner to believe that there must be two lesions responsible for this combination of signs. Further evidence for this innervation pattern is to be found in patients suffering a focal motor seizure: the head turns towards the convulsing limbs (see also Figure 7.4), pulled there by the action of the ipsilateral sternomastoid.

The Sensory Pathways (Fig. 11.8)

Dorsal Column Sensation (accurate light touch, two point discrimination sense and joint position sense)

Fibres from the dorsal columns of the spinal cord ascend to the gracile (leg) and cuneate (arm) nuclei in the dorsal medulla. The leg fibres lie medially in the dorsal column, but as the fibres decussate in the medulla through the internal arcuate fibres the leg fibres come to lie laterally, to parallel the motor fibre arrangement. The new tract that is formed by the decussation (the medial lemniscus) is at first vertically disposed and then flattens and spreads laterally, merging finally with the spinothalamic tract in the mid-brain, just below the thalamus.

Spinothalamic Sensation (pain and temperature sensation)

Fibres conveying these sensations have already decussated in the central part of the spinal cord, usually two to three segments above their level of entry. They then ascend into the medulla, lying in a lateral position with the leg fibres lying laterally and the arm fibres lying medially (see Chapter 13). The tract maintains its dorsolateral position throughout the brain-stem until the medial lemniscus merges with it in the midbrain. Throughout its course in the brainstem it lies in close association with the descending sympathetic pathways. This leads to the frequent association of a Horner's syndrome on one side, with pain and temperature loss on the opposite side of the body, whenever the dorsolateral brainstem is damaged at any level.

Trigeminal Sensory System (Fig. 11.9)

The very complex central pathways subserving facial sensation are also discussed in detail in Chapter 15, as they are even better understood when considering the anatomy of syringomyelia. All sensory information from

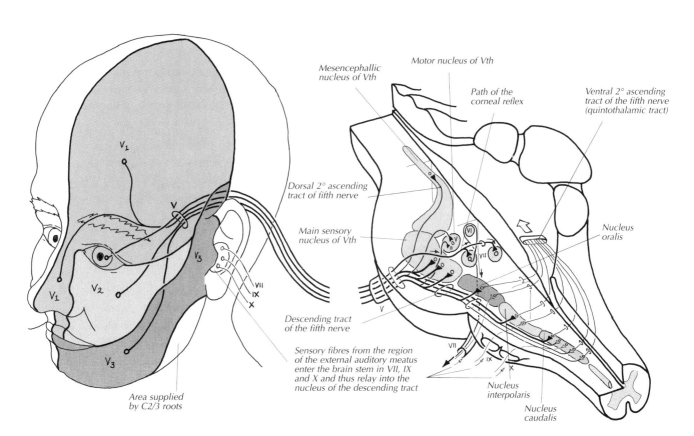

11.9 Trigeminal sensory supply and sensory supply to the face.

The sensory areas of the face are laminated in a forwards direction quite different from the vertical ophthalmic, maxillary and mandibular distribution of the peripheral branches of the trigeminal nerve

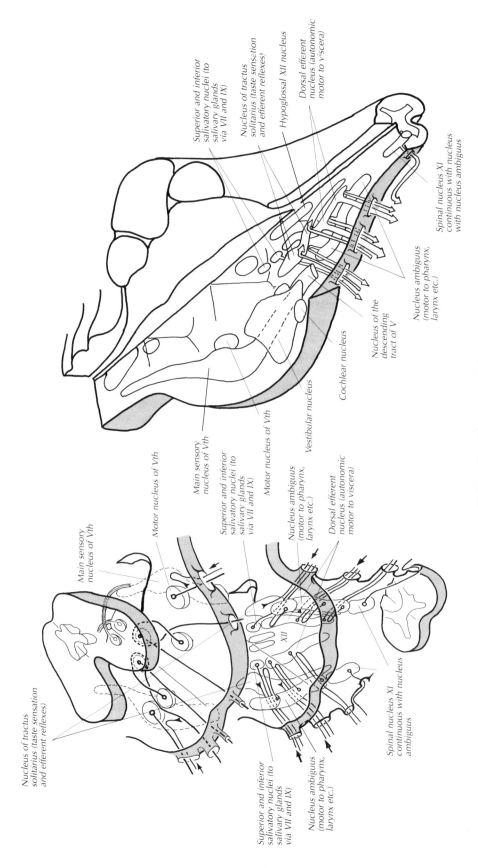

11.10 Cranial nerve nuclei.

the right side of the face enters the brain stem in the right fifth nerve at midpontine level. The fibres subserving the corneal reflex and simple tactile sensation immediately enter the nucleus of the fifth nerve in the pons, and decussate at midpontine level to the opposite side of the pons.

Fibres subserving pain and temperature sensation do not enter the nucleus but **descend** parallel to the descending nucleus of the fifth nerve and enter it to relay to the opposite side in the lower medulla and upper cervical cord. The crossed fibres then become the secondary ascending tract of the fifth nerve (the quintothalamic tract), lying adjacent to the medial lemniscus as both ascend through the brain stem. The levels at which fibres decussate are of practical importance and are detailed in the figures.

Because of this complex and extensive anatomical pathway a lesion in the dorsolateral lower pons and medulla on the left side will result in numbness of the left side of the face and numbness of the right side of the body. This crossed sensory loss is typical of a dorsolateral brainstem lesion, at any level between the mid-pons and C2 cord level.

The Cranial Nerve Nuclei (Figs. 11.3 and 11.10)

The clinical features of individual cranial nerve lesions have already been covered in previous chapters. The anatomical arrangement of the cranial nerve nuclei is not haphazard, and an understanding of their embryological development greatly facilitates learning.

The motor nuclei are derived from two nuclear columns, clearly indicated by different tones in figure 11.3.

1. The nuclei of the third, sixth and twelfth cranial nerves are derived from a paramedian nuclear mass. The third and fourth nuclei retain a close relationship in the midbrain but the sixth nerve nucleus is pulled down into the pons when the pontine flexure develops (see Chapter 15). The twelfth nerve nucleus is a long column of cells lying ventral to the obex and central canal of the cord at cervicomedullary level.

2. The ninth, tenth and eleventh nerve nuclei arise from a ventrolateral column of cells that is splayed laterally by the development of the fourth ventricle, as illustrated in Figure 11.3.

The positions of the nuclei within the brain stem influence the fascicular course of the cranial nerves. Fascicles are those parts of the nerve that course through the substance of the brainstem. The fascicles of the third, sixth and twelfth nerves must traverse the entire depth of the brain stem to exit just lateral to the midline on the ventral surface. The fourth nerve exits in a unique way by emerging from the dorsal aspect of

the brain stem after decussating in the superior medullary velum, and then passes forwards around the cerebral peduncles. The fifth nerve passes laterally to exit from the anterolateral surface of the pons.

The seventh nerve fasciculus follows a peculiar course, at first heading towards the floor of the fourth ventricle, where it passes round the sixth nerve nucleus, and then turns back on itself to cross the entire depth of the brain stem to exit from the ventral surface. This peculiar arrangement means that a brainstem lesion in this area will usually damage both the sixth and seventh nerves (see Figure 11.7).

The ninth, tenth and eleventh cranial nerves have very complicated nuclei. The main motor nucleus of all three is the nucleus ambiguus. The main parasympathetic secretomotor nuclei, to the lacrimal and salivary glands, are the inferior salivatory nucleus to the ninth nerve and its anatomical continuation, the dorsal efferent nucleus to the tenth nerve.

Gustatory reflex activity and taste sensation are relayed through the long spoon-shaped nucleus of the tractus solitarius.

The vestibular nuclei occupy almost the entire lower lateral pons, with ramifications over the entire brain stem from the midbrain down to the cervical spinal cord. For this reason vestibular symptoms and signs are almost always present in brainstem disease but are therefore of limited localizing value (for further discussion of the relationship of the vestibular and other cranial nerve nuclei, see Chapter 7).

The Blood Supply of the Brain Stem (Figs 11.11 and 11.12)

Vascular lesions have always been important causes of brainstem disease. Syphilitic vascular disease was extremely common 40 years ago when numerous eponymous brainstem syndromes were first described. Syphilis is now a rare cause, but degenerative arterial disease has assumed increasing significance and produces the syndrome known as 'vertebrobasilar ischaemia'. There is a continuing need to have a basic knowledge of the blood supply of the brain stem in order to understand the constellations of symptoms and signs that may result from a brainstem vascular accident.

The blood supply of the medulla is derived from the paired vertebral arteries which join at the pontomedullary junction to form the basilar artery. From its medial side each vertebral artery gives origin to a branch that joins with its fellow to form the anterior spinal artery. This vessel supplies part of the central medulla and the bulk of the spinal cord down to T1. On its lateral side each vertebral artery gives off a variable branch, the posterior inferior cerebellar artery. This vessel is absent in 25% of people. When the vessel is

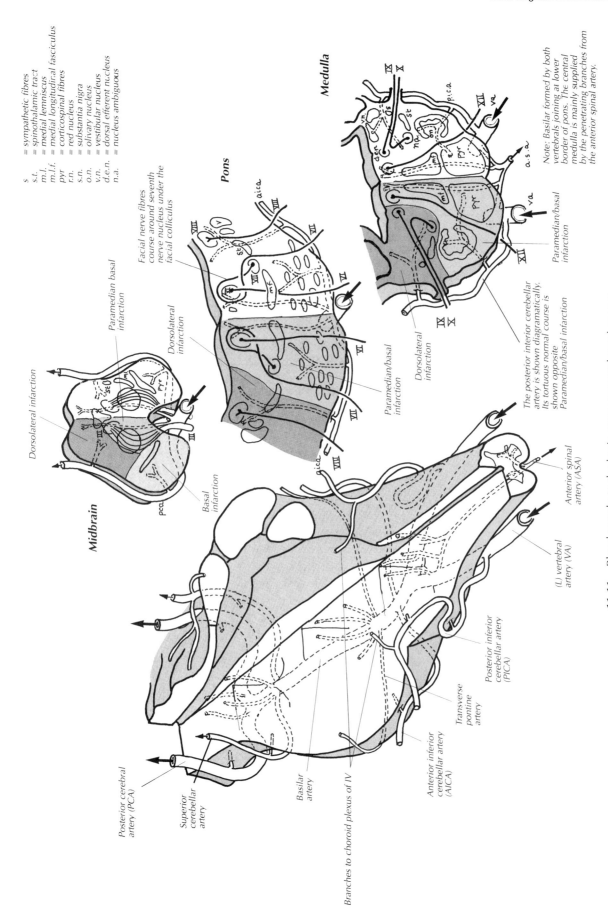

Midbrain

Pons

Medulla

s   = sympathetic fibres
s.t.   = spinothalamic tract
m.l.   = medial lemniscus
m.l.f. = medial longitudinal fasciculus
pyr   = corticospinal fibres
r.n.   = red nucleus
s.n.   = substantia nigra
o.n.   = olivary nucleus
v.n.   = vestibular nucleus
d.e.n. = dorsal efferent nucleus
n.a.   = nucleus ambiguous

Facial nerve fibres course around seventh nerve nucleus under the facial colliculus

Note: Basilar formed by both vertebrals joining at lower border of pons. The central medulla is mainly supplied by the penetrating branches from the anterior spinal artery.

Dorsolateral infarction

Paramedian basal infarction

Basal infarction

Dorsolateral infarction

Paramedian/basal infarction

Paramedian/basal infarction

Dorsolateral infarction

Paramedian/basal infarction

The posterior inferior cerebellar artery is shown diagramatically. Its tortuous normal course is shown opposite

Anterior spinal artery (ASA)

(L) vertebral artery (VA)

Posterior inferior cerebellar artery (PICA)

Transverse pontine artery

Anterior inferior cerebellar artery (AICA)

Basilar artery

Branches to choroid plexus of IV

Superior cerebellar artery

Posterior cerebral artery (PCA)

11.11   Blood supply to the brain stem: posterolateral aspect

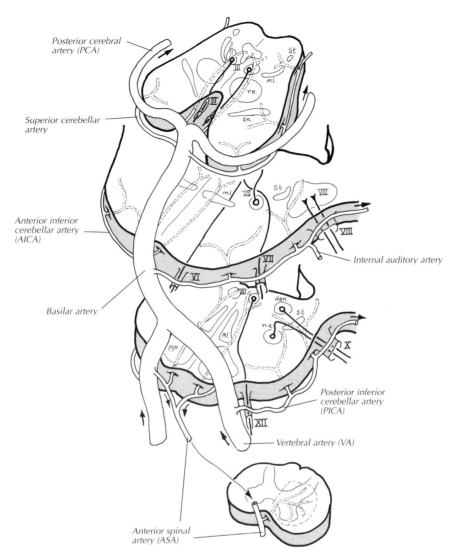

11.12   Blood supply to the brain stem : Anterior aspect

present it runs a tortuous course along the posterolateral surface of the medulla, which it supplies.

Higher up the brain stem vessels follow the same pattern of distribution. These vessels arising from the basilar artery are, from below upwards: the anterior inferior cerebellar artery, the transverse pontine arteries, the superior cerebellar arteries and the posterior cerebral arteries. Each gives off a long penetrating paramedian branch that supplies the central area of the brainstem to the floor of the fourth ventricle, and a series of short branches that supply the basal area of the brain stem, while the main trunk of the vessel passes round the brain stem to supply the dorsolateral quadrant and then part of the cerebellar hemisphere. The superior cerebellar artery supplies all the deep structures of the cerebellum, including the nuclei. The anterior inferior cerebellar artery usually gives off a named branch, the internal auditory artery, that supplies the inner ear and the vestibular apparatus.

Clinical Aspects of Brainstem Disorders

Brainstem disorders unfortunately represent one aspect of neurology in which an often-voiced criticism – that neurologists make the diagnosis but have no treatment to offer – has some substance. Thanks to the pinpoint accuracy of MRI scanning, clinical uncertainty may be resolved and direct and stereotactic surgical approaches to brainstem lesions are now feasible. There are also some other relatively rare and treatable conditions. As so often in neurology, it is the ability to recognize the unusual features or signs that do not make anatomical sense, that enables such cases to be identified.

The differential diagnosis of brainstem disease is complicated by a specific feature of the symptomatology. All the common symptoms, such as diplopia, dysarthria, vertigo, nausea and vomiting, are by their very nature acute. For example, a patient either has double vision or he does not, and although it may vary in degree the onset will be abrupt. Unless this fact is recognized, all lesions will appear to be due to vascular disease because of the abrupt, stroke-like onset of symptoms. Progression of a brainstem lesion can only be established if new acute symptoms or signs appear. Without MRI scanning the necessary period of observation, which was required to indicate the progressive nature of the neurological disorder, often proved a harmful or even fatal course of action. Even with MRI there is still a need to have a clear idea of the typical symptoms, signs and behaviour of various brainstem lesions for diagnostic precision.

Vascular lesions produce a defined area of damage in an identifiable vascular territory. If the lesion appears to be patchy, or to involve both sides of the brainstem, a vascular lesion becomes much less likely. Vascular syndromes will be considered first and then the clinical pictures produced by multiple sclerosis, pontine gliomas and other brainstem disorders can be compared and contrasted.

Brainstem Vascular Syndromes

In the diagrams of the midbrain and pons three vascular territories are indicated and in the medulla only two. This is because the central area of the medulla is supplied by penetrating branches derived from the vertebral, basilar and anterior spinal arteries. Occlusion of any of these main vessels, with consequent blockage of their penetrating branches, may lead to extensive unilateral or even bilateral infarction at central medullary level, producing confusing, patchy brainstem lesions.

Midbrain Vascular Lesions (Figs 11.11a and 11.12)

Dorsolateral Infarction

Infarction of the dorsolateral area will cause a Horner's syndrome on the same side and total loss of sensation on the opposite side of the body, as all the sensory pathways have come together at this level. This will be associated with a cerebellar deficit on the **same** side if the superior cerebellar peduncle is also damaged. If the lesion is extensive enough to interfere with the third nerve nucleus, the combination of a third nerve lesion and ipsilateral cerebellar lesion is known as Nothnagel's syndrome.

Paramedian Infarction

A third nerve lesion will occur if there is damage to the nucleus itself or the nerve fascicle. Because of the long vertical extent of the oculomotor nucleus in the midbrain, incomplete third nerve lesions may occur. Damage to the red nucleus interrupts the dentatorubrothalamic tract from the opposite cerebellar hemisphere, and this will result in cerebellar signs in the limbs **opposite** the third nerve lesion. This is referred to as Benedikt's syndrome.

Basal Infarction

The third nerve fascicle will be damaged, resulting in a complete third nerve palsy. The damage to the cerebral peduncle will result in hemiplegia of the opposite limbs, including the face. This combination is called Weber's syndrome. This combination of a third nerve lesion and hemiplegia of the opposite side can very accurately mimic a developing tentorial pressure cone (see Chapter 23). This situation can now be readily resolved by CT scanning but in the past, when combined with the inevitable drowsiness, this syndrome presented a difficult diagnostic challenge.

Pontine Vascular Lesions (Figs 11.11b and 11.12)

Dorsolateral Infarction

As usual, a Horner's syndrome on the side of the lesion will be found in nearly all cases, often coupled with loss of pain and temperature sensation in the limbs on the opposite side of the body. Above midpontine level facial sensation should be spared and touch and proprioception should be intact, as the medial lemniscus is too deeply placed at this level to be involved.

Below midpontine level there is an increased likelihood of finding loss of sensation over the face on the **same** side, because the lesion can damage the entering and descending sensory fibres of the fifth nerve. At all pontine levels some degree of cerebellar involvement will be found on the same side.

At midpontine level the lateral pontine reticular formation will be affected, with loss of conjugate lateral gaze towards the side of the lesion. At lower pontine level the vestibular and cochlear nuclei are likely to be damaged, causing vestibular symptoms, nystagmus and deafness. This will frequently be combined with loss of pain and temperature sensation over the face on the side of the lesion, and loss of the same modalities on the opposite side of the body. This is the classic location of the lesion causing this 'crossed sensory loss'.

Paramedian Infarction

The most readily identifiable lesions occur at the level of the sixth nerve nucleus. There will be a sixth nerve palsy, often combined with a conjugate gaze palsy to the same side as the connections to the opposite third nerve will also be damaged. The seventh nerve fibres will also be interrupted as they sweep round the sixth nerve nucleus. If the medial lemniscus is affected there will be loss of touch and proprioception on the opposite side of the body.

Basal Infarction

The fascicles of the sixth and the seventh nerve will be damaged, together with the pyramidal pathways. In an extensive lesion a full hemiplegia will result and this coupled with the sixth and seventh nerve lesions, is known as Millard–Gubler syndrome. If only the sixth nerve is affected, with a hemiplegia on the opposite side, it is known as Raymond's syndrome. As the pyramidal pathways are still dispersed at this level the hemiplegia may be incomplete. In most cases conjugate gaze will be intact. Therefore, although the eye on the side of the lesion will be unable to abduct because of the sixth nerve palsy, the opposite eye will move normally on attempted lateral gaze towards the side of the lesion. Occasionally more extensive infarction of the ventrolateral pons may occur, resulting in a conjugate gaze palsy to the side of the lesion, facial numbness, facial palsy, Horner's syndrome and deafness, all on the same side. This is called Foville's syndrome.

The facial weakness in pontine lesions may be extremely complicated. The facial nerve on the side of the lesion may be damaged at fascicular level, causing a lower motor neuron lesion on that side. If, in addition, the upper motor neuron fibres to the opposite seventh nerve are affected as they decussate, an upper motor neuron seventh nerve lesion will occur on the opposite side. Bilateral asymmetrical facial weakness of this sort can be very hard to detect and may be readily overlooked (see Fig. 11.7).

Medullary Vascular Lesions (Figs 11.11c and 11.12).

Dorsolateral Infarction

The clinical picture resulting from damage in this area is known as Wallenberg's syndrome. Because of the variability of the blood supply to this area it is incorrect to regard this as necessarily synonymous with posterior inferior cerebellar artery occlusion. In many cases it is an occlusion of the parent vertebral artery that is responsible. The major features are an ipsilateral Horner's syndrome and contralateral loss of pain and temperature sensation. Because the descending tract and nucleus of the fifth nerve are invariably affected, there will be loss of pain and temperature sensation over the face on the side of the lesion.

The lower vestibular nuclei are usually involved, resulting in severe vertigo, nausea, vomiting and nystagmus. Damage to the inferior cerebellar peduncle will cause ataxia of the limbs on the side of the lesion. The ninth and tenth cranial nerves are affected, causing intractable hiccups and serious difficulty in swallowing. It is sometimes claimed that sixth, seventh and twelfth nerve lesions and hemiplegia can occur as part of the syndrome. Anatomically, this combination of signs would indicate infarction of the entire half of the medulla and is inconsistent with a pure dorsolateral medullary lesion, and to use the term Wallenberg's syndrome for such a combination of signs renders the eponymous syndrome invalid as a synonym for dorsolateral medullary infarction.

Paramedian/Basal Infarction

Due to the slightly different pattern of blood supply of the central medulla much more extensive unilateral or even bilateral infarction of the central medulla can occur. In the upper brain stem vascular lesions produce strictly unilateral damage that does not transgress the midline – an important diagnostic point. A central lesion in the medullary area will typically cause a twelfth nerve palsy on one side, with hemiplegia and sensory loss to touch and joint position sense on the opposite side. Bilateral infarction can occur, producing bilateral twelfth nerve lesions, bilateral loss of touch and position sense and a quadriplegia. This renders the patient mute and paralysed. This has been called the 'locked-in' syndrome, as the patient is quite unable to communicate although fully conscious. There may also be bilateral loss of sensation over the face, as the decussating fibres of the trigeminal system may be damaged as they cross to their respective quintothalamic tracts.

Transient Brainstem Ischaemic Attacks

Transient brainstem ischaemic attacks occur when either a large embolus traverses the main arterial tree or microemboli pass through the smaller branches. This may result in very generalized brainstem dysfunction or very brief episodes of ischaemia that can be clearly localized to one of the many arterial territories discussed above. Because the brainstem vessels are end arteries the risk of a small embolus causing infarction is quite high. It seems likely that the majority of transient attacks are due to more major emboli traversing the vertebral and basilar arteries. The most frequent symptoms are vestibular. It has been suggested that this is because the vestibular nuclei have a precarious blood supply, but it seems much more likely, when the full extent of the vestibular representation in the brain stem is considered, that it is impossible for some part of the vestibular system **not** to be affected wherever the ischaemia occurs. There is a danger that any elderly patient feeling dizzy in a crowded shop on a hot day will be incorrectly diagnosed as having suffered a brain stem ischaemic episode. There is also a tendency to attribute any giddiness noted by the patient to be related to extending their head, to temporary blockage of the vertebral artery by degenerative cervical spine disease. This not only suggests a serious design fault, but is a concept for which there is remarkably little anatomical support. In most instances it is due to benign positional vertigo (see Chapter 7).

The symptoms of brainstem ischaemic episodes may include vertigo, dysarthria and tingling around the mouth, all indicating central medullary dysfunction. At pontine levels vertigo, hearing abnormalities, tingling, unilateral numbness or weakness of the limbs and diplopia are frequent symptoms. Mesencephalic ischaemia may cause diplopia, sudden loss of consciousness, unilateral weakness of limbs and complete blindness or transient hemianopia, if the calcarine cortex becomes ischaemic from impaired flow in either posterior cerebral artery. The following case is an interesting example, in which the passage of an embolus through the vertebral basilar territory to the posterior cerebral artery can be followed.

CASE REPORT I

A 63-year-old man visited his son in Cyprus. During a meal in a mountaintop restaurant at 5000 feet he suddenly felt very dizzy and his speech became slurred. He thought it was the effect of altitude and staggered outside for fresh air, but found he could barely walk and his right leg became increasingly weak. He was driven down the winding mountain road with steadily increasing vertigo, slurred speech, diplopia and vomiting. He made a steady recovery over the next 48 hours, but when he became mobile he noticed that he was bumping into things on his right side. When examined a week later, the only residual physical sign was a right macular-sparing hemianopia, typical of a posterior cerebral artery occlusion.

Brainstem Dysfunction Caused by Intracranial Haemorrhage

There are several ways in which intracranial haemorrhage can affect brainstem function. An acute haemorrhage into the pons itself causes a very characteristic clinical picture. The patient complains of a severe headache and rapidly becomes unconscious, and then develops periodic respiration, pinpoint pupils, loss of 'doll's-head' eye movements and a spastic tetraplegia. This immediate spasticity is a striking feature of brainstem haemorrhage. There seems to be no stage of 'shock' with flaccidity, and decerebrate posturing may quickly follow. Death may ensue within hours, but should the patient survive for several days the body temperature typically steadily rises before death.

Haemorrhage into the basal ganglia or internal capsule often tracks down into the cerebral peduncle

and produces a midbrain lesion. If the haematoma ruptures into the ventricular system, the rapid rush of blood down into the fourth ventricle may produce acute brainstem dysfunction with cardiac and respiratory arrest.

A primary haemorrhage into the cerebellum produces its lethal effect by brainstem distortion. Surgical evacuation offers a significant chance of recovery and prompt diagnosis is critical. The onset is acute, with sudden occipital headache, vomiting and ataxia. Within a variable period consciousness becomes impaired, with the onset of gaze palsies, bilateral pyramidal signs and periodic respiration. Death will follow rapidly unless surgical evacuation of the clot is attempted. The clinical picture can mimic a subarachnoid haemorrhage and the risk of a diagnostic lumbar puncture in this precarious situation is only too obvious. This particular syndrome is also a frequent presentation of a 'benign' cerebellar haemangioblastoma, and examples of this condition are included in Chapters 7 and 12.

Subarachnoid haemorrhage may produce an identical picture. The onset is heralded by sudden headache, usually associated with acute nausea, vomiting and vertigo. These brainstem features occur so frequently that the bleeding is often mistakenly thought to be due to an aneurysm in the posterior fossa. The similarity between this and intracerebral haemorrhage should indicate why it is unwise to rush into performing a lumbar puncture in a case of suspected subarachnoid haemorrhage. An intracerebral haematoma is 'space occupying' in the same way as a tumour. The risks of lumbar puncture are the same, and in the case of a cerebellar haematoma the risk is considerable. Lumbar puncture is never a life-saving procedure in subarachnoid haemorrhage, and should **never** be allowed to become a life-threatening investigation. CT scanning will usually clarify the diagnosis and only rarely would a lumbar puncture be considered necessary. It is safer to move the patient to a facility where scanning is available than perform a lumbar puncture, especially if they are rapidly deteriorating. Rapid clinical deterioration in subarachnoid haemorrhage indicates either a coexisting intracerebral haematoma or massive infarction in the territory supplied by the artery containing the aneurysm. In both situations the damaged area acts as a rapidly expanding space-occupying lesion, and the prognosis for survival is poor. Subarachnoid haemorrhage is discussed further in Chapters 9 and 22.

Multiple Sclerosis and the Brain Stem

Multiple sclerosis commonly affects the brain stem and in a known case of multiple sclerosis the cause of a brainstem attack is obvious. If it is the first event, the diagnosis can be more difficult to establish. Fortunately, there are certain features that would strongly suggest that the cause of a brainstem lesion is multiple sclerosis. The medial longitudinal bundle is extremely vulnerable and any form of internuclear ophthalmoplegia is likely to be caused by demyelination and, if bilateral, multiple sclerosis is almost certain to be the cause. Involvement of the (Vth) fifth nerve in the brain stem may cause unilateral facial numbness which recovers over 6-9 weeks. Sometimes after recovery the patient may develop trigeminal neuralgia as a later complication. Isolated sixth nerve palsies are another common manifestation of multiple sclerosis and this is the only common **lower** motor neuron lesion that occurs in this disease. Bilateral vestibular pathway damage with rotatory nystagmus on lateral gaze and vertical nystagmus on upward gaze is unlikely to be caused by any other disorder. The subsequent spontaneous recovery over 6–10 weeks makes the diagnosis almost certain. The hallmark of brainstem multiple sclerosis is the combination of bilateral cerebellar and pyramidal signs. The patient may complain only of ataxia and slurring of speech, but physical examination will reveal that in addition to the anticipated cerebellar signs there are bilateral pyramidal signs, including a brisk jaw jerk, pathologically brisk reflexes and bilateral extensor plantar responses. Although any of the signs discussed above strongly suggest the diagnosis of multiple sclerosis, it is always worth remembering that nothing can be regarded as absolutely pathognomonic of this condition.

MRI scanning will sometimes demonstrate the actual brainstem lesion if sufficiently large, but in many instances it is extensive white matter lesions in the hemispheres that will confirm the diagnosis and allow the safe presumption that the lesion in the brain stem is also due to demyelinating disease.

Pontine Glioma

If a young child or a patient with neurofibromatosis develops brainstem signs the possibility of a brainstem glioma should be considered. In other situations or age groups this diagnosis is extremely rare, and multiple sclerosis is usually suspected. Delay in diagnosis may be potentially serious, as pontine gliomas are moderately radiosensitive and early diagnosis and radiotherapy may offer some hope of a prolonged remission. Many of these tumours start in the region of the sixth nerve nucleus, and any combination of a sixth and seventh nerve palsy should be regarded with suspicion. Minimal motor signs, brisk reflexes and extensor plantar responses are often present, but hemiplegia is not an early symptom. The sensory pathways also seem to be extremely resistant to infiltration by these tumours, and patients may die of the disease without developing detectable sensory loss. In spite of gross

enlargement of the pons – the condition used to be called 'pseudohypertrophy of the pons' – blockage of the aqueduct is unusual and headache is not a feature of the clinical picture.

Previously careful documentation of the signs and the recognition of new lesions in the brainstem was often the only way of confirming that the diagnosis was correct if there was any initial uncertainty after air encephalography. MRI scanning with gadolinium enhancement can now confirm the diagnosis with certainty.

Other Posterior Fossa Tumours

The two major types of cerebellar tumour in childhood produce rapidly progressive cerebellar signs and raised intracranial pressure. Medulloblastomas may directly infiltrate the brain stem via the cerebellar peduncles. Cystic astrocytomas do not invade the brain stem but may threaten its viability by mechanical distortion if the diagnosis is long delayed. In adults ependymomas arising in the floor of the fourth ventricle produce unheralded vomiting and the presence of papilloedema usually excludes the diagnosis of a primary pontine tumour.

Posterior fossa tumours, other than metastases, are relatively rare in adulthood. They also tend to be slow-growing, producing a much less dramatic clinical picture than in childhood, and differential diagnosis may be extremely difficult. Pineal tumours produce raised intracranial pressure and evidence of upper mid-brain compression, such as Parinaud's syndrome. Acoustic nerve tumours usually produce signs of a cerebellopontine angle lesion, but sometimes the signs of brainstem distortion may dominate the clinical picture (see Chapter 6).

Chordomas, cholesteatomas and meningiomas may arise in front of the brain stem, and examples are included in Chapters 6 and 12. A rare condition which can produce either a relentlessly progressive or intermittent brain stem syndrome is ectasia of the basilar artery. In this condition, arteriosclerotic aneurysmal dilatation and tortuosity of the basilar artery acts as a large space-occupying lesion on the front of the brainstem.

CASE REPORT II

A 45-year-old man presented with complex partial seizures which were successfully treated with carbamazepine. The EEG showed non-specific findings. Five years later he developed a slowly progressive left facial palsy, increasing deafness in the left ear and ataxia. An acoustic nerve tumour was suspected, although it was recognized that the sequence of onset of symptoms was atypical. Vertebral angiography revealed an enormously ectatic basilar artery, the upper end of which had pushed laterally into and was deeply indenting the medial aspect of the left temporal lobe. This was almost certainly the cause of the original symptom.

CASE REPORT III

A 58-year-old man presented with classic trigeminal neuralgia, which was successfully treated by stereotactic thermocoagulation of the trigeminal ganglion. He returned 7 years later with a mild facial palsy and slurring of speech of acute onset, and a brainstem vascular lesion was suspected. Over the next few months he developed increasing difficulty in swallowing, wasting weakness and fasciculation of the tongue and increasing ataxia. An MRI scan revealed a serpentine basilar artery with massive backward displacement of the brain stem.

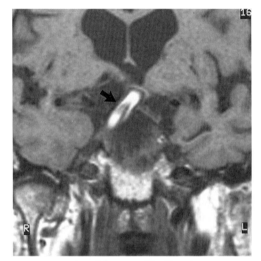

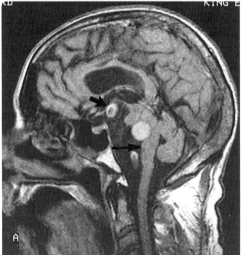

CRIII. *Ectasia of the basilar artery producing gross distortion and backwards displacement of the medullar and pons.*

In both these instances the presenting symptom was suggestive of common benign conditions and the long delay before other symptoms appeared is surprising, but this is typical of the behaviour of basilar ectasia. There is no treatment available for this condition, for obvious reasons, but the long time course and the

extent of distortion of the brain stem and its blood supply are amazing.

All the posterior fossa lesions discussed above may produce intermittent brainstem symptoms mimicking multiple sclerosis or transient ischaemic attacks. Transient sixth nerve palsies, ataxia and pyramidal signs may be found. Even vertical nystagmus, often held to be diagnostic of an intrinsic brainstem lesion, can occur with extrinsic compression of the brain stem. Tumours in the region of the foramen magnum, usually meningiomas or neurofibromas, are notorious for producing recurrent episodes of tetraparesis and ultimately tetraplegia. Many of these cases were in the past incorrectly diagnosed as multiple sclerosis for 20 years or longer, until sudden progressive symptomatology prompted re-evaluation. Once again, CT and MRI scanning have made investigation of these lesions safe and usually diagnostic.

Metabolic Brainstem Dysfunction

The toxic effects of alcohol and many drugs are caused by reversible metabolic effects on the brain stem. Severe vertigo ataxia, dysarthria and nystagmus are common side-effects of nearly all anticonvulsant drugs. Diphenylhydantoin, (Epanutin) (Dilantin USP), carbamazepine (Tegretol) and lamotrigine (Lamictal) can even cause a reversible internuclear ophthalmoplegia. The diagnosis of deliberate or accidental overdose of diphenylhydantoin or other anticonvulsants should be suspected in any patient having repeated attacks of drowsiness, ataxia, dysarthria and nystagmus. An overdose of glutethimide causes drowsiness, widely dilated pupils and brisk reflexes, stimulating a brainstem lesion. Extensor plantar responses may occur transiently during drug overdosage and deflect attention from the desirability of obtaining blood samples for drug levels in any drowsy or unconscious patient.

CASE REPORT IV

A 3-year-old child had been repeatedly admitted to hospital with unexplained episodes of coma since she was 1 year of age. This had been diagnosed at two hospitals as a rare form of epilepsy without EEG abnormality. By chance, she went into one of these attacks shortly after recovering from an episode, while still in the hospital. In this emergency situation the child was seen for the first time by a different neurologist. The striking features were the normality of the pupil responses, the profound depression of the reflexes and the flexor plantar responses in a comatose child. As she recovered, nystagmus was observed. It was suggested that the picture was due to sedative drug poisoning rather than epilepsy. A drug level estimation detected barbiturate even though the child was not taking a barbiturate anticonvulsant. The suggestion that this was due to non-accidental administration of the agent by the mother was treated with a certain amount of disbelief. Fortunately for the child, the mother chose to do it again and was caught with a straw containing tuinal capsules (a composite barbiturate sedative), which she was feeding to the child. It subsequently transpired that the only times the child had gone into coma during previous admissions to a paediatric hospital was on two occasions when the mother had been allowed to take her for a walk in a pram!

This is a classic example of Munchausen syndrome by proxy, and emphasizes the reason that this diagnosis is made with such reluctance even when it is obvious. It is difficult for even medical personnel to understand the motivation that may lead to the death of a child, and even harder when the cause is a member of the medical team itself, as recently happened in the UK.

Wernicke's encephalopathy is a serious complication of alcoholism. In addition to the characteristic mental change of gross confusion with memory loss, there is also a potentially fatal disturbance of brainstem function. Extraocular nerve palsies, usually sixth nerve palsies, conjugate gaze palsies, nystagmus and ataxia are the main features. These signs are readily reversible following parenteral therapy with Vitamin B_1, although the mental changes are more persistent. It should be remembered that this condition can also occur in patients who are malnourished for medical reasons, such as malabsorption or following postoperative vomiting.

Central pontine myelinolysis is a rare and potentially lethal condition closely related to Wernicke's encephalopathy, occurring in the same clinical setting and with the similar signs. In the past the diagnosis was usually made at post mortem, when the patient had failed to respond to Vitamin B_1 therapy. The lesion is now demonstrable by MRI scanning, showing brainstem demyelinating lesions. The clinical picture is of the rapid evolution of a tetraplegia with brainstem involvement at all levels, which may produce a 'locked-in' syndrome. Non-alcohol-related cases are usually due to severe electrolyte disturbance, complicating sepsis, burns, malnutrition, liver disease and adrenal failure. Severe hyponatraemia is a constant feature of these conditions and there is some evidence that the mechanism is related to the too rapid restoration of sodium levels, which should be avoided.

Brainstem angiomas and brainstem encephalitis are exceptionally rare and are usually given more prominence in differential diagnostic discussions than they deserve. In the majority of cases where either diagnosis is entertained the patient is ultimately found to have another condition. A lethal encephalitis of the brain stem can be caused by herpes simplex virus. A rhomboencephalitis associated with *Listeria monocytogenes* meningitis is a rare condition occurring in neonates and immunocompromised patients. Very rarely, herpes zoster affecting the fifth cranial nerve may be associated with a brainstem encephalitis which, unlike the former conditions, carries an excellent prognosis for recovery.

Congenital malformations of the foramen magnum may lead to the development of brainstem problems in later life. The syndrome of vertebrobasilar ischaemia may be caused by an anomalous odontoid peg, basilar invagination or platybasia. Syringomyelia and syringobulbia are related to congenital abnormalities of the foramen magnum and associated neural maldevelopment. These conditions are fully discussed in Chapter 15.

Brainstem lesions are quite common and may represent an immediate threat to the patient's life or a delayed threat from complications, such as aspiration pneumonia. Prompt accurate diagnosis is essential, and this can best be achieved with a sound anatomical knowledge and an understanding of the common causes of brainstem disease and their clinical behaviour.

In the past, the investigation of a lesion within or distorting the brain stem was extremely difficult, even with CT scanning, because the cup-like shape of the bony margins of the posterior fossa produce extensive bone artefact in most tomographic cuts, particularly down towards the foramen magnum. MRI scanning has overcome this difficulty, with its unique ability to avoid bone artefact, and the incredibly precise sagittal views possible with this technique has transformed our ability to image this anatomically complex area. Distinctions between haemorrhage and infarction, Multiple Sclerosis and glioma, and aneurysmal dilatation of the basilar artery have become relatively simple, but management has unfortunately not improved in parallel.

12. The Extrapyramidal System and the Cerebellum

Although it is an unconventional approach, there are anatomical, pathological and clinical reasons for considering disorders of the extrapyramidal system and cerebellum together, and this unusual combination has been retained in this edition.

Anatomical knowledge of the architecturally homogeneous cerebellum has always been in advance of clinical knowledge of cerebellar function. There are relatively few physical signs of cerebellar disease and direct clinicoanatomical correlation is rarely possible. Often the resulting physical signs and symptoms are secondary to distortion of the brain stem and interference with the circulation of the CSF. Multiple sclerosis commonly affects the cerebellum but coincidental involvement of brainstem pathways makes clinical distinction impossible.

In contrast, many disorders have long been known to be due to damage in the extrapyramidal system and yet pathological findings were minimal or absent. Even now the anatomical extent of the extrapyramidal system is uncertain, hence the expression 'extrapyramidal system', rather than the more restrictive older term 'basal ganglia disease'.

With the knowledge that many of these disorders have a neurochemical basis, an entirely different concept of the functioning of the system has emerged. It is now apparent that, far from the cerebellum being the 'head ganglion of the proprioceptive system', with direct control over movement, it serves as an integrating centre for postural information, which it relays to the cerebral cortex and the basal ganglia and, via the gamma loop system, controls the basic tone in muscles via the intrafusal muscle fibres. This explains the similarities of the symptoms and signs of extrapyramidal and cerebellar disease, which cause such diagnostic confusion in beginners. Disease in both areas causes abnormalities of gait, movement and tone and unwanted additional movements that occur either at rest or on attempted movement.

Unfortunately, such dynamic clinical disorders do not readily lend themselves to an illustrative approach. Instead, an attempt has been made to provide clear descriptions of the various clinical signs and a disease classification based on clinical similarities and the age of the patient. The latter is particularly important to cerebellar disease in which the diagnostic possibilities are quite different in the child and adult.

Anatomical Considerations (Fig. 12.1)

Movement is initiated through the direct corticospinal or pyramidal system, which is at its most highly developed in man. At the same time, the continual postural adjustments that underlie smooth and coordinated movement are initiated by the corticopallidal system, which projects mainly into the putamen. To complete the volitional side of activity there are the important cortico-pontocerebellar projections, which enter the cerebellum through the very large middle cerebral peduncle (the brachium pontis). Therefore, all three parts of the CNS concerned in movement are simultaneously alerted to the onset, intended direction and ultimate objective of a movement. It is only in disease states that the extent and importance of the nonpyramidal mechanisms become apparent.

The main sensory input to the system comes from the muscle, tendon and joint position sense receptors, mainly via the spinocerebellar tracts, and from the vestibular apparatus via the vestibular nuclei. Information from both sources enters the cerebellum mainly through the inferior cerebellar peduncle, the restiform body in older terminology.

The cytoarchitecture of the cerebellar cortex is uniquely arranged to allow the projection of a vast amount of information on to the extensive dendritic net of each Purkinje cell, and models explaining this in computer and mathematical terms have been made. The large axon from each Purkinje cell projects to the central cerebellar nuclei, mainly to the dentate nucleus on the same side. This nucleus relays the information to the opposite ventrolateral thalamus and to the cortex via the dentatorubral, rubrothalamic, dentatothalamic and thalamocortical projections. These pathways leave

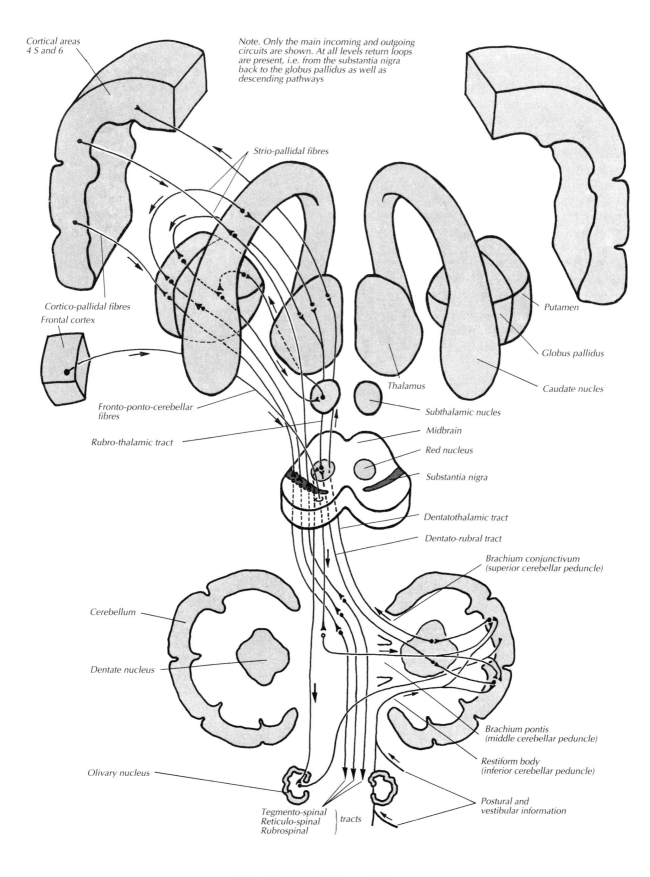

12.1 Extrapyramidal cerebellar system.

the cerebellum through the superior cerebellar peduncle, the brachium conjunctivum, and decussate through the region of, or relay in, the red nucleus. The information reaching the thalamus is then projected to the extrapyramidal cortical areas and direct to the basal ganglia, particularly to the putamen, caudate and external globus pallidus. This completes a group of circuits involving the cortex, basal ganglia and cerebellar components. The cortex initiates the activity and the cerebellar input provides the necessary feedback information.

In addition to these outer circuits there is a very important inner loop which has an inhibitory feedback effect on the globus pallidus. This is a relay through the subthalamic nucleus of Luys. Damage to this circuit literally unleashes one of the most dramatic conditions in neurology, the syndrome known as hemiballismus.

The other efferent pathways from the basal ganglia remain uncertain. The critically important pathway to the substantia nigra is well established but the exact routes of extrapyramidal activity below this level are unknown. The projections probably include the tegmentospinal, rubrospinal, reticulospinal and olivospinal tracts. The relay through the olivary nucleus includes a circuit back into the cerebellum. Damage in this pathway has been implicated in the disorders characterized by myoclonic phenomena.

The pathways described and illustrated represent only a fraction of the total neuronal circuitry involved in normal extrapyramidal function. Those included provide the best framework for clinical discussion.

Pathological and Biochemical Considerations

Parkinsonism was the first recognized and is certainly the most studied disease of the extrapyramidal system. In spite of intensive pathological study over 50 years, the only constant finding was depigmentation and loss of neurons in the substantia nigra and the later recognition that the other pigmented neurons in the CNS were also affected. In the period 1918–1927 a pandemic of a viral disorder known as encephalitis lethargica (Von Economo's encephalitis) occurred. This was associated with very gross disturbances of sleep, behaviour and every possible combination of abnormal movement. In patients dying of the disorder no constant pathological findings that could account for the physical signs were found. In the 1960's the severe and occasionally irreversible facial dyskinesias and dystonias caused by phenothiazines provided further evidence of obvious clinical disease in the absence of any pathological abnormalities.

In the last 30 years, histochemical studies of the brain have produced the dramatic breakthrough that indicates that these conditions are due, initially at least, to neurochemical disorders, and later complicated by progressive neuronal damage. The initial normality of the underlying neural pathways has been adequately confirmed clinically by the dramatic restoration of near normal function to patients immobilized by parkinsonism for decades, by the oral administration of transmitter precursors such as levodopa or amantadine hydrochloride, which may release residual dopamine. Some of the manifestations of Parkinson's disease would appear to be related to the relative overactivity of cholinergic pathways unmasked by the reduced activity in dopaminergic pathways. It would also seem that it is not a simple matter of stimulatory and inhibitory transmitters in balance. There is evidence that both acetylcholine and dopamine have stimulant effects in some areas and inhibitory effects in others.

It is possible to make some broad generalizations as to the possible relationship of the two systems, as revealed by clinical observations of the effect of drugs in the treatment of Parkinson's disease.

Normal extrapyramidal function would seem to require a balance between cholinergic and dopaminergic pathways, whether these be inhibitory or stimulatory. A decrease in activity in the cholinergic pathway or an increase in dopaminergic pathway activity results in choreiform movements. In Huntington's chorea, which is pathologically characterized by severe degeneration of the caudate nucleus, in which most cholinergic neurons are concentrated, choreiform movements are the prominent feature. Identical movements can be produced in patients with Parkinson's disease if they are treated with excessive doses of levodopa, and the advent of such movements late in the course of the disease is a major dose-limiting factor in treatment.

Theoretically, an increase in cholinergic activity could cause Parkinson's disease but this condition seems not to exist, although efforts to enhance cholinergic activity are currently the main thrust of research into the possible treatment of Alzheimer's disease. Idiopathic Parkinson's disease is due to a decrease in dopaminergic activity and the clinical manifestations are a combination of tremor, rigidity and slowness of movement. Hence atropine-like drugs which block cholinergic neurons are of some benefit in Parkinson's disease, particularly in the relief of tremor, although often at the cost of producing hallucinations and confusion. Drugs such as reserpine, the phenothiazines, tetrabenazine and butyrophenones, which deplete or block dopaminergic neurons, will worsen or cause parkinsonism.

It follows from these therapeutic and biochemical observations, and the observation that depression often complicates parkinsonism and that antipsychotic drugs may produce parkinsonism, that there is high probability that many mental disorders are related to similar but as yet unidentified alterations in the neurotransmitters. The complexity of these pathways, which are actually closed loops with different transmitters at different synapses, certainly explains the peculiarities and paucity of pathological findings. For example, histochemically and clinically it is clear that in parkinsonism the main problem lies in the dopaminergic synapses in the pallidum, and yet the main pathological change is found in the synaptic area of the substantia nigra. It also explains why a lesion in one site does not necessarily indicate a specific function for that area. For example, it would be incorrect to assume that because chorea occurs if the caudate is damaged, the normal function of the caudate is to prevent chorea. However, the assumption that damage to one circuit leads to an imbalance that could be corrected by deliberately destroying another, formed the theoretical basis for the moderately successful stereotactic operations for parkinsonism which enjoyed a vogue before the introduction of levodopa. These operations almost became obsolete, although by 1975 it seemed likely that there would still be a place for such surgery in Parkinson's disease and some other conditions where tremor was a major feature. This has proved to be the case, particularly with the recognition that antitremor drugs have limited effectiveness and unacceptable side-effects, and stereotactic surgery has enjoyed something of a renaissance. Computer-guided stereotactic lesions have improved the effectiveness, but careful patient selection is still necessary and the risk of unwanted deficit still limits its usefulness.

Clinical Features of Extrapyramidal Disease

There are a wide range of movement disorders and physical signs associated with disease in the extrapyramidal system. To avoid lengthy descriptions, a terminology of these signs has been developed which ought to have simplified their documentation. Owing to the varying use of these terms the situation has become more confused, and attempts are now being made to combine certain signs into fewer major groups. It is probably best to define carefully all terms in current use to enable the beginner to find his way through this particularly difficult neurological 'jargon'. Table 12.1 indicates the major clinical causes of the various movement disorders, which will be amplified in later discussion. Many of these are extremely rare diseases. From the novice's point of view the main problem is recognizing that a movement disorder is organic: early

choreiform movements are often misdiagnosed as habit spasms, or thought to be of non-organic origin.

Tremor

The most important feature of tremor is that the rhythm is constant, producing a steady oscillation, although the amplitude of the movement may vary. From the outset it is important to stress that tremor is not always due to parkinsonism. Although parkinsonism often starts as a tremor there are numerous other diagnostic possibilities.

There are three clinically distinct forms of tremor.

Rest Tremor

Tremor due to any of the causes shown in Table 12.1 may be present at rest, and is often accentuated when the hands are held outstretched, but in Parkinson's disease, because the tremor often diminishes on action, holding the hand straight out usually lessens the tremor. In Parkinson's disease the tremor is often best observed when the patient is distracted while giving the history, or while walking along, when the non-swinging arm may start to tremble, often unnoticed by the patient.

Action Tremor (Intention Tremor)

It is so often stressed that action tremor is typical of cerebellar disease that the observation that nearly all types of tremor tend to be worse on action is frequently overlooked. The feature that distinguishes cerebellar action tremor on finger/nose testing is the inaccuracy of the movement and the tendency for the tremor to be accentuated just before the finger touches the nose. This is called terminal intention tremor. A parkinsonian tremor may stop on movement but, if it continues, the direction of movement remains accurate and the tremor is constant throughout the range. The most extreme degree of terminal intention tremor is seen in Wilson's disease, and has been called a 'batswing tremor' because the oscillations are so violent and over such a wide range that there is a real risk that the patient will injure their face or eyes.

Peduncular or Red Nuclear Tremor

This is a violent form of action tremor and most often occurs in patients who have multiple sclerosis or who have suffered midbrain vascular accidents. The tremor may be present at rest and can cause jerking extension movements of the head and inarticulate speech. The slightest attempt to move the arm is followed by severe wide-amplitude tremor. For example, the patient may take several minutes to release the handbrake of

Table 12.1   Movement disorders

Disorder	Disease responsible	Pathology
Tremor At rest	Parkinsonism	Failure of dopamine synthesis
	Anxiety	
	Alcohol or drugs (valproate)	Increased physiological tremor
	Thyrotoxicosis	
	Benign essential tremor	Unknown, often familial
	Wilson's disease	Abnormal copper metabolism
	Mercury poisoning	Basal ganglia damage
	Neurosyphilis	Infective or vascular lesion responsible
On action	Severe parkinsonism	
	Severe essential tremor	
	Cerebellar disease	
	Lesion of cerebellar connections	Lesion in region of the red nucleus
Chorea Localized	Sydenham's chorea	Rheumatic fever
	Posterior capsular CVA	Lesion in posterior thalamic region
	Tumour in basal ganglia	
	Post thalamotomy	
Generalized	Sydenham's chorea	Rheumatic fever
	Contraceptive pill chorea	Related to previous
	Chorea gravidarum	rheumatic fever
	Thyrotoxicosis	
	Disseminated lupus erythematosus	Unknown
	Polycythaemia rubra vera	
	Huntington's chorea	Heredofamilial degeneration
	Senile chorea	Associated with dementia
	Hypercalcaemia	Metabolic
	Phenytoin toxicity	Unknown
Hemiballismus	Haemorrhagic damage	Lesion in the subthalamic nucleus
	Embolic infarction	
	Post traumatic	
Athetosis	Cerebral palsy	Neonatal jaundice
	Wilson's disease	Abnormal copper metabolism

	Juvenile Huntington's
	  chorea (rigid form)
		Heredofamilial disease
		  (very rare type)

	Hallevorden–Spatz disease	Demyelinating condition
	Alper's disease	Demyelinating condition
	Following cerebral anoxia	Anaesthetic accident or drowning
	Ataxia telangiectasia	Inherited neurocutaneous disorder
Dystonias Generalized	Encephalitis lethargica	Viral infection
	Lesch–Nyhan syndrome	Abnormal uric acid metabolism
	Phenothiazine sensitivity	Idiosyncratic drug reaction
	Butyrophenones	Idiosyncratic drug reaction
	Dystonia musculorum deformans	Inherited metabolic disorder
	Paroxysmal choreoathetosis	Inherited disease
	Levodopa	Drug sensitivity or overdose
Localized	Post– hemiplegia	Basal ganglia damage
	Post–thalamotomy	(rare complication)
	Post– traumatic	(rare complication)
	Spasmodic torticollis	Probably neurotransmitter defect
	Writer's cramp	Probably neurotransmitter defect
	Blepharospasm	Probably neurotransmitter defect
	Oral facial dyskinesias	Phenothiazines acute or tardive Senility Mental subnormality

the wheel chair, often bruising their arm in the process. They are quite unable to feed themselves and attempts to open the mouth are often accompanied by such violent head jerking that the food or drink is spilled. This type of tremor may respond to stereotactic surgery, but careful evaluation by MRI to avoid making an operative lesion symmetrical to an existing multiple sclerosis plaque is essential to avoid causing a pseudobulbar palsy. The lesion causing this tremor can be anywhere along the dentatorubrothalamic tract, and is not specifically located in the red nucleus itself.

CASE REPORT I

A 79-year-old man was brought to the A and E department because of dramatic uncontrolled movements of his left limbs. These were so violent that he had actually injured his elderly wife while trying to help her get out of bed, because

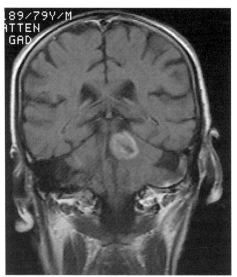

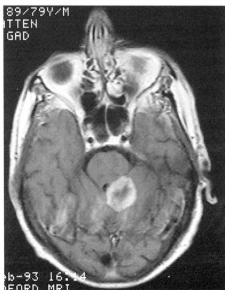

CRI. *Peduncular tremor due to presumed metastatic lesion in superior cerebellar peduncle.*

his arm flew into her face. At rest there was little or no movement but on attempted movement there were wild oscillations of almost ballistic severity. The leg was similarly affected, making walking almost impossible. The house physician on call was convinced that this was non-organic, as there were no other physical findings. This was thought to be unlikely in an octogenarian and an MRI scan revealed a solitary discrete lesion in the left superior cerebellar peduncle, confirming that this was a tremor due to a lesion in the dentatothalamic pathway. Its severity was modestly reduced when the patient was given tetrabenazine, but the dose required to control the movements caused unacceptable sedation. Screening tests revealed no obvious primary tumour and the patient was transferred to a nursing home where he collapsed and died 2 weeks later. Unfortunately, the hospital was not informed of his demise until several days later and the opportunity to confirm the exact site and nature of the lesion was lost.

Hemiballismus

This rare condition is considered at this point because it is so similar clinically to peduncular tremor and, if persistent, may also be improved by stereotactic surgery. It is very rare and is usually of abrupt onset following haemorrhage, infarction or damage to the subthalamic nucleus. Is the patient lies at complete rest the movements may be minimal, but any attempt to move is followed by wild flinging movements, particularly of the upper limb.

CASE REPORT II

A 38-year-old patient was in the surgical ward awaiting aortic valve surgery for aortic stenosis secondary to rheumatic fever. She quite suddenly developed violent flinging movements of the left arm, fracturing her radius and ulna against an adjacent radiator. When seen a few minutes later, the violent flinging movements of the arm – with devastating effects on the fracture – and to a lesser extent, of the left leg, had provoked angina. An intravenous injection of chlorpromazine 25 mg controlled the movements within minutes. It is presumed that they were due to an embolus from the aortic valve, which was later successfully treated.

Chlorpromazine 25 mg intravenously usually produces almost immediate relief and oral chlorpromazine will subsequently control the condition, with a tendency for the movements to subside over several weeks. If it fails to subside stereotactic surgery may be successful. Some classify this disorder as severe hemichorea, but the clinical features and the discrete pathological lesion responsible seem to warrant its classification as a separate entity.

Chorea

Choreiform movements are sudden rapid involuntary and purposeless jerks or fragments of movements that continually intrude into the patient's normal activity.

They are particularly prominent in the face and distal muscles, and the overall impression obtained of a patient with mild chorea is that they are 'fidgety'. The eyebrows may raise and lower, the mouth distort to produce half-smiles and half-grimaces. Patients repeatedly cross and uncross their legs and may sit with their arms tightly folded. Occasionally an arm may jerk out of place, the patient attempting to disguise the movement by stroking the chin or smoothing their hair. When fully developed the gait may be modified by abrupt sudden jerks of the trunk and flinging movements of the arms and legs. The movements are exhausting and are minimal while the patient is lying quietly. Any active movement will provoke further jerking. In an extremely mild case the movements are best seen in the outstretched hands or in the feet as sudden flexion or extension movements of the fingers or side-to-side movements of individual fingers or toes, which are virtually impossible to imitate. Hemichorea may occur following cerebrovascular accidents affecting the basal ganglia, and respond well to tetrabenazine.

Athetosis

Athetoid movements are slow writhing sinuous movements of the arms and legs. There is an increasing tendency to include athetosis with dystonia, but from a descriptive point of view there is some advantages describing what is still referred to in the majority of texts as athetosis. In common with many of the movement disorders, the condition occurs on attempted movement. Typically, on holding the arms outstretched the arm becomes extended and internally rotated, the wrist hyperextended or fully flexed and the fingers extended. The foot is inverted and plantar flexed and the leg is extended. These peripheral movements are often associated with dystonic movements of the trunk. It occurs most often in children with an infantile hemiplegia following cerebral palsy and typically develops between 5 and 10 years of age (Fig. 12.2).

A combination of bilateral chorea and athetosis is the classic type of cerebral palsy produced by neonatal jaundice due to any cause. This is often associated with sensorineural deafness, and may be further complicated by epileptic events starting in the teens.

Dystonia

Dystonic movements are due to slow prolonged contractions of the trunk muscles which may be regarded as proximal athetosis (Fig. 12.3). They may cause retraction of the head and hyperextension, twisting or lateral flexion of the spine, eventually pulling the patient into an extremely uncomfortable, unnatural and maintained posture.

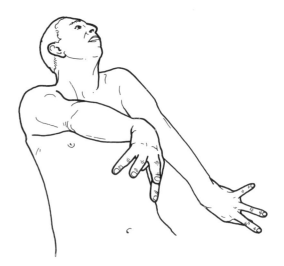

12.2   Athetoid posture.

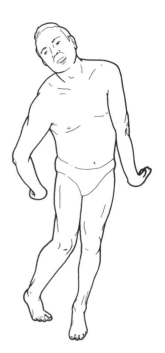

12.3   Dystonic posture.

Included in the dystonic group disorders are localized slow contractions of different muscle groups. These include the conditions known as spasmodic torticollis, in which the head is pulled to one side (Fig. 12.4), writer's cramp in which the shoulder muscles go into spasm as the patient attempts to write; blepharospasm, in which the eyes shut tightly and remain closed for minutes at a time (Fig. 12.5); and various facial distortions, including forced tongue protrusion with contraction of the facial muscles and platysma. This latter variety may occur as an acute reaction to phenothiazines and is easily mistaken for tetanus.

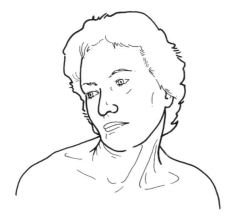

12.4 Spasmodic torticollis.

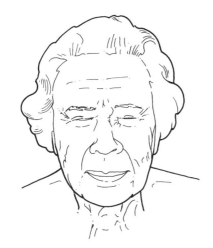

12.5 Blepharospasm.

Myoclonus

Myoclonus consists of sudden brief shock-like jerks in a group of muscles, a single muscle or part of a muscle. In its most severe form the violence of the movement may throw the patient to the ground, especially if the jerk is followed by an equally brief inhibition of muscle contraction. If continual, such myoclonus may stimulate cerebellar ataxia. At the opposite extreme minute myoclonic twitches in relaxed muscles may be mistaken for fasciculation. Myoclonus may occur physiologically as 'sleep starts' or indicate the onset of severe progressive brain disease. The causative conditions are fully discussed in a later section.

Tics

Tics are defined as brief contractions of a muscle or group of muscles, repetitive in the same place. The patient is usually able to mimic the movement and suppress it by intense concentration. They usually occur in children and may take the form of sniffing, grunting, snorting, pouting, clearing the throat, shoulder shrugging, winking, grimacing or appearing to try and bite one or other shoulder, and become so frequent that medical advice is sought. A typical feature is that from time to time the movement alters and for a few months persists in another form. Eventually recovery occurs and no consistent psychopathology is responsible.

The most dramatic tic is known as the syndrome of Gilles de la Tourette. In these patients the tic movements are accompanied by the utterance of a four-letter word. This particular variant may respond to phenothiazines or haloperidol, suggesting an organic basis for the disorder.

Other physical signs of extrapyramidal disease including rigidity, reflex changes and associated specific signs of certain disorders will be discussed in the appropriate clinical section.

Disease Affecting the Extrapyramidal System

Benign Essential Tremor

This condition occurs sporadically or is inherited as an autosomal dominant. It may start at any age, but in the inherited varieties the onset is typically in the teens in some families and senility in others.

The upper limbs are most severely affected by a fine tremor which is present at rest but dramatically increased by stress or embarrassment. One of the most striking and often diagnostic features of the disorder is a dramatic response to alcohol. This may be so effective at controlling the symptoms that some sufferers have become alcoholics. Half the patients also suffer from titubation (a nodding movement of the head) and a third have some movement of the trunk and legs. A tremulous voice may occur in others.

In many patients the disability is mainly social, and most sufferers deliberately avoid social functions and may become very depressed. The main importance of the condition lies in the frequency with which it is mistaken for parkinsonism. In the elderly the use of antiparkinsonian drugs for senile familial tremor may cause gross confusion and compound the diagnostic error. Diazepam, chlordiazepoxide, propanolol and primidone are helpful in severe cases, but in mild cases the social use of alcohol will often control the symptoms adequately. The differential diagnosis includes simple anxiety states, thyrotoxicosis and alcohol-induced tremor. Parkinsonism is excluded by the absence of any other signs of the disorder. Some families with benign essential tremor also appear to have an inherited form of Parkinson's disease that may develop after 30 years of tremor with no other parkinsonian features in the earlier years.

Parkinson's Disease

There are four features common to idiopathic, postencephalitic and drug-induced parkinsonism. So-called arteriosclerotic parkinsonism is discussed separately.

Tremor

Tremor has already been described. In parkinsonism it may involve the facial, jaw and tongue muscles, but primarily affects the hands, producing the very characteristic 'pill-rolling' tremor. This results from the posture of the hand – it is flexed at the wrist with the fingers extended and the thumb abducted. The oscillations of the fingers and thumb in two planes produces the 'pill-rolling' effect (Fig. 12.6). The tremor is worse during anxiety and is supposed to decrease on activity, but in many patients with well-developed tremor it persists, producing an intention tremor easily mistaken for cerebellar disease.

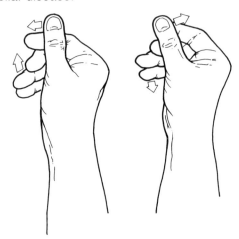

12.6   Pill-rolling posture of hand.

Rigidity

All muscle groups in the affected limbs are rigid in parkinsonism, producing stiffness of movement throughout the entire range. This has been likened to the sensation experienced when bending a lead pipe. In most patients phasic decreases in tone produce 'cog-wheel' rigidity, a sensation as if turning a sticking cogwheel. This is best felt while passively flexing and extending, or supinating and pronating, the patient's wrist. It is markedly increased if the patient clenches the opposite fist while the test is performed. It is difficult to detect cogwheel rigidity in the legs in a mild case, but it is sometimes first detectable at the hip by gently rolling the leg from side to side.

Bradykinesia

Bradykinesia is the most disabling component of the disease, affecting mainly the face and axial muscles

which, when combined with rigidity and tremor, makes simple tasks such as writing, dressing or doing up buttons almost impossible. It is responsible for the fixed facial expression, reduced blinking, reduced swallowing with consequent dribbling, the slow monotonous speech, lack of arm swinging, rigidity of the trunk when walking and the lack of associated movements when performing any tasks.

The ultimate expression of bradykinesia is so-called 'freezing', where the patient will suddenly be rooted to the spot, quite unable to walk forwards, as if their feet were glued to the ground. This typically happens when the patient first stands from a chair, attempts to change direction while walking along, goes through a doorway or walks from one surface to another. This problem can often be overcome by the patient imagining that they have to step over a brick, but if this is unsuccessful the spouse may offer a foot for them to step over, hoping that bystanders do not notice, particularly if the patient succeeds in tripping over the proffered foot!

The slowness of postural adjustments coupled with the forward-flexed posture and shuffling of the feet greatly increases the risk of the patient tripping and falling. This is known as a 'festinant' gait. Patients often find they can run more easily than they can walk once they get moving (Fig. 12.7).

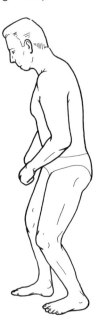

12.7   Parkinsonian posture.

Loss of Postural Reflexes

Patients complain bitterly that they are 'off balance' all the time, but they have simply stumbled upon the fact that standing up is in reality the art of not falling over, and they are suddenly aware of the constant imperceptible postural adjustments that normally occur. The patient will notice that they just cannot stand up straight, and when they attempt to move forwards the head and trunk move off with the feet somewhat reluctantly following just in time to prevent them falling. They dare not attempt to change direction without stopping and regaining their starting posture, and then repeating the whole process.

Simple tasks such as turning in the toilet to reach the toilet-roll or the flushing handle become almost impossible, and may result in falls. Any manoeuvring in confined spaces presents immense problems. Getting in and out of the bath, unless there is something to pull on, may prove completely impossible. When getting into bed patients tend to fall back in the same flexed posture adopted when standing, and are then unable to achieve a comfortable position or even adjust the bedclothes around them. They are quite unable to use their body weight to advantage and, when trying to sit up, repeatedly fall back and can only turn by being pulled. They cannot swing the arm and leg across to set the trunk rolling. Quite often, minor versions of all these symptoms have been present for a year or more before the patient actually seeks advice, usually when a more obvious symptom such as tremor intrudes.

Clinical Presentations of Parkinson's Disease

The presenting symptoms are varied and frequently dismissed as being due to 'old age', 'arthritis', 'rheumatism', 'depression' or 'one of those things'. If one side is predominantly affected, particularly by bradykinesia, the patient may be suspected or having suffered a stroke or of developing a cerebral tumour. Sometimes the presenting symptom may be head injury or a fractured hip resulting from one of the many falls. The disease may be first recognized when the patient's rehabilitation proves slow or difficult.

In some patients slurring or hesitation of speech are prominent features. Excessive salivation and dribbling may be a major problem and may suggest the diagnosis of dementia. In fact, the production of saliva is no greater than in the normal patient, it is the infrequency of swallowing that allows saliva to accumulate and dribble from the mouth. Infrequent blinking also occurs and is one of the most useful confirmatory diagnostic clues. It gives the patient rather an intense staring look. The loss of facial expression and infrequent smiling – the 'mask faces' – is often indistinguishable from the uncompromisingly miserable face of a patient with severe retarded depression, and this is another diagnostic trap, compounded by the fact that many patients with parkinsonism actually are severely depressed.

A series of very useful questions will often confirm the diagnosis:

1. What has the patient noticed about their writing? Sometimes it has become so difficult that they have stopped writing altogether, but they always mention that their writing become very small and tended to run up the page before they gave up.

2. Can they manage to get in and out of the bath? This is usually a serious problem and many patients relate being stuck in the bath on many occasions while waiting for help.

3. Can they turn over in bed? This apparently simple but technically very difficult manoeuvre is an early problem, and the spouse will usually recall being woken up to assist the patient.

4. Can they continue to roll pastry, beat eggs, do the ironing, peel potatoes or wring out washing or use a screwdriver, saw or hammer effectively? It will be realized that most of these tasks require a rhythmic series of repetitive movements, and the patient may volunteer that they get stuck each time they attempt to change direction, the egg whisk barely moving or the saw constantly snagging in the wood.

5. Does the patient have any difficulties walking? Have they ever found themselves 'stuck to the floor'? Sometimes patients may notice that they can walk better on uneven ground, where walking is a deliberate 'pyramidal' function, than on the flat where walking is a purely automatic 'extrapyramidal' function. One patient likened this difficulty to his 'automatic pilot being switched off'.

Other Conditions With Parkinsonian Components

The features discussed above are applicable to parkinsonism in general and especially the idiopathic variety, which is now known to be due to an abnormality of dopamine synthesis and release, particularly in the globus pallidus.

Drug and Chemical-Induced Parkinsonism

Parkinsonism occurs in patients exposed to manganese (an industrial problem in manganese miners) and following carbon monoxide poisoning (leaking car exhaust, unsuccessful suicide bid).

CASE REPORT III

A 22-year-old man, a talented musician of depressive disposition, attempted suicide in his car. He was found at 7 a.m., the car engine having stalled, and it was estimated that he had started the engine about 2 a.m. Although deeply unconscious with fixed pupils, he recovered consciousness over 48 hours in the intensive care unit without treatment with hyperbaric oxygen. Following recovery he had completely forgotten his musical skills, which he had to regain and which never matched his former skills. Some 18 months after these events, over a period of weeks he developed profound brady-

kinetic Parkinson's disease which responded well to amantadine hydrochloride and dopamine. Nine months later he had his first epileptic fit. The epileptic events proved harder to manage than the Parkinson's disease but when last seen, some 10 years after the original carbon monoxide poisoning, both conditions were controlled.

Drug-induced parkinsonism generally causes little tremor but is dominated by considerable cogwheel rigidity and bradykinesia. Although it is widely recognized that the long-term use of chlorpromazine and depot injections of major tranquillizers can cause overt extrapyramidal side-effects, probably the chronic use of prochlorperazine in elderly women who have had a 'dizzy turn' often many years before, is the most frequently encountered cause of drug-induced parkinsonism.

On rare occasions parkinsonism can follow a head injury, The rarity probably reflects the fact that a head injury of sufficient severity to damage the basal ganglia is likely to prove fatal. Cerebral tumours may produce extrapyramidal features but there are very few published cases. The following are two interesting examples of this association.

CASE REPORT IV

A 63-year-old woman presented with right-sided signs of Parkinson's disease. There was little tremor but marked rigidity and bradykinesia. There were no pyramidal signs at presentation. She responded reasonably well to the use of dopamine supplements, particularly when amantadine was added to the regimen. After some 9 months she started to deteriorate, with increasing drowsiness and occasional difficulty with speech, and she developed a right extensor plantar response. CT scanning revealed an extensive tumour with patchy widespread calcification in the left basal ganglia. It had all the appearances of an oligodendroglioma and biopsy was not attempted. She continued to deteriorate, the parkinsonian signs being overwhelmed by the increasing pyramidal deficit.

CASE REPORT V

A 56-year-old aeronautical engineer and WWII right lower limb amputee had been seen some years previously with migraine. In his spare time he had been instrumental in several advances in artificial limb construction based on aeronautical knowledge. He was re-referred because he suddenly had difficulty operating his artificial right leg. He could not explain what was wrong, except that he had suddenly lost the ability to balance on it and its movement had again become unnatural. He had clear-cut evidence of right-sided Parkinson's disease with cogwheel rigidity and bradykinesia of the right upper limb. There was no tremor. Amantadine hydrochloride produced a rapid improvement and he reasserted control over his artificial limb. Dopamine was then added and for several months he remained well. He then developed headaches indistinguishable from his previous migraines, but accompanied for the first time by transitory

dysphasic speech. This rapidly worsened and he became increasingly drowsy. CT scanning revealed a large left middle cranial fossa meningioma. This was successfully resected, with complete clearance of his parkinsonian syndrome.

Both these cases were seen within 6 months of each other in 1982, and a literature search revealed surprisingly few similar cases, although tumours are always included in the differential diagnostic list of Parkinson's disease. Perhaps the absence of tremor in both cases is worthy of comment, although a great many patients without tremor are seen and this is sometimes a feature of unilateral presentations. In both instances, in spite of anatomical defects, a convincing response to appropriate medication over several months was surprising. In both cases it was the development of unanticipated features that led to the recognition of the underlying lesions, another example of the need to follow patients carefully, although probably not justification for routine CT scanning in all patients with Parkinson's disease.

Postencephalitic Parkinsonism

This condition occurred as an immediate and delayed complication of Economo's encephalitis. The peak incidence was between 1918 and 1928, but isolated patients manifesting some of the features very typical of the postencephalitic variety are still seen. Historically, there have been several pandemics of the disorder over several hundred years and it may well appear again. The features of this form of Parkinson's disease are:

Reversed Argyll Robertson pupils (see Chapter 2)
Oculogyric crises (see Chapter 7)
Seborrhoeic dermatitis of the forehead and face
Severe sialorrhoea (drooling of saliva)
Respiratory tics, intractable hiccups
Behavioral disturbances

Survivors of the last epidemic are now very few and the condition has become extremely rare. In some cases the encephalitis was extremely mild and the Parkinson's disease occurred 30–40 years later. A patient who was seen in the 1960s with classic postencephalitic Parkinson's disease denied that he had had any previous illness, but when carefully questioned remembered that in 1928 he had been dismissed from his first job as a solicitor's clerk because over a period of 6–8 weeks he was repeatedly found asleep on his desk, and recollected that he had over the same period been unable to sleep at night. This reversal of the sleep – wake pattern was a feature of the condition and it is very likely that this was a mild attack of encephalitis lethargica, the other name for the condition.

Arteriosclerotic Parkinsonism

This is not true parkinsonism and arteriosclerotic rigidity is a better term. The patient or a relative usually gives a history of the surprisingly abrupt onset of mental and physical slowing, coupled with slurred speech, drooling of saliva, difficulty chewing and swallowing and loss of mobility. There is no tremor and the main physical findings are very marked rigidity and slowness of movement, without other features typical of parkinsonian bradykinesia such as the feet getting stuck. In fact, the gait consists of quick, short shuffling steps known as 'marche au petits pas'. On physical examination pseudobulbar dysarthria, a brisk jaw jerk, brisk reflexes and bilateral extensor plantars usually provide adequate evidence of diffuse cerebral damage. In idiopathic parkinsonism the reflexes are unaffected and the plantar responses are usually flexor.

This diagnosis has great practical significance. The use of antiparkinsonian drugs in these patients almost invariably provokes severe confusion and visual hallucinations, without any beneficial effect on the physical disabilities.

Normal Pressure Hydrocephalus

Although this condition was recognized prior to the advent of CT scanning, its use in elderly patients has led to the increasing recognition or suspicion of this rather inexplicable but potentially important condition. The patient, usually elderly, will present with a combination of a 'tottery' gait, which can be very similar to that of Parkinson's disease, intellectual deficit dominated by memory disturbance, and urinary incontinence. The overall picture can mimic Parkinson's disease, Alzheimer's disease or multiple cerebral vascular accidents, and there is no absolutely typical clinical picture. Only a high index of suspicion and the routine use of CT scanning in such patients will detect the condition.

Unfortunately, the distinction between massive ventricular dilatation due to intraventricular pressure and dilatation due to brain atrophy is not easily made, and the frequent coexistence of cerebral cortical atrophy, given the elderly age range of these patients, makes the decision to proceed to ventriculoperitoneal shunting very difficult. This procedure is not without hazard, with a risk of subdural haematoma, septicaemia or meningitis, and may prove ineffectual, but a successful shunt procedure in such patients can be one of the most dramatic events in neurology.

CASE REPORT VI

A 68-year-old man was referred with a 4-year history of generalized slowing down and a tendency to scuff his feet. He walked with his knees slightly bent, shuffling the feet forward, resulting in numerous falls. It was particularly dangerous for him to lean forwards to stir the embers of a fire or unplug the TV, as he would pitch forwards uncontrollably in this position. He had shown a little intellectual deficit and memory impairment but there was no micturition disturbance. There was a past history of two severe head injuries, 30 and 14 years previously, and on the first occasion his survival was thought unlikely. On examination all reflexes were remarkably brisk and both plantar responses were extensor. There was no sensory deficit and no extrapyramidal signs, although his gait could be described as typically parkinsonian. An MRI scan revealed severe hydrocephalus. As he had not developed the full triad of symptoms shunting was delayed for 6 months, but further decline in memory prompted the insertion of a ventriculoperitoneal shunt, which caused quite severe headaches but a dramatic improvement in his gait and memory. The post-shunt problems eventually resolved and a CT scan 3 weeks postoperatively showed a dramatic change in the size of the ventricles which paralleled the clinical improvement. He remained completely well for 4 years. He then represented complaining that his 'centre of gravity had shifted', he was starting to shuffle again and his memory had become impaired. This was even more striking than previously and he was intermittently quite confused. Physical examination confirmed that there were no extrapyramidal features, although his gait again looked parkinsonian, but apart from a slight tone increase in both legs and extensor plantar responses, there were no signs. Rescanning (see below) demonstrated severe hydrocephalus; the shunt was found to be blocked and was replaced, with an immediate improvement in gait and restoration of intellectual function to near normal within 7 days.

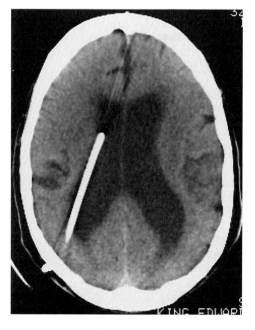

CRVI. *Recurrent normal pressure hydrocephalus (shunt in situ in right lateral ventricle).*

The cause in most cases is obscure, and although called 'normal pressure' hydrocephalus even this integral part of the name of the syndrome is disputed. Very few patients give a history of previous meningitis, head trauma and subarachnoid haemorrhage to explain the blockage of CSF circulation at the level of the arachnoid granulations, which is theorized to be the cause of the condition. In the case cited above it is hard to ignore the serious head injury 30 years previously as a potential cause of this syndrome, although if the cause was subarachnoid blood blocking the CSF circulation it is difficult to explain the 30-year delay in presentation. Nevertheless, this case, with a dramatic response to shunting on two occasions, is as certain an example of this condition and its ability to mimic Parkinson's disease with dementia as could be imagined, and was worth quoting in detail.

Intellectual Function and Depression in Parkinsonism

It was originally claimed that parkinsonism was not associated with intellectual deterioration. Since the advent of the marked physical improvement produced by levodopa it has become apparent that at least half the patients with parkinsonism have a moderate to severe degree of intellectual impairment. The majority eventually develop intellectual impairment with increasing age. This is often heralded by the onset of visual hallucinations, at first only at night and then throughout the day. Initially these are rarely frightening and usually consist of imaginary domestic animals, such as cats and dogs, in the house, or bushes and trees in the garden may seem to be populated by hundreds of cats and dogs, or become giant figures. Unless the drugs are immediately reduced more psychotic, delusional features start to appear, causing a severe confusional state requiring hospital admission.

From then on, management is on a therapeutic knife-edge for control of the patient's mobility and mentality. Sadly, the patient then becomes either highly mobile but grossly confused or completely immobile but quite rational. The speed with which this situation can develop after years of excellent control is frightening. The use of phenothiazines to control the confusion clearly carries the risk of worsening the parkinsonian state. There is evidence to support the use of clozapine, a novel antipsychotic agent that does not produce extrapyramidal side-effects in this situation. Unfortunately, there is a 1:300 risk of agranulocytosis and this drug is currently only available for use under stringent control but it at least offers the possibility that in the future this dreadful problem – almost inevitable if the patient lives long enough – may become manageable. The following case is a striking example of this particular problem in evolution, and documents a dramatic response to the use of clozapine.

CASE REPORT VII

A 60-year-old accountant was referred in 1986 with clumsiness of the left arm and shuffling gait. He had become rather depressed and emotional. His mother had had Parkinson's disease. On examination left arm swing was impaired while walking and he scuffed the left leg. On the couch, there was bilateral cogwheel rigidity with mild bradykinesia, more marked on the left. There was an immediate marked improvement when amantadine hydrochloride was started, and he cited the ability to climb over stiles while walking his dog, a feat that had become impossible over the previous year. He was able to continue on amantadine alone for 1 year before his golf deteriorated, and on a walking holiday his gait again became impaired. Dopamine was introduced, with an immediate improvement that allowed him to resume all normal activities, including golf, within a month. He remained extremely well for 3 years. His family then noticed a sudden deterioration in his intellectual skills. Psychometric testing revealed clear evidence of early dementia. Fortunately, this appeared not to progress rapidly, and 5 years after diagnosis he was still able to play a full round of golf without difficulty. Six years after diagnosis he started to have very vivid dreams, and occasionally became quite confused. Bromocriptine was introduced with benefit and amantadine was discontinued. There were some problems with postural hypotension. A year later, while walking his dog, he had hallucinations that everyone he saw was 'a giant', and thought that 'all the trees were covered in flags'. When he returned home he thought that the back garden was 'covered in furniture'. His medication was reduced, the confusion cleared and he was allowed to go on a Rhine cruise. Unfortunately, during one of the coach trips he suddenly thought that they should be in Bridgewater, and was very incensed that the driver had taken them to Cologne cathedral. This confusion persisted and his wife had to stay with him in the cabin throughout the rest of the trip. He was admitted to hospital immediately on his return and was found to be psychotic with paranoid delusions and non-stop visual hallucinations. Withdrawal of all medication produced a complete resolution of these symptoms but a dramatic decline in his physical abilities. Dopamine in small doses was gradually reinstated and an acceptable degree mobility attained. A year later, a further, much more severe episode occurred. He was admitted to hospital, all drugs were withdrawn, but he remained confused, frightened and hallucinated, convinced that his wife had left him, all his belongings had been stolen and that the nurses were trying to poison him. On this occasion total bradykinesia and immobility required drip and nasogastric feeds and became life-threatening. With some difficulty, as the drug is not licensed for this indication, the use of clozapine was permitted and within 5 days of starting 6.25 mg daily he was lucid, and having said nothing coherent for 3 weeks suddenly asked if I had anticipated bringing him back from this situation 'when we started the long trek together' (his actual words). Dopamine was cautiously reintroduced, his mobility improved and 4 weeks later he was able to walk his dog at the venue of previous hallucinations without trouble. He remains on the combined medication with the situation at present under control.

The 8-year course in this patient is fairly typical of the behaviour of Parkinson's disease starting in middle age. The disease appeared modest at onset and responded well to simple medication. Some unexpected intellectual difficulty indicated the possibility of a more serious turn of events at a time when the patient was physically still well controlled. He had been intermittently depressed over those years but had been able to remain at work and proceed to retirement as originally planned. The advent of the hallucinatory phenomena was dramatically sudden and was very severe demonstrating the sinister significance of the advent of visual hallucinosis in the parkinsonian patient on treatment. From that stage, a sequence of events as documented above was almost inevitable.

Depression has always been recognized as a part of the parkinsonian syndrome; in some instances it is an integral part of the disease and in others a reaction to it. When a part of the syndrome itself, it does not necessarily recover in parallel with the improvement in mobility when treatment is commenced. In some patients it actually deteriorates. Depression in parkinsonian patients can have a profound effect on their physical disabilities, perhaps more marked than the effect of depression in any other neurological condition. Identification and treatment of the depression in parallel with the use of antiparkinsonian drugs is a very important part of management. In patients who have significant tremor imipramine may have a special place, as its anticholinergic effect may also benefit tremor, but in elderly males its other disadvantages may preclude its use, with urinary retention being a major hazard.

The Parkinson's Plus Syndromes

This is a collection of disorders that include parkinsonian features among their clinical manifestations. They are notable not only in that the parkinsonism is poorly responsive to treatment but that the attempted treatment may actually aggravate the other features of the conditions concerned. This may prove to be the first clue that the patient has not got simple Parkinson's disease. All these disorders are progressive and ultimately fatal.

Multisystem Atrophy (MSA)

There are four main variants of this disorder.

Striatonigral Degeneration The picture is that of Parkinson's disease without tremor and a very minimal response to medication, with a tendency to develop all the side-effects of any agent tried. This is probably the commonest cause of drug-unresponsive Parkinson's disease. It is very hard to distinguish this variant from arteriosclerotic pseudoparkinsonism.

Shy–Drager Syndrome This consists of Parkinson's disease combined with severe autonomic neuropathy.

Sometimes the parkinsonian component responds well to medication at first, but is often complicated by postural hypotension which eventually forces the withdrawal of medication. In many instances the autonomic neuropathy is responsible for the presenting symptoms, which in the male are usually impotence and micturition difficulties. In some cases the development of dementia and a motor neuron disease component may further complicate the condition. The following are examples the behaviour of this unpleasant disorder.

CASE REPORT VIII

A 48-year-old woman had been admitted to hospital with a history of unsteadiness of gait, severe constipation, urinary retention and syncopal attacks. She was discharged with the diagnosis of hysteria. When referred to the neurology clinic only 6 months later she had obvious parkinsonism, with gross bradykinesia, a postural hypotensive drop from 120/80 to 60/0 and severe sphincter disturbance. She deteriorated steadily over the next few months, developing widespread muscle wasting and fasciculation, and died 18 months after the onset.

CASE REPORT IX

A 68-year-old man was referred with a 6-year history of impotence, a 5-year history of severe constipation, and urgency with both occasional incontinence and difficulty initiating micturition. Apart from some aching in the neck there were no other symptoms, but on examination he had brisk reflexes and extensor plantar responses. There were no extrapyramidal signs. Myelography and MRI scanning, CSF examination and full haematological and biochemical studies revealed only degenerative change in the cervical region but insufficient to explain his difficulties. By that stage he was requiring intermittent self-catheterization. A year later he presented with several episodes of sudden collapse while standing. He went white, his eyes became glazed and he fell to the ground. If he stood up immediately it would recur. Lying/standing blood pressures revealed a fall from 120/80 to 90/50 without symptoms. He was admitted to hospital, where frequent severe postural hypotension was demonstrated, so severe that on one occasion that he collapsed while washing at the hand basin and flooded his room. He was started on fludrocortisone, with excellent control. This treatment proved satisfactory for 6 months, during which time he completed a cruise to Alaska without incident. He then developed cold puffy hands and difficulty walking, and minimal cogwheel rigidity was defected in the upper limbs. Within 2 months he was clearly parkinsonian and improved rapidly on a combination of amantadine and dopamine. This was surprising, because he now had all the features of Shy–Drager syndrome. The postural hypotension caused further problems and he was admitted to a nursing home. The control of his Parkinson's disease became more and more difficult and the postural hypotension so severe that he could even faint sitting up in bed. He died during one of these collapses 10 years after onset of the syndrome.

These two cases demonstrate the extremes of these conditions. It may be very rapidly fatal or develop slowly and piecemeal, as in the second case. The very severe constipation is a major diagnostic clue and is one of the earliest symptoms noted by most patients. Impotence and micturition disturbance tend to be the dramatic features in the male, and the lethal feature is the severe autonomic neuropathy. In both the cases above, the Parkinson's disease was initially surprisingly responsive to medication. As a general rule, a poor response is a feature of the degenerative forms of Parkinson's disease.

Olivopontocerebellar Atrophy Syndrome(OPCA)   This is another condition with a bewildering variety of presentations, depending on whether the cerebellar ataxic features or the extrapyramidal parkinsonian features predominate. It may also be complicated by autonomic neuropathy and ventral horn cell degeneration. The following is an example of this condition in a relatively young man.

CASE REPORT X

A 49-year-old oil company executive was referred with progressive gait disorder, incoordination and slurring of speech. He had noted difficulty in passing urine. On further questioning he had noticed that to keep his balance he had to deliberately make himself sway slightly, but he was still able to play squash. He had developed erectile impotence 4 months previously. His writing had become illegible. He had an identical twin brother who was unaffected. On examination he was extremely ataxic with a severe cerebellar speech disturbance. There was no nystagmus and no jaw jerk. All reflexes were brisk but the plantar responses were flexor. There was severe limb incoordination and he could only stand with his feet 12" apart and his eyes open, and swayed uncontrollably on eye closure. He was unable to walk on a line and staggered without lateralization. The diagnosis of olivopontocerebellar atrophy was suspected and an MRI scan revealed cerebellar cortical atrophy, but the brain stem appeared normal. A fall resulted in fracture of the left elbow and caused an ulnar nerve lesion. His previously normal blood pressure had dropped to 90/60 without postural fall. Unfortunately, his condition continued to deteriorate, the autonomic neuropathy and cerebellar features dominating the picture with later impairment of gaze, and he died some 3 years after the onset.

Parkinsonism and Motor Neuron Disease   This is the rarest of the disorders, in which a modest parkinsonian picture is associated with a rapidly overwhelming generalized form of motor neuron disease.

As is apparent from these descriptions, these disorders overlap and some patients may progress from one variant to another, making exact classification difficult and altering the prognosis, usually in a less favourable direction.

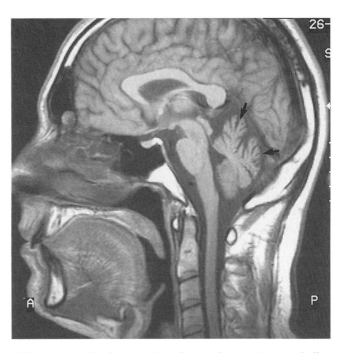

CRX.   *Cerebellar degeneration due to olivopontine cerebellar atrophy.*

Progressive Supranuclear Palsy (Steele–Richardson–Olzewski Syndrome)

In this condition the presenting symptoms mimic Parkinson's disease but the patient may be very obviously mentally slowed and arteriosclerotic rigidity may at first be suspected, a suspicion apparently confirmed by the absence of response to levodopa. However, careful examination of eye movements will usually detect impaired up gaze at presentation and, within a few months, loss of all extraocular movements. Pseudobulbar palsy develops insidiously, with loss of speech, impaired swallowing with the risk of aspiration, and a relentless and ultimately fatal progression.

Corticobasal Ganglionic Degeneration

A patient with this disorder presents as typical Parkinson's disease with severe unilateral rigidity and often with early speech disturbance. The asymmetry of signs may suggest underlying cerebrovascular disease. Walking becomes severely impaired, with numerous falls and a supranuclear gaze palsy is a not uncommon later development. In some patients myoclonus and sensory disturbance have been reported. The following case is a probable example of this condition, seen 15 years ago before the more recent classification of these disorders.

CASE REPORT XI

A 61-year-old man was referred with a 6-month history of difficulty in writing. His hand would shake violently, the print had become smaller and it tended to run up the page. His wife said that he had become a 'lazy walker' in the past year and occasionally scuffed his right foot. His posture when writing was typical of writer's cramp. Very exhaustive examination revealed no other evidence of extrapyramidal disease. Nevertheless a small dose of dopamine was used, with a slight improvement in his writing and a definite improvement in gait, although he and his wife had now noted that it was only the first two strides that were abnormal and that once he was walking he progressed normally. He was kept under review and over the next 2 years became more obviously parkinsonian, but the difficulties remained strictly right sided, with cogwheel rigidity only demonstrable in the thumb. Maximal doses of dopamine produced no improvement. He continued to deteriorate and a year later would frequently fall over while attempting to put his shoes on; and his gait had by then assumed the characteristics of a right hemiparesis, although the reflexes were symmetrical and both plantars remained flexor. The dopamine was supplemented with selegiline, amantadine and later with bromocriptine, up to 30 mg t.d.s., with no improvement. Two years after the onset he had become impotent. CT and MRI scanning revealed no abnormality. Three years after the onset a mild degree of postural hypotension developed but continence remained normal and eye movements remained full. He sought numerous second opinions and was restarted on antiparkinsonian medication in different formulations on three occasions without any discernible response. He then developed retention of urine, which was not relieved by resection of his prostate, and he required permanent catheterization. He continued to deteriorate and died some 6 years after the onset. Unfortunately, postmortem examination was not performed.

Unilateral Parkinson's disease presenting as writer's cramp would usually be a relatively benign condition, indeed with minimal features of the condition at presentation the prognosis seemed excellent. The total failure of medication to influence the relentless progression of strictly unilateral findings characterizes the condition. The degree of overlap with the other variants is apparent, in that impotence and sphincter disturbance with hypotension developed later, but there was no intellectual disturbance or eye movement disorder to indicate that this was a Steele–Richardson–Olzewski syndrome.

Parkinsonism/Dementia Complex

A variety of disorders combine dementia with the parallel development of parkinsonian features. This includes Guam disease, Creutzfeld–Jakob disease and some patients with senile dementia of Alzheimer's type. The first two conditions are prion-related disorders. There is as yet no evidence that Alzheimer's disease has an infectious basis but the possibility that some cases of this type have an underlying infective disorder to which they are genetically predisposed is one recently identified possibility.

Treatment of Parkinson's Disease

As will be apparent from the previous discussion, Parkinson's disease is not always a straightforward diagnosis and the failure of the patient to respond to appropriate medication may be the first clue to a more sinister disorder. Confusingly, some patients may appear to respond but the effect is short-lived and the addition of other agents produces no further benefit – indeed, a catalogue of side-effects dominates the history in the follow-up clinic. The original favourable prognosis given to the patient may then have to be quickly reappraised. Even if the patient is suffering from straightforward chemically based Parkinson's disease there can still be difficulties, and a recent comment that the 'skill in Parkinson's disease management has become the management of the complications of treatment' is unfortunately extremely accurate.

The method of treatment outlined below is based on extensive personal experience over the last 35 years, including the period during which the modern medications have gradually become available.

Anticholinergic Agents

These drugs have been in use since the 1950s and their main value is in the treatment of tremor. They have minimal effect on rigidity and no effect on bradykinesia. They are notorious for causing confusion, hallucinations and nightmares, especially in the elderly, and even patients in their 40s have been known to develop serious problems of this sort. They can also cause blurred vision, dry mouth and bladder difficulties, and for all these reasons enjoy limited use. Their use is only really justified with caution in patients whose tremor is a major disabling factor. They should be withdrawn the moment a patient develops hallucinations.

Amantadine Hydrochloride

This unusual drug, originally synthesized as an antiviral agent against influenza, was discovered to have a beneficial effect in Parkinson's disease at the same time as levodopa was introduced, and unfortunately has remained in its shadow ever since. Although it is said to have its beneficial effect as a weak anticholinergic agent, this cannot explain the dramatic response of severely bradykinetic patients, which matches anything reported with levodopa. It is likely that part of its action includes the facilitation of dopamine release. The following method of use supports the suggestion. Many patients given amantadine hydrochloride 100 mg b.d. (8 a.m. and 4 p.m.) report a dramatic improvement in their physical condition within hours of the first dose. In some this effect persists for months, but in others it wanes within weeks but is immediately restored if levodopa is then added to the regimen. Its continued use may permit lower doses of dopamine to be used with advantage. Its major disadvantages are a hallucinogenic potential similar to anticholinergic drugs, particularly nightmares, and this is the reason for taking the second dose early in the day. Some patients develop an itchy rash over the lower legs with ankle oedema, called livedo reticularis, which may necessitate withdrawal of the agent. The maximum dose is 100 mg b.d. A higher dose may trigger epileptic fits and for this reason it should not be used in patients known to have epilepsy. It should also be used extremely cautiously in patients over 70, as even 100 mg in the morning may produce severe confusion. It should also be the first drug to be dropped from the regimen if a patient becomes confused.

Dopamine Precursors

Levodopa, combined with a dopa-decarboxylase inhibitor, is now the standard treatment used in Parkinson's disease. The two formulations available are Sinemet, with carbidopa as the inhibitor, and Madopar, with benserazide the inhibitor. Both are available in a variety of soluble, quick-acting and long-acting formulations, in a wide range of doses.

In the early days of treatment two or three doses a day, conventionally taken at mealtimes, will usually suffice. As the years pass the dose required increases and the duration of action shortens, so that five or six doses a day at 2–3 hour intervals may become necessary to achieve the same benefit. The major disadvantages are that as the dose increases the likelihood of dyskinetic movement disorder increases in parallel, and this, combined with reduced effectiveness, results in variable control with good and bad patches and eventual 'on–offing'. In this situation the patients are highly mobile at the expense of non-stop choreiform movements, or alternatively almost completely immobile for variable periods.

Which ever dosing schedule is used, patients spontaneously volunteer that they are often surprised how good they are in the middle of the night or first thing in the morning for periods of 10–30 minutes. In contrast, they also notice how bad they tend to be either in the late morning or early afternoon. There is often a surprisingly good patch in the evening. These fluctuations seem to be an inherent part of the condition and are very hard to modify by varying the drug dosage or timing, and it is possible that in some patients overdosage results from ineffectual attempts to modify these built-in fluctuations. Sometimes encouraging the patient to plan their day around the 'bad' patches is a more successful approach than altering the dosage to suit – a policy which may also further delay the onset of side-effects.

There also seems to be little obvious advantage in using a high dose last thing at night. There is no chance that this dose will last through until the following morning, and unless the patient needs to spend a great deal of their night getting in and out of bed there is no advantage. Many patients express surprise that they are briefly better in the night, when they have gone longer without medication than at any other time of the day! The original reason for taking levodopa with meals was that the very high doses involved produced nausea and sickness unless taken with food. It is now claimed that if it is taken with a high-protein meal absorption is reduced, and fluctuating responses may be related to this problem but this rarely seems to be of practical significance.

There is a real advantage in patients taking the first dose of the day on awakening, as the benefit is often discernible within 30 minutes. Many patients wake up, wash, shave, dress and prepare their breakfast – some 75% of their daily activity – completely without the benefit of medication, if they delay the first dose until they are eating their breakfast. Very few patients find the modern preparations cause problems if taken with a glass of milk first thing in the morning. As a general principle, contriving to use the lowest dose that is effective, timed to suit that particular patient's needs, until forced to increase the dosage, may delay the almost inevitable onset of dose–response fluctuations and uncontrollable dyskinesia. Perhaps the fact that some of the worst examples of these problems are seen in younger patients with Parkinson's disease reflects the over-generous use of levodopa because of unrealistic targets for an acceptable level of functional control. Older patients, whose ambitions for physical activity are more modest, seem less likely to run into this problem.

Dopamine Agonists

There are two generally available agonists, bromocriptine (Parlodel) and pergolide (Celance). The best use of these agents is still controversial. Some recommend their early use to limit the dopamine intake, but others prefer to wait until dopamine requirements start to escalate before adding dopamine agonists, which is the author's preference. The major disadvantage of these agents is postural hypotension, which may not only limit the dosage and usefulness but sometimes raise the spectre of an autonomic neuropathy, associated with the more malevolent parkinsonism-plus syndromes discussed above. The effective dose range of these agents is wide and the dose should be very gradually increased while monitoring the blood pressure, both standing and lying.

Apomorphine is another agent with dopamine agonist properties which can only be used by subcutaneous infusion. It can be helpful in younger patients who were severely 'on–offing', during immobile periods. It is not without hazard, is indicated in relatively few patients, and is probably best reserved for use in specialist centres.

Selegiline Hydrochloride

This interesting monoamine oxidase-B inhibitor, is available as Eldepryl in the UK and as Deprenyl in other countries. Its original use was as an adjuvant drug to inhibit dopamine breakdown. Following the demonstration that it could prevent the onset of Parkinson's disease caused by MPTP in illicit narcotic use, rather extravagant claims were made for its value. It was suggested that Parkinson's disease itself may be due to damage caused by breakdown products of dopamine metabolism, and that by inhibiting dopamine metabolism the disease might be arrested or, even more, the onset could be delayed or prevented by pretreatment with selegiline. No clear benefit of this type had ever emerged from the extensive trials over 15 years in Europe and the very dramatic claims made after only 2–3 years' availability in the USA were surprising. Some of these claims have had to be modified in the light of longer experience, and the final view on the value of this agent in Parkinson's disease still awaits further clarification.

In some patients a dopamine-sparing effect is obvious but in many patients its addition to the regimen produces no discernible difference. The dosage used is 10 mg taken in the morning.

It is a sad fact that, however impressive the patient's initial response to treatment and however carefully the drugs are used, if the patient lives long enough, in due course, dose–response fluctuations, 'on–offing', confusion, nightmares, hallucinations and frank psychosis may eventually appear. All the drugs are capable of aggravating these problems, so that a policy of reducing or discontinuing the drugs and allowing the disease to assert itself in an effort to reduce the side-effects, is not always successful. Attempts to control the symptoms with major tranquillizers will make the situation worse. Thioridazine in a dose of 12.5–25 mg t.d.s. seems to be the drug least likely to worsen Parkinson's disease. The future use of clozapine or derivative drugs, if the dangers can be reduced, offers hope for the future. Twenty-five years ago, with the discovery of the effectiveness of levodopa, Parkinson's disease was regarded as a curable condition. As will be realized from the above discussion, the problems of this disorder are far from resolved.

Choreiform Disorders

Sydenham's Chorea

This condition is a cerebral complication of rheumatic fever and has become a rare disease. It typically occured within 3 months of an attack of ß-haemolytic streptococcal infection or rheumatic fever in patients between 5 and 20 years of age. It had an insidious onset and in half the patients was unilateral. It was often dominated by an emotional upset that very easily led to a mistaken diagnosis of hysteria. The typical choreiform movements subsided in 3–6 months. Occasionally an unusual variant of this condition in younger children produced a flaccid hemiparesis.

Chorea gravidarum is thought to represent a recurrence of Sydenham's chorea during a subsequent pregnancy, and has therefore also declined in frequency. Some doubt has been thrown on this explanation by the recognition of typical chorea syndromes produced by the contraceptive pill. An intriguing example of both 'pill' chorea and chorea gravidarum in sequence with no evidence of associated rheumatic fever is to be found in the case report (Case Report VII) in Chapter 24 under 'Complications of pregnancy'.

Another patient developed chorea due to the pill 3 months after the completion of a chorea-free pregnancy, making an underlying neural deficit an unlikely explanation.

Rare Causes of Chorea

Chorea has been reported in association with systemic lupus erythematosus, polycythaemia rubra vera, thyrotoxicosis, diphenylhydantoin intoxication, phenothiazine hypersensitivity, hypercalcaemia, Wilson's disease, and as a complication of excessive doses of levodopa. Some elderly patients develop choreiform movements spontaneously, which raises the possibility of Huntington's chorea, but in most instances this is senile chorea, without genetic significance. Unilateral chorea may rarely occur as a consequence of cerebral vascular accident and subside spontaneously.

Huntington's Chorea

Huntington's chorea is a most unpleasant disease, not only because it is inherited as an autosomal dominant with complete penetrance, but also because of the nature of the disease itself.

A childhood onset of the disorder is extremely rare and it is then somewhat atypical, with considerable rigidity and even parkinsonian features rather than chorea, and may even be associated with epilepsy. Family studies have suggested a high incidence of anti-social, alcoholic or psychopathic behaviour as a premorbid personality feature in patients with this disease, but it is possible that these phenomena merely reflect their knowledge of the possibility that they will develop the disease that has devastated their family. When one realizes that the death often involves 10 years of relentless generalized choreiform movements with progressive dementia, this alternative explanation seems reasonable. For this reason, it is not unusual to discover that a positive family history has been deliberately concealed until an apparently sporadic case is closely investigated.

CASE REPORT XII

A woman in her 30s was first seen as the wife of a patient who was dying of motor neuron disease. She always appeared very 'fidgety', but her movements were not recognized as choreiform at that time. She was seen again 4 years later, when she was referred because of widespread choreiform movements and there was clear evidence of intellectual decline. She had already had two children by a previous marriage, two children by the husband who died of motor neuron disease and one child by her present partner, and was again pregnant at the time she was referred. She denied that there was any family history of choreiform movement disorder, but had always been led to believe that her mother died in a mental hospital of complications of a head injury. Eventually her eldest sister revealed that her mother had died of Huntington's chorea, but she had concealed this information from her younger siblings. A copy of the death certificate and postmortem findings of the mother confirmed this diagnosis. The patient had the baby, but within 6 months it was quite clear that she was not physically or mentally capable of looking after the child, who was made a ward of court. The very unpleasant duty of detailing the mother's prognosis, in open court, was a necessary part of these proceedings and extremely distressing for all concerned.

All six children clearly carry an equal risk of developing Huntington's chorea, in spite of the three different fathers. They have been offered genetic probe testing when old enough.

When patients are aware of their family history they usually first seek advice either when they are contemplating having a family or because they are frightened that they have detected the onset of choreiform movements. In the past they almost never sought advice before getting married, but now that genetic testing is common knowledge more patients are coming forward even though they dread the early knowledge of their future that a positive result will bring.

At first the movements consist of typical little choreiform jerks especially involving the hands and feet, affecting individual fingers and toes in a random way that is very difficult to imitate. Trunk involvement causes shoulder shrugging and constant position changes while sitting. Facial involvement produces fleeting changes in facial expression, such as wrinkling of the forehead, snarling movements of the nose and mouth and sudden generalized facial grimaces. In the earliest stages the general impression is that the patient is 'fidgety'. By the time the disorder is fully developed, the patients will appear to hug themselves when sitting as they attempt to prevent the unwanted movements. The legs will constantly cross and uncross, often quite noisily as they kick the chair or table. When they walk, the head and trunk and jerk forwards or twist and the arms flail. They will stagger but almost never fall. Eventually walking becomes so precarious that it may be safer to be in a wheelchair, but the constant writhing movements continue and may even throw them from the chair unless they are strapped in. Relief from the movements only comes with sleep.

Apart from the movement disorder and dementia, which usually begins in the third decade, there are no other physical signs. The reflexes are usually normal, the plantar responses are flexor and continence is only impaired with the onset of the final severe phases of dementia. In some cases severe psychological disturbance or dementia may precede the movement disorder by several years.

CASE REPORT XIII

A 38-year-old nurse had been an inmate of a mental hospital for 5 years with severe behavioural disturbance and loss of intellectual skills. She had formerly been extremely highly qualified and had been in charge of intensive care units in the USA and UK prior to her illness. She had developed a movement disorder which was initially thought by the psychiatrists to be due to phenothiazine medication. She had typical choreiform movements and the overall clinical picture was diagnostic of Huntington's chorea. Delicate enquiries of her family revealed that she had been born during the war, only 6 months after her father returned from the services, and had been led to believe that she was a premature baby. The family had always suspected otherwise, and in the total absence of a positive family history it seemed likely that this was not a spontaneous mutation but the result of an extramarital affair. Her parents were deceased by this time. Unfortunately, this was in the early 1980s before genetic testing was available.

Genetic Probe Testing

Certainly one of the most dramatic scientific advances of the last decade has been the detection of the location of the genetic defect in Huntington's chorea and the development of the specific probe test that no longer requires specimens from affected family members. This sometimes proved difficult when other members of the family did not wish to participate. This means that isolated cases can now be diagnosed with certainty, but when the younger family members discover the seriousness of the illness many choose not to take advantage of the test, preferring, in the absence of any specific treatment, not to know. The complete reassurance that a negative test can give someone at risk is more than balanced by the certainty of future events in the case of a positive test, and many prospective patients cannot face this choice. Until specific treatment becomes available the hoped-for eradication of the illness in affected families will remain unachievable.

Some symptomatic relief from the movements may be achieved with tetrabenazine in a dose of 12.5–25 mg t.d.s., but both relentless progression of the movements and declining intellectual skills is the rule, with death usually occurring within 10 years of the onset.

Athetoid and Dystonic Diseases

Dystonia is a feature of many rare diseases and their rarity justifies only a brief description of some of the clinical and biochemical features.

Kernicterus

Children who have had kernicterus due to neonatal jaundice of any cause, may demonstrate developmental delay with floppy tone. Choreiform movements with athetoid components on attempted action only become fully manifest when the pyramidal pathways myelinate at 18–24 months of age. It is often associated with sensorineural deafness, and a surprising number of patients seem to develop epilepsy in their teens. This problem has been greatly reduced by the prompt recognition and management of all causes of neonatal jaundice and the prevention of rhesus incompatibility.

Wilson's Disease

This is a rare inborn error of copper metabolism in which copper is deposited in the basal ganglia and liver. In children the disorder may present as liver disease, but at the opposite extreme some patients may present as late as 40 years of age with an extrapyramidal movement disorder, and Wilson's disease must be excluded in all patients presenting with abnormal movement disorder under 40 years of age. A remarkably wide range of movements, including tremor, athetoid posturing and dystonic movements, may develop. Cirrhosis of the liver is the life-threatening component if the disorder is not recognized and treated. The classic clinical sign is a fine brown dust-like ring of copper around the edge of the limbus of the cornea, called a Kayser–Fleischer ring. The serum copper may be misleadingly normal, reduced or increased; the diagnostic test is the serum caeruloplasmin level. This is the copper transport protein and the blood levels are markedly decreased. The disorder is now treatable by a low-copper diet and penicillamine in a dose of 1–2g per day. Early recognition of the disorder is essential to prevent irreversible hepatic and cerebral damage occurring. Some patients develop problems on penicillamine (see Chapter 19) and triethylene tetramine may be used as an alternative.

Hallevorden–Spatz Disease

This is a rare degenerative disease which causes progressive dystonia and hyperkinetic movements in children and is associated with retinitis pigmentosa. It may rarely present in adulthood as a Parkinson's disease-like syndrome. The aetiology is unknown, but pathological examination has revealed the deposition of iron in the basal ganglia. The course of the disease is one of progressive physical and mental deterioration.

Lesch–Nyhan Disease

Lesch–Nyhan disease is a rare disorder. The presentation is dominated by severe athetoid and dystonic movements and a striking tendency to self-mutilation. The latter is not uncommon in mentally defective children but is particularly severe in this disorder, in which the children will eat their lips, tongue and fingers unless all their teeth are removed. It is associated with very high serum uric acid levels, but the relationship of this finding to the movement disorder is unknown.

Neuroacanthocytosis

This a another very rare familial syndrome characterized by an onset in the third decade. It is associated with a wide variety of movement disorders, including facial dyskinesia, chorea and parkinsonian components. A peripheral neuropathy and epileptic seizures may further complicate the disorder. Acanthocytes are found in the blood film but the ß-lipoproteins in the serum are normal, unlike in Bassen-Kornsweig syndrome (see Chapter 19).

Dystonia Musculorum Deformans

This condition may be inherited either as an autosomal recessive or as a dominant gene. The recessive variety is particularly common in Jewish families and usually produces severe disability. The dominant variety demonstrates variable penetrance, with very mild disability in some affected members. In the fully developed form the patient's body is pulled into grossly abnormal dystonic postures and jerked by constant choreiform movements.

Paroxysmal Choreoathetosis (Reflex Epilepsy)

This can also be inherited as an autosomal dominant. In typical form sudden brief choreoathetoid posturing or movements follow any sudden movement.

CASE REPORT XIV

A 14-year-old cathedral choirboy was referred because of peculiar movements that occurred when he was processing in the cathedral. As the choirboys turned the corner to go into the choir stalls, the right side of his body would go into peculiar contortions, with the arm twisting inwards and the fingers and wrist flexing, and he would half buckle at the knee and his foot would drag on the ground. Within two strides he was walking normally again, and he had been accused of performing these movements deliberately. It transpired that while fielding in cricket, whenever he broke into a run to chase the ball, the same movements occurred, often resulting in his completely missing the ball. His mother had had a similar disorder in her teens and his younger brother subsequently developed the same condition. They both grew out of this by their late teens. The movement disorder responded to the use of primidone.

This condition is quite rare but readily identifiable. If the patient is observed, just getting up out of a chair may result in choreiform movements down one side of the body for a few seconds, before walking commences. If the patient changes direction or suddenly tries to speed up, the movements recur, again for only a few seconds. Although the EEG is typically normal, the condition may respond to anticonvulsants and primidone seems particularly effective in an acceptably low dosage.

Segmental or Localized Dystonias

The commonest types of dystonia are known as the segmental torsion dystonias, as opposed to the disorders discussed above which involve all or most of the body. This is another group of disorders where the movements are dystonic in type but confined to a limited anatomical area. They are known as the segmental or localized dystonias.

Spasmodic Torticollis

This is an extremely unpleasant and disabling condition which may occur at any age. In torticollis the head is turned to one or other side by the obvious action of the sternomastoid, and typically the upper fibres of the trapezius on the opposite side hunch the shoulder up, as if to meet the chin. At first the movement is spasmodic but later the spasm becomes continual, with severe cramp-like pain in the contracting muscles and diffuse aching in the muscles attempting to resist the abnormal movements. The typical posture is shown in Figure 12.4. In some cases the patient can get the head back into a normal position by gentle pressure applied to the side of the chin. The condition is now universally accepted as an organic disorder of neurotransmitter origin, although it was previously regarded as a functional disorder. The condition usually stays limited to the one side and does not progress to a more generalized movement disorder.

In the second commonest variant the sternomastoid on both sides contracts and jerks the head forwards. This is called antecollis, and is often accompanied by similar contractions of the platysma and the lower facial musculature, producing webbing of the neck and grimacing of the lower face. Much less frequently the neck extensors may be involved, jerking the head backwards – the condition known as retrocollis.

Considerable relief can now be achieved by the use of small doses of botulinum toxin injected into the major dystonic muscles. Repeated injections at 1 or 2 monthly intervals are necessary to maintain the benefit and it is still uncertain whether the effectiveness can be sustained indefinitely. Some patients are developing antibodies to the toxin, which reduces its usefulness. Unfortunately, although it is easy to paralyse the most obviously affected muscles, the abnormal movement is generated centrally and includes a great deal of dystonic spasm in the deep cervical and occipital muscles, which are less amenable to injection. Attempts to treat the precervical muscles in particular may cause temporary but disabling dysphagia, and although patients are generally delighted with the results of this treatment it still falls far short of perfection.

Writer's Cramp

Writer's cramp was also previously regarded as a neurotic syndrome in preretirement clerical workers. It is now recognized that this is another organic extrapyramidal syndrome, and some of these patients do go on to develop parkinsonism or other dystonic syndromes.

The classic feature of the condition is that the patient starts writing normally but then quickly loses control of the pencil, which may fly from their hand. The diagnosis can be readily made by observing the patient's attempts to write. The immediately obvious feature is that they 'strangle' the pencil, the index finger and thumb are hyperextended and the knuckles turn white (see Fig. 12.8). It is at this stage that the pencil may fly from their grasp if it twists slightly. The arm will then flex at the wrist, adopting a similar position to a left-hander who, when writing, flexes the wrist in this way in order to see what they have just written. Both the elbow and shoulder will then be seen to tense up and the entire arm is now stiffened and becomes involved in the attempts to move the pencil. This is quite unlike the normal writing action, where the pencil is held lightly between the finger and thumb and the main movements occur at the forearm and the upper arm merely moves the hand across the page. If an unaffected person holds a pencil in this position and tries to write like this, they will quickly appreciate why the condition is called 'writer's cramp'!

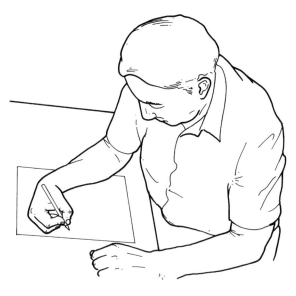

12.8 Writer's cramp.

Some patients find that if they hold the pencil between the knuckles of the index and middle finger they are able to write more easily. Tranquillizers are of minimal help and some patients are now being treated with botulinum toxin. Some patients have had success learning to write left-handed, others have had to resort to tape recorders and typing, which is usually unaffected by the condition.

Blepharoclonus and Blepharospasm

These conditions usually occur in the over-50 age group and may either consist of a tendency to blink very fast; blepharoclonus or alternatively, the patient may blink and then be unable to open the eyes; this is called blepharospasm. The frequent and prolonged episodes of forced eye closure render the patient virtually blind. Driving is particularly hazardous, as both problems may be provoked by flashes of light. Blepharospasm sometimes occurs in association with Parkinson's disease and may be a presenting symptom of this disorder. (See Fig. 12.5.) It can be readily treated with botulinum toxin and this was the first licensed use of this agent.

Unfortunately, eye closure has two components, the passive ptosis of the lid to cover the eye that occurs in a normal blink, and a more dramatic eye closure in response to threat, involving the use of the periocular muscles. It is only these latter muscles that can be treated with botulinum. A major problem with the injections is occasional unwanted ptosis. Some patients with long-standing blepharospasm are left with what is, in effect, a prolonged blink rather than a spasm, and reach a stage where the injections are no longer of value. In these patients the provision of old-fashioned ptosis props fitted on the spectacles may be of some help.

Facial Dyskinesias

This group of disorders has been increasingly recognized as a complication of chronic phenothiazine therapy in schizophrenic patients, but the chewing, chomping movements of the face, lips and tongue can also occur in elderly, demented or mentally subnormal patients. In addition to the facial movements repeated swallowing or tongue protrusion may occur. These are centrally generated movements. Benign hemifacial spasm which is due to irritation or degeneration of the seventh nerve is not a related disorder and is fully discussed in Chapter 6.

Meige's Syndrome

Meige's syndrome is a combination of severe facial grimacing with blepharospasm. It is a spontaneously occurring condition similar to drug-induced facial dystonias, and indeed may respond to phenothiazine treatment. Dramatic chewing, chomping or mouth opening with forced tongue protrusion are dominant features and may be so severe that the patient may spontaneously dislocate the jaw.

Drug-Induced Dystonias

The commonest causes of dystonic syndromes are drug hypersensitivity, drug overdosage or prolonged drug use. The drugs responsible include all the phenothiazines, butyrophenones, tricyclic antidepressants, dopamine and dopamine agonists. It was the recognition that all the dystonic syndromes described above, which had in the past been thought to be neurotic, could be produced by any of these drugs, that completely altered medical opinion to the general acceptance that these are organic disorders.

Drug-induced disorders include blepharospasm, oculogyric crisis, facial spasms, tongue protrusion, webbing of the neck due to muscle contraction, torticollis, antecollis, retrocollis, hyperextension of the back, lateral flexion of the spine, dystonic postures of the limbs and fine jerking restless movements of the limbs, which is correctly referred to as peripheral akathisia.

Although drug therapy is generally ineffective in the organic disorders, in drug-induced cases increasing the dose of the offending drug or treatment with an alternative phenothiazine may prove as effective as withdrawing the drug. In many instances the movement disorder develops long after the offending drug is withdrawn. This is known as tardive dyskinesia and is often the cause of facial dystonia.

There are important differences between the different types of phenothiazine and extrapyramidal syndromes. Piperazine side-chain drugs, trifluoperazine (Stelazine), fluphenazine (Modecate), perphenazine

(Fentazine) and prochlorperazine (Stemetil), are particularly likely to produce acute-onset dystonia, often after a single dose in young females. It is interesting that it is the antiemetic effect that is often the indication for the use of the drug and that metoclopramide (Maxolon), an antiemetic drug unrelated to the phenothiazines, can also produce acute dystonic syndromes of this type. These are hypersensitivity reactions. The chloro substituted agents such as chlorpromazine are more likely to produce parkinsonian syndromes after many years of use, and are often responsible for the tardive dyskinesias. These movements are due to chronic alterations in neurotransmitters and not to drug hypersensitivity.

Disorders Associated With Myoclonus

Myoclonus is defined as a brief shock-like jolt in a muscle, producing a very quick jerky movement. It can be dramatic and frequent enough to make a whole limb shake or consist of a single jolt. The latter is well known as the normal sleep startle or hypnogogic myoclonic jerk that has happened to almost everyone as they drop off to sleep. It is normally a positive phenomenon but can be seen as a negative phenomenon in asterixis, in liver failure, when the patient's outstretched arms jerk in a myoclonic way as tone is restored after a brief collapse of resting tone. The classification of myoclonic disorders is extremely difficult and the range of disorders is briefly summarized in Table 12.2. Only those disorders of major clinical significance are discussed below.

Infancy and Childhood

Myoclonic jerking associated with epilepsy is a feature of several conditions in infancy and childhood. These range from the benign remitting conditions such as benign myoclonus of infancy in which brief shock-like muscle contractions follow startle or attempted movement, to the lethal conditions such as the progressive lipoidosis of Krabbe, causing dementia and ultimately death.

Salaam Attacks

Infantile myoclonic spasms or 'salaam' attacks are much more serious and associated with a classic EEG appearance known as hypsarrythmia. The attacks start in the first year of life and consist of a cry followed by truncal flexion or a brief 'lightning jerk' of the entire body with extension of the legs and upturned eyes. These attacks cease after 2–3 years, but by that stage it is usually apparent that the child has considerable cerebral damage and severe mental subnormality. The commonest identifiable cause of this syndrome is now known to be tuberous sclerosis, which can be identified in infancy by the demonstration of subependymal lesions on CT scanning (see below). Tuberous sclerosis can occur in the absence of previous salaam attacks in childhood and in the presence of normal intellect. An instructive case report is to be found in Chapter 24 in the section on tuberous sclerosis. (Case Report XXI.)

Table 12.2   Causes of myoclonus and myoclonic epilepsy

Generalized	Localized
Idiopathic epilepsy	Subacute spinal neuronitis
Familial essential myoclonus	Spinal cord tumours
Progressive myoclonic epilepsy	Palatal myoclonus
Familial type	Hemifacial spasm
Lafora body type	Facial myokymia
Lipoidosis	
System degenerations	
Spinocerebellar degeneration	
Ramsay Hunt syndrome	
Myoclonic encephalopathy of infancy	
Infantile spasms (hypsarrythma)	
Epilepsy partialis continua	
Jones–Nevin syndrome	
Postcerebral anoxia	

Many of these disorders are extremely rare. This list has been prepared to show the wide range of underlying disorders and to emphasize the need for skilled evaluation of all patients with myoclonus

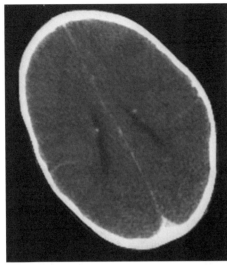

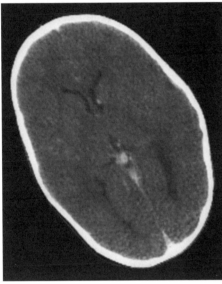

CT scan appearances of tuberous sclerosis in 2-year-old boy with salaam attacks.

Epilepsy with Myoclonus

Myoclonus may also be associated with other forms of epilepsy. Idiopathic grand mal epilepsy may be associated with morning myoclonus, a series of little jolts occurring at breakfast time and often proceeding to a generalized convulsion later (see Chapter 22). Myoclonus may also occur in patients with petit mal as a series of myoclonic jolts involving the eyelid, but the eye normally continues to look straight ahead. These episodes are known as myoclonic absences. A specific variant of epilepsy is photosensitive myoclonic epilepsy. The child (and eventually the parents) discovers that flickering light produces a series of jolts and fluttering of the eyelids. This is usually noticed when travelling through trees in bright sunlight. The child's eye may roll up and the episode may culminate in a major seizure. Sometimes children are seen following a first witnessed epileptic attack who relate that for years they have been aware of this phenomenon when travelling by car. A contemporary variant of this flicker-sensitive epilepsy is seen in children using computers. Episodes occur while scrolling or playing computer games with vivid flashing. In some instances, if the attack occurs when the child is still playing computer games at 3 a.m., sleep deprivation may be as important a factor as the flickering screen! The modern 625-line television screen with a dot matrix pattern seems to have dramatically reduced the incidence of television-triggered epilepsy.

Progressive Cerebral Disease Associated With Myoclonus

In the teens, in addition to the possible continuation of epilepsy-associated myoclonic attacks as described above, another group of disorders occur which are unfortunately progressive and, in many instances, lethal conditions.

Subacute Sclerosing Panencephalopathy (SSPE)

This is a rare but important fatal disorder and is due to an abnormal immune response to the measles virus. It occurs in the age range 5–20 years. The affected patient usually has a history of measles occurring very young, typically before 2 years of age. Many years later the condition suddenly appears. The onset may include intellectual or behavioural problems, myoclonic jerking, spasticity and rigidity. The condition is then dominated by increasing dementia, usually leading to death over a period of 1–2 years, although occasionally survivals of 10–15 years are reported. The diagnostic laboratory findings are a marked elevation of CSF globulins and very high antimeasles antibodies. It is thought that an abnormal immune response to intraneuronal measles virus is responsible. The EEG is characterized by an extremely flat tracing with occasional bursts of high-voltage spikes associated with simultaneous myoclonic jerks.

CASE REPORT XV

A 16-year-old boy presented following an epileptic fit on the first morning of his GCSE examinations. He had seemed somewhat dulled in affect over the previous 3 weeks but this was attributed to studying hard. He was admitted and an EEG showed changes diagnostic of subacute sclerosing panencephalitis. The epileptic fits were easily controlled but over the next few months rapid intellectual decline occurred, and although he was able to stay at home with his parents for 2 years, he then required admission to a long-term care facility. He is still alive 10 years later but is severely demented and totally dependent on nursing care.

Lafora-Body Disease

This is a lethal condition. What starts as myoclonic epilepsy is rapidly complicated by the development of cortical blindness and progressive dementia. Lafora bodies are found on cerebral biopsy and consist of mucopolysaccharide cellular inclusions. They are also found in the suprarenal glands and kidneys. All patients die within 2–3 years of the onset. The condition is inherited as a recessive.

Adult

Myoclonic jerking preceding an epileptic fit occurs in some 10% of epileptic patients and is discussed above and in detail in Chapter 22. Myoclonic jerking occurs in some families with Friedreich's ataxia, and this variant was formerly classified as Ramsay Hunt cerebellar degeneration (dyssynergia cerebellaris myoclonica). This condition is now thought to be part of a heterogeneous groups of degenerative cerebellar disorders, and two of the original patients described clearly had Friedreich's ataxia.

Some families have been reported in which parkinsonism and myoclonus appear in different members, and some patients with myoclonic epilepsy may develop a parkinsonian state in later life. These associations not only indicate the uncertain classification of these disorders but also indicate an overlap with some of the multisystem atrophies discussed earlier. It is because of this confusion and these associations that these disorders have been somewhat unconventionally grouped in this chapter.

Creutzfeldt–Jakob Disease

The most important adult acquired condition associated with myoclonus is Creutzfeldt–Jakob disease. It is characterized by a rapidly progressive dementia associated with myoclonic jerking and a typical EEG appearance. It is the first disease in man to be identified as being due to a prion (proteinaceous infectious particle). It is transmissible and cases due to corneal grafting, dural grafting, stereotactic EEG electrodes and in particular human growth hormone prepared from human pituitary glands, have been identified. In the majority of cases the mode of transmission is unknown. There is an inherited predisposition to the disease, but with only 1–2 cases per annum per million of population, exactly how and why the disease develops is unclear. The characteristic pathological finding is a spongiform vacuolar change in the affected nerve cells with rapidly developing atrophy. The condition is fatal within 3–12

months. The relationship to bovine spongiform encephalopathy (BSE) in cattle is unclear and transmission by ingestion has not been demonstrated, but the similarity of the pathology has prompted anxiety in some quarters. A similar familial condition also due to a prion is the Gerstmann–Straussler syndrome, which is extremely rare. The following is an example of the disease at its most malevolent, with an unusual presentation.

CASE REPORT XVI

A 63-year-old man presented with numbness of both legs and slight numbness of the fingers. Four weeks later he became unsteady when walking. There was no significant past history. On examination there was bilateral nystagmus, depressed arm reflexes, absent leg reflexes and flexor plantar responses. There was marked ataxia, more severe on the left. Pinprick sensation to both knees was impaired. He was unable to stand tandem. All biochemical and haematological studies and CSF examination were normal. Nerve conduction studies showed prolonged distal latencies but normal velocities with small sensory action potentials. Four weeks later he was barely able to walk and had developed evidence of rapidly progressing dementia. An MRI scan showed cerebellar atrophy and diffuse white matter lesions, consistent with cerebral ischaemic changes. He continued to deteriorate, with increasing confusion, dysarthria, dysphagia and increasingly severe incoordination. Occasional myoclonic jerks were seen and fasciculation was noted in the right arm and both legs. An EEG at that stage showed minimal residual alpha rhythm and widespread low voltage theta activity, but no repetitive or generalized discharges. He continued to deteriorate and died 12 weeks from presentation. Post mortem revealed typical spongiform changes that were most striking in the cerebellum, brain stem and basal ganglia. The changes in the cerebral cortex were relatively mild and no abnormality was found in the region of the white matter lesions seen on the MRI scan.

The unusual features in this case were the presentation with neuropathy and the very severe cerebellar involvement. The diagnosis was tentatively suspected when the myoclonic jerking appeared, but this was a very minor feature in this case. At the time of his death the possibility that this would prove to be a peripheral neuropathy and cerebellar degeneration, with limbic encephalopathy all secondary to an undetected carcinoma, was thought to be a more likely diagnosis.

There are many other disorders in which myoclonic jerking may occur of even greater rarity than those already discussed. In view of the possible serious implications, any patient with myoclonic jerking should be referred for an expert opinion. It is also important to recognize that myoclonus as a reversible phenomenon is seen in uraemia, hypomagnesaemia and liver failure, and metabolic causes should always be excluded when myoclonus is of sudden onset.

The Cerebellum

For clinical purposes there is little to be gained by attempting to learn the detailed anatomy of the cerebellum with its confusing double nomenclature, but a knowledge of the basic structure and the main nuclei is essential to understand the conditions discussed in this section.

Basic Anatomy

The anatomy of the cerebellum and its connections is detailed in Figures 12.9–12.10, 12.11 and 12.12. There are two basic regions, the midline structures and the cerebellar hemispheres. The midline groups include the lingula anteriorly, the vermis in the middle and the flocculonodular lobe posteriorly. The lobes are divided into a small anterior lobe and a large posterior lobe. Each hemisphere contains a large main nucleus, the dentate, through which the bulk of efferent cerebellar information passes. There are smaller roof nuclei which are mainly concerned with vestibular reflexes and ocular movements.

The major cerebellar input derives from the massive frontopontocerebellar projections which are relayed by the transverse pontine fibres to the opposite cerebellar hemisphere. The importance of this pathway can be judged from its size. It is responsible for the shape of the pons. It programmes the cerebellum as to the intended next movement of the trunk and limbs.

The cerebellar inputs from below are of major clinical importance, providing instant feedback information as to the current posture, position and movement of the limbs and trunk. The disruption of these functions in diseases specifically affecting these pathways, such as Friedreich's ataxia, attests to their importance.

The dorsal spinocerebellar tract has a laminar pattern and contains rapidly conducted proprioceptive information relayed via Clarke's dorsal nucleus. It enters the cerebellum through the inferior cerebellar peduncle and is distributed to all areas.

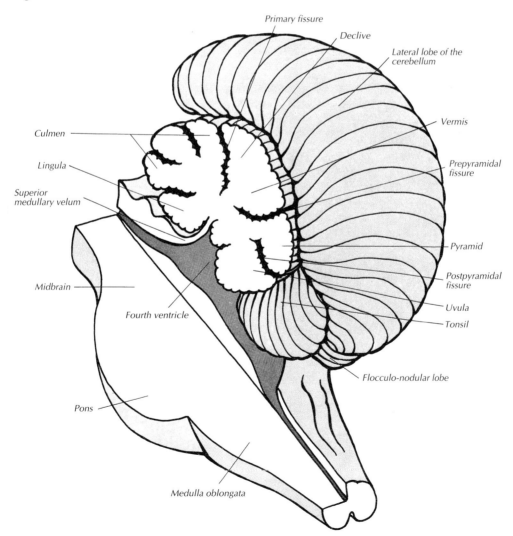

12.9   Schematic diagram of the cerebellum in relation to the brain stem.

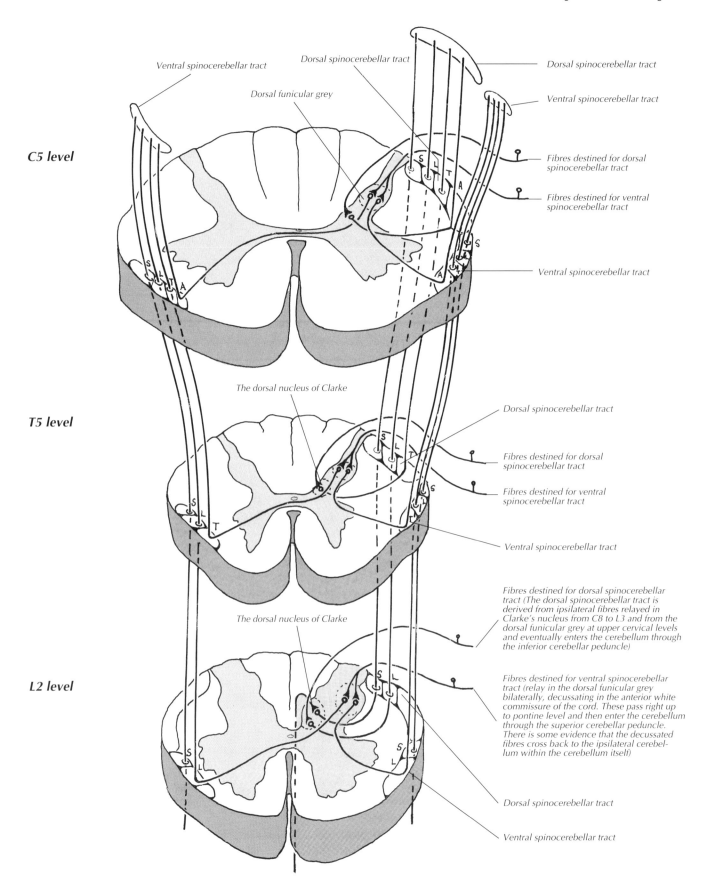

C5 level

T5 level

L2 level

Ventral spinocerebellar tract

Dorsal spinocerebellar tract

Dorsal funicular grey

Dorsal spinocerebellar tract

Ventral spinocerebellar tract

Fibres destined for dorsal spinocerebellar tract

Fibres destined for ventral spinocerebellar tract

Ventral spinocerebellar tract

The dorsal nucleus of Clarke

Dorsal spinocerebellar tract

Fibres destined for dorsal spinocerebellar tract

Fibres destined for ventral spinocerebellar tract

Ventral spinocerebellar tract

Fibres destined for dorsal spinocerebellar tract (The dorsal spinocerebellar tract is derived from ipsilateral fibres relayed in Clarke's nucleus from C8 to L3 and from the dorsal funicular grey at upper cervical levels and eventually enters the cerebellum through the inferior cerebellar peduncle)

Fibres destined for ventral spinocerebellar tract (relay in the dorsal funicular grey bilaterally, decussating in the anterior white commissure of the cord. These pass right up to pontine level and then enter the cerebellum through the superior cerebellar peduncle. There is some evidence that the decussated fibres cross back to the ipsilateral cerebellum within the cerebellum itself)

The dorsal nucleus of Clarke

Dorsal spinocerebellar tract

Ventral spinocerebellar tract

12.10 The spinocerebellar pathways.

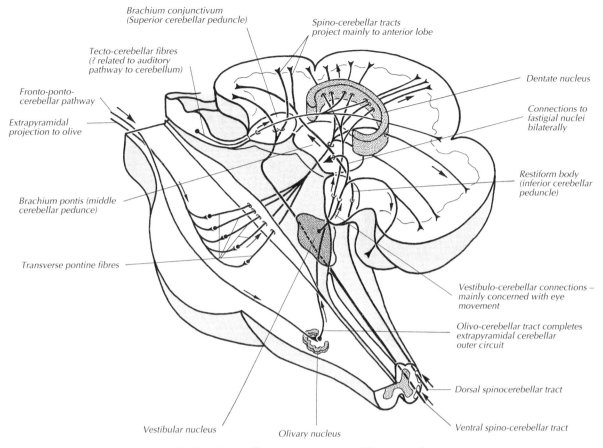

Brachium conjunctivum
(Superior cerebellar peduncle)

Spino-cerebellar tracts
project mainly to anterior lobe

Tecto-cerebellar fibres
(? related to auditory
pathway to cerebellum)

Fronto-ponto-
cerebellar pathway

Extrapyramidal
projection to olive

Dentate nucleus

Connections to
fastigial nuclei
bilaterally

Restiform body
(inferior cerebellar
peduncle)

Brachium pontis (middle
cerebellar peduncle)

Transverse pontine fibres

Vestibulo-cerebellar connections –
mainly concerned with eye
movement

Olivo-cerebellar tract completes
extrapyramidal cerebellar
outer circuit

Dorsal spinocerebellar tract

Vestibular nucleus

Olivary nucleus

Ventral spino-cerebellar tract

12.11 Main afferent connections of the cerebellum.

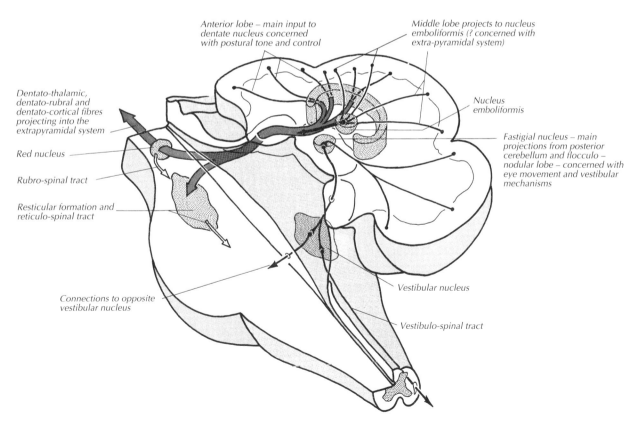

Anterior lobe – main input to
dentate nucleus concerned
with postural tone and control

Middle lobe projects to nucleus
emboliformis (? concerned with
extra-pyramidal system)

Dentato-thalamic,
dentato-rubral and
dentato-cortical fibres
projecting into the
extrapyramidal system

Nucleus
emboliformis

Red nucleus

Fastigial nucleus – main
projections from posterior
cerebellum and flocculo –
nodular lobe – concerned with
eye movement and vestibular
mechanisms

Rubro-spinal tract

Resticular formation and
reticulo-spinal tract

Connections to opposite
vestibular nucleus

Vestibular nucleus

Vestibulo-spinal tract

12.12 Main efferent connections of the cerebellum.

The ventral spinocerebellar tract is crossed. The relay occurs in the dorsal funicular grey, decussation occurs in the anterior white commissure and the pathway ascends and enters the cerebellum through the superior cerebellar peduncle. There is considerable clinical and anatomical support for further decussation of this information within the cerebellum itself, back to the side of origin, so that cerebellar input is essentially homolateral.

Midline Lesions

Clinically, lesions affecting the midline group produce severe ataxia of gait. Neoplastic lesions in the lingula extend into the superior medullary velum producing fourth nerve palsies, or into the superior cerebellar peduncle producing severe tremor of the arm on the same side. Lesions in the vermis cause severe truncal ataxia, often making it impossible for the patient to sit or stand unsupported. Lesions in the flocculonodular region cause ataxia, vertigo (due to damage to vestibular reflex pathways) and vomiting if they extend into the floor of the fourth ventricle. Tumours at all midline sites tend to cause early obstruction of the aqueduct or fourth ventricle, resulting in headache and papilloedema.

Cerebellar Hemisphere Lesions

The signs of a lesion in the cerebellar hemisphere depend on the symmetry. A unilateral lesion produces classic cerebellar signs in the limbs on the same side (see later). Symmetrical involvement of both hemispheres, as happens in some of the cerebellar degenerations, may produce quite mild symmetrical signs with moderate gait ataxia.

The most dramatic 'cerebellar' signs are found in diseases which damage cerebellar connections in the brain stem, either the main efferent pathways in the superior cerebellar peduncle or the inflow pathways in the inferior and middle cerebellar peduncles. One of the most difficult false localizing signs in neurology may result from a lesion affecting the frontopontocerebellar pathway. (See Case Report XX in Chapter 8.)

Clinical Signs of Cerebellar Disease

The most important physical sign of cerebellar disease is ataxia. This is best defined as incoordinated or inaccurate movement which is not due to paresis, alteration in tone, loss of postural sense or the intrusion of involuntary movements. For this reason the majority of neurologists do not test cerebellar function until they are certain that the patient has normal power, tone and sensation.

Diagnostic Pitfalls

In children there are three common findings that may easily be mistaken for ataxia. These are the intrusion of choreiform movements, the presence of myoclonic jerks and petit mal status epilepticus. In the latter condition the child will sit drooling with a blank expression on its face, and all voluntary movements are performed with little pauses and sudden jolts. The EEG will be diagnostic.

In the adult there are also three potential clinical errors. Mild pyramidal weakness may easily produce 'ataxia' on cerebellar testing unless allowances are made for the weakness. Many extrapyramidal disorders in their early stages produce 'pseudoparesis' or 'pseudoataxia' unless the underlying rigidity and involuntary movements are identified, and finally extremely anxious patients perform very badly on formal cerebellar function tests, owing to their tense state.

Gait Ataxia

A patient with gait difficulty due to a cerebellar disorder becomes frightened to stand. They will preferentially stand with the feet wide apart and will hold on to any support that is available. They will not fall, but may reel from side to side even when supported, and consistently to the same side if a unilateral lesion is present. Minimal degrees of gait ataxia are best detected by asking the patient to walk on a line. After one or two inaccurate steps the patient often refuses to go further and reverts to a wide-based stationary stance. Although patients in this position tend to wobble even more when they close their eyes, they do not fall. This is often described as Rombergism but, as discussed in Chapter 6, this is not strictly accurate. Romberg's test was originally intended as a test for intact joint position sense.

The 3F Syndrome (Fear of Further Falling)

This is an important gait abnormality that is often misdiagnosed as cerebellar ataxia in elderly and usually female patients. It has been called the 3F syndrome. It often occurs after an elderly patient has had an attack of vertigo, syncope, a drop attack, or after a fall. The patient will only walk in a bizarre posture, pushing one foot forward tentatively while leaning back on the other. The arms are held forwards with the hands facing downward. The patient insists on a relative, however elderly or frail, walking behind them. This has been called the 3G syndrome (grabbing great grandmother). When they finally reach their chair they will dive forward much too soon, the 3P syndrome (precipitate premature perching). This seems to be an entirely functional disorder that is extremely difficult to treat. Even prolonged physiotherapy seems to provide little reassurance, and as soon as the patient attempts to walk alone they revert to the classic and bizarre posture. In spite of all the apparent difficulty they do not fall: they are just overwhelmed by the fear that they might.

Truncal Ataxia

Truncal ataxia is a particular feature of midline cerebellar lesions. The patient may be unable to sit or stand without support, with a tendency to fall backwards. Unless the flocculonodular lobe is involved there may be no other definite symptoms or signs. Limb ataxia is minimal or absent, It is usually an ominous physical sign indicative of either midline cerebellar degeneration with no likelihood of recovery, or a midline cerebellar tumour such as a medulloblastoma or metastasis. It is a very striking feature of the post-chickenpox cerebellar syndrome of childhood, which normally recovers completely over 4–6 weeks.

Limb Ataxia

Cerebellar function in the limbs is tested in several ways. In Chapter 8 the value of observing the patient's outstretched hands as a screening test for disorders of pyramidal and proprioceptive function was discussed. In cerebellar disease the outstretched hand on the affected side tends to hyperpronate, so that the palm faces outwards, and rises above the level of the other hand. This is known as Riddoch's sign. If the examiner then presses down gently on the outstretched hands and suddenly releases the pressure, the hand on the affected side will fly up completely out of control and the patient is unable to return it to the start position, the limb oscillating up and down as they attempt to do so. This is called the rebound phenomenon. The ability of the patient to touch their index finger tips together in front of them with their eyes closed should also be tested. This is difficult to do perfectly, even in the absence of any disease process. The abnormality of both range and direction is referred to as dysmetria.

When these tests have been performed the patient's ability to touch the tip of their nose and then the examiner's index finger is tested. This is known as the finger/nose test. If postural sense has already been tested there is no need for the patient to attempt the test with the eyes closed. The value of the test is greatly enhanced if the examiner moves the target finger, varying both the direction and distance from the patient's nose. In this finger/nose/finger test quite mild incoordination, terminal intention tremor and dysmetria can be more readily detected.

The equivalent test in the legs is the heel/knee/shin test. The patient is asked to place the tip of the heel (not the sole of the foot) on the tibial tubercle of the other leg and run the heel down the front of the shin. The heel is then lifted off and replaced on the tibial tubercle. The foot is not rubbed up and down the shin. If the sole of the foot is allowed to sit astride the shin the foot slides up and down with the tibia acting as a guide. Some mild incoordination is within normal limits for this test, particularly in the elderly with painful hips or knee joints, and normal children seem to have surprisingly poor coordination on this particular test. The test must be performed properly and over-interpretation of minor abnormalities should be avoided.

Unilateral ataxia should be reliable indicator of disease affecting the cerebellar hemisphere on the same side. However, if severe it could indicate disease affecting the cerebellar input on the same side, a lesion of the dentatorubrothalamic pathway, or even damage in the opposite frontal pole. It can also be modified by a coexistent pyramidal deficit or impairment of posture sense. When all these possibilities are taken into account the difficulty occasionally experienced in diagnosing a cerebellar lesion with confidence is understandable. Perhaps the commonest error made by a beginner is to misinterpret clumsiness due to a mild pyramidal deficit as ataxia due to a cerebellar lesion.

Rapid Alternating Movements

On completion of the ataxia tests a variety of simple rapid movement tests are performed. These detect fragmentation of movement or inaccuracy of movement, which is accentuated by the speed at which the movement is attempted. This is known as dysdiadochokinesia. The most useful tests are those in which the patient taps himself on the back of one hand as fast as he can, or taps his foot on the floor or against the examiner's hand. This test is also subject to the proviso that there should be no pyramidal deficit. The patient is then asked to make a fist, and with his elbow half flexed tries to pronate and supinate the forearm as fast as possible. In abnormal situations the movement is slow and irregular and the shoulder joint will start to abduct and adduct wildly as the whole arm becomes involved in the effort.

Tremor

A major feature of cerebellar disease is the non-rhythmic tremor that appears on action, which is also known a kinetic or intention tremor. At rest the limbs are still but in action tremulousness appears, which is maximal at the beginning and end of the range of movement and is sometimes referred to as terminal intention tremor.

Truncal tremor can also occur and here the situation is different. When sitting or standing these muscles are already in action, and a tremor of the trunk will appear and may become so violent that constant jerking movements of the head and body may occur, which may be backwards and forwards or even include lateral flexion or rotational movements.

Other Signs

The signs already discussed, difficult as they are to elicit, are definite evidence of cerebellar dysfunction. There are a variety of other signs that are occasionally even more difficult to elicit and less certain in their interpretation.

Tone

In cerebellar disease the tone in the muscles is reduced on the side of the lesion. Reduced tone is a highly subjective phenomenon and although occasionally it is unequivocally reduced, this is not always the case. In many instances no definite tone change will be detected.

Reflexes

In parallel with the decrease in tone, the reflexes tend to be less brisk and rather slower in rise and fall producing what is known as a pendular jerk. Again, this is highly subjective and in the majority of patients no definite abnormality of the reflexes is found.

Nystagmus

A bewildering variety of eye movement abnormalities, including nystagmus, are seen in cerebellar disease, particularly midline cerebellar lesions in those areas most intimately associated with occular movements in relationship to head posture. Disease in the cerebellar hemispheres produces less clear-cut disorders, with impairment of smooth tracking as a major feature, and any resulting nystagmus will be maximal towards the side of the lesion. In any patient with cerebellar disease nystagmus is not necessarily a feature, and subtle abnormalities of saccadic movement and tracking may be overlooked by a cursory clinical examination. These problems are discussed in greater detail in Chapter 7.

Dysarthria

Cerebellar disease affects the autoregulation of breathing, and particularly its integration with speech. This tends to produce spluttering staccato speech. So-called scanning dysarthria is more typical of combined pyramidal–cerebellar lesions, and usually occurs in multiple sclerosis. There is some evidence that speech coordination is mainly controlled by the left cerebellar hemisphere.

Writing

Writing is often affected and typically the patient enlarges the writing to make it more legible – quite the reverse of parkinsonism, in which the writing becomes smaller.

Head Posture

There are three ways in which head posture may be altered by cerebellar disease. All produce a head tilt to one side. Lesions in the superior medullary velum may cause a fourth nerve palsy which results in a head tilt to compensate for diplopia. A cerebellar hemisphere lesion may unbalance postural tone, leading to a head tilt towards the side of the lesion. Lesions in the flocculonodular lobe may directly irritate the dura in the posterior fossa, causing neck stiffness and tilting and retraction of the head to one side. This is not necessarily lateralizing.

Vomiting

In view of the difficulties encountered in making a definite diagnosis of cerebellar disease on clinical evidence, the considerable significance of vomiting in patients with cerebellar tumours deserves special mention. The characteristic features may be remembered as another 3P syndrome (postural, positional and projectile). The vomiting typically occurs on movement, particularly on sitting up from a lying position, is of very sudden onset without preliminary nausea, and hence tends to be projectile. Vomiting with these characteristics is virtually diagnostic of a posterior fossa tumour, even in the absence of other physical signs.

CASE REPORT XVII

A 36-year-old self-employed builder had been under great deal of pressure and developed mild headaches and attacks of sudden vomiting. There were absolutely no physical signs but if he suddenly sat up from lying he almost invariably vomited. An CT scan revealed a cystic midline tumour, confirmed by operation. The patient and his original medical advisers had thought his symptoms were due to anxiety.

CASE REPORT XVIII

A 38-year-old woman was seen on the gastroenterology unit with a diagnosis of psychogenic vomiting. For several weeks she had been subject to sudden effortless vomiting with minimal nausea. There were no other symptoms or signs and extensive upper intestinal investigation had revealed no cause. The additional feature in the history of neurological importance was that position change was often critical in initiating the vomiting, which was not only effortless but sometimes projectile. A posterior fossa tumour was suspected but a CT scan was reported normal. On review it was felt that the fourth ventricle was not clearly demonstrated, and it was decided to examine the region of the foramen magnum and fourth ventricle using contrast with metrizimide. During the myelographic phase of this investigation, a tongue of tissue was seen projecting through the foramen magnum and down into the upper cervical canal. The fourth ventricle could not be demonstrated. At surgery the lesion was found to be an ependymoma of the fourth ventricle, which had protruded through the foramen of Magendie and extended down into the upper cervical canal. The vomiting ceased following surgery.

The significance of headache accompanied by vomiting has been stressed in previous discussions. In particular, the features of positional projectile vomiting were emphasized. In neither of the cases above was headache an important feature, but the vomiting itself was nevertheless diagnostic of 'cerebral' vomiting. Once again, it is worth repeating that vomiting on position change, without preliminary nausea and catching the patient unawares, should be regarded as a very ominous symptom until proved otherwise.

In summary, pure cerebellar disease may produce very definite symptoms, particularly unsteadiness of gait, but remarkably subtle physical signs, often dominated by a single feature such as truncal ataxia. Patients with very florid physical signs usually have involvement of cerebellar connections in the brain stem. For the same reason extensive surgical resection of part of the cerebellum may produce remarkably little residual deficit, and even metastatic lesions may be treated surgically in anticipation of an acceptable end result.

Cerebellar Disease in Childhood

In childhood there are five main categories of disease that may affect the cerebellum. Some of these are detailed elsewhere and will not be discussed in detail here.

Congenital Lesions

These conditions include various maldevelopments of the cerebellum, often associated with Arnold–Chiari malformation or the Dandy–Walker syndrome (see Chapter 15). Often the associated meningocoele or hydrocephalus gives rise to the presenting symptoms, but mild cases of Arnold–Chiari syndrome may not produce symptoms until adulthood, and a minor degree of the malformation often underlies syringomyelia.

As in the case of extrapyramidal disorders, it should be remembered that ataxia cannot become manifest until the pyramidal system becomes fully functional. Therefore, apparently 'acute' disorders of movement or gait, starting in the second year of life, are frequently found to be due to congenital abnormalities or neonatal brain damage. Congenital aqueduct stenosis is another

condition that may cause a delayed presentation, dominated by ataxia. Some patients with this condition may present as late as 35 years of age with symptoms which may include ataxia, sixth nerve palsies, deafness, papilloedema with visual failure and declining intellectual function. The onset may be very insidious and the condition is readily misdiagnosed as a cerebellar tumour. Fortunately, CT scanning has now made this diagnosis relatively easy. Previously ventriculography was the only way of confirming the diagnosis.

Metabolic Disorders

There are several metabolic disorders which may cause cerebellar dysfunction and ataxia. These include metachromatic leukodystrophy, Bassen–Kornsweig disease and Refsum's syndrome, which are discussed in Chapter 18. There are also the mitochondrial disorders, Leigh's syndrome and Kearns–Sayre syndrome, which include acute cerebellar ataxia triggered by intercurrent infection as one of their clinical manifestations.

There are five additional disorders with metabolic implications following the removal of lead from white paint.

1. Ataxia in children may be due to drugs, especially anticonvulsants and in particular diphenylhydantoin, carbamazepine and primidone. Occasionally acute ataxia and drowsiness may be found to be due to alcohol if the child has had access to the family drinks cabinet!

2. Ataxia, papilloedema and drowsiness may be due to lead poisoning and consequent cerebral swelling. This is easily misdiagnosed as a cerebellar tumour. This has fortunately become an extremely rare condition following the removal of lead from white paint.

3. Maple syrup urine disease is one of the rare disorders of amino-acid metabolism in which episodic ataxia occurs, often precipitated by infection. During attacks increased amounts of valine, leucine and isoleucine are excreted in the urine. Between attacks there is no abnormality.

4. Hartnup disease is due to impaired absorption of tryptophan. Episodic ataxia precipitated by infection, and usually associated with a dry, scaly red pellagra-like skin rash, occurs. Variable amino-aciduria is found even between attacks.

5. Ataxia telangiectasia (Louis–Barr syndrome) is extremely rare. The main features of this fatal progressive disorder are telangiectasia of the conjunctivae (usually misdiagnosed as chronic conjunctivitis), progressive cerebellar degeneration and a tendency to infection in those patients who have associated agammaglobulinaemia. The usual course of the disease is progressive ataxia and mental impairment, with early death due to infection. For further discussion see Chapter 24.

Infectious Disorders

Acute viral infection of the cerebellum has been reported, or at least patients in whom the evidence of viral encephalitis has been dominated by ataxia.

An acute ataxic syndrome may occur after **any** of the exanthemata of childhood and infectious mononucleosis. There is a specific association with chicken pox, in which severe ataxia may start within 3 weeks of the initial infection and subsides over several months. Chicken pox 'cerebellitis' usually occurs in children under 2 years of age and is less common in older children. In all cases of 'postinfectious' ataxia in childhood it is important to exclude the metabolic disorders that can triggered by infection (see above).

Children with Guillain–Barré syndrome may appear to be ataxic on initial examination. This is due to proximal motor weakness and/or sensory loss, and re-emphasizes the importance of being certain that 'ataxia' is not due to complex combinations of weakness and sensory deficit.

Degenerative Disorders

The commonest inherited form of spinocerebellar degeneration is Friedreich's ataxia, which usually causes symptoms between the ages 5 and 10. It is fully discussed in Chapter 14. The majority of inherited cerebellar degenerations present in adulthood and certainly constitute the longest delayed in onset of all inherited disorders; the possibility of inherited disease may not even be considered in view of the age of the patient.

CASE REPORT XIX

A 37-year-old railway guard was admitted for investigation of suspected multiple sclerosis. He was certainly ataxic, because his presenting symptom was that while attempting to clip a passenger's ticket the ataxia intruded and he clipped a piece out of the passenger's finger instead! On examination he had depressed reflexes, extensor plantar responses, intact abdominal reflexes and marked bilateral pes cavus. Further history revealed that his father had had similar feet and had frequently been suspected of being drunk on duty when he was a railway guard, because he would be seen staggering in the train corridor. The father unfortunately was deceased, but there was no doubt that the patient had a similar inherited condition. No evidence was found to support a diagnosis of multiple sclerosis.

Two varieties may cause symptoms in childhood. The olivopontocerebellar atrophy group, which is discussed in detail later, which tends to start as ataxia and dysarthria in the adult, confusingly may cause progressive spastic paralysis and death in the child. Another Ramsay Hunt syndrome (dentatorubrothalamic degeneration) in childhood causes a mild progressive ataxia complicated by sudden myoclonic jerking, which may be sufficiently severe to throw the child to the ground, in addition to falls directly related to the ataxia. Opsoclonus may also be a feature.

Tumours

It is pertinent to recall that the majority of cerebral tumours in childhood occur in the cerebellum, and that there are two types: the highly malignant medulloblastoma, which produces a 'midline' picture with gross truncal ataxia, and the benign cystic astrocytoma, which may start in the midline but later spreads laterally as a large cystic extension into one or other hemisphere, and is more likely to produce a unilateral cerebellar syndrome.

The first symptom of a cerebellar tumour in the child is usually ataxia, closely followed by headache, vomiting and diplopia. Papilloedema may develop very rapidly and it is unusual to see a child who has had symptoms for longer than 7–10 days before presentation. The main differential diagnoses are lead poisoning and aqueductal stenosis. Pontine gliomas do not cause CSF obstruction and are more likely to produce multiple cranial nerve palsies or retention of urine (see Chapters 11 and 15).

Cerebellar Disease in the Adult

In the adult the causes of cerebellar disease are quite different. Cerebellar infarction due to vascular disease is a relatively rare cause of cerebellar dysfunction. Giddiness and ataxia are usually due to involvement of the cerebellar pathways in a brainstem vascular lesion. Potentially fatal acute intracerebellar haemorrhage has been described in Chapter 11. Several hereditary disorders typically cause their first symptoms in adulthood. Tumour in the cerebellum and posterior fossa are rare if one excludes acoustic nerve tumours, and are usually metastatic. The one exception is the cerebellar haemangioblastoma. Finally, there are several metabolic causes of cerebellar disease, alcohol and anticonvulsant toxicity being the main offenders.

Inherited Cerebellar Disease

Most of the cerebellar ataxias begin in middle age; they have recently been extensively reclassified and many of the previous eponymous syndromes have disappeared and been incorporated into a general groups of what are now called the dominantly inherited ataxias. Three major groupings that account for roughly a third of all inherited ataxias have now been defined. They are Friedreich's ataxia, dominant inherited ataxia and the recessively inherited ataxic disorders.

Friedreich's Ataxia

Friedreich's ataxia is discussed in Chapter 14. It is worth emphasizing again that not only is the ataxic component mainly due to spinal cord and peripheral nerve damage, but that the disorder is part of a much more generalized degenerative condition. A majority of patients have scoliosis, sometimes sufficiently severe as to compromise respiration. Cardiac conduction defects, atrioseptal hypertrophy and cardiac muscle degeneration occur in 90% of patients, and are usually responsible for death. There is also islet-cell atrophy in the pancreas, resulting in frank diabetes in 20% of patients and subclinical diabetes in another 20%.

Dominant Inherited Ataxias

Many variants of late-onset ataxia, with slightly different clinical pictures, were identified by the giants of neurology. These include the conditions previously classified under the names of Dejerine, Thomas, Marie, Sanger-Brown and Holmes. All these disorders are now regarded as variants of olivopontocerebellar atrophy (OPCA). The different variants merely reflected the wide range of additional degenerative features and the sequence in which they appeared that modified the clinical picture. It was the realization that the end result in all cases was so similar that prompted the reclassification.

Ataxia of gait is the universal feature. At first increased reflexes and pyramidal signs including even spasticity may occur, but later the reflexes disappear to be replaced by cerebellar hypotonia. Dysphagia and dysarthria tend to be early and prominent symptoms. Sphincter disturbance and impotence occur and may be surprisingly early. In some cases sensory features later intrude, and in a great many extrapyramidal signs and dementia are later developing features that finally disable and destroy the patient. The time course of the disease is extremely variable, some patients progressing to death in 1–2 years and others developing a relatively incomplete version and surviving for many years.

MRI scanning has become the diagnostic test of choice for these disorders, demonstrating the atrophy of both the pons and the cerebellum in most instances.

Recently a dominantly inherited paroxysmal ataxia has been identified. In affected females the episodes of ataxia are specifically related to periods, pregnancy and the use of oral contraceptives. For reasons that are far from clear, attacks may be modified by the use of acetazolamide.

Recessive Inherited Ataxias

In addition to Friedreich's ataxia, which is by far the commonest of these disorders and therefore classified separately, all the inherited metabolic disorders discussed earlier under childhood ataxias are included here, and for completeness we should add the cerebellar components seen in Wilson's disease, Refsum's syndrome, Bassen–Kornsweig syndrome and those conditions involving abnormal vitamin E metabolism. Many of these disorders are potentially treatable by dietary and metabolic means, and their recognition is therefore important. The rarity of the conditions is such that expert opinions are essential for their accurate identification.

In all these disorders some decline in intellectual function is common, even though the brunt of the damage falls on the cerebellum. The familial nature may initially be obscured by the early death of parents (before they could develop the disease) or long separation from siblings by the time the disease occurs. Careful family tracing may reveal several siblings in different parts of the world with the same disease masquerading under several different diagnostic labels.

Metabolic Cerebellar Disease

There are a variety of possible metabolic causes of cerebellar degeneration, characterized by loss of Purkinje cells and in some cases confined to fairly discrete areas of the cerebellum. Alcohol is the commonest cause and may produce very severe but reversible acute ataxia during intoxication, slowly worsening ataxia or severe acute irreversible ataxia during an attack of Wernicke's encephalopathy. The brunt of the damage falls on the anterior lobe and severe gait ataxia is the result.

Anticonvulsant drugs cause reversible ataxia in acute overdosage but there is no doubt that chronic and occasionally acute overdoses of diphenylhydantoin can produce irreversible cerebellar damage.

Carbon monoxide poisoning and severe hyperthermia may produce acute destruction of the cerebellar cortex.

CASE REPORT XX

A elderly man attempted suicide in a coal-gas oven. He was found and taken to hospital semiconscious. He was given oxygen and within 24 hours appeared normal. Ten days later be became acutely ataxic, dysarthric and dysphagic. He was tube fed but his condition deteriorated and he died a few days later. A post mortem the cerebellum had a jelly-like consistency and was completely destroyed.

Malignant disease usually causes metastatic cerebellar disease but cerebellar degeneration as a remote complication of carcinomas, and malignant lymphomas without metastasis does occur, although rather less often than the impression that is sometimes given in discussion. Most patients with malignant disease who develop cerebellar signs will have a metastasis in the cerebellum rather than a remote non-metastatic complication of their tumour.

A slowly progressive cerebellar ataxia is a rare but clearly defined complication of myxoedema and is responsive to treatment if identified early. Cerebellar degenerative components have also been identified in B_{12}, folate and vitamin E deficiency in malabsorption.

Neoplastic Involvement

Metastatic malignant disease accounts for the majority of cerebellar tumours in the adult. Carcinoma of the lung and breast is usually responsible but a surprisingly high proportion are metastatic from large bowel tumours, particularly those in the descending and rectosigmoid colon. It has been suggested that these tumours metastasize directly to the cerebellum via the paravertebral plexus of veins up the spine and into the posterior fossa.

Primary tumours are rare, although occasionally medulloblastomas may occur in the adult. Primary gliomas are very rare. The most frequent tumour is the benign haemangioblastoma, often a very small vascular nodule associated with a large cyst. The prognosis is excellent, although recurrences may occur. Occasionally these tumours produce erythropoietin and are associated with polycythaemia.

Extrinsic compression of the cerebellum by acoustic neuromas has been considered in Chapter 6.

Multiple Sclerosis

Cerebellar signs in multiple sclerosis are common, but in the majority of cases the responsible lesions are in the brainstem cerebellar pathways and the cerebellar signs are almost always associated with internuclear opthalmoplegia, long tract signs and evidence of bilateral pyramidal lesions. MRI scanning often reveals white matter lesions in the cerebellum, which may be both asymptomatic and not accompanied by any of the physical signs of cerebellar disease discussed in this chapter.

Cerebellar disease can surprisingly difficult to diagnose, but having established that there is involvement of the cerebellum there are a wide range of diagnostic possibilities. In the ataxic child urgent investigation to exclude a tumour should take priority. Some of the recessive inherited disorders may be responsive to specific treatment, so that attempts to define the disorders are important.

In the adult a very detailed family history should be taken however old the patient, and a thorough enquiry into drug and alcohol intake is essential. Congenital malformations of the posterior fossa or aqueduct should always be considered in the differential diagnosis of an apparent posterior fossa lesion at **any** age.

13. The Anatomy, Physiology and Clinical Features of Spinal Cord Disease

Gross Anatomy of the Spinal Cord

The spinal cord is approximately 45 cm long and extends from the top of C1 vertebra to the bottom of the body of L1 vertebra. At birth the conus of the spinal cord has already been pulled up to L3 level and the final position is established at the latest by the age of 10. The spinal cord is not a perfect cylinder but has two major enlargements at cervical and lumbar level. These are the areas of the motor neuron pools that supply the arms and the legs and the result is a considerable expansion of the grey matter in these areas. They extend respectively from C3 to T2 and from L1 to S3 (Fig. 13.1).

At its upper end the cord is continuous with the medulla oblongata and at the lower end the conus medullaris becomes the filum terminale, a fibrous band containing very little neural tissue that extends down to attach to the bony canal at S4 level, within the sacrum. It lies in a tube of dura and is surrounded by pia mater down to S2. This is called the sacral sac.

Within the entire spinal canal down to S2 level the spinal cord and filum terminale is surrounded by a thick tube of dura mater, which is loosely separated from the fine arachnoid mater by the potential subdural space. The arachnoid mater is separated from the pia mater which invests the spinal cord and the nerve roots by the subarachnoid space, which contains the cerebrospinal fluid. As the spinal cord ends at L2 level and the dural sac at S2 level there is a large space which contains only the lumbar, sacral and coccygeal roots, which constitute the cauda equina. This space allows sampling of the spinal fluid by lumbar puncture without risk to the spinal cord, and the technique for achieving this is described fully in Chapter 14.

Basic Internal Structure of the Spinal Cord

The Central Grey (Fig. 13.2)

The central grey consists of an H-shaped area present at all levels. It is joined across the midline by the grey commissure, within which lies the small central canal. The grey matter is referred to anatomically as the anterior and posterior columns (or horns). Unfortunately, neurologists prefer to use the terms dorsal and ventral horns, rather than columns, which can cause confusion. They refer to the gracile and cuneate fasciculi as the dorsal columns and the sensations conveyed within them are called dorsal column sensations. Similarly, conditions affecting the motor cells in the anterior column are referred to as ventral horn cell diseases rather than anterior column cell diseases. Throughout this volume, the neurological terminology is used. The area at the tip of the dorsal column (known to neurologists as the dorsal root entry zone) is a relatively translucent area known as the substantia gelatinosa, an area of great importance in central pain mechanisms.

Architecture of the Central Grey Matter

The anterior grey column (the ventral horn) contains the large cells of the α motor neurons a large number of smaller interneurons and the small motor cells of the γ fibre system. The cells are grouped into motor neuron pools, which control a group of muscles having similar actions and are functionally grouped into flexor and extensor actions.

The posterolateral grey consists of the dorsal root entry zone, the cell bodies and fibres of Lissauer's tract, the substantia gelatinosa and the dorsal funicular grey, which contains more specific nuclear masses at different levels.

The intermediate grey consists of the autonomic preganglionic cells. These are in two major groupings, the intermediolateral group and the intermediomedial group. The column that extends from C8 to L1 contains the cells of the thoracolumbar outflow, which controls the sympathetic nervous system. A less defined group of cells in the intermediate grey of the cord at S2, S3 and S4 are the preganglionic parasympathetic cells of the pelvic splanchnic nerves.

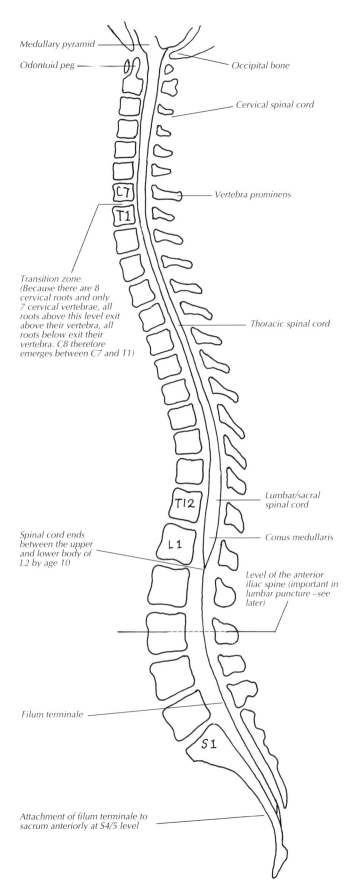

Medullary pyramid

Odontoid peg

Occipital bone

Cervical spinal cord

C7

T1

Vertebra prominens

Transition zone
(Because there are 8
cervical roots and only
7 cervical vertebrae, all
roots above this level exit
above their vertebra, all
roots below exit their
vertebra. C8 therefore
emerges between C7 and T1)

Thoracic spinal cord

T12

Lumbar/sacral
spinal cord

L1

Conus medullaris

Spinal cord ends
between the upper
and lower body of
L2 by age 10

Level of the anterior
iliac spine (important in
lumbar puncture –see
later)

Filum terminale

S1

Attachment of filum terminale to
sacrum anteriorly at S4/5 level

13.1   Gross anatomy of the spinal cord.

The embryological development of the spinal cord and vertebrae is described in Chapter 15 and the vascular supply of the spinal cord in Chapter 14.

Practical Anatomy of the Spinal Cord Pathways

The Motor Pathways (Fig. 13.3)

Motor pathway damage is the most easily recognized part of the clinical picture produced by conditions affecting the spinal cord. Clinically, the constellation of findings is known as 'pyramidal signs', although it is likely that many of the typical features are produced by damage to non-pyramidal pathways. With the exception of the vestibulospinal tract the exact anatomy of these other extrapyramidal pathways – the reticulospinal rubrospinal and tectospinal tracts – below cervical cord level is uncertain. The pyramidal pathway (the corticospinal tract) is easily identified in the cord at all levels, including the conus. The corticospinal tract gets progressively smaller as it passes down the cord as fewer and fewer fibres are required to supply the remaining ventral horn cells. The corticospinal pathway starts at the cervicomedullary junction, just below the decussation of the medullary pyramid opposite the top of C1 vertebra, as shown in Figure 13.1. The fibres conveying information to the motor neuron pools supplying the arm are then lying in a medial position and the fibres destined to supply the motor neuron pools of the leg decussating slightly lower down and assuming a lateral position in the tract (see Fig. 11.5).

Sensory Pathways (Figs 13.4 and 13.5)

The sensory pathways are more complicated than is generally appreciated, but for clinical purposes the traditional descriptions form a practical framework for discussion.

Tactile Sensation

Tactile sense includes accurate localization of a light touch, two-point discrimination and poorly localized touch sensation. Accurate touch and two-point discrimination (referred to as 2 PD in discussion) are relayed to the brain in the gracile (leg) and cuneate (arm) fasciculi on the same side of the spinal cord. As the leg fibres enter the cord lower down they are pushed medially as incoming fibres join the cord at progressively higher levels, forming a laminated pattern, the dorsal columns getting larger as they ascend the cord. Clinically the gracile and cuneate fasciculi are referred to as 'the dorsal columns', and the sensations conveyed in them as 'dorsal column sensation'.

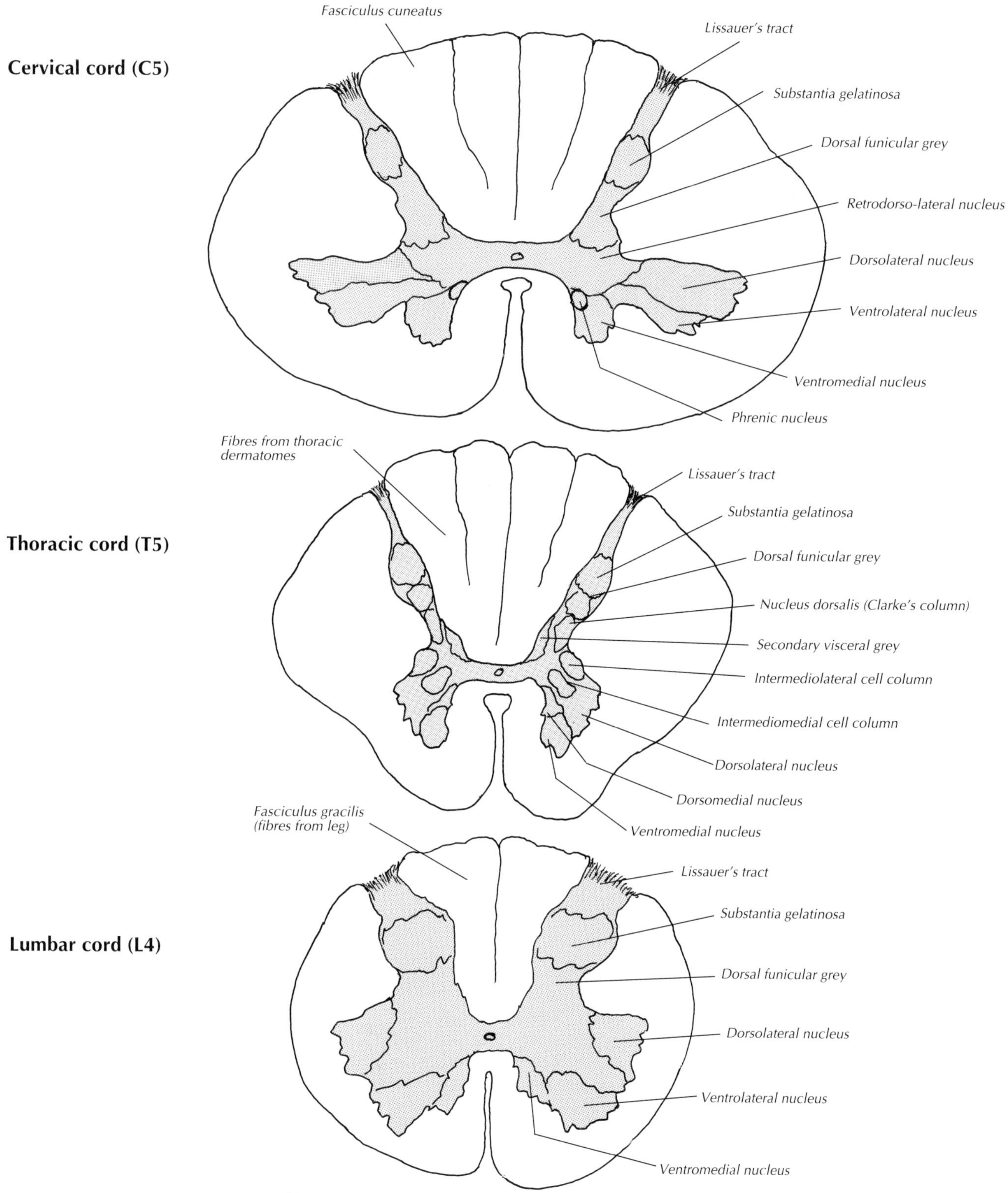

Cervical cord (C5)

Fasciculus cuneatus

Lissauer's tract

Substantia gelatinosa

Dorsal funicular grey

Retrodorso-lateral nucleus

Dorsolateral nucleus

Ventrolateral nucleus

Ventromedial nucleus

Phrenic nucleus

Thoracic cord (T5)

Fibres from thoracic dermatomes

Lissauer's tract

Substantia gelatinosa

Dorsal funicular grey

Nucleus dorsalis (Clarke's column)

Secondary visceral grey

Intermediolateral cell column

Intermediomedial cell column

Dorsolateral nucleus

Dorsomedial nucleus

Ventromedial nucleus

Lumbar cord (L4)

Fasciculus gracilis (fibres from leg)

Lissauer's tract

Substantia gelatinosa

Dorsal funicular grey

Dorsolateral nucleus

Ventrolateral nucleus

Ventromedial nucleus

Note:

a *The relatively large grey matter at lumbar level as the ascending tracts are only just forming and the descending tracts diminishing*

b *The relatively large anterior horn concerned with motor function in the leg*

c *The relatively sparse grey matter at thoracic level due to the modest amount of musculature innervated by each anterior horn*

d *The large amount of white matter present at cervical level as both the ascending and descending tracts contain most fibres at this level*

13.2   The central grey.

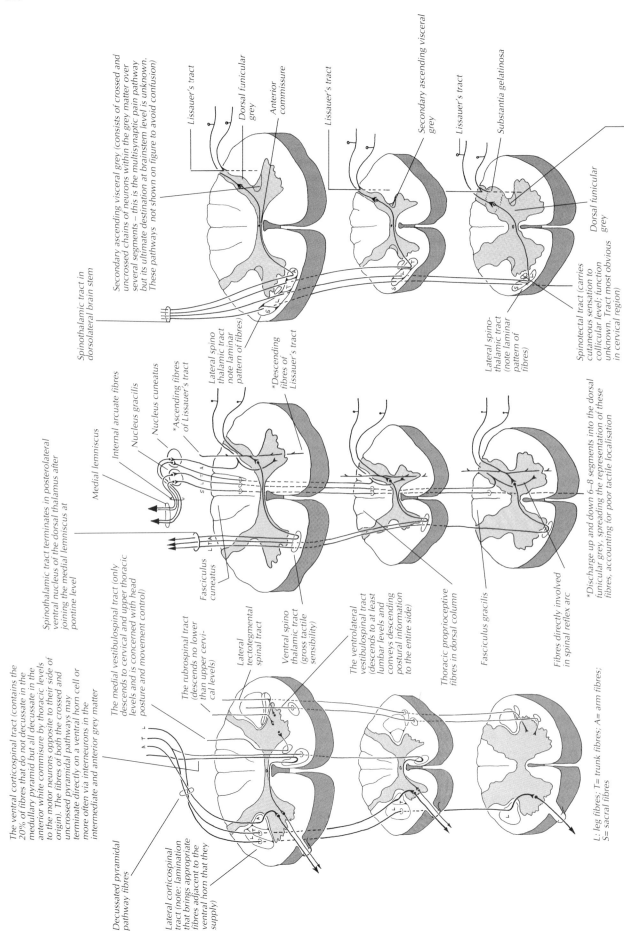

The ventral corticospinal tract (contains the 20% of fibres that do not decussate in the medullary pyramid but all decussate in the anterior white commisure by thoracic levels to the motor neurons opposite to their side of origin). The fibres of both the crossed and uncrossed pyramidal pathways may terminate directly on a ventral horn cell or more often via interneurons in the intermediate and anterior grey matter

Decussated pyramidal pathway fibres

Lateral corticospinal tract (note: lamination that brings appropriate fibres adjacent to the ventral horn that they supply)

The medial vestibulospinal tract (only descends to cervical and upper thoracic levels and is concerned with head posture and movement control)

The rubrospinal tract (descends no lower than upper cervical levels)

Lateral tectotegmental spinal tract

Ventral spino thalamic tract (gross tactile sensibility)

The ventrolateral vestibulospinal tract (descends to at least lumbar levels and conveys descending postural information to the entire side)

L: leg fibres; T= trunk fibres; A= arm fibres; S= sacral fibres

13.3   Descending tracts of the spinal cord.

Spinothalamic tract in dorsolateral brain stem

Spinothalamic tract terminates in posterolateral ventral nucleus of the dorsal thalamus after joining the medial lemniscus at pontine level

Medial lemniscus

Internal arcuate fibres

Nucleus gracilis

Nucleus cuneatus

*Ascending fibres of Lissauer's tract

Fasciculus cuneatus

Thoracic proprioceptive fibres in dorsal column

Fasciculus gracilis

Fibres directly involved in spinal reflex arc

*Discharge up and down 6–8 segments into the dorsal funicular grey, spreading the representation of these fibres, accounting for poor tactile localisation

13.4   Tactile and dorsal column sensation.

Secondary ascending visceral grey (consists of crossed and uncrossed chains of neurons within the grey matter over several segments – this is the multisynaptic pain pathway but its ultimate destination at brainstem level is unknown. These pathways not shown on figure to avoid confusion)

Lissauer's tract

Dorsal funicular grey

Anterior commissure

Lissauer's tract

Secondary ascending visceral grey

Lissauer's tract

Substantia gelatinosa

Lateral spino thalamic tract note laminar pattern of fibres)

*Descending fibres of Lissauer's tract

Lateral spino-thalamic tract (note laminar pattern of fibres)

Dorsal funicular grey

Spinotectal tract (carries cutaneous sensation to collicular level; function unknown. Tract most obvious in cervical region)

Secondary ascending visceral grey

13.5   Pain and temperature sensation pathways.

Poorly localized sense of touch is relayed across the spinal cord to the opposite ventral spinothalamic tract, which ultimately joins the accurate touch pathway, the medial lemniscus, in the brain stem. Because there are two pathways for touch, unless the cord is totally transected it is unusual for gross touch sensation to be completely abolished in any form of cord disease.

Joint Position Sense

Joint position sense (clinically referred to as JPS) is also carried in the dorsal columns and is often impaired in spinal cord disease. This only applies to that part of joint position sense that reaches consciousness. Most joint position sense information is utilized in the reflex control of posture and is conveyed to the cerebellum via the dorsal and ventral spinocerebellar pathways (see Fig. 12.10). The considerable importance of this insensible joint position information is seen in Friedreich's ataxia, a disease in which the pathological process specifically affects spinocerebellar pathways, causing gross ataxia.

Vibration Sense

This is a man-made sensory modality that for many years was thought to be conveyed in the dorsal columns. There is now much evidence that it is conveyed in several pathways. For this reason impaired vibration sense cannot be regarded as specific evidence of a dorsal column lesion, although severe impairment is a feature of diseases that are known to primarily affect the dorsal columns. Its main value lies in the very early loss of vibration sense that may be detectable in peripheral neuropathy.

Pain and Temperature Sensation

Pain and temperature sensation are traditionally considered together, although only one of the several pain pathways also conveys temperature sensation. Pain is conveyed in fast pathways, allowing immediate and accurate appreciation of a painful stimulus, and in slow multisynaptic pathways which relay in the dorsal grey in Lissauer's tract, in the substantia gelatinosa and in the central grey matter of the spinal cord. These latter pathways are of great yet incompletely understood importance in several serious and painful clinical disorders, including causalgia, the pain that may follow a peripheral nerve lesion.

The classic pain pathway is the lateral spinothalamic tract, and this is the pathway that also carries temperature sensation. Pain afferents enter the spinal cord and ascend two to three segments before they cross the cord anterior to the central canal. This may cause misleading clinical signs. For example, a lesion at T3 level may only damage fibres from as low as T6, three seg-

ments lower down, causing false localization of the level of the lesion. If there is a central lesion in the cord it may only interrupt the fibres crossing over at the affected segments and produce a band of numbness perhaps extending over three to four segments and often unilateral, even though a symmetrical bilateral sensory loss would be anticipated on purely anatomical grounds. These features are described in detail in Chapter 14.

As the fibres reach the opposite spinothalamic tract the lowest entering fibres are progressively pushed laterally, as more and more fibres join the tract at higher levels, producing a laminated tract with the lowest entering sacral fibres lying in the most lateral position.

Fibres from the lateral spinothalamic tract may then project back into central grey matter after crossing the cord. This further accounts for the failure of surgical transection of the spinothalamic tract to completely block pain sensation from the opposite side of the body, especially pain of the deep visceral type. Such pain could only be blocked by complete transection of the cord – not a practical form of treatment!

Temperature sensation is also conveyed in the lateral spinothalamic tract, although there is some doubt as to whether the topographical anatomy of the temperature fibres is identical to that of the pain fibres. Hence different sensory levels to pain and temperature sensation may be found when the lateral spinothalamic tract is damaged, although it is obvious that there is a considerable difference between the precision of pinprick perception and the more diffuse temperature stimulus, which may account for some of this apparent difference.

Symptoms of Motor Pathway Damage

Lower motor neuron lesions which damage the ventral horn cells or ventral nerve roots cause wasting and weakness in the muscle groups supplied by those cells and their nerve fibres. When the spinal cord is damaged the local motor units, arranged as pools of ventral horn cells, are affected. The ventral horn cells are arranged in groups that work together to perform specific movements. This was most strikingly seen in poliomyelitis, where groups of muscles performing a movement, rather than single muscles, were affected. Whether this is clinically detectable depends on the location of the damage. For example, if the damage is at T1 level the weakness and wasting of the small hand muscles is readily appreciated by the patient, and at L5 level a foot drop can scarcely escape notice. Yet at almost all other levels the earliest evidence of damage may pass unrecognized by the patient and be detected only by the most diligent examiner. Wasting or fasciculation in a segment of the abdominal wall or in an individual intercostal muscle may be difficult or impossible to detect. Segmental abdominal weakness may be best observed with the patient standing, when a bulging band will appear around the trunk like a 'Michelin man'. Weakness in an intercostal muscle is best seen during full inspiration, when the intercostal space will draw in. In most instances evidence of a lower motor lesion will be found by the examiner when unnoticed by the patient, and this is quite the reverse of an upper motor neuron lesion, in which the patient may notice symptoms long before any definite clinical abnormality can be found.

Damage to the descending corticospinal tract is usually responsible for the first symptoms of a spinal cord lesion, particularly when the lesion causes spinal cord compression. The earliest symptom is a subtle stiffening of the legs, often noticed by the patient as a tendency to trip over minor undulations and difficulty walking on rough ground. The patient may find it impossible to walk quickly or break into a run. Patients often use the expression 'tripping over matchsticks' to describe this symptom. The patient may notice increasing difficulty climbing stairs, due to weakness of hip flexion and dorsiflexion of the foot.

Spontaneous ankle clonus may be experienced while stepping down a kerb or step due to spasticity of the plantar flexors of the foot. The patient may describe the foot as 'vibrating'. Eventually the patient notices that their feet are dragging and that they have developed a stiff-legged gait, keep tripping over and are scuffing the tips of their shoes. They often comment that they can 'hear' their feet walking when in a corridor.

In cord compression due to a neoplasm this whole sequence may develop to its full extent over a matter of hours to days, but for example in spondylotic myelopathy the symptoms may develop insidiously over 1 or 2 years. The early symptoms of cord compression or degenerative spinal cord disease are often dismissed as being due to 'normal ageing' or 'arthritis'.

The symptoms of an upper motor neuron lesion may occur long before definite clinical evidence is detectable. It is extremely dangerous to attach facile explanations to such symptoms, and the patient should be kept under close observation until the situation is resolved by recovery or the development of physical signs. Eliciting these physical signs is a major neurological skill.

Physical Signs of Motor Pathway Damage

Muscle Wasting and Weakness

Lower motor neuron lesions are extensively covered in Chapters 16, 17 and 19, and are not considered further here other than to point out that a lower motor neuron lesion causes wasting and weakness of muscles and loss of the local reflex.

If a patient with cord compression presents with bilateral weakness of the legs due to an upper motor neuron lesion, and on examination the triceps muscle on one side is found to be wasted and weak and the triceps jerk absent, there is a strong probability that the compressive lesion is simultaneously damaging the lower motor neuron at C7 level. Hence the importance of clearly identifying the relationship of the different muscles in the arm to the root origin of their nerve supply (see tables in Chapters 16 and 17).

Upper motor neuron lesions produce the signs of a 'pyramidal lesion'. The doubtful accuracy of this term has already been mentioned but for clinical purposes it is a useful abbreviation, indicating as it does a standard constellation of symptoms and signs. These signs usually occur in combination and in a sequence which consists of reflex changes, then tone changes and finally weakness developing in specific muscle groups, as discussed in a later section.

Reflex Changes

In the early stages the reflexes below the level of the lesion are enhanced. This finding is always difficult to evaluate as reflexes are so often enhanced by anxiety. In an extremely anxious patient a few beats of clonus may also occur, further compounding the difficulty. It is traditional to document the reflexes + (normal), ++ (enhanced) and +++ (very brisk). This scale is subject to personal interpretation and experience. In many instances the unequivocal **absence** of a single reflex may carry more certain clinical significance, as there should always be an explanation. A brisk reflex may merely indicate that the patient is very anxious. If there is marked asymmetry of reflexes it is easier to be certain that there is an abnormality.

For more certain evidence of a pyramidal lesion the abdominal reflexes and plantar responses are invaluable. These are two of the most difficult signs in neurology to elicit and interpret correctly.

Abdominal Reflexes

The abdominal reflexes are cutaneous reflexes elicited by gently stroking the skin over the abdominal wall and observing the contraction of the underlying muscles. These reflexes are abolished by an upper motor neuron lesion above T9 level. In practice they are often difficult or impossible to detect in obese, multiparous or multiscarred abdomens. Only in the young, slim unscathed abdomen can absent abdominal reflexes be regarded as definitely pathological. The abdominal reflexes are therefore best used as a cross-check on a possible extensor plantar response. For example, if the right plantar response appears to be extensor and the right abdominal reflexes are absent, and those on the left can be easily elicited, this is certain evidence of a pyramidal lesion affecting the corticospinal pathway on the right side. In this setting, if the abdominal reflexes were intact this would either indicate that the lesion damaging the spinal cord is below T12 level or would cast some doubt on the validity of the extensor plantar response, which should then be checked again.

Plantar Reflexes

The plantar responses are often referred to incorrectly as 'Babinskis'. The Babinski response is the pathological extension of the big toe produced by stroking the sole of the foot. There is no such thing as a 'negative' Babinski response. In neurological discussion the Babinski response is also frequently referred to as an 'upgoing toe'. The reflex is difficult to elicit correctly. It is said that a skilled neurologist can make the big toe extend or flex as he wishes, and this is certainly possible using incorrect technique. If the very tender sole of the foot is stimulated the big toe will almost always flex and the whole leg will withdraw. If the stimulus is applied to the lateral side of the foot and then across the pad and allowed to touch the flexor aspect of any of the toes, especially the big toe, extension of the big toe will almost always be produced, mimicking a Babinski response (see Fig. 13.6).

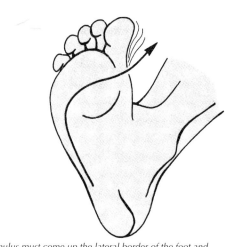

Stimulus must come up the lateral border of the foot and not touch flexor crease of toes.
not touch big toe at all
In a classical reponse the big toe extends as the stimulus leaves the foot

13.6   Eliciting the plantar response.

The correct way to elicit the reflex and avoid inadvertently producing a misleading response, is to scrape gently along the lateral border of the sole and then across to the ball of the foot and off without touching the toes. The normal response is flexion of the big toe and an abnormal response (a Babinski reflex) is extension of the big toe. What the other toes do is not important: it is usually difficult enough to see which way the

big toe is moving without worrying about them. It is also the first movement of the big toe that matters. In patients with extremely sensitive feet the initial normal flexion response is quickly followed by a mass extension of the toes and withdrawal of the entire leg. This is not a Babinski response. Other techniques involving squeezing the Achilles tendon or compressing the anterior compartment – Gordon and Oppenheim responses – are difficult to elicit and not reliable.

These problems have been dealt with at length as many think that the only real skill in neurology lies in confirming an extensor plantar response and that it is a very ominous sign in neurological disease, and, most worrying of all, the conclusion that a flexor plantar response virtually excludes neurological disease. None of these views is correct, and when one considers the difficulty of performing the test reliably the potential danger of misdiagnosis is obvious. Perhaps it is safest to regard the plantar response as the 'ESR' of the nervous system. If it is extensor it certainly indicates a problem, but if flexor it does not necessarily mean that all is well. As so often in neurology the response has to be correlated with the history and other physical findings before apportioning its full significance.

Tone

In parallel with the development of the above signs the tone in the affected limbs increases: in clinical terminology, 'the limbs become spastic'. This means that there is an increased resistance to passive movement of the limbs. Evaluation may be difficult in a very tense or elderly patient. The elderly in particular have great difficulty in relaxing and often try to move the leg to help the examiner. This can make the evaluation of the tone extremely hard work and often quite impossible. The more the patient is asked to relax the more he fights the examiner! A useful trick is to continue to talk to the patient and very gently roll the leg from side to side with a hand placed under the knee, and when the leg is rolling freely quickly flick the knee up in the air. The normal leg will passively flex at the knee, a mildly spastic leg will remain stiff and jerk up into the air.

Tone in the arm can be tested by holding the patient's hand as if shaking hands, and by gently flexing and extending the elbow and wrist joints and then rotating the arm at the elbow. The earliest sign of increased tone in the arm is often detected on this last movement, with a slight catch as the arm is passively supinated.

Tone is increased in those muscles that remain strong. In the arm these are the shoulder adductors, elbow flexors, wrist flexors and finger flexors. The ultimate expression of this tone increase is that the patient has an arm which is fully flexed at the elbow, wrist and fingers. In the leg spasticity of the hip extensors, knee extensors and plantar flexors of the foot results in a stiff extended leg, with forced plantar flexion of the foot (Fig. 13.7).

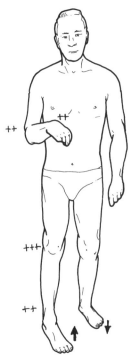

13.7 Spastic hemiparetic posture. Note increased reflex responses and extensor plantar response on the affected side.

Weakness

At some stage in the evolution of a pyramidal lesion weakness will develop. This will be maximal in those groups that are **not** spastic. In the upper limb these will be the shoulder abductors, the elbow extensors and the wrist extensors, and in the leg the hip flexors, knee flexors (hamstrings) and the dorsiflexors of the foot.

In the very early stages of pyramidal weakness, the secret of the neurological examination is knowing **where** to look for the weakness. Non-neurologists are usually content to test the hand grips and quadriceps muscles and, if no weakness is detectable, assume that power is normal. In almost all neurological disorders these two functions are the **least** likely to be affected.

As the pyramidal lesion evolves the patient's gait will become progressively abnormal. At first there may merely be a tendency for one or other foot to scuff the ground; later the leg will clearly drag, until finally the patient can barely move one leg past the other. This abnormality is most easily observed when the patient comes into the room. This very important observation is a good reason for personally calling the patient in from the waiting room, taking the opportunity to observe them getting out of the chair and walking across the

waiting area. Sometimes the diagnosis is already obvious before the patient has entered the consulting room.

Once on the examination couch a useful initial screening test for pyramidal function is the ability of the patient to hold their arms extended and play a piano in mid-air. In the legs the ability to wiggle the toes fast and symmetrically serves the same purpose. Very early pyramidal motor deficit may be indicated by slowing of these movements.

In a pyramidal lesion the weakness will be found in the extensor groups of the arm and the flexor groups of the leg. This is most easily remembered if a patient with a spastic hemiparesis is visualized. They walk with the elbow flexed and the arm and fingers flexed across the chest. The leg is extended and circumducts in an effort to prevent the toe scuffing as it moves forwards. This posture is imposed on the patient by the strength of the spastic muscles and the weakness of the opposing groups.

To facilitate evaluation of weakness by a series of doctors or to document recovery, a scale has been devised which grades muscle strength.

It is more helpful to grade movements rather than individual muscles in the present context. The grading system is as follows:

Grade 0 – No muscle action.
Grade 1 – Muscles seen to contract but no movement.
Grade 2 – Movement occurs if gravity eliminated.
Grade 3 – Movement occurs against gravity.
Grade 4 – Movement against gravity and up to 75% resistance.
Grade 5 – Movement against gravity and maximum resistance.

All the difficulties discussed above may develop in a different sequence and the discussion is only broken into sections for clarity. A fully developed pyramidal lesion will eventually include all the features described.

Symptoms of Sensory Pathway Damage

Radicular or root symptoms may occur at the level of a spinal cord lesion, especially in those diseases that specifically affect the nerve roots. These are very important symptoms as they often indicate the level of the disease process extremely accurately.

Radicular or root symptoms are readily recognized as such when they affect the arm or the leg. When radicular pain occurs in the thoracic dermatomes it is usual for irritation of the nerve roots to be the **last** diagnosis considered. Heart or lung disease is suspected when the pain is in the thorax and gallbladder, or renal disease when the pain is in the abdominal dermatomes. It is important to remember that the T12 dermatome lies just above the inguinal ligament and it is the lumbar dermatomes that supply the legs. Because the roots sweep down and forwards, the pain will mimic gallbladder and renal disease very convincingly. There are several case reports in the subsequent chapters which emphasize this very important consideration.

The sensations described may vary widely, from a dull ache to a severe knife-like pain or from a warm glow to a sensation like an icy-cold bandage around the area. Sometimes soreness or hypersensitivity of the affected area may be described by the patient as a sensation as if the skin were being 'rubbed by sandpaper' or being 'sprayed with scalding water'. The important clue is that the pain extends round from the back and along an identifiable dermatome. The description and the localization of the pain should make recognition possible. Bilateral dermatome pain should be more readily identified, with the exception of T3 or T4 root pain, which is usually misdiagnosed as cardiac in origin.

Damage to the central pathways also causes typical but variable symptoms.

Symptoms of Dorsal Column Pathway Damage

Dorsal column pathway damage causes fine tingling paraesthesiae in the extremities below the level of the lesion. At times these may assume a vibrating quality that is likened to touching an electric typewriter, or like the vibration felt when standing on the deck of a ship. Dorsal column lesions are also probably responsible for the well-recognized 'band sensations'. These are sensations described by the patient as if a cold or warm wet bandage or towel was being pulled tight around the lower thorax or lower abdomen. The affected area may also feel hypersensitive and the brassière or briefs may feel too tight or uncomfortable. Similar sensations may occur at the knee or ankle joints, but are then often more localized and may feel more like a ligature or a steel clamp wrapped round the limb. These sensations may be excruciatingly severe.

Disordered touch and joint position sense may also produce some bizarre disorders of body image. A limb may feel as if it is twice the normal size or as if it is encased in wet clothing which is shrinking. A sensation as if the leg were in a long wellington boot filled with icy-cold water may be contrasted with a sensation as if the leg were badly sunburned and swollen. Either the hands or the feet may feel as if they had been plunged into stinging nettles or a hornet's nest, and when touching objects patients may describe a sensation as if a thick felt pad were interposed between the skin and the object touched.

Symptoms of Spinothalamic Pathway Damage

This causes very different but equally unpleasant symptoms. The earliest symptoms consist of very deep, poorly localized aching pains with a nagging quality. This may persist for years and is very often regarded as functional because of its persistence and, at first sight, non-anatomical distribution. Patients who have syringomyelia, or spinal cord tumours may have symptoms of this sort for years before their organic nature is recognized. Several case reports in the subsequent chapters typify this difficulty. As the condition progresses the sensations become more dramatic. They may be likened to 'being kicked in the shin' 'as if the flesh were being torn from the bones', 'as if my bones were on fire' or 'icicles being stuck in my leg'. These are all entirely characteristic descriptions, but because they are somewhat bizarre may be regarded as functional and the patient suspected of having a vivid imagination or malingering. This is a particularly unfortunate diagnostic error if these symptoms later prove to be the first evidence of an intrinsic spinal cord tumour. This is undoubtedly the reason that the average delay from first symptom to correct diagnosis of intrinsic spinal cord tumours is some 3–4 years.

CASE REPORT I

A ward consultation was requested on a 58-year-old woman who presented with a 3-year history of constant burning pains and soreness below the waist. She had seen general physicians and was recommended to have psychiatric treatment, which she had refused. On physical examination there were no neurological findings but the patient gave a very straightforward history suggestive of bilateral spinothalamic pain and a myelogram was recommended. Her medical advisers, however, felt that this was unnecessary and recommended that she proceed with psychiatric treatment. This proved unavailing and she was referred again 2 years later by her GP. The symptoms were unchanged, as was the physical examination, and there were no findings, but on this occasion she agreed to myelography. She was examined and no abnormality found 15 minutes prior to the myelogram and myelography using sodium iodophenylate revealed near complete block at T7 (see plates). She was held head-down for 15 minutes, and enough contrast got past the tumour to demonstrate the upper limits and the appearances were characteristic of an intradural extramedullary lesion, almost certainly a meningioma. She was re-examined 1 hour after the myelogram and there were still no physical findings. The tumour was successfully removed but sadly her symptoms persisted until her death some 8 years later.

It seems very likely that the symptoms were related to the presence of the tumour but the complete failure of the symptoms to remit postoperatively remains inexplicable.

Patients sometimes complain that an area has gone 'numb'. When patients use this expression they nearly always mean the heavy sensation that occurs when a

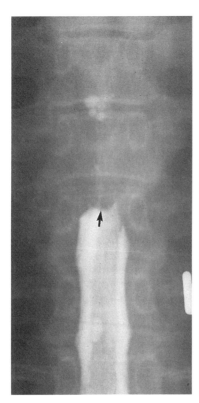 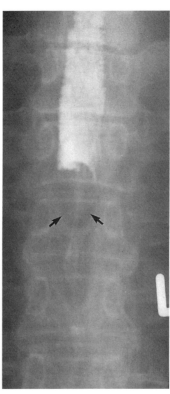

CRI.   Spinal meningioma with near complete block on myelography but no physical findings.

limb is weak. This is a descriptive term that should never be accepted as indicating sensory loss until the meaning has been carefully discussed with the patient, and after careful examination to confirm sensory loss has been performed.

Physical Signs of Sensory Pathway Damage

The finer points of sensory examination are discussed in the next chapter. At this stage discussion will be confined to general points.

Because there are dual sensory pathways a casual examination of the 'can you feel me touching your leg?' type has little value and might as well be dispensed with altogether. It is worth emphasizing as a general rule that patients often have sensory symptoms in the absence of detectable sensory signs, whereas motor signs may be found in the absence of motor symptoms. It follows that if there are no sensory symptoms it is extremely unlikely that any sensory signs will be detected.

Pain Sensation

When testing pain sensation it is important to test **pain**. In conditions specifically affecting pain sensation, touch sensation is usually preserved. Unless the patient happens to cut or burn themselves by accident they may be quite unaware of extensive areas of loss of pain sensation. During formal testing the patient must

be aware of the requirement to sense both the touch of the pin **and** the pain produced by it. It is not sufficient merely to ask if the patient can feel the pin. They should also be asked to specify that it was painful. This of course presumes that the patient knows what pain feels like. There are patients who are congenitally insensitive to pain and they have no concept as to what pain actually is. The following are two typical examples of this situation.

CASE REPORT II

An 11-year-old boy was referred by his GP because of swelling and deformity of the foot that prevented him wearing his shoe, but he had no discomfort. His legs were covered in bruises. Physical examination revealed a perfectly normal nervous system except that he did not flinch from a pinprick, although he could feel the touch. The corneal responses were absent and his foot was quite painless on movement, even though there were two recently fractured metatarsals. The bruises were the result of his schoolfriends activities, who had discovered that he did not cry if punched or kicked, and had repeatedly confirmed this observation!

CASE REPORT III

The neurologists were asked to review a 60-year-old man in the ENT ward who had been diagnosed 30 years previously as having syringomyelia. He was admitted to have his stenosed oesophagus bougied for the umpteenth time. The stenosis was a consequence of numerous bets during his national service that he could drink hot cocoa made direct from a boiling kettle. He always won the bet, but at some cost to his oesophageal mucosa! Examination revealed none of the usual features of syringomyelia but clear evidence of total body anaesthesia to pain and temperature.

Another classic presentation of pain sensation loss is the Charcot joint. This typically occurred in patients with tabes dorsalis who developed gross destructive arthropathy of the knee and ankle joints, but is now seen mainly in severe diabetic neuropathy. A Charcot joint at the shoulder is almost exclusively a consequence of syringomyelia, with loss of pain sensation in the cervical dermatomes.

Temperature Sensation

Accurate temperature sense testing is unnecessary on a routine basis as it is unlikely to be affected if pain appreciation is normal. It is formally tested by filling either glass test tubes or copper tubes with warm and cold water. These need only be a few degrees above and below normal skin temperature: if too hot or too cold, pain fibres may well be stimulated, thereby invalidating the tests! During routine examinations the coldness of a metal tuning fork may be used as a simple screening test.

Vibration Sense

Vibration sense has limited clinical value, not only because of the anatomical uncertainty of the pathways involved but also because many patients over 70 years old have impaired vibration sense below the knees. Vibration sense testing is really of most value in young patients where multiple sclerosis is suspected, or in any patient suspected of suffering from a peripheral neuropathy. In peripheral neuropathy vibration sense may be one of the earliest modalities to be impaired (see Chapter 19). A 64 or 128 Hz tuning fork should be used, applied successively to the tip of the big toe, the medial malleolus, the tibial tubercle, the anterior iliac spine, the lower costal margin and the clavicle, and the result is documented as the lowest bony point at which the vibrating fork was appreciated. It is readily apparent that a tuning fork applied to one side of the sternum will produce a transmitted impulse which will be perceived on the other side. If unilateral total sensory loss of non-organic origin is suspected, the patient's failure to detect the tuning fork placed to one side of the midline of the sternum is strong evidence of a non-organic sensory deficit. The same applies to claimed loss of vibration sense over one half of the skull.

Joint Position Sense

Joint position sense testing can be quickly performed and is a very reliable test of dorsal column function.

Correct technique is important. The terminal interphalangeal joint of either the finger or the toe being tested should be held at the sides and the tip of the digit in the same way. It is wrong to hold the tip of the digit by the nail and pulp. This provides a push–pull stimulus and will give a clue as to the direction of movement. If the finger or toe is held at the sides, only the movement of the joint can be detected (see Fig. 8.1). It is helpful to show the patient what is required with their eyes open before proceeding to formal testing with the eyes closed or averted. Very small movements over a range of 2–3 mm should be detectable at the fingers and larger movements of 3–5 mm at the toes. With severe impairment even movements of the wrist and ankle joints may not be detected.

Testing Posture Sense in the Presence of Spastic Weakness

Testing posture sense in a spastic limb can present special problems. It is obviously important to look for coexistent sensory deficit, especially in spinal cord lesions. Even in the normal situation some information about the position of a joint in space is gained by the patient from stimulation of the muscle and tendon stretch receptors around the joint, particularly at the extremes of movement. If the hand or foot is spastic, movement against the pull of the spastic muscle may be sensed by its stretch receptors and movement away from the pull will not be perceived. The clue to this situation will be that movements will only be detected in one direction. In the hand only extension movements of the fingers will be detected, and in the foot only dorsiflexion will be perceived and movement in the opposite direction will be missed.

Testing for a Sensory Level

The detection of a sensory level is critical in indicating the level of a spinal cord lesion.

Only light touch and pinprick appreciation can be tested inch by inch up the body and are the modalities normally used when looking for a sensory level. When sensation is only mildly impaired it may be very difficult to distinguish a genuine level from a physiological difference in sensation. Those physiological areas of suddenly increased sensitivity, which may falsely suggest a sensory level, are indicated in Figure 13.8. These can readily be experienced by self-testing. The marked sensitivity across the inguinal ligament, just below the breasts and just above the clavicle, is very striking. A comparison with the normal dermatomes at those levels is shown in Figure 13.9. By the time a sensory level is complete, where there is a transition from total loss of sensation to normal sensation, irreversible damage may have been sustained.

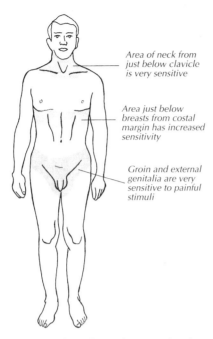

13.8 Physiological sensory levels.

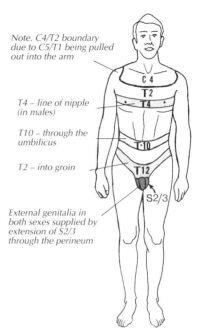

13.9 Normal dermatomes.

Deciding when a minor transition from mild sensory impairment to normality is abnormal requires considerable experience. This is a situation where routinely testing the appreciation of pinprick sensation up the trunk of every patient will condition the examiner to appreciate these normal variations and lessen the likelihood of missing a significant abnormality when it is encountered.

Brown–Séquard Syndrome

This is a classic neurological syndrome which is very rarely seen in a pure form, and is the consequence of hemisection of the spinal cord. It is appropriate to consider it here, both as an anatomical exercise in localization and as an object lesson in knowing what other physical signs to look for when confronted by a patient who cannot understand why they have a weak right leg which feels otherwise perfectly normal and cannot feel pain or temperature in the perfectly functioning left leg. Incomplete forms of the syndrome are extremely common and are usually the result of compression of the spinal cord. It is likely that it is impaired venous drainage of one half of the cord that produces the clinical picture, with sparing of the dorsal columns which have a separate vascular supply. Therefore, the main feature of the incomplete syndrome is that dorsal column sensation is spared, so that it is more accurately described as an anterior half hemisection of the cord (Fig. 13.10).

The resulting clinical picture consists of a spastic weak leg with brisk reflexes and an extensor plantar response and, because the lateral spinothalamic tract

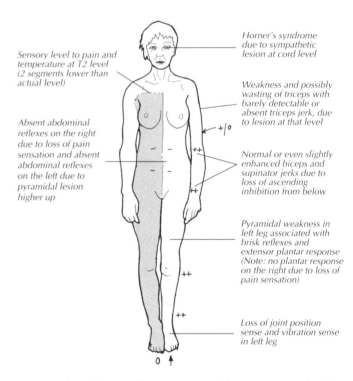

13.10 Clinical signs of Brown–Sequard lesion (at C7–8 level on left side).

on that side is conveying information from the opposite leg, loss of pain and temperature sensation in the opposite leg will be detected. This will extend up to a level which may be two or three segments below the level of the lesion. If the dorsal column on the same side **is** actually affected, which is very rare, the patient will be found to have impaired joint position sense in the weak leg. The commonest causes of the syndrome are cord compression due to degenerative spine disease or multiple sclerosis. As a unique example of a pure lesion the following case is of interest.

CASE REPORT IV

*A 38-year-old man was referred for further evaluation of a long-standing Brown–Séquard syndrome. Five years previously he had been involved in a fight and had been stabbed in the neck from behind. The knife had broken off after penetrating through the spinal canal into the body of the vertebra. The neurosurgeons involved at the time had decided that the risk of attempted removal carried greater hazard than leaving it in situ. The patient had all the features of **complete** hemisection of the spinal cord at C4 level, including even a Horner's syndrome on the affected side, which had been achieved with almost surgical precision by this injury.*

The correct application and interpretation of all the techniques discussed in this chapter will be amplified in the subsequent chapters and their correct use in arriving at an accurate clinical diagnosis will then be appreciated.

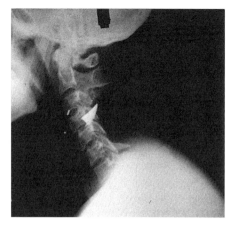

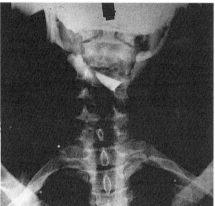

CRIV. *Knife broken off in vertebra.*

14. Metabolic, Infective and Vascular Disorders of the Spinal Cord

The discussion of spinal cord disease in many textbooks centres around classic conditions such as tabes dorsalis and subacute combined degeneration of the cord. These conditions are now so rare that to base a whole chapter on them would be misleading. In this chapter the disorders of the spinal cord will be considered in relationship to their clinical importance. In spite of the uncertainty as to its cause, the rather poorly understood condition of progressive cervical myelopathy remains an important condition, which in many instances is associated with cervical spondylosis. Cord lesions related to fracture dislocations of the spine are covered in Chapter 23.

Progressive Cervical Myelopathy

This condition may be encountered in either sex, usually between the ages of 30 and 70. It remains a negative diagnosis where all investigations have failed to demonstrate any specific alternative pathology. The clinical picture is suggestive of mild spinal cord compression, and owing to the age range in which it occurs, coexistent degenerative spondylosis of the cervical spine is to be anticipated. The advent of MRI scanning has made it easier to exclude spinal cord compression of severe degree, but the role of lesser degrees of canal encroachment due to disc degeneration remains to be established, particularly considering the highly mobile nature of the neck, where the possibility of dynamic cord stretching across osteophytes on neck flexion and compression from behind by the ligamentum flavum on head extension may play a role, and a dynamic rather than static lesion of the spinal cord may be the cause.

It was previously suspected that many of these cases were due to late-onset multiple sclerosis, and CSF taken during myelography would occasionally provide support for this diagnosis. Nowadays, in those patients where no convincing cord compression has been demonstrated, the MRI scan of the spinal cord may reveal a possible inflammatory lesion and a scan to demonstrate MS white matter lesions in the brain and, possibly, CSF examination may be necessary. The age range in which this condition occurs makes even MRI scanning of the brain difficult to interpret as in this older group white matter lesions thought to be of vascular origin may mimic the appearances of multiple sclerosis and lead to incorrect diagnosis. There is no doubt that MRI scanning has certainly supported the long-held view that many cases of progressive cervical myelopathy were actually cases of MS in an older than anticipated age group.

Typically the patient's presenting symptoms consist of a mild to moderate spastic paraparesis. This may have evolved over several years and may initially have been attributed to age alone. It is only when the patient discovers that they cannot hurry for a bus, or starts to trip or fall, that they seek advice. In most instances there are no sensory symptoms and bladder function is unimpaired. The signs are often confined to the motor system; all reflexes are brisk and both plantar responses are extensor. The weakness is of pyramidal type but is confined to the legs. Weakness of the arms is a late and relatively minor problem. In patients over 60 years old, physiological impairment of vibration sense to the knees may be an additional feature and is often the only sensory finding.

There is no doubt that severe cervical spondylosis can cause this clinical picture, and in any patient with severe changes on MRI scan the condition should correctly be called spondylotic myelopathy; decompression by anterior discectomy may be indicated and is often beneficial. The previous operative approach utilizing posterior decompression by multilevel laminectomy was relatively unsuccessful, perhaps because of the fact that major compressing lesions lie anterior and the cord is stretched across the spondylotic bars. The mechanism and management of spondylotic myelopathy is discussed in greater detail in Chapter 15.

Motor neuron disease may occasionally present as a pure upper motor neuron lesion of relatively slow progression, and cause diagnostic difficulty until other features appear. This is discussed later in the chapter.

This diagnosis should always be borne in mind when there is no convincing evidence to support any other specific diagnosis responsible for a pure spastic paraparesis.

It would seem wise to follow any patient who has been diagnosed as having progressive cervical myelopathy by exclusion and to reinvestigate if significant deterioration occurs. If anything, modern investigational techniques have made the exact status and cause of this condition even more obscure.

There is no convincing evidence that the use of a cervical collar has any beneficial effect in these patients, and in many instances the added discomfort seems to make them less able to cope with the problems presented by the paraparesis. Full investigation by myelography, or preferably MRI scanning if available, should always be performed for reasons exemplified by the following case reports.

CASE REPORT I

A 53-year-old man developed a slowly progressive paraparesis over 2 years. There were no signs to indicate damage to the nervous system outside the spinal cord. His plain cervical spine X-rays were normal and myelography was performed with considerable reluctance on the part of the radiologist because the plain films were normal. Complete spinal block at C7 was demonstrated, which proved to be due to a neurofibroma. Surgery cured all his symptoms.

CASE REPORT II

A 58-year-old woman had been observed in the neurology clinic for nearly 3 years as a case of cervical spondylosis with myelopathy. On routine review it was felt that the spondylosis was relatively mild as judged from the plain X-rays, and that the signs were those of a spastic tetraparesis with fine lateral nystagmus and a very brisk jaw jerk, suggestive of a very high cord compression – higher than is normally the case in degenerative cervical spinal disease. Myelography was therefore performed and a meningioma in the foramen magnum was demonstrated.

These cases have historical significance as they show the considerable reluctance of clinicians to embark on myelography in the days when this was the only definitive investigation. However skilled the clinician, there were no clinical features that allowed confident exclusion of spinal cord compression to be made on clinical grounds alone. During this time it became obvious that normal cervical spine X-rays were perhaps one of the strongest indications for myelography, as they did not provide an adequate explanation for the patient's symptoms. Myelography was therefore mandatory, even if the result led to the rather unsatisfactory diagnostic label of progressive cervical myelopathy. MRI scanning, with its brilliant ability to demonstrate the cervical anatomy in both sagittal and transverse planes, has transformed the investigation

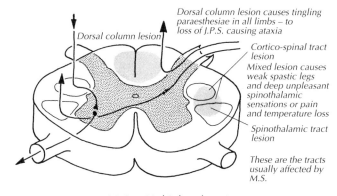

14.1   Multiple sclerosis.

and management of many of these patients, but myelography to exclude cord compression should still be used in such cases where MRI is still not available.

Multiple Sclerosis (Fig. 14.1)

Multiple sclerosis is the major cause of spinal cord disease in Europe and North America. As with progressive cervical myelopathy, the clinical picture may be indistinguishable from spinal cord compression and before the advent of MRI scanning usually required myelography to exclude this possibility. This was always a difficult decision to take, because there is little doubt that myelography occasionally led to an acute deterioration in patients who actually had multiple sclerosis. The reverse situation is equally unfortunate. On one occasion in the same ward of a neurological hospital there were three young female patients with paraplegias and severe bed sores. None had had myelography because a confident clinical diagnosis of multiple sclerosis had been made. All three had subsequently been shown to have operable compressive spinal cord lesions, which were unfortunately irreversible by the time they were eventually demonstrated. In the 1970s the arrival of visually evoked responses and CSF immunoglobulin assays appeared to offer alternative methods of investigation and a way of avoiding myelography. Unfortunately, this proved not to be completely foolproof.

CASE REPORT III

A 28-year-old woman presented with a 2-year history of mildly progressive difficulty in walking, which proved to be due to a mixture of a mild spastic paraparesis and ataxia, a combination strongly suggesting a diagnosis of multiple sclerosis in this age range. However, there were no cerebellar signs or evidence of visual pathway lesions and the ataxia seemed to be due to mild impairment of joint position sense. She was admitted for myelography, but on admission mild nystagmus was found and a simple CSF examination was substituted for the intended myelogram. This revealed an ele-

vated CSF protein but no diagnostic immunoglobulins were identified. She appeared to respond to a 10-day course of ACTH (adrenocorticotrophic hormone) injections. She was kept under outpatient review and no deterioration was observed until her husband's transfer to another part of the country, when she would have been lost to follow-up. Continuing diagnostic unease prompted direct referral to the neurologist at her new location. A few months later sudden deterioration led to a myelogram being performed which revealed a meningioma at C2 level which was successfully removed.

It is possible that the nystagmus observed was due to distortion of the upper cervical cord, which is a rare but recognized diagnostic trap.

There are three main patterns of clinical presentation of cord lesions in multiple sclerosis. In order of ascending severity these are the 'neuropathic' type, subacute cord compression type and acute transverse myelitis.

'Neuropathic' Type

In this type sensory symptoms predominate and consist of fine, tingling peripheral paraesthesiae. These may be spontaneous or provoked by touch. They are similar to the symptoms occurring at the onset of a peripheral neuropathy. Sensory loss is minimal and the patient may complain that there is no actual numbness, but that the tingle seems to 'blot out' normal sensation. When touched by the examiner the patient often has difficulty in describing exactly what is abnormal about the sensation. They may say that they can feel but it feels as if there is a layer of cotton wool between the touch and the skin. The tingling symptoms will usually be confined to the distal arms and legs and do not involve the area around the mouth. This is an important differential diagnostic point when the differential diagnosis between multiple sclerosis of this type and the symptoms of hyperventilation are being considered.

This type of presentation is frequently associated with L'hermitte's phenomenon (sometimes known in the USA as the 'barber's chair' sign). This consists of a slight exaggeration of the existing tingling, a sudden sensation as if an electric shock had been passed into all four limbs, or a sensation as if the spinal column were being plucked 'like a violin string' when the neck is flexed. This symptom is undoubtedly most often seen in multiple sclerosis, but can occur with any compressive or inflammatory lesion affecting the cervical cord. Occasionally these symptoms will be associated with other evidence of minimal cord damage, such as micturition disturbance or stiffness of the legs, but the clinical picture is often exclusively sensory.

The clue to the diagnosis is often to be found in the reflexes. Patients who have peripheral sensations of this type due to peripheral neuropathy will have decreased or absent reflexes and usually well-marked

peripheral sensory loss. In multiple sclerosis the reflexes are not only preserved but are almost invariably extremely brisk, the abdominal reflexes may be absent and the plantar responses may well be extensor, even in those patients without definite motor symptoms. If there is any sensory deficit it may amount to no more than loss of vibration sense to the level of the costal margins.

Hyperventilation syndrome is the most important differential diagnosis. This occurs in anxious patients and produces extremely variable tingling paraesthesiae in all four limbs. These symptoms may be present for minutes only and then clear completely, occurring many times in the day – behaviour quite unlike the paraesthesiae of multiple sclerosis. These patients also usually notice tingling and numbness around the mouth. Because of anxiety, the reflexes may be quite brisk but pathological reflexes will not be found. Unfortunately, these symptoms frequently occur in patients who have read about multiple sclerosis in the popular press. They then become very anxious and promptly develop these symptoms, reinforcing their own view that they have this disorder. It can be almost impossible to reassure them that they do not, and they spend the rest of their lives waiting for something else to happen and seem positively incensed that so many doctors seem unable to confirm their self-made diagnosis. Many find solace in the self-made diagnosis of ME syndrome (myalgic encephalomyelitis), a diagnosis that is usually made by the patient looking up a list of symptoms in a leaflet.

The prognosis for multiple sclerosis of this 'neuropathic' type is very good, and although the symptoms may continue for months they usually remit without sequelae although motor signs, if present, tend to persist. This is very much a feature of young patients with multiple sclerosis in the 18–30 age group, and often heralds the onset of the disease, but many patients never develop any other manifestations.

Subacute Cord Compression Type

This mode of onset is very similar to progressive cervical myelopathy and it is highly likely that some cases of this condition are actually a variant of multiple sclerosis, occurring in an older age group. This can now be confirmed in many instances by MRI scanning.

Some patients with a history of previous attacks of the disease and clear evidence of multiple sclerosis in other areas of the central nervous system develop a slowly progressive spastic paraparesis, manifest as stiffness affecting one or both legs over a period of months or years. There may be no new sensory symptoms and the picture becomes essentially an asymmetrical progressive spastic paraparesis. This is very commonly the way patients with long-standing MS ultimately become disabled, and nearly all patients in a wheelchair relate this type of history.

The possibility of making a serious diagnostic error is at its greatest in this slightly older age group, where compressive lesions are more likely. Because of the age range there is also the problem of coexistent degenerative cervical disc disease, which may play a role, and the decision to treat the coexistent disc lesion surgically is difficult when there is also clear evidence of inflammatory spinal cord disease.

CASE REPORTS IV

A 43-year-old man was admitted for investigation of a 9-month history of tingling, numbness and clumsiness in both hands, pins and needles in the left leg and a band of tingling and burning around the right costal margin on neck flexion and a sensation as if his trousers were wet. VERs, BAERs, CSF IgG and myelogram were all negative. Several years previously he had been admitted to a hospital elsewhere with a band of chest pain which was initially thought to be angina, which was not confirmed. There were some similarities with the present chest pain. A diagnosis of transverse myelitis was made and he was given a 10-day course of ACTH injections with no improvement. Six months later he had a further episode where the left arm and leg both became clumsy and the discomfort on neck flexion had recurred.

A diagnosis of multiple sclerosis seemed certain but an MRI scan of the brain was normal. The MRI scan of the neck showed not only a high signal in the C3/4 segment of the cord but also severe degenerative changes at C4/5 and C5/6, which were compressing the spinal cord. He is still under observation, as even with the most modern technology the role played by the spondylotic changes in his ongoing symptoms is hard to quantify, and there is concern that surgery might aggravate the unequivocal demyelinating lesion in the cord.

In complete contrast, as an example of the occasional benign behaviour of demyelinating disease of this type over many years, the following case may be cited.

CASE REPORT V

A 58-year-old former nurse complained of tingling, numbness and heaviness of the left leg for 6 weeks. She denied any other significant previous illness. Examination revealed spinothalamic sensory disturbance affecting the entire left leg and brisk reflexes in both legs, with a left extensor plantar response. There was slight pyramidal weakness of the left leg. While dressing she asked whether the following symptom had any significance. She had first noticed it at the age of 18, when she started nursing, and it had been present continuously for 40 years. Whenever she flexed her neck she developed a fine tingling in all four limbs clearly indicating L'hermitte's sign. Further questioning confirmed that there had been no other episodes of neurological dysfunction over that entire period. MRI scanning revealed not only an inflammatory lesion in the cervical cord, but also extensive white matter lesions throughout both hemispheres. By the time the scans had been performed her symptoms had cleared, leaving her with only mild pyramidal deficit in the left leg.

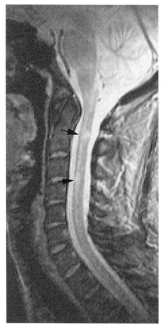

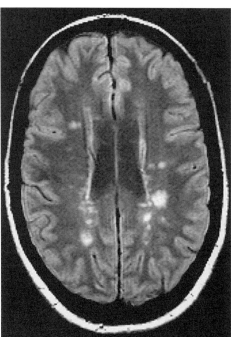

CRV. *Multiple sclerosis presenting at 58 years of age with a 40-year history of L'hermitte phenomenon.*

There can be no doubt that this is an example of multiple sclerosis at its most benign.

Spinal cord lesions in MS tend to be symmetrical, although the symptoms experienced by the patient are often more marked on one side, to the extent that a Brown–Séquard syndrome can occur with spinal cord demyelination. It is also a feature of MS that the symptoms can be aggravated by a rise in body temperature, a finding often exaggerated if the temperature rise is due to strenuous exercise. This is known as Uhtoff's phenomenon. The following case is a good example of both these features.

CASE REPORT VI

A 36-year-old Greek Cypriot male related that 4 months previously, after playing energetic squash, he developed a sensation as if a nail had been hammered up through his left heel. This subsided but was replaced by a sensation as if he had pulled his calf muscle very severely. A few days later, while using a scythe in his left hand, he noticed that his left arm was incoordinated and heavy. Two months later, after swimming in warm sea, he sat down heavily on the sand and developed a sensation as if a nail had been hammered in alongside the left anal margin and up his spine to mid-thoracic region. He had a sickening dull ache between the shoulder blades and in the subsequent weeks developed an ongoing sensation as if a tight elastic band were stretched between his left upper thorax and the sole of his left foot. The whole left side below the mid-thorax felt extremely unpleasant if lightly touched, in striking contrast to the inner feeling that the area was numb. Hot and cold water in the shower produced extremely unpleasant exaggerated temperature effects. On physical examination there was loss of pain and temperature sensation to T2/3 level on the left. A pin dragged on the left leg or trunk felt as if the flesh were being laid open with a scalpel. There was no dorsal column sensory deficit, the reflexes were symmetrical and brisk and the right plantar response was extensor. A compressive cord lesion was suspected because of the rarity of demyelinating disease in patients from the Mediterranean area. An MRI scan revealed an intrinsic inflammatory lesion in the right side of the cord at C5/6 level, correlating perfectly with his partial Brown–Séquard lesion. No specific treatment was attempted and the symptoms subsided. When reviewed 2 years later he had made a complete recovery, with the exception of short-lived recurrent symptoms when he exercised in the heat in Cyprus.

Acute Transverse Myelitis

This presentation is in every way the most difficult to diagnose and the most serious presentation of spinal cord demyelination. The clinical picture is identical to acute cord transection, as a result of either spinal trauma, tumour or a vascular lesion of the spinal cord. The onset may occur over 2 or 3 days or be almost instantaneous. It usually occurs at mid-thoracic cord level, which can produce a band of pain around the chest which mimics intrathoracic or cardiac disease, and myocardial infarction is often suspected before the onset of weakness.

The acute onset is marked by flaccid paralysis of the lower limbs, with retention of urine and a sensory level which is usually an accurate guide to the level of the lesion. If the onset is less acute a rising sensory level may cause confusion until progression stops, often at a level very much higher than indicated at the onset. This is of particular concern where a compressive lesion has to be distinguished because delaying the diagnosis until the sensory level is established may permit irreversible cord damage to occur. If the condition occurs in a setting of known multiple sclerosis the diagnosis may be secure on clinical grounds, but if it is the first

episode immediate further investigation is necessary. Even the advent of MRI scanning has not provided complete protection against misdiagnosis.

CASE REPORT VII

A 53-year-old woman from New Zealand, where she had lived until 3 years previously, was admitted with a 24-hour history of a rapidly evolving flaccid paraplegia with retention of urine and a sensory level to T10. There was no past history of any illness. She had been under a great deal of stress because her husband had recently had a malignant melanoma removed from his shoulder, and the dangers of this lesion were well known in the Antipodes. The clinical picture suggested transverse myelitis and an MRI scan was obtained with great difficulty (this was in 1987). The scan obtained 10 days after her admission showed findings consistent with a inflammatory lesion of the spinal cord at T8 level. There was no expansion of the spinal cord. All other investigations were normal. No recovery occurred. She and her husband were due to return to New Zealand and she left hospital, her clinical condition unaltered after some 3 months. A few weeks after her return to New Zealand she suddenly deteriorated and became anaemic and jaundiced, with evidence of severe liver damage. Investigation demonstrated metastatic malignant melanoma in the liver. At post mortem the spinal cord lesion was found to be a melanoma metastasis within the spinal cord itself. The primary melanoma was not found.

The specific association of an attack of acute transverse myelitis with bilateral retrobulbar neuritis is known as Devic's disease. The onset may be simultaneous or both lesions can occur in either order, several months apart. The prognosis for recovery for both the retrobulbar neuritis and the transverse myelitis is good and, by definition, no other manifestations of MS should appear. It is a rare condition and is said to be more frequent in children and patients of Asian descent. If other manifestations appear later, it is probably incorrect to use this diagnostic label but knowledge of this association can occasionally be of diagnostic value.

CASE REPORT VIII

A 56-year-old man was referred via the ophthalmology department with asymmetrical bilateral visual failure and optic atrophy which was acute in onset but then slowly progressive. VERs had revealed marked slowing in the optic nerves and MRI scanning had shown no evidence of a compressive lesion or cerebral demyelinating disease. No improvement was seen following intravenous methylprednisolone, but his vision did improve marginally over the next 9 months. He then returned with a 4-day history of stiffness and weakness in both legs, difficulty in initiating micturition and numbness of the legs and trunk. A rather indefinite sensory level at upper thoracic level was demonstrated, both plantar responses were extensor and there was mild bilateral pyramidal deficit. In view of his previous poor response to methylprednisolone this was withheld, and over the next 6 weeks his new symptoms recovered completely. There was no change in his visual difficulties during this time. An MRI scan of the spinal

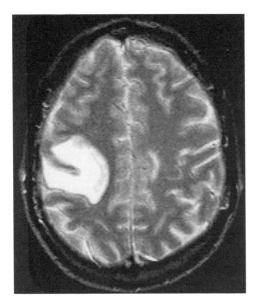

CRVIII.   *Multiple sclerosis – cerebral lesion.*

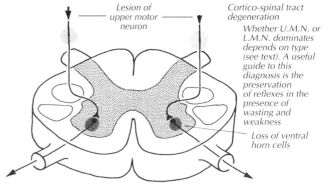

14.2   Motor neuron disease.

cord did not detect an inflammatory lesion but a tentative diagnosis of Devic's disease seemed justified on the evidence available. Nine months later he developed an acute left hemiparesis with sensory deficit and hemianopic field defect. The diagnosis of a cerebral vascular accident in the absence of the previous history would have been inescapable, but the possibility of acute cerebral demyelination required consideration. An MRI scan revealed extensive confluent white matter lesions with normal architecture of the overlying cortex in the right parietal region. No treatment was given and an almost complete recovery occurred over the next 6 weeks.

The diagnosis of multiple sclerosis seems inescapable with an extraordinary combination of unusual features, each typical in their behaviour of demyelinating disease, with an acute onset, dramatic physical signs and complete recovery over a period of 6 weeks, the only exception being the visual disturbance, which can remain severe particularly in patients who present with acute bilateral retrobulbar neuritis. MRI scanning is not infallible in the diagnosis of demyelinating lesions and failed to demonstrate two of the three specific lesions in this patient.

Motor Neuron Disease (Fig. 14.2; see also Fig. 19.2)

Motor neuron disease can produce a variety of clinical pictures as it is a process which affects both the ventral horn cells and the upper motor neuron. Some patients may have overwhelming evidence of a lower motor neuron lesion, while others develop a purely upper motor neuron picture with a spastic paraparesis simulating cord compression. These variants are also discussed in Chapter 19.

The classic variant, amyotrophic lateral sclerosis, consists of a combination of both upper and lower motor neuron lesions.

In a classic case the hands are affected first, with progressive wasting and weakness, and then a mild spastic paraparesis develops insidiously in the legs. This may closely simulate the findings of cervical spondylosis, and as this is also a disease of the older age group the coexistence of cervical spondylosis often presents diagnostic problems. In some cases associated lumbar spondylosis may further confuse the clinical features by producing lower motor neuron findings in the legs. Where sensory phenomena such as root pain in the arms or legs are a major feature, the diagnosis of spondylosis should present little difficulty, but extensive painless, spondylotic change can produce a picture almost indistinguishable from motor neuron disease, especially if the cervical cord compression is sufficient to produce additional upper motor neuron signs.

The single most important clue to spondylotic upper limb wasting is the **loss** of reflexes. Motor root lesions will produce wasting, weakness and fasciculation, but the reflex arcs are also interrupted. If wasting and weakness are due to ventral horn cell disease, the reflex arc is not disrupted and the simultaneous upper motor neuron lesion will enhance the reflexes. **The hallmark of motor neuron disease is wasting and weakness in the presence of preserved or brisk reflexes**. It should also be noted that fasciculation, the flickering movements visible in a denervated wasted muscle, will be seen with **any** disease process that damages the lower motor neuron. As a solitary finding it is not diagnostic of motor neuron disease. If the entire musculature of the arm or all the shoulder girdle muscles are seen to be fasciculating, it is highly likely that motor neuron disease is the cause, but very localized fasciculation in the distribution of one peripheral nerve or one nerve root is not necessarily indicative of motor neuron disease.

At the onset of motor neuron disease, remarkably localized weakness may appear and violate this rule. For example, in the leg, wasting and weakness of the anterior compartment may simulate an L5 root lesion or peroneal nerve lesion, and only the development of identical changes and progressive involvement of other. muscle groups will indicate the correct diagnosis. Similarly, wasting and weakness of the intrinsic muscles of one hand may simulate an ulnar nerve or T1 root lesion, until more widespread changes occur.

CASE REPORTS IX

A 45-year-old airline pilot presented with progressive weakness of the right leg. Two years previously he had torn his right gastrocnemius and the leg had remained slightly weak ever since. Over 4 months he had developed wasting and weakness of the right thigh and his wife had noticed wasting of the right buttock. This had not responded to extensive physiotherapy. There were no other symptoms and there had been no pain. His mother had died of bulbar motor neuron disease at 65 years of age. On examination there was wasting of the glutei, quadriceps, adductors and hamstrings of the right leg. The knee jerk was slightly depressed but all other responses were normal. EMG studies revealed chronic partial denervation in all the affected muscles. An MRI scan of the lower spinal canal showed striking wasting of the retroperitoneal psoas muscle. He was informed of the diagnosis of motor neuron disease, which rapidly progressed. He had to give up flying almost immediately and within 18 months was breathing purely with the accessory muscles of respiration. He was admitted for 3 days to familiarize himself with the hospital ward to which he would be admitted for terminal care, but suddenly collapsed and died of a pulmonary embolism just before his intended discharge.

This is a good example of a remarkably localized initial presentation in an atypical area and also of the familial nature of this disorder, which is found in some 5% of patients. The malevolence of the condition in this case was surprising, as patients whose symptoms start in the legs as a lower motor neuron lesion usually have a rather better long-term prognosis.

The diagnosis of motor neuron disease is a death sentence for the patient and every effort should be made to exclude alternative diagnoses, sometimes to the extent that an incorrect diagnosis may be made until the evidence becomes overwhelming. The following are examples of the type of problems encountered.

CASE REPORT X

A 73-year-old woman was referred by her cardiologist with weakness of the pincer movements of the left hand over 12 weeks. At first sight this appeared to be an anterior interosseous nerve lesion, but there was wasting and weakness of the intrinsic muscles of the hand and a suspicion of weakness in other forearm muscles. The reflexes in the left arm were intact and the left leg was normal. Nerve conduction studies showed no evidence of conduction delay in the

anterior interosseous nerve, and EMG studies showed evidence of chronic partial denervation in the intrinsic hand muscles and other forearm groups. A diagnosis of motor neuron disease was made. She sought a second opinion and because of the asymmetry of involvement a negative myelogram was performed without complication. She continued to deteriorate and 6 months later started to have unexplained falls, even though the only new findings in the left leg were brisk reflexes and an extensor plantar response. A CT scan revealed an extensive right hemisphere glioma. Biopsy revealed only a very oedematous brain with abnormal astrocytes in several areas. Over the next 3 months, until her death from the glioma, more extensive evidence of motor neuron disease appeared which included lower motor neuron involvement of both legs.

This is another example of a very localized presentation, and even though the electrophysiological evidence was overwhelming, others were sufficiently impressed by the localized nature of the lesion to perform a myelogram. Careful follow-up detected early upper motor neuron signs on the same side, which at first mimicked progressive motor neuron disease, but the degree of disability seemed in excess of the physical evidence, justifying a CT scan which revealed the otherwise asymptomatic cerebral tumour.

CASE REPORT XI

A 56-year-old spinster who had devoted her life to caring for her mother, who had severe multiple sclerosis, presented with a mild spastic paraparesis, 3 months after her 80-year-old mother's death. There were no ocular or sensory symptoms and the signs consisted of generally brisk reflexes, mild spastic weakness of both legs and extensor plantar responses. An MRI scan of the brain and spinal cord were normal. This was surprising, as the likelihood that this was familial multiple sclerosis seemed high. She went for a second opinion and was not seen again for 10 months. In that time further scans were normal but the diagnosis of demyelinating disease was accepted. When next seen, she was barely able to walk and had developed dramatic atrophy of the intrinsic muscles of both hands, and re-examination revealed generalized muscle atrophy with widespread fasciculation and a severe spastic tetraparesis. She was bedbound within 2 months. The electrophysiological evidence at that stage confirmed motor neuron disease. She died of her disease 3 years after the onset.

CASE REPORT XII

A 21-year-old man developed very severe pain across the right shoulder 2 days after sitting fishing all day in cold wet weather. A few days later he became aware of weakness of the right shoulder. He had suffered mild flu-like symptoms during that time. On examination, within days of the onset, there was surprisingly extensive wasting and weakness of the entire right shoulder musculature, in muscles innervated by three separate cervical roots. The pain had cleared. Neuralgic amyotrophy (brachial neuritis) seemed to be the obvious diagnosis but very brisk reflexes throughout the right arm, including a clonic finger jerk, caused concern. Over the next 3 months, the development of further wasting and weakness throughout the right arm and the appearance of similar findings developing in the same sequence in the left arm, left no doubt that the diagnosis was motor neuron disease. He died 11 months after the onset.

These cases demonstrate the problems caused by localized presentations of the illness and the ease with which other diagnostic possibilities may be suspected and even seem to be confirmed. The feature that emerges throughout is the reliability of reflex enhancement, in the presence of localized wasting and weakness, as a diagnostic physical sign.

In the absence of any specific treatment, failure to make an immediate correct diagnosis does not disadvantage the patient. It is essential to be sure of the diagnosis before revealing it to the patient and their relatives. Reluctance to make a dogmatic diagnosis may be misinterpreted as being due to clinical uncertainty or incompetence, so it is advisable to suggest a second opinion the moment that the diagnosis is certain, to avoid misunderstanding and recriminations later if the relatives incorrectly assume that the diagnostic delay worked to the patient's disadvantage.

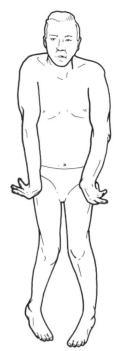

14.3 Posture in spastic tetraparesis. Note inversion of forearms, flexion of wrist and extension of fingers; flexion at hip and knee, adduction of hip; plantar flexion and inversion of feet.

Familial Spastic Paraplegia

This is a relatively rare condition which is inherited either as a dominant or a recessive gene. The recessive variety tends to have an earlier onset (7–10 years of age) and runs a more severe course, whereas the dominant type often starts after the age of 20 and has a benign course. Even those cases that start in childhood tend to have a slower course if they are inherited in a dominant way.

The disease is progressive and starts with increasing stiffness in the legs; arm involvement is late and relatively minor. Significant bladder involvement is very unusual until very late in the course of the disease, and if present would be strong evidence against this diagnosis. Furthermore, although called a 'paraplegia' in fact 'spastic' is the dominant feature. The patient's power is often near normal but it is the gross spasticity of the extensor groups that is so disabling. Not only are the legs rigid, adducted and plantar flexed, but the active muscles have to overcome the spasticity in order to move the limbs, hence the very peculiar dragging type of gait, the patient often appearing to be about to topple forwards as he drags one leg past the other (Fig. 14.3).

The reflexes are very brisk but in some patients the spasticity is so great that they cannot be elicited at all because the muscles are already maximally contracted, and they are then incorrectly documented as being absent. The plantar responses are strongly

extensor and the big toe may wear a hole in the top of the patient's shoe, due to its permanently extended position even at rest. The abdominal reflexes are usually preserved and this, coupled with normal bladder function, is an almost certain indication that a spastic paraplegia is of familial type. Sensory loss may occur but is usually a late feature and consists of modest vibration and joint position sense loss. Relatively few patients become confined to a wheelchair until late in life, and most are able to cope with surprisingly severe disabilities and hold down a job or run normal households for the bulk of their lives.

In recent years a number of variants of this condition have been described, with additional features including amyotrophy, optic atrophy, athetosis, chorea, sensory neuropathy and mental changes. They are all very rare disorders.

Friedreich's Ataxia (Fig. 14.4)

Friedreich's ataxia is included in this section as, although many of the clinical findings are due to degeneration of the peripheral nerves and brainstem pathways, atrophy of the spinocerebellar pathways is the major component of the condition. The disease is familial and usually inherited as a recessive with an incidence of 1:100 000. In a given family the age of onset is usually constant and ranges from 8 to 16 years of age.

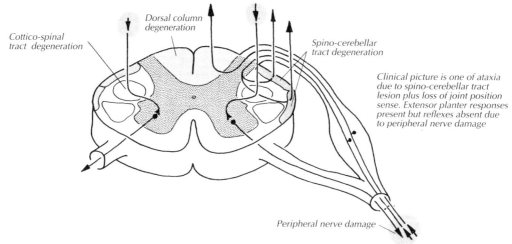

14.4   Friedreich's ataxia.

The clinical picture may be extremely variable, but is usually similar for each family. In childhood a high arched foot with hammer toes may be found; this is known as 'Friedreich's foot', and may also be found in family members who do not develop the full-blown picture, which is then regarded as 'forme fruste' of the disease. A scoliosis developing in childhood may be another forerunner of the disease and any child with the combination of a scoliosis and a high arched foot should be regarded as a candidate for the later development of any of the spinocerebellar disorders.

The cerebellar component of the illness produces cerebellar dysarthria and ataxia, although nystagmus is uncommon. Some 20% of patients develop diabetes mellitus. ECG abnormalities are common and may be an important diagnostic early feature in uncertain cases. Inverted T waves and evidence of left ventricular hypertrophy are the usual findings.

The other lesion that dominates the physical signs is the degeneration of peripheral nerves and a total absence of reflexes (areflexia) is a constant finding. The plantar responses are usually extensor, owing to damage to the corticospinal pathways, but the reflexes are unable to become brisk as they are abolished by the peripheral nerve damage. This condition is one of several that can cause this combination of absent reflexes and extensor plantar responses. The others are noted below. Because the onset is insidious and the condition is inherited recessively, the clinical picture may be surprisingly fully developed by the time the patient seeks advice.

CASE REPORT XIII

A 29-year-old woman was worried that she had multiple sclerosis. For years she had been aware of progressive slurring of speech, particularly when fatigued, progressive clumsiness and difficulty walking in a straight line. She denied any family history but related that her youngest sister had recently been referred to an ENT surgeon for a disorder of balance. On

examination she had staccato slurred speech and an extremely ataxic gait, having to hold on to the wall. On formal testing the left side was more ataxic than the right. There was no optic atrophy or nystagmus. The arm reflexes were absent, the knee jerks could just be elicited, the ankle jerks were absent and both plantar responses were extensor. She had a striking thoracic scoliosis convex to the left but perfectly normal feet. Nerve conduction studies revealed prolonged distal latencies and small delayed sensory action potentials. An MRI scan of the cerebellum and cervical spinal cord was normal and the ECG showed changes consistent with Friedreich's ataxia Her sister has refused to be examined.

Sub acute Combined Degeneration of the Spinal Cord (Fig. 14.5)

This is a classic disease, a metabolic disorder of the spinal cord due to vitamin B_{12} deficiency. It was a frequent complication of pernicious anaemia before effective treatment with raw liver or vitamin B_{12} became available. In recent years it has become a rare condition owing to earlier recognition and treatment of pernicious anaemia, but patients may present with the neurological syndrome and it is always important to consider this possibility in the differential diagnosis of patients with spinal cord lesions. It has also been shown that some 25% of patients who have CNS damage due to vitamin B_{12} deficiency do not have haematological abnormalities. A serum vitamin B_{12} estimation is justified if the clinical picture is suspicious.

Vitamin B_{12} deficiency can complicate total gastrectomy, blind loop syndrome, infestation with fish tapeworm (*Diphyllobothrium latum*) and Crohn's disease, which damages the region of the small bowel where B_{12} is normally absorbed. Strict vegetarians (vegans) may also develop serious B_{12} and other nutritional deficiencies.

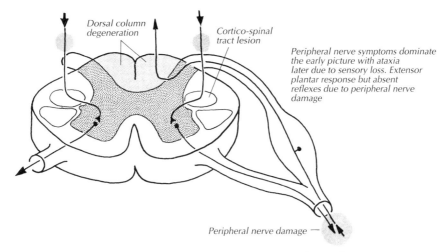

14.5 Sub-acute combined degeneration of the cord.

The earliest symptoms and signs are related to damage to the peripheral nerves, rather than the spinal cord. Non-stop tingling peripheral paraesthesiae are often the first manifestation, and is the symptom most likely to respond to vitamin B_{12} therapy. Areflexia is the major motor finding and is also due to the peripheral nerve damage.

The first evidence of the underlying spinal cord lesion is the detection of extensor plantar responses. As in Friedreich's ataxia, the development of the full picture of an upper motor neuron lesion is prevented by the pre-existing peripheral nerve damage. In a full-blown case subsequent degeneration of the corticospinal tract and dorsal columns leads to paraplegia, in addition to the peripheral weakness and very severe ataxia due to loss of joint position sense. There is also considerable micturition difficulty owing to loss of awareness of bladder filling, and painless retention of urine occurs. The bladder problems are discussed further in Chapter 15.

A mild dementing type of illness and optic atrophy are other less common presenting symptoms of vitamin B_{12} deficiency, and serum B_{12} estimation should be part of the routine investigations in both dementia and progressive visual impairment.

Unfortunately, the spinal cord damage is not significantly benefited by vitamin B_{12} therapy and may be made dramatically worse if folic acid is given instead of B_{12}. Early diagnosis is therefore essential before significant cord damage has occurred, and vitamin B_{12} studies should be performed routinely in patients with persistent peripheral paraesthesiae and **absent** reflexes. If the reflexes are intact it is extremely unlikely that the paraesthesiae are due to any form of neuropathy.

This is another condition in which absent reflexes are found in association with extensor plantar responses. Folate deficiency may produce a similar clinical picture but whether it can cause similar spinal cord damage is disputed.

Tabes Dorsalis (Fig. 14.6)

This classic neurological disorder has virtually vanished owing to better epidemiological control and effective

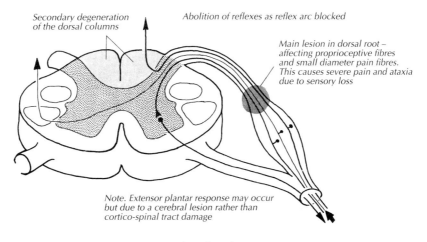

14.6 Tabes dorsalis.

treatment of syphilis. The exact relationship of the disease to the syphilitic process has never been clearly established, although it is undoubted. Spirochaetes were never demonstrated in the dorsal roots or dorsal columns and typically the disorder occurred some 10 or 20 years after the primary infection, at a time when all other evidence suggested that the disease was 'burnt out'. The serological tests in the blood were often negative before more specific testing for treponemal antibodies became available.

Progressive meningeal fibrosis enveloping and damaging the spinal roots was thought to be the basic pathology, producing secondary damage to the dorsal columns. The pain fibres seemed to be particularly vulnerable and damage to these fibres was probably the cause of the classic 'lightning' pains of this disorder, which were described as excruciating 'electric shock' – like sensations, which could occur in the limbs, rectum, stomach or throat, culminating in what were known as tabetic crises. Later, loss of deep pain sensation occurred and the classic finding was that the patient's Achilles tendon or testis could be squeezed hard without discomfort. As the root damage continued the reflex arc became blocked, leading to areflexia and hypotonicity of the muscles. The combination of extreme hypotonicity, allowing an excessive range of joint movement, coupled with loss of deep pain sensation, led to the progressive joint destruction known as 'Charcot's joints' (described in Chapter 13). They may also occur in patients with hereditary insensitivity to pain and syringomyelia.

In the later stages of the disease severe secondary degeneration of the dorsal columns caused total loss of joint position sense. Patients then complained that they could only hear their feet hitting the ground and felt as if they were walking on cotton wool. A high-stepping gait was the result, with the feet slapping the ground. This characteristic gait would now only be seen in patients with Dejerine–Sottas disease (hypertrophic polyneuritis), Charcot–Marie–Tooth disease (H.M.S.N. I and II) or recovering Guillain–Barré syndrome. This problem, caused by severe loss of joint position sense, is greatly accentuated in the dark or with the eyes closed, and is the basis of one of the classic tests in neurology.

Romberg's test   Patients standing with their eyes closed sway slightly. This has the effect of increasing the sensory input to the cerebellum. In cerebellar disease this swaying is greatly accentuated and the patient may swing wildly from side to side, but will not fall. In the presence of gross posture sense loss, while standing with the eyes open the patient is perfectly stable, but the moment they shut their eyes they will fall because the cerebellum is suddenly deprived of all sensory input. Romberg's test is therefore more a test of dorsal column disease than cerebellar disease. A posi-

tive test (the patient falls over when his eyes are closed) is known as Rombergism. The test has been adapted to vestibular function testing and its alternative use is fully discussed in Chapter 8.

Patients with tabes dorsalis usually had evidence of disease elsewhere in the CNS. Nearly all had Argyll Robertson pupils and many had optic atrophy with peripheral visual field loss. Damage to the upper motor neuron produced extensor plantar responses, the combination of signs known as taboparesis. This is another cause of extensor plantar responses with absent reflexes.

The condition has been included in some detail as it may well make an unwelcome return to the diagnostic scene, as the incidence of syphilis is again increasing and there is uncertain evidence that effective treatment inevitably prevents this particular complication, although the current rarity of the condition would suggest that it does.

AIDS and the Spinal Cord

Encephalopathy and myelopathy commonly coexist in patients with AIDS. The myelopathy may be the first evidence of the disorder and produces a spastic paraplegia, often combined with evidence of a peripheral neuropathy which modifies the physical findings so that combinations of pyramidal weakness, peripheral paraesthesiae, absent reflexes and extensor plantar responses may be found. The brunt of the pathological change occurs in the posterolateral columns, producing an ataxic component, the end result being a clinical picture with remarkable similarity to subacute combined degeneration of the spinal cord. Appropriate investigations for this disorder now have to be regarded as part of the investigational battery in appropriate patients with progressive spinal cord lesions of this type.

Tropical Spastic Paraparesis

For many years a form of subacute or chronic progressive spastic paraparesis was identified in patients of Afro-Asian origin. The picture is similar to multiple sclerosis, a condition that is extremely rare in these ethnic groups. When first identified, efforts to find a neurotoxic compound that could be responsible for the condition were unsuccessful and it is only since the identification of the retroviruses that the condition has been identified as being due to HTLV-1 infection. The changes seen on MRI are similar to those of multiple sclerosis. Some cases, particularly those of acute onset, reportedly respond to the use of steroids. It is an obvious differential diagnostic consideration in a patient of appropriate ethnic origin with evidence of a spinal cord lesion.

Radiation Myelopathy

This is a subject of considerable importance. It is a complication of radiation to the cervical thoracic and lumbar regions where the spinal cord inevitably lies in the centre of the radiation field. It may be secondary to radiation treatment of carcinoma of the larynx, palliative radiotherapy for carcinoma of the bronchus or oesophagus, and in the routine treatment protocol for Hodgkin's disease. In some of these conditions the prolonged survival of the patient greatly increases the chance of such damage becoming apparent. It typically occurs some 9–18 months following treatment, although onset as early as 1–2 months or as late as 24 months has been reported. Spinothalamic sensory symptoms dominate the acute clinical picture in many instances. The patient may notice coldness and numbness of the legs on both sides and then the rapid development of stiffness and weakness in both legs. The sensory symptoms tend to be more severe than the motor difficulties, which is the reverse of what would be anticipated were the new symptoms due to spinal cord compression, which is the major differential diagnosis. MRI scanning has made the exclusion of this other diagnostic possibility relatively simple. The condition may arrest after several weeks' progression and may produce modest disability, or can be slowly relentlessly progressive, producing severe disability if the patient's survival is prolonged.

A relatively recently recognized variant has been identified in very long-term survivors of radiation to the para-aortic lymph nodes in the treatment of malignant seminoma of the testicle. The condition is very hard to distinguish from motor neuron disease of the progressive muscle atrophy type. Wasting, weakness and fasciculation in the affected muscles is the dominant feature. All muscles supplied by the lumbar and sacral motor neurons are involved, producing slowly progressive damage over several years. Sensory findings are modest and this feature makes it difficult to see why this should be regarded as a fibrotic process in the retroperitoneal tissues. There are no upper motor neuron findings. The reflexes are not enhanced and may disappear under observation. This is a major differential diagnostic feature. The condition may be due to radiation damage to the ventral horn cells in the lumbar enlargement of the spinal cord. It is likely that more cases of this condition will be seen because of the excellent survival rate following treatment.

CASE REPORT XIV

A 46-year-old man presented with painful cramp in the left calf, which was noted to be wasting. He had had a malignant teratoma of the testes 14 years previously and had had post-operative radiotherapy to the para-aortic lymph nodes. Physical examination revealed weakness and wasting in the

L4, L5 and S1 root distribution, more on the left than the right. All reflexes were depressed and the plantar responses were flexor. There was uncertain sensory alteration to pinprick from L1 downwards. He had a normal myelogram and EMG studies showed evidence of chronic partial denervation in L4, L5 and S1 root distribution. The possibility of radiation myelopathy was considered. He has been kept under yearly review for 10 years and has developed progressive symmetrical weakness and wasting of all groups previously affected, but no significant sensory loss, sphincter disturbance or involvement of other neural structures has developed.

This clinical picture is similar to other reported cases and seems to represent a specific complication of radiation to the lumbar sacral spinal cord.

Spinal Cord Compression

Spinal cord compression may be caused by lesions arising on the nerve roots, the coverings of the spinal cord, in the extradural fat or from lesions of the vertebral column itself. At this stage, we will consider only the features of the history and the clinical signs which suggest that the patient is suffering from spinal cord compression.

The clinical feature of early cord compression that must be stressed is that the symptoms and signs are dominated by motor pathway damage. The reasons for this are not entirely clear, but may be related to the blood supply of the spinal cord and in particular to the venous drainage. This is discussed in more detail later in this chapter, but basically any impairment of venous drainage will tend to lead to oedema and poor capillary circulation in the watershed zone of the spinal cord, an area which includes the corticospinal pathways.

The earliest symptoms are those of a mild spastic paraparesis. The patient may complain of slight dragging of the feet and heaviness of the legs, as described in the previous chapter. These symptoms may develop over a period of months in some instances, or in a matter of hours in the case of acute lesions, and occasionally instantaneously. Impending irreversible cord damage is indicated by either the onset of micturition disturbance or sensory symptoms. Difficulty in initiating micturition or urinary retention may occur quite suddenly, and usually indicates that rapidly progressive deterioration is about to occur.

Sensory symptoms have a similar significance and may start as a tingling sensation in the soles of the feet, which then ascends. This may reach a fixed level in a matter of hours or advance slowly over several days. In either event it is unwise to delay action until the level becomes static, typically two to three segments below level of the compression.

In summary therefore, spinal cord compression is dominated in the early stages by motor symptoms and signs and the onset of sensory features heralds a phase of rapid deterioration leading to irreversible cord damage. The clinical sequence and signs at the various stages are summarized in Figure 14.7. To give some idea of the range of presentations of spinal cord compression, three examples are included below.

Note: Although sensory loss is shown developing in anatomical sequence, it must be stressed that in most cases the motor signs dominate the early clinical picture, and the evolution of these sensory signs may be very rapid when motor deficit is already well established.

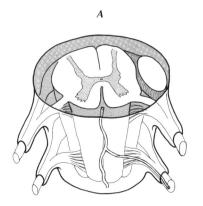

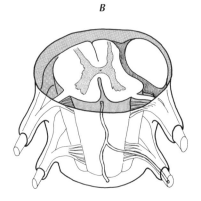

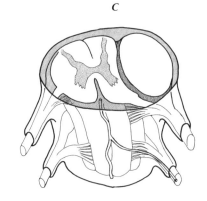

A	B	C

A neurofibroma on the left T9 dorsal root is shown. The root is irritated, causing root pain at T9

The cord is now seriously distorted and definite sensory loss may be detected in the root zone and in the opposite spinothalamic distribution

The terminal stage of cord compression has been reached.
Total paralysis of the legs.

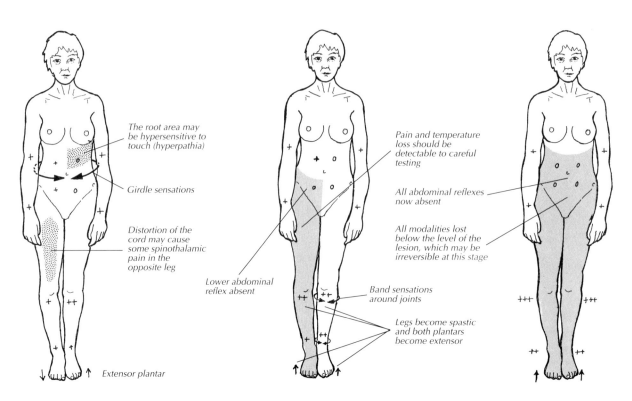

The root area may be hypersensitive to touch (hyperpathia)

Girdle sensations

Distortion of the cord may cause some spinothalamic pain in the opposite leg

Extensor plantar

Pain and temperature loss should be detectable to careful testing

All abdominal reflexes now absent

All modalities lost below the level of the lesion, which may be irreversible at this stage

Lower abdominal reflex absent

Band sensations around joints

Legs become spastic and both plantars become extensor

Root pain may be worse on coughing
Tight band or cold bands around abdomen noticed

Root area now numb. Band sensations occur in legs

Final stage: may be acute after long stages A and B or can go from A to C over a matter of hours

14.7   Evolution of spinal cord compression.

CASE REPORT XV

A 50-year-old coal miner who was a heavy smoker became paraplegic at a funfair. He was asymptomatic prior to the event. He had elected to try his strength by attempting to ring a bell by hitting a block with a heavy wooden mallet. As he swung the mallet down with all his strength, he shouted out and fell to the ground, paralysed from the waist down. When seen in A and E 30 minutes later, he had a flaccid paraplegia and a sensory level to T9. A lateral thoracic spine X-ray showed a total collapse of T7 vertebra and a chest film revealed a large asymptomatic carcinoma of the lung.

CASE REPORT XVI

A 60-year-old woman presented with an 8-month history of pain in the neck radiating down the inner aspect of the left arm and associated with some wasting of the intrinsic muscles of the left hand. Her admission was prompted by increasing stiffness of the legs over 3 or 4 weeks and increasing discomfort in her arm. On examination both arms were areflexic, with a combination of both radicular and pyramidal weakness in the lower cervical segments. The reflexes were brisk in both legs and the left plantar response was extensor. Pain sensation was impaired from C5 to T8. Plain X-rays revealed loss of the left pedicle of T1 vertebra and myelography revealed a complete block at T1 due to an extramedullary tumour. Spinal cord decompression was achieved and histology revealed a plasmacytoma. Further investigation confirmed myelomatosis. Subsequent subluxation was eventually treated by excision of the bodies of C7, T1 and T2 and replacement by an iliac crest bone graft. Within 6 weeks of this second operation the patient was able to walk with two sticks. During the next year several opportunistic bacterial infections and herpes zoster blighted her survival, and she died of the myeloma some 18 months after presentation.

CASE REPORT XVII

A 36-year-old bank manager was referred for a course of steroid injections after a diagnosis of spinal cord demyelination following a vaccination procedure had been made after a reportedly normal myelogram performed in a hospital in Scotland. He had been vaccinated 3 months previously, 1 month before travelling to Singapore. About 4 weeks after the vaccination his legs became progressively weaker and he developed a cold sensation in his feet. He also became impotent. There had been no back pain or sphincter disturbance and on his return he drove himself to Scotland for New Year. On New Year's Day, he realized that he had become numb from the chest down and that his legs were very stiff and rapidly becoming weaker. A sensory level at T7/8 was documented at the hospital but a myelogram reportedly revealed no abnormality. Although CSF and visual evoked responses were normal a diagnosis of multiple sclerosis was made. He was allowed to return home after 2 weeks, during which his symptoms progressed. Examination at that time, 8 weeks after the onset, revealed no abnormality in the cranial nerves or arms. The abdominal reflexes were absent and both legs were so spastic that passive movement at the hip and knee was almost impossible. The reflexes were very brisk and the

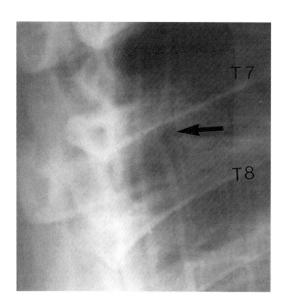

CRXVII. *Metrizimide myelogram showing mid-thoracic disc lesion with cord compression*

plantars extensor. The sensory findings were unusual. Vibration sense was completely intact, posture sense was slightly impaired in the right leg, but pain and temperature were severely impaired to T7 bilaterally. It was felt that the history and clinical signs were atypical and that an intrinsic cord tumour required exclusion. He was admitted for repeat myelography. The initial myelogram was thought to be normal but a CT scan at T7/8 was suspicious, and a repeat myelogram the next day confirmed unequivocal cord compression by a degenerate disc at that level. This was successfully removed via a costotransversectomy, with a very rapid improvement in his clinical condition. On review, 6 years following surgery, apart from slight impairment of cold appreciation in the left leg and a left extensor plantar response, there were no demonstrable abnormalities. He had resumed playing squash and golf.

These three cases demonstrate acute, subacute and chronic cord compression and its varied presentations. The third case emphasizes the considerable problems of myelography in demonstrating mid-thoracic lesions, and failure to detect this lesion would undoubtedly have resulted in eventual paraplegia. The sensory findings were those of a central cord lesion rather than the more typical effects of extrinsic compression, and only dogged persistence eventually led to the correct diagnosis. It is a very brave patient who agrees to a third myelogram 48 hours after his second, and diagnostic conviction was required by the neurologist to inflict this on the patient.

Spinal Epidural Abscess

It is appropriate to consider this rare condition at this point because of the overlap between the symptoms of a cord-compressive and an intrinsic spinal cord lesion.

Epidural infections are extremely rare and are usually haematogenous in origin. Over 30% of recorded cases occur following non-penetrative trauma to the spinal column. Some are complications of medical conditions such as diabetes, subacute bacterial endocarditis and septicaemia, and the risk is higher in immunocompromised patients. Epidural abscess is very rarely the result of direct infection such as surgical trauma, epidural anaesthesia or a lumbar puncture. The organism is nearly always *Staphylococcus aureus*. The commonest location is on the dorsal aspect of the thoracic spinal cord, where the loose attachment of the dura permits rapid spread of infection.

The pathological basis of the cord damage is an admixture of direct compression by the mass effect and secondary infarction due to thrombophlebitis of the local venous channels. This leads to a complex combination of signs of both cord compression and intrinsic spinal cord disease and, allied to the rarity of the condition, accurate diagnosis is almost impossible. The most frequently suspected clinical diagnosis is transverse myelitis. Only in those patients where there is a clear infection risk would this condition immediately enter into the differential diagnosis.

Myelography may merely indicate an extradural lesion but the CSF obtained at the procedure may point to an infective process, although organisms are unlikely to be identified and the CSF findings are not those of meningitis. An MRI scan indicating the extent and location of the lesion is the only way to make a definitive diagnosis. The combination of great rarity and atypical clinical presentation makes this a diagnostic minefield, and over half the reported cases were incorrectly diagnosed until surgical exposure revealed the diagnosis.

Intrinsic Lesions of the Spinal Cord

The clinical history and signs of an intrinsic lesion in the spinal cord are usually quite the reverse of cord compression. The anatomical feature that determines the sequence of events is the course of the pain and temperature pathways in the central spinal cord. These are the fibres most likely to be damaged in the early stages. A lesion in the central spinal cord (ependymoma, glioma or syringomyelic cavity) will irritate and destroy pain and temperature fibres as they cross the cord, but only at the level of the lesion in the early stages.

Little or no long tract damage may occur at this stage, so that a narrow segment of pain and temperature loss is produced. The pain is of deep spinothalamic type, but the sensory loss may not be detected unless pain sensation is carefully tested. Occasionally, a patient accidentally discovers the sensory loss when they drop a lighted cigarette on the skin or notice an area of impaired temperature sensation while bathing in warm water. Later, as the lesion extends laterally, the reflex arc is blocked and the segmental reflexes disappear. This rarely produces any motor symptoms, but any patient with spinothalamic symptoms should be carefully checked for loss of reflexes. Reflex loss applies only to lesions affecting the standard reflex arcs in the arms and the legs, and of course the abdominal reflexes which are also segmental. Although the provoked muscle contraction will be fairly generalized to the upper or lower quadrants of the abdominal wall, the provoking stimulus can be very accurately applied to specific dermatomes from T8 down to T12, and it is occasionally possible to accurately identify the afflicted nerve root by the abolition of the abdominal reflex when stroking the skin of the appropriate dermatome.

In the cervical spinal cord the sympathetic pathways may be affected at this stage, producing a unilateral or bilateral Horner's syndrome. If the lesion extends into the anterior horn cells focal wasting and weakness may occur, typically affecting the intrinsic muscles of the hand. The location of these new signs will depend on the site of the lesion. If the lesion is in the mid-thoracic cord it is very unlikely that the patient will notice wasting and weakness of individual intercostal muscles, although this should certainly be looked for in a patient with spinothalamic symptoms localized to the thoracic region. This may be detected by noting indrawing of the intercostal space when the patient takes a deep breath. If abdominal segments are affected, the patient may develop a bulge around the abdomen like a 'spare tyre' in the affected myotome.

It is only when the cord becomes markedly expanded that the long tracts become involved. This may take several years to develop, even when the underlying cause is an intrinsic tumour of the spinal cord. The average time from first symptom to diagnosis of intrinsic spinal cord tumours is 3–4 years. Bilateral pyramidal signs then appear, with brisk reflexes in the legs and extensor plantar responses. The inner part of the spinothalamic tract may be damaged, causing descending spinothalamic sensory loss. In the final stages of the process only the peripheral fibres carrying sensation from the sacral area will survive and the patient develops what is known as sacral sparing, a rare but diagnostic feature of an intrinsic lesion of the spinal cord. The dorsal columns seem very resistant to infiltration or distortion by tumours, and in general dorsal column signs are a late feature of intrinsic lesions. The sequence and anatomical correlation of the signs at various stages are illustrated in Figure 14.8.

14.8 Evolution of central cord lesion.

This picture would be seen in syringomyelia, ependymoma, and intrinsic glioma or astrocytoma. The progress of the signs relates directly to degree of involvement shown in the cord sections

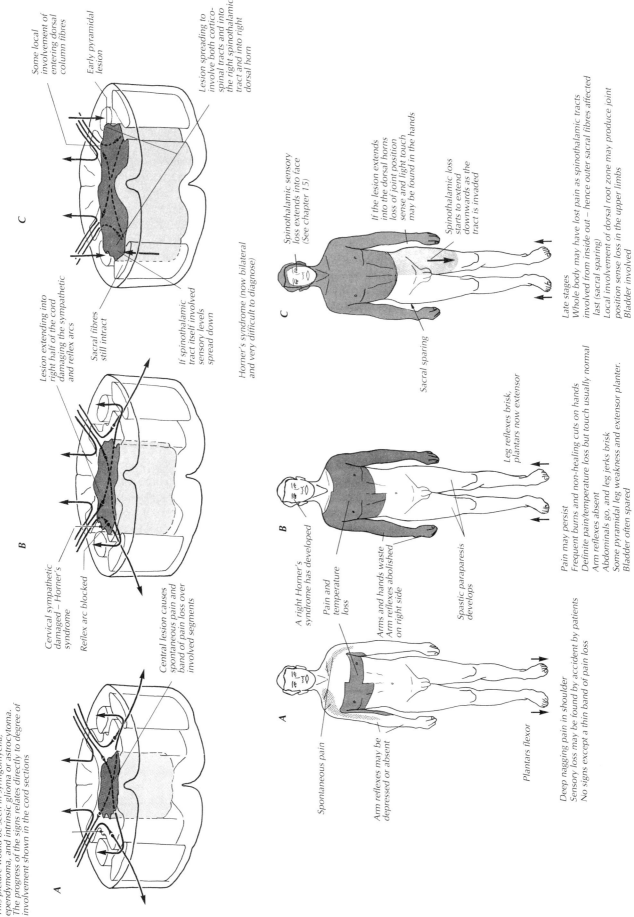

Some local involvement of entering dorsal column fibres

Early pyramidal lesion

Lesion spreading to involve both cortico-spinal tracts and into the right spinothalamic tract and into right dorsal horn

Lesion extending into right half of the cord damaging the sympathetic and reflex arcs

Sacral fibres still intact

If spinothalamic tract itself involved sensory levels spread down

Cervical sympathetic damaged – Horner's syndrome

Reflex arc blocked

Central lesion causes spontaneous pain and band of pain loss over involved segments

C

B

A

Spinothalamic sensory loss extends into face (See chapter 15)

If the lesion extends into the dorsal horns loss of joint position sense and light touch may be found in the hands

Spinothalamic loss starts to extend downwards as the tract is invaded

Horner's syndrome (now bilateral and very difficult to diagnose)

Sacral sparing

C

A right Horner's syndrome has developed

Pain and temperature loss

Arms and hands waste Arm reflexes abolished on right side

Spastic paraparesis develops

Leg reflexes brisk, plantars now extensor

B

Spontaneous pain

Arm reflexes may be depressed or absent

Plantars flexor

A

Deep nagging pain in shoulder
Sensory loss may be found by accident by patients
No signs except a thin band of pain loss

Pain may persist
Frequent burns and non-healing cuts on hands
Definite pain/temperature loss but touch usually normal
Arm reflexes absent
Abdominals go, and leg jerks brisk
Some pyramidal leg weakness and extensor planter.
Bladder often spared

Late stages
Whole body may have lost pain as spinothalamic tracts involved from inside out – hence outer sacral fibres affected last (sacral sparing)
Local involvement of dorsal root zone may produce joint position sense loss in the upper limbs
Bladder involved

CASE REPORT XVIII

A 44-year-old woman gave a history of numbness in the left thigh over 18 months. The leg felt heavy and weak but was not painful on walking, but when resting there was an extremely unpleasant, deep discomfort in the leg and unpleasant aching round the left costal margin. She was said to have had a slipped disc at the age of 14, which had been treated with bed rest. Physical examination revealed no abnormality although the reflexes were extremely brisk in all four limbs, probably due to anxiety as the plantar responses were flexor. Motor power testing was difficult because of severe pain in the left leg, which was worse on movement, but power was thought to be normal. There was variable impairment of pinprick sensation from just above the left knee to just below the left costal margin. Temperature sensation and proprioception were normal but vibration sense was lost, to the costal margins. A myelogram revealed a large intramedullary defect from T7 to T12. A CT scan confirmed expansion of the spinal cord over those segments. At operation a partially cystic lesion was resected which proved to be a myxoid spinal ependymoma. Ten years later she walks with a stick, but unfortunately still has considerable central pain which is refractory to all treatment.

CASE REPORT XIX

A 14-year-old girl was referred for a neurological opinion before the insertion of Harrington rods for increasing scoliosis that had developed over the previous 5 years. She was otherwise asymptomatic. On physical examination the only unequivocal findings were bilateral extensor plantar responses. There was no motor or sensory deficit. Cord tethering was suspected and she was admitted for myelography. When the contrast was inserted it was arrested at L2 vertebral level by a 'sausage-like' expansion of the terminal cord. Further contrast was inserted at cervical level and the normal cervical spinal cord suddenly expanded to a similar shape at T3 level. CT scanning confirmed an intramedullary lesion extending from T3 to the conus, the expanded cord totally occupying the spinal canal. During a lengthy neurosurgical procedure a 12" long ependymoma was removed from the cord through a dorsal rhizotomy and multiple laminectomies. On recovery she had a flaccid paraplegia. She subsequently required Harrington rods for the combination of scoliosis and kyphosis due to the laminectomies, and remains wheelchair bound 9 years later.

These cases will at first sight appear atypical, given the foregoing discussion which detailed the typical progression of the symptoms of an intrinsic lesion of the spinal cord. Fortunately, intrinsic lesions are relatively rare and gliomas and astrocytomas which do produce the more typical findings are extremely rare. These two cases are included to emphasize several important points. Provided the development is slow, the lesion may reach massive size with minimal physical evidence of its presence. The first case emphasizes the central pain syndrome that could easily have defied diagnosis for several years, had its nature not been immediately identified, because the physical findings were minimal. The second case again emphasizes the potential sinister significance of scoliosis as a marker of underlying neurological disease, and how a high index of suspicion in the absence of very dramatic clinical findings is still a major requirement in neurological practice.

The Blood Supply of the Spinal Cord
(Figs 14.9 and 14.10)

The spinal cord is not supplied by segmental arteries or by a continuous vessel running down its length. There is a fairly constant territorial distribution of blood supply in the transverse plane. The central area is supplied by the sulcal arteries, which are given off alternately from each side of the anterior spinal artery which lies in the ventral sulcus of the cord. The anterior spinal artery also gives off circumferential arteries which lie on the surface of the cord, forming a surface plexus by anastomosing with branches of the posterior spinal arteries and supplying the periphery of the cord.

The paired posterior spinal arteries form a plexus over the dorsal columns, which they supply. The posterior spinal arteries are less clearly defined than the anterior spinal artery, although even the latter vessel is often incomplete and may end at lower dorsal cord levels and reappear below as a new vessel. Although these small vessels are affected by microvascular disease processes such as syphilis, diabetes, arteritis, epidural infection, subacute bacterial endocarditis, poly-

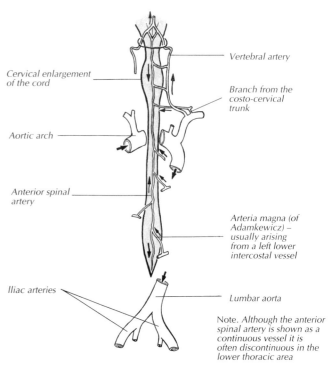

14.9   Blood supply of the spinal cord.

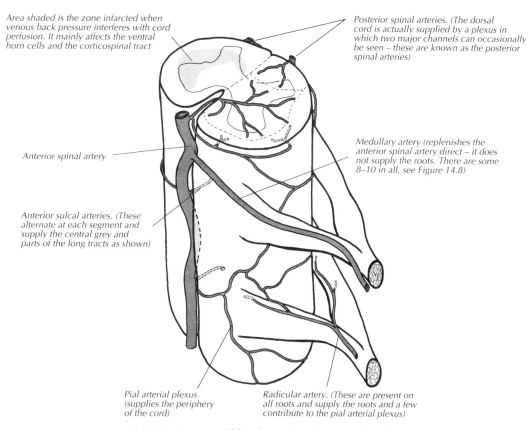

Area shaded is the zone infarcted when venous back pressure interferes with cord perfusion. It mainly affects the ventral horn cells and the corticospinal tract

Posterior spinal arteries. (The dorsal cord is actually supplied by a plexus in which two major channels can occasionally be seen – these are known as the posterior spinal arteries)

Anterior spinal artery

Medullary artery (replenishes the anterior spinal artery direct – it does not supply the roots. There are some 8–10 in all, see Figure 14.8)

Anterior sulcal arteries. (These alternate at each segment and supply the central grey and parts of the long tracts as shown)

Pial arterial plexus (supplies the periphery of the cord)

Radicular artery. (These are present on all roots and supply the roots and a few contribute to the pial arterial plexus)

14.10   Segmental blood supply to the spinal cord.

arteritis nodosa and arteriosclerosis, clinical disorders of the cord circulation are usually due to disease in the feeder vessels which replenish the artery at various points along its course.

The anterior spinal artery arises from the vertebral arteries in the foramen magnum as two vessels that join to become a single vessel opposite the odontoid peg. It is replenished by a fairly constant vessel which enters the canal on the C3 or C4 root and comes off the left thyrocervical trunk, which may be damaged in surgical procedures in the neck. This upper part of the vessel supplies the cord down to about T4

The thoracic spinal cord segment of the artery is replenished by a variable branch from one of the intercostal arteries, usually at T5 or T6. This vessel is vulnerable in operations through the bed of the sixth rib, such as intrathoracic hiatus hernia repair. The main feeder vessel is the arteria magna of Adamkewicz. This arises from the left T10, T11 or T12 intercostal artery in 75% of the population. This critical vessel is also easily damaged during thoracic operations through the left side of the chest, lumbar sympathectomy, left nephrectomy, splenectomy, adrenalectomy and intercostal nerve blocks. In any of these procedures damage to the vessel may cause infarction of the thoracic spinal cord, usually up to T3/4 level, which is the upper extent of this feeder supply.

The lower spinal cord and the nerve roots of the cauda equina are supplied by a variable vessel entering the canal on one of the upper lumbar roots. Damage due to occlusion of this vessel is rare, but impaired vascular supply to the lumbar spinal cord and nerve roots is responsible for the condition known as claudication of the cauda equina.

Vascular Syndromes

The surgical causes of vascular cord disease have been indicated above. Medical causes are dominated by atheromatous changes in the feeder vessels and, in particular, disease of the vertebral arteries occluding the origin of the anterior spinal artery, which causes infarction of the central medulla and upper cervical cord, producing a flaccid tetraparesis (see Chapter 11).

At any cord level, diabetes mellitus, meningovascular syphilis, any thrombotic haematological disease, hyperviscosity syndromes, embolic phenomena (subacute bacterial endocarditis, atrial fibrillation, myocardial infarction), dissecting aneurysm of the aorta, intravascular air bubbles in decompression sickness, microangiopathies and sickle-cell disease are all notable causes of feeder vessel occlusion.

When the arteria magna is occluded by any of these processes, the ultimate level of the lesion is usually found at T4–T6. The entire anterior half of the spinal cord is infarcted, producing an acute flaccid paraplegia with retention of urine and spinothalamic sensory loss to the level of the lesion, but often with complete preservation of touch and joint position sense. The onset of acute infarction is usually accompanied by severe localized pain in the back.

The lumbar feeder vessel may be involved in the syndrome of 'intermittent claudication of the cauda equina' which occurs in patients with congenitally narrowed lumbar canals or patients with severe multilevel degenerative lumbar disc disease causing canal stenosis, but rarely seems to produce a primary occlusive picture with infarction of the lumbar cord.

Claudication of the Cauda Equina

This important and common condition is characterized by the onset of severe pain, numbness and weakness in one or both legs during exercise, which brings the patient to a stop. This typically occurs after walking only 50–100 yards and the recovery time is as brief as 20–30 seconds, although the patient will usually have to sit down to recover: standing still may not suffice. The patient can then walk another 50–100 yards before being brought to a stop again. This must be distinguished from the Leriche syndrome, which is due to claudication of the gluteal muscles owing to severe arterial disease at the aortic bifurcation. In this condition it is the buttock muscles that cramp and hurt, and the recovery time is much longer.

Claudication of a Lumbar Nerve Root

A modification of this syndrome is seen when a single nerve root is trapped by a degenerate disc. Instead of ongoing root pain and numbness, the patient only develops root symptoms when walking and if the L5 root is involved may develop a transient foot drop, which rapidly recovers when they stop walking. If the S1 root is affected pain and tingling in the calf and weakness of plantar flexion has to be distinguished from intermittent claudication of the calf itself. The location of the pain and weakness may mimic S1 root claudication but the longer recovery time should make the distinction relatively straightforward.

Both these 'vascular' conditions are usually encountered in patients who give a long history of recurrent attacks of backache and root pain which have been called 'lumbago' and 'sciatica' and have been successfully managed conservatively. It is now well recognized that even when large permanent disc prolapses have occurred the patient may recover fully from the acute attack and enjoy long asymptomatic periods, but in the future it is possible that MRI and the increasing use of microdiscectomy may not only give more effective relief

from the acute symptoms but may also prevent the later development of these claudicating complications when the patient is much older and at greater risk from surgical complications.

Posterior spinal artery occlusion is less likely to produce classic signs as the vessel is part of a plexus and does not have a constant territory to supply.

The effects of spinal cord compression are initially due to vascular factors and it seems likely that impaired venous drainage leads to back pressure and capillary stasis. This will be maximal in the watershed areas of the central cord indicated in Figure 14.10. This would also account for the fact that signs of corticospinal tract damage dominate the early findings in cord compression.

There are some other rare, but interesting vascular lesions that may affect the spinal cord:

1. Spinal cord angiomas, usually found in the lower mid-dorsal segment of the cord, may cause repeated attacks of paraparesis with severe back pain. An associated angioma in the skin of the back may be found on careful examination.

CASE REPORT XX

A 59-year-old man was referred for investigation of incontinence of urine, loss of bowel control and impotence of 6 years' duration. The urinary incontinence had become worse following prostatic surgery. He was known to have hereditary haemorrhagic telangiectasia. He had been aware of numbness of his right foot for many years, which had previously been attributed to a lumbar disc lesion. In the last 2 years both hands had tingled and occasionally became numb, and although left-handed he found he was increasingly forced to use his right hand. His biggest embarrassment was that he could quite suddenly, in mid-stride, be incontinent of both urine and faeces without any warning. He denied any symptoms referrable to the cervical spine. On physical examination there was dramatic facial evidence of telangiectasia. In the upper limbs there was a marked enhancement of reflexes in the right arm but no wasting or weakness. Two-point discrimination in both hands was markedly impaired. His abdominal reflexes were absent, the knee jerks were very brisk, the ankle jerks were absent and both plantars were extensor. Vibration and joint position sense were markedly impaired and the right leg was ataxic on formal testing. Myelography was not without incident: when tipped head-down he had a massive epistaxis but insisted that the procedure continue. The myelogram revealed massive tortuous blood vessels starting at T3. Because of the severe epistaxis the procedure was abandoned at that stage and a spinal angiogram, performed later, revealed a massive arteriovenous malformation filling at T1/2 level. At operation the lesion was found to be an intramedullary high-flow malformation and the enlarged vessels were venous. A limited procedure was performed, giving considerable improvement in his walking and continence. The patient was reluctant to consider a more aggressive procedure. He remains well 10 years later. The full extent of his lesion can be seen on recently obtained MRI scans.

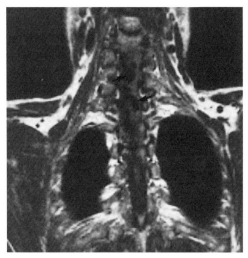

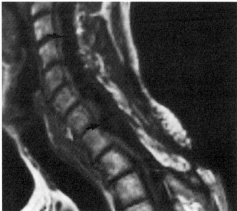

CRXX. *MRI demonstrating massive intramedullary and dural arteriovenous malformation of cervical spinal cord (vessels show as black flow voids on MRI scans).*

This case is included for several reasons. It is not only an excellent example of the late presentation of a congenital lesion but is notable for the very long history of sphincter disturbance with relatively modest evidence of spinal cord damage. It is unlikely that there is any connection between his telangiectasia and the presence of the spinal arteriovenous malformation.

2. Telangiectasia of the spinal cord may cause spontaneous haemorrhage into the substance of the spinal cord or spinal subarachnoid haemorrhage with cord compression.

3. Coarctation of the aorta is sometimes associated with massive enlargement of the mid-thoracic feeder vessel, which may be large enough to compress the spinal cord.

4. Haemangioblastomas of the cord are dense vascular tumours usually found in the upper dorsal cord, often continuous with a syringomyelic cavity. They are

usually found in patients with retinal and cerebellar haemangioblastomas (Von Hippel–Lindau disease).

5. Vertebral haemangiomas are vascular malformations of the vertebral body or arch. They may cause vertebral collapse or produce an extradural mass due to gross thickening of the vertebral arch. The differential diagnosis is metastatic malignant disease because these malformations usually cause symptoms in adulthood; the X-ray appearance may suggest osteolytic or osteosclerotic metastases.

As a final example of all the problems that spinal cord lesions may present diagnostically, and as further evidence of the dramatic improvement in imaging, the following case, which just spanned the two investigational eras, is very instructive.

CASE REPORT XXI

A 35-year-old architect was admitted to a district general hospital with the sudden onset of paraparesis, loss of sensation down the left side of the body and urinary retention. He was referred to a neurosurgical unit, where a normal myelogram was performed. He was transferred to the local neurological unit for further management, with a diagnosis of transverse myelitis. On admission there was a sensory level to pain and temperature from T5 to T7, a spared area from T7 to T12 and loss of pain and temperature below T12. Light touch, posture sense and vibration were completely intact. The left knee jerk was brisk both plantars were extensor and he was unable to stand or walk. VERs and BAERs were normal and a further CSF examination showed no oligoclonal IgG. Following a course of ACTH injections he showed a gratifying improvement, mobilized with physiotherapy, and became able to walk with a frame. Bladder sensation returned and the catheter was removed. He had a pulmonary embolus requiring anticoagulation before his discharge 6 weeks later walking with a stick.

A year later he was walking without aids but had some residual urgency of micturition. Over 2–3 weeks his left leg started to drag again and he was readmitted. On this occasion there had been some pain over the upper thoracic spine at the onset. Sensation was impaired to T4 level but only on the left side. All other modalities were normal. Both legs showed increased tone; the weakness on this occasion was more marked in the right leg. A repeat lumbar puncture was negative for IgG. A 7-day course of intravenous methylprednisolone was given with rapid improvement, but it was thought that this clinical picture was sufficiently atypical, with no hard evidence of demyelination, to justify an MRI scan. This was performed a month later and revealed a haemorrhage into the lower cervical and upper thoracic cord. He was referred for surgery, where the lesion was found to be a cavernous intramedullary angioma extending from C4 to C7. Following surgery, he was able to walk with one stick for short distances and had severe urgency of micturition. He continued to improve but was unable to resume his former employment.

It is difficult to see how this diagnosis could have been made without MRI scanning. The original myelogram was normal, even on subsequent review. The odd clinical features on the first occasion were the band of segmental spinothalamic loss with an area of sparing below, suggesting a central cord lesion, and the sparing of the dorsal columns which are usually involved in cord lesions due to multiple sclerosis. Transverse myelitis is not inevitably due to MS but recurrent transverse myelitis at the same level should always arouse comment. Once again, the normality of the ancillary tests, which failed to support the diagnosis of MS, proved to be valuable in raising further doubts. The apparent response to steroids on two occasions seemed to provide some support for an inflammatory lesion even though the value of steroids in MS is disputed. It is possible that the clinical course was merely the natural history of two haemorrhages into the spinal cord, or that the steroids reduced the oedema around the haemorrhage and were beneficial by that mechanism. The MRI scan findings were therefore not totally surprising and permitted surgical treatment of this lesion, which might only have been eventually diagnosed when it had destroyed the spinal cord. He was one of the first patients to be scanned on the first MRI scanner service available to the neurological unit. It is sad that the ultimate outcome was not as successful as was hoped when the lesion was demonstrated.

15. The Spinal Cord in Relation to the Vertebral Column

Developmental Anatomy of the Nervous System

It is impossible to understand the developmental malformations of the CNS and their delayed complications without some knowledge of the embryology. This section is not intended to replace the superb available textbooks but merely attempts to summarize the information in a dynamic way. Because many of the developments occur in parallel it is difficult, in a limited number of illustrations, to define each component as accurately as the standard staging classifications. The following text and the illustrations are given on a rough timescale at which the developments occur. All the illustrations are drawn from the same angle of view, so that the orientation and sequence of events is more readily followed.

The Development of the Spinal Cord

1. When the embryo has reached the stage of separation into a clear-cut upper amniotic sac and a lower yolk sac, the upper sheet of cells becomes the ectoderm and the lower sheet of cells the endoderm. By day 15, the ectodermal cells migrate to the centre of the disc to form the primitive streak. At the head end, the primitive node with its central pit appears. From its base a rod of cells, the notochordal process, develops and extends to the head end, and in so doing separates the ectoderm and endoderm. From either side of the notochordal process, the mesoderm develops and pushes laterally, anteriorly and posteriorly in a butterfly pattern, leaving two areas where it does not separate the ectoderm and endoderm, the oral membrane at the head end and of the cloacal membrane at the tail end. This process pushes the primitive node further towards the tail end of the embryo (Fig. 15.1, 15.2).

2. The notochord fuses with the endoderm and the primitive pit is then in open communication between the amniotic and yolk sacs, forming the neurenteric canal. By day 21 this canal is normally obliterated by the further development of the notochord. This stage may be important in the development of diastatomyelic deformity (split

spinal cord). If the notochord is removed from an embryo, two separate spinal cords and vertebral canals form on either side of the midline. If the neurenteric canal persists, each half of the centrum of the vertebral body tries to form a complete vertebra and the pedicle formation on the midline aspect of each produces a bony spur, splitting the midline with a separate section of spinal cord on each side. This will cause problems later when the spinal cord is pulled up the canal. Support for this postulated mechanism can be found in that such defects are usually accompanied by a split in the ectoderm leading to tethering of the skin to the vertebral spine at the level of the defect (Fig. 15.2, 15.3).

3. The mesodermal layer now lies on either side of the notochord and is only absent at the head and tail ends and where the notochord occupies the midline (Fig. 15.3 and 15.4). At its periphery the mesoderm starts folding in on itself to form a peripheral ridge. At this stage (days 17–19) the nervous system starts to develop by neuralization. The notochord partially folds to form a tube, which becomes fully formed by 28 days. This starts the neuralization process in the overlying ectoderm. In parallel, the mesoderm on either side thickens to form two columns, the paraxial mesoderm. Laterally this differentiates into the intermediate and lateral mesodermal plates, which form the organs and will not be discussed further. The medial paraxial mesoderm then undergoes segmentation into somites, starting on day 20 and first appearing in what will become the occipital area and extending downwards, so that by day 35 there are 42 somites. The hollow centre is called the myocoele. The mesoderm differentiation also proceeds from above downwards. The dorsolateral components become the dermatomes, the medial cells become the dorsal musculature and the ventromedial cells become the sclerotome. It is these latter cells, with their migratory capacity, that move towards and surround the notochord and neural tube to form the vertebrae and the discs (Fig. 15.5).

4. Neuralization, the first stage of formation of the cord and brain, starts at day 17. The midline cells become the neuroectoderm and the centre sinks

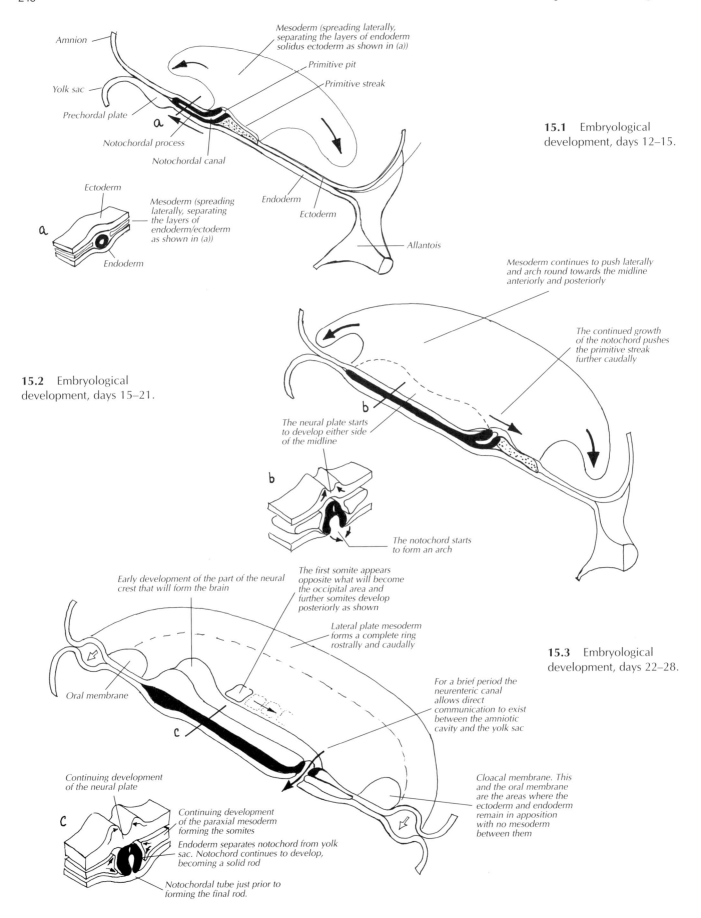

Amnion

Yolk sac

Prechordal plate

Notochordal process

Notochordal canal

Mesoderm (spreading laterally, separating the layers of endoderm solidus ectoderm as shown in (a))

Primitive pit

Primitive streak

15.1 Embryological development, days 12–15.

Ectoderm

Mesoderm (spreading laterally, separating the layers of endoderm/ectoderm as shown in (a))

Endoderm

Endoderm

Ectoderm

Allantois

Mesoderm continues to push laterally and arch round towards the midline anteriorly and posteriorly

The continued growth of the notochord pushes the primitive streak further caudally

15.2 Embryological development, days 15–21.

The neural plate starts to develop either side of the midline

The notochord starts to form an arch

Early development of the part of the neural crest that will form the brain

The first somite appears opposite what will become the occipital area and further somites develop posteriorly as shown

Lateral plate mesoderm forms a complete ring rostrally and caudally

15.3 Embryological development, days 22–28.

For a brief period the neurenteric canal allows direct communication to exist between the amniotic cavity and the yolk sac

Oral membrane

Continuing development of the neural plate

Continuing development of the paraxial mesoderm forming the somites

Endoderm separates notochord from yolk sac. Notochord continues to develop, becoming a solid rod

Notochordal tube just prior to forming the final rod.

Cloacal membrane. This and the oral membrane are the areas where the ectoderm and endoderm remain in apposition with no mesoderm between them

15.4 Continued development of the CNS days 15–17.

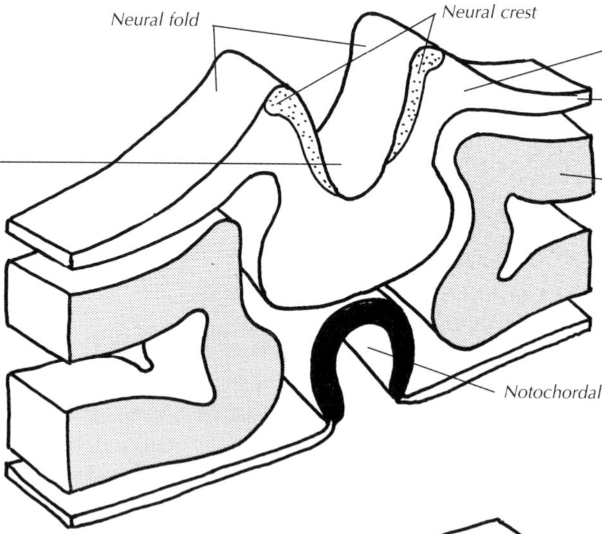

Neural fold

Neural crest

Neuroectoderm

Ectoderm

Neural plate

Paraxial mesoderm

Notochordal process

15.5 Continued development of the CNS days 17–19.

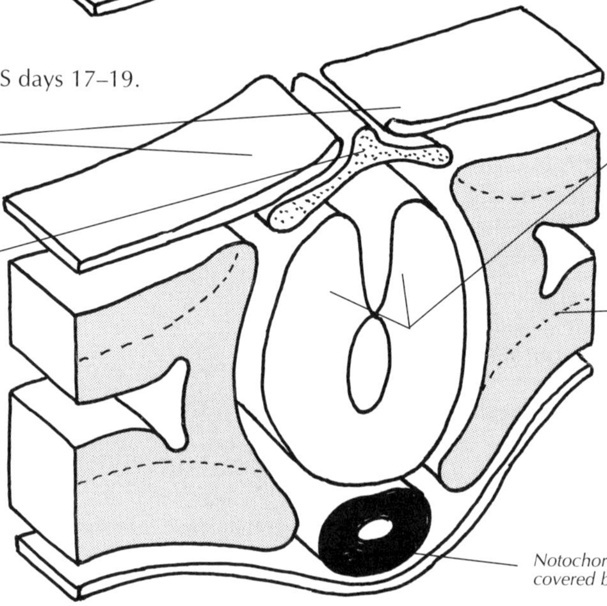

Neural folds starting to meet in midline

Neural folds meeting in midline to form neural tube

Cells of the neural crest form a separate layer under the ectoderm, which segments under the influence of the developing mesoderm

Developing mesoderm condensing and segmenting into somites

Notochord now a tubular rod covered by endoderm

15.6 Continued development of the CNS days 20–28.

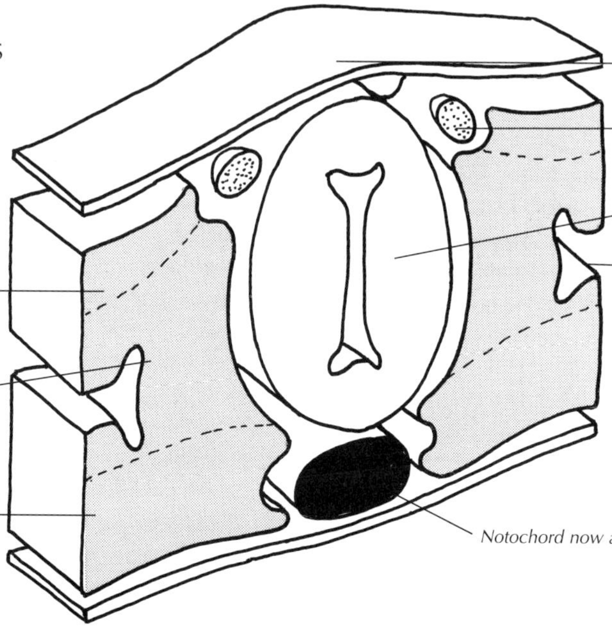

Ectoderm now complete

Neural crest segmenting to form ganglia and nerve fibres

Neural tube now complete with large central cavity

Myelocoele (cavity within the myotome)

Dermatomyotome containing the cells that will become the dermis

Dermatomyotome containing cells that will become the dorsal musculature

The sclerotome, which will give rise to the vertebrae and ribs by surrounding the notochord

Notochord now a solid rod

inwards as the neural plate. The lateral margins curl over and join in the midline, forming a tube covered by the ectoderm. The first fusion occurs at the level of the third and fourth somites, and proceeds up and down. The anterior neuropore closes first at 24 days, and the posterior neuropore at 26 days. The neural crest is the precursor of the formation of a varied range of important structures. These include the pia, the arachnoid mater, the dorsal root ganglia, the Schwann cells of the peripheral nerves, the autonomic ganglia, the chromaffin tissue, the skin pigment and the cartilage in the branchial arches. Abnormalities of neural crest differentiation may be important in conditions where underlying neural maldevelopments are associated with pigmentary and other abnormalities of the skin, such as neurofibromatosis, Sturge–Weber syndrome and tuberous sclerosis. The neural crest contains the cells of origin of the malignant ganglioneuromas of childhood. The cells of the neural crest also form the spinal ganglia, down to L1/2 level (Figs 15.5 and 15.6). At this stage the lower lumbar, sacral and coccygeal cord and vertebrae are **not** present.

5. The development of these lower components occurs by a process of canalization. Cells in the tail section of the embryo aggregate at day 22 to form around vacuoles, which coalesce to form a cyst-like structure which connects to the distal end of the neural tube, forming a small caudal extension (Fig. 15.7). This area then further modifies by a process of organized dedifferentiation. The embryonic tail disappears and the centre of the distal neural tube narrows to become the central canal, leaving a definite cavity in the lower lumbar and sacral region called the ventriculus

terminalis. This lies opposite what will become the S2 vertebral level. At this stage the cord extends down to S2, but from day 70 the cord is pulled up to a level opposite L5, as the longitudinal development of the vertebrae outstrips the length of the spinal cord, and by day 160 the cord ends opposite L2, its normal position at birth. The distal neural tube atrophies and becomes the filum terminale. This remains attached to the S2 vertebral body and this completes the development of the spinal cord.

Anomalies of Spinal Cord Development

There are three major anomalies of spinal cord development and one of them, diastatomyelia, has already been described. The others are myelodysplasia and spinal dysraphism.

Myelodysplasia

This malformation is due either to the failure of the neural tube to close, or to closure followed by reopening owing to excessive pressure within the central canal. It is thought that the former is the correct explanation, as there is often abnormal proliferation of the neural ectoderm at the edges of an open spina bifida. This would not be expected if development had been complete and then disrupted afterwards. There are varying degrees of severity. At its worst the whole neural tube may fail to close, usually associated with anencephaly. If it only affects the posterior neuropore, varying degrees of spinal bifida occur in three grades: a myelocoele, in which the whole lower back is open,

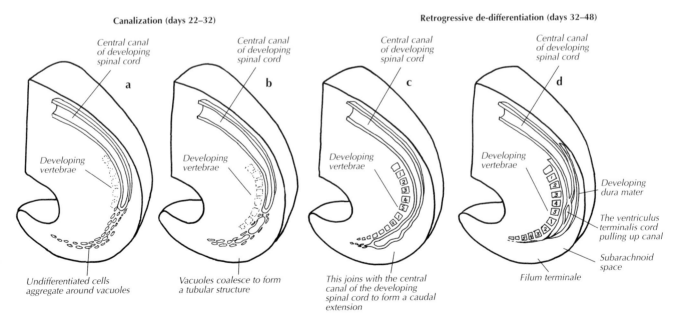

15.7   Development of sacral segments.

neural remnants are on the surface and there is an open leakage of CSF; a myelomeningocoele, in which the skin is closed but abnormal neural components lie within a large cyst; and a meningocoele, where there is a cystic cavity containing CSF but the underlying neural elements are relatively normal, although other associated anomalies may coexist and cause problems later. The more severe spina bifida lesions are usually associated with an Arnold–Chiari malformation, a congenital anomaly at the level of the anterior neuropore and consequently hydrocephalus. Cervical meningocoeles are quite rare but occur over the occipitocervical region and are related to more severe closure defects at the anterior neuropore.

An example of severe spina bifida is shown in the MRI scan below.

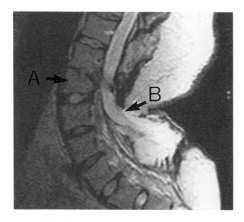

MRI of lumbar spine in a 28-year-old patient with severe spina bifida. Shows compression fracture of L1 body and spinal cord and roots tethered within the meningocoele

Spinal Dysraphism

This is a spinal abnormality resulting from defects in dedifferentiation during the formation of the sacral spinal cord. The overlying skin may be abnormal, with telangiectasia, a naevus or a dermal sinus. Underlying bone defects are common and spina bifida occulta with an intracanalicular lipoma (a lipomeningocoele) is common (see Case report VI). Intraspinal and subcutaneous dermoids, teratomas, pilonidal cysts and chordomas all occur in this area and are of developmental origin. Rarely, the ventriculus terminalis may remain enlarged and produce a syringomyelic cavity in the sacral spinal cord. Spinal cord tethering due to a short thick non-stretching filum terminale also reflects incomplete dedifferentiation. The neural arch of S1 fails to close in some 5% of the population and represents the mildest closure defect found.

Development of the Vertebral Column (Figs 15.8 and 15.9)

1. At 23 days, in parallel with the formation of the neural tube, the mesenchymal tissue derived from the medial paraxial mesoderm becomes migratory, attracted by the developing notochord and neural tube. The notochord is first surrounded by the cells that will become the vertebrae and the intervertebral disc. This begins in the cervical region and extends up and down. The cells that will form the neural arches and the transverse processes surround the neural tube and others migrate laterally to form the anlage of the ribs.

2. The formation of the vertebrae and intervertebral discs is very complicated but explains important features of adult anatomy. The segment of sclerotome derived from a somite evolves into a less cellular upper part and an increasingly cellular lower part, with a marked condensation of cells at its upper end which is destined to become the disc and the annulus fibrosus. The costal processes develop from the lower end of the dense component. The lower dense component then fuses with the upper less dense component of the sclerotome below, forming the centrum of the vertebra. During this process the notochord within what has now become the vertebral body is squeezed almost to nothing, and persists in the fully formed vertebra as the mucoid streak. In the region of the disc it persists and some of the vertebral notochord migrates into that area to become the nucleus pulposus of the intervertebral disc.

3. When complete this process leaves the segmental artery that originally lay between the somites – now opposite the centre of the vertebral body – and the developing segmental nerve, formerly in the middle of the somite, now lies opposite the newly formed disc space. The segment of muscle derived from the somite does not split and is therefore supplied at its centre by the segmental nerve. This is the membranous stage of vertebral development.

4. The cartilaginous phase starts at day 40, when chondrification centres appear either side of the notochord, in the arches and in the costal processes. The inner layer of the arch, the closure membrane, becomes the dura and the anterior and posterior longitudinal ligaments develop from the residual mesenchyme. The anterior ligament attaches to the body of the vertebra and the posterior ligament is only adherent to the edge of the disc. The final ossification process starts at 20–24 weeks and starts in the arches of the vertebrae and the other processes in the cervical region and progresses up and down. The ossification of the bodies starts at the lower thoracic and upper lumbar levels and extends first down towards the tail and then up towards the head. The first complete closure of the arches during ossification occurs in the

15.8   Development of the vertebral column and intervertebral discs.

[This stage starts at day 23 and over 10 days cells of the sclerotome surround the notochord, those migrating dorsally form the neural arches and those migrating ventrolaterally form the transverse processes and ribs. The sclerotome around the notochord condenses to form the ultimate vertebral body. At day 24 resegmentation takes place and the first stage is shown in Figure 15.8a.]

a. Resegmentation

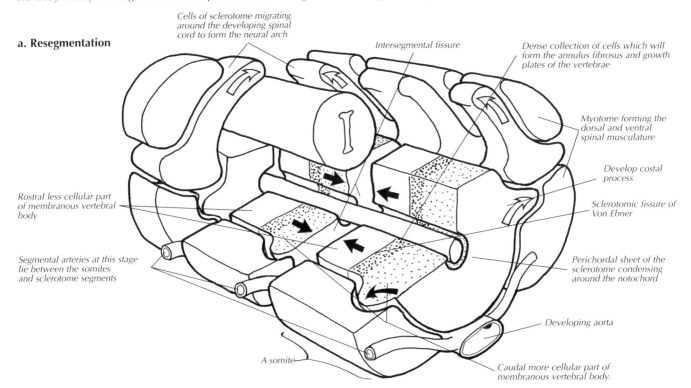

Cells of sclerotome migrating around the developing spinal cord to form the neural arch

Intersegmental fissure

Dense collection of cells which will form the annulus fibrosus and growth plates of the vertebrae

Myotome forming the dorsal and ventral spinal musculature

Develop costal process

Sclerotomic fissure of Von Ebner

Perichordal sheet of the sclerotome condensing around the notochord

Rostral less cellular part of membranous vertebral body

Segmental arteries at this stage lie between the somites and sclerotome segments

Developing aorta

A somite

Caudal more cellular part of membranous vertebral body.

The dense caudal half of the segment above joins the less cellular rostral part of the segment below, to form the new vertebral body

b. Final disposition of nerve roots, intervertebral arteries, discs and vertebrae

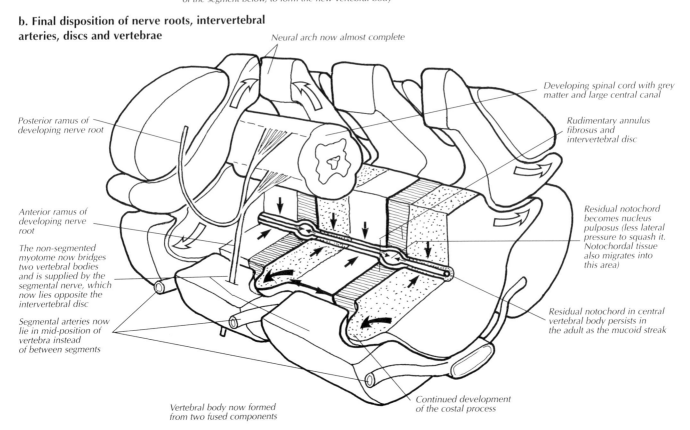

Neural arch now almost complete

Developing spinal cord with grey matter and large central canal

Rudimentary annulus fibrosus and intervertebral disc

Posterior ramus of developing nerve root

Anterior ramus of developing nerve root

The non-segmented myotome now bridges two vertebral bodies and is supplied by the segmental nerve, which now lies opposite the intervertebral disc

Segmental arteries now lie in mid-position of vertebra instead of between segments

Residual notochord becomes nucleus pulposus (less lateral pressure to squash it. Notochordal tissue also migrates into this area)

Residual notochord in central vertebral body persists in the adult as the mucoid streak

Vertebral body now formed from two fused components

Continued development of the costal process

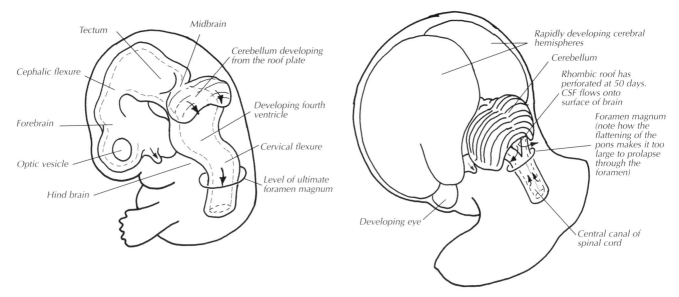

15.9   Brain at 3.4 mm and 7.5 mm embryo stages.

lumbar area. The body of the vertebra ossifies, leaving only the cartilaginous annulus to which the disc is attached.

Anomalies of Vertebral Development

The basic defects are the result of failure of bone growth at the enchondral growth areas at the upper and lower end plates of the vertebrae or of the articular processes posteriorly. Anterior lesions will cause a flexed spine (kyphosis), anterolateral lesions introduce a tilt (kyphoscoliosis) and, if purely lateral, a sideways tilt (scoliosis) occurs.

Notochord Abnormalities

If the notochord persists a split vertebra results. Conversely, if it degenerates completely no disc will form and the vertebrae will fuse, and if no growth occurs anteriorly, the normal growth of the arches will produce a severe localized kyphosis.

Non-Segmenting Arches

As the vertebral arches form a gap develops between them to permit flexion and extension movements of the spine. If the arches fail to segment the arch and pedicles fuse, preventing growth and movement.

Failure of Somite Migration

Because the vertebrae form from two halves of adjacent somite mesenchyme it is essential that the split meets precisely in the midline, particularly in view of the subse-

quent dramatic reorganization of the two components. If they are out of alignment, the formation of half-vertebrae above and below with incomplete intervertebral discs between them will produce an immobile segment with unequal growth and severe scoliotic deformity.

Vertebral Body Malformation

If a somite fails to develop properly there will be a defect of half the vertebra, the arch, the spine, the transverse process and the rib. This may result in a very small or very large wedged half-vertebra with scoliotic deformity. Other problems may occur when the ventral or dorsal part of the vertebral body fails to develop or to chondrify or ossify. All these abnormalities lead to severe alterations in growth potential and subsequent spinal deformity.

Cervical and Lumbar Ribs

The costal processes at cervical and lumbar level normally become part of the transverse process. Occasionally they continue to grow, forming a rib-like structure at cervical or lumbar level. At lumbar level they are of no great significance but a cervical rib may trap the subclavian artery or the lower components of the brachial plexus (see Chapter 16).

Development of the Brain

Brain development is less well understood and considerably more complex, and only requires consideration in this chapter because of the association of some cranial anomalies with spinal abnormalities.

1. At 24 days the neural tube becomes fully closed and at the head end is rapidly subdivided by the development of three main vesicles, which divide the neural tube into the forebrain, midbrain and hindbrain, known embryologically as the prosencephalon, the mesencephalon and the rhomboencephalon. The neural crest only extends as far as the midbrain as it contributes to the formation of cranial nerves III–XII. The olfactory and optic nerves develop as direct extensions of the forebrain.

2. As the embryo flexes, the first flexion occurs between the cervical cord and the hindbrain. The cephalic flexure then develops between the forebrain and the mesencephalon and the very rapid growth of the cerebral hemispheres envelops what now becomes the brain stem. From a practical point of view, the most important flexure is the third, the pontine flexure, which occurs at the mid-hindbrain, flattening the neural tube at this point and turning it into the beginnings of the fourth ventricle. This occurs between 30 and 36 days.

3. During the rapid development of the hemispheres, the remnants of the central cavity of the forebrain become divided into the two lateral ventricles and the midline third ventricle, which is normally separated into two halves by two layers of pia mater, with a potential space between them. Sometimes this space is filled with CSF, forming in effect a midline ventricle between the two lateral third ventricles, and this is known as a cavum septum pellucidum. Since the advent of CT scanning it has become clear that this is a very common anomaly. The commissures joining the two hemispheres are the anterior commissure, the corpus callosum and the posterior commissure. The anterior

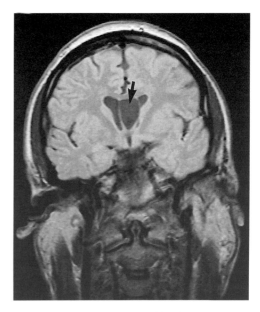

Cavum septum pellucidum.

commissure is a very important pathway linking the olfactory bulbs and the temporal lobes. All other areas link through the corpus callosum. The very small posterior commissure is of less importance. The corpus callosum may fail to develop (agenesis) or can be replaced by a large lipoma. These abnormalities are not necessarily associated with clinical disability.

4. At day 56 the anterior roof of the fourth ventricle thickens to become the rhombic lip, which then rapidly enlarges to form the cerebellum and, rather like the cerebral hemispheres, extends backwards and upwards to arch over the roof of the fourth ventricle.

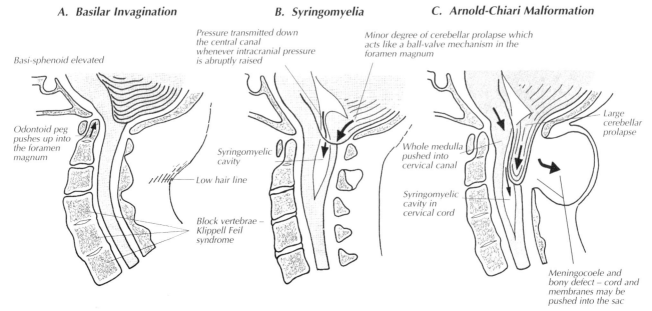

15.10 Common cervicomedullary abnormalities.

The roof plate of the fourth ventricle becomes thinner and perforates to allow CSF to communicate with the subarachnoid space through the foramina of Luschke and Magendie. If this membrane fails to perforate a giant cystic fourth ventricle forms, which is known as the Dandy–Walker syndrome and is one of the causes of hydrocephalus. Another major cause is aqueductal stenosis, sometimes associated with forked maldevelopment of the aqueduct; it is of uncertain origin but is important clinically in that patients may present with hydrocephalus due to this defect as late as the third decade.

5. The Arnold–Chiari malformation consists of varying degrees of ectopia of the cerebellum and medulla through the foramen magnum (Fig. 15.10C). A minor degree may consist only of the cerebellar tonsils lying in the posterior canal down to C1 level. In its most severe form, part of the medulla and long thin cerebellar tonsils extending down to the mid-cervical level may be found. There is a common association between the more severe deformities and spina bifida, and it has been suggested that the cerebellum is either pushed into the cervical canal by the hydrocephalus or is pulled down into it by the developmental malformation at the bottom of the back, which prevents the cord pulling up. Minor degrees of Arnold–Chiari malformation have become important clinically in that the majority of cases of syringomyelia are associated with it. It is still unclear whether there is a direct dynamic connection, as discussed later, or whether both are coincidental malformations. The multilocular nature of many cavities is inconsistent with a simple ballooning effect in some cases, and surgical decompression of the prolapsing tonsils is not always successful in treating syringomyelia, although in most cases further progression seems to be prevented.

6. Bony abnormalities in the region of the foramen magnum and cervical spine occur and the embryological mechanism is uncertain. They may lead to a small posterior fossa, basilar invagination with the odontoid peg through the foramen magnum (Fig. 15.10A), or cervical vertebral fusion, the Klippel–Feil syndrome. All these anomalies may be associated with a short neck. Abnormalities of the skull base tend to produce progressive posterior fossa complications which may not occur until middle age. Klippel–Feil syndrome is associated with severe degenerative change in the remaining mobile segments of the neck, leading to atypical nerve root irritation or spinal cord compression.

7. Lesser degrees of cervical meningocoele, analogous to the minor degrees of spinal bifida, may occur. A midline naevus or telangiectatic patch on the skin over the nape of the neck and occiput is not uncommon. An extremely important defect is a dermal sinus, which can occur in the midline of the nape of the neck and which may be in communication with the meninges. This can be a cause of recurrent meningitis and a dermal sinus in the hairline should be sought in any patient with recurrent meningitis, or if the meningitis is due to atypical organisms.

Although these malformations are relatively rare, they cause considerable clinical and ethical problems.

Previous enthusiasm in the 1950s and 1960s for major surgery to repair lumbar myelomeningocoeles and shunting procedures for hydrocephalus has now been tempered by appreciation of a subsequent lifetime spent undergoing shunt revisions, orthopaedic surgery for vertebral instability and the problems of the increasing disparity between the size of the upper and lower halves of the body and the complications of a wheelchair existence that resulted from such aggressive management. The tragic legacy of this former enthusiasm has left many young adults with multiple neurological abnormalities, both from their malformations and from the treatment they have received, and is an object lesson for those who regarded warning voices raised at the time as unethical. The technical ability to perform procedures is not always in the patient's best interest in the longer term. Fortunately, intrauterine ultrasound has considerably reduced the frequency of children born with severe abnormalities of this type. Those who have had to care for such patients are greatly relieved that this era of unbridled surgical enthusiasm has passed.

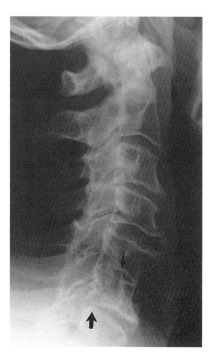

Radiograph of block vertebra.

An example of a mild segmentation defect leading to a block vertebra at C5/6. A vestigeal intervertebral disc (small arrow) is seen with marked degenerative change (large arrow) at C6/7. The patient presented with severe radicular pain from the lesion at C6/7.

It is very important to recognize that although many of these abnormalities are congenital, symptoms may not occur until late middle age in many instances. Perhaps the best example is syringomyelia.

Syringomyelia

Syringomyelia has already been mentioned in Chapter 13 in relation to the clinical signs of an expanding lesion in the cervical cord. The recent recognition that the cavitation of the cord is associated in the majority of cases with a congenital abnormality at the foramen magnum was mentioned above. This usually consists of a mild degree of Arnold–Chiari malformation, with the cerebellar tonsils lying in the posterior foramen magnum (see Fig. 15.10B). It is postulated that throughout life pressure rises during coughing or straining impact the cerebellar tonsils in the foramen magnum and this transmits the increased CSF pressure into the grey matter of the cord, instead of the pressure rise being dissipated into the spinal CSF. Occasionally patients will develop acute syringomyelia during a cough or a sneeze; this is called hydromyelia.

Operations to decompress the posterior foramen magnum and drain the cavity at its lower end may relieve the situation and improve the patient's clinical status. MRI scanning is necessary to demonstrate the lesion as bony abnormalities are not always present. In addition to the symmetrical dilation of the central canal, slit-like cavities adjacent to but in continuity with the central canal can produce asymmetry of the physical signs. Why the cavitation begins at C7–D1 level is not clear. The cord may expand with greater ease in the cervical enlargement. The mechanism may be compared to the way a balloon made with expanded sections inflates to a series of bulges. As the lesion expands upwards into the region of the fourth ventricle the condition known as syringobulbia develops, and progressively higher sensory loss occurs as the decussating pain fibres from the descending tract of the fifth nerve become affected. The sensory loss spreads from the back of the head, forwards on to the face like a balaclava helmet. This is shown in detail in Figure 15.11. The earliest cranial nerve nuclei to be affected are the hypoglossal nuclei in the floor of the canal under the obex. This causes bilateral wasting and weakness of the tongue. There is also disruption of vestibular afferents from the neck muscles, and nystagmus is usually present by the time the sensory loss extends on to the face. This is of the downturning type on lateral gaze, typical of an anomaly in the region of the foramen magnum.

Although this is a classic neurological disorder it is often completely misdiagnosed for years. The main reason is the failure to realize that cutaneous sensation is normal, and unless pain sensation is specifically and carefully tested over the arms, upper thorax, back of the head and face no sensory loss will be documented. Multiple sclerosis, motor neuron disease and cervical spondylosis are the alternative diagnoses that are usually suspected. Accidental painless injury to the upper limbs is a frequent presenting symptom but it is important to recognise this condition as a cause of severe pain, often present for years before sensory deficit is detected. In most instances correct examination technique is the only way to confirm the clinical suspicion, and even then, until the advent of MRI scanning the diagnosis was extremely difficult to confirm. Patients who had gross anomalies with the cerebellar tonsils prolapsed well into the cervical canal could sometimes be diagnosed by myelography, but because of the head-down position required to demonstrate this area, it was suspected that the cavity would collapse at the critical moment, so that the expanded cervical cord could not be demonstrated.

The following case is an excellent example of a clinically confident diagnosis made 9 years before an MRI scan provided diagnostic confirmation after symptoms had been present for 29 years, and the clinical picture to this day is far from classical.

CASE REPORT I

A 44-year-old woman with a history of epilepsy since the age of 7 presented (in 1976) with a 16-year history of severe intermittent pain down the inside of her right arm in the ulnar nerve distribution. An exploration of the ulnar nerve at the elbow in 1975 had been unhelpful. The only abnormalities

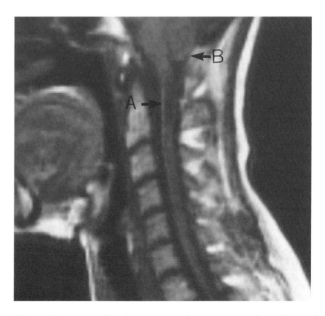

CRI. *Syringomyelia demonstrated 15 years after diagnosis first made, Arnold–Chiari malformation not previously detected by myelography.*

were some impairment of two-point discrimination and pin-prick over the right ulnar nerve or C8 distribution. There was no reflex change or other sensory deficit. Nerve conduction studies were normal. In 1981 she related a sensation as if there were a giant burn involving the entire inner aspect of the right arm up to the scapula and round on to the right breast. She had noticed that her right hand did not sweat and there were some trophic changes in the right fingers. There was no Horner's syndrome. The left triceps jerk was now absent and there was sensory change to pinprick over C8–T2 on the right-hand side. Vibration sense was impaired to the costal margins and joint position sense was impaired in the right leg. A myelogram, taking the contrast into the foramen magnum, was normal. The CSF protein was slightly elevated. A CT scan of the foramen magnum and posterior fossa was normal. A clinical diagnosis of syringomyelia was suggested but unproven. In 1983 she developed a mild left Horner's syndrome but no other change was documented and she was not reviewed again in detail until 1989, when the trophic changes in the hands were even more striking but there were no other new findings. Fortunately, MRI scanning was by then available, which confirmed an Arnold–Chiari malformation with a syrinx extending down to T1 level. A posterior

fossa decompressive operation was performed in 1989, which unfortunately has not relieved her symptoms although there has been no further progression.

This case emphasizes the very long history of poorly localized unpleasant pain, which often dominates the early symptomatology of syringomyelia and is frequently suspected as being non-organic in origin. A more classic presentation is the accidental discovery of severe loss of pain appreciation.

CASE REPORT II

A 40-year-old hospital carpenter presented because he had discovered that he had lost pain sensation in both arms. He had realised for years that cuts on his hands took several weeks to heal and he was never free of inflamed lacerations, but they never seemed to hurt. On one occasion he had put a chisel through his hand and removed it himself. He decided to seek advice when he suddenly found that a long piece of wood that he was planing was covered in blood and he could not see where this had come from. When he inspected the underneath of his arm he found that he had rubbed the skin

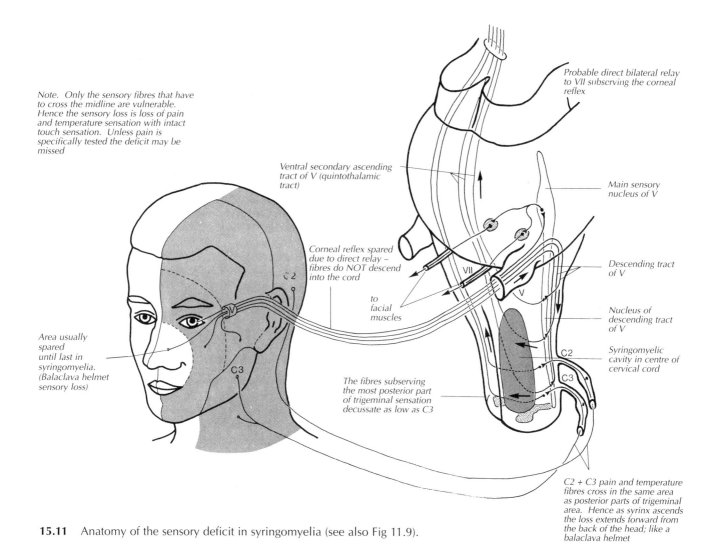

Note. Only the sensory fibres that have to cross the midline are vulnerable. Hence the sensory loss is loss of pain and temperature sensation with intact touch sensation. Unless pain is specifically tested the deficit may be missed

Ventral secondary ascending tract of V (quintothalamic tract)

Corneal reflex spared due to direct relay – fibres do NOT descend into the cord

to facial muscles

Area usually spared until last in syringomyelia. (Balaclava helmet sensory loss)

The fibres subserving the most posterior part of trigeminal sensation decussate as low as C3

Probable direct bilateral relay to VII subserving the corneal reflex

Main sensory nucleus of V

Descending tract of V

Nucleus of descending tract of V

Syringomyelic cavity in centre of cervical cord

C2 + C3 pain and temperature fibres cross in the same area as posterior parts of trigeminal area. Hence as syrinx ascends the loss extends forward from the back of the head; like a balaclava helmet

15.11 Anatomy of the sensory deficit in syringomyelia (see also Fig 11.9).

off his elbow, which was bleeding profusely. He had not felt any discomfort. Physical examination revealed the classic features of syringomyelia, with total sensory loss to pain and temperature over the upper half of the body and marked wasting and weakness of the intrinsic muscles of the hand and arm, which had forced him to modify his working techniques and undoubtedly contributed to the heavily traumatized state of his hands and forearms.

The hardest situation in which to detect syringomyelia is at the stage when the patient clearly has what at first sight appears to be a non-organic pain syndrome. Being aware of the diagnostic possibility and knowing exactly what to look for is critical if a diagnostic error is not to be perpetuated. The following case is an excellent example of this situation.

CASE REPORT III

A 17-year-old girl was referred for a fifth opinion on a pain syndrome that had taken her to paediatricians, orthopaedic surgeons and rheumatologists over 5 years. The consensus view was that this was psychologically based, with an element of school refusal. At the age of 11, while her mother was fitting a new suit, she shouted at her to stand up straight because the skirt was hanging too far down on one side. She burst into tears and said that she was, and they then realized that she had a severe scoliosis. Two years later she developed a severe pain in the right arm, particularly when doing homework. It was so severe that it reduced her to tears and she described it as having a gnawing quality deep in her arm. It was not related to movement or posture and got steadily

*worse over the next 2 years, and she developed a similar sensation in the right leg. There were no other symptoms and the only organic diagnosis suggested was that she had hemiatrophy syndrome because her right foot was slightly smaller. On examination she had a marked thoracic scoliosis. The cranial nerves were normal, the right arm reflexes were barely present and the left were normal. The abdominal reflexes were absent, the leg reflexes were all brisk with clonus on the right, but the plantar responses were normal. Power and coordination were normal in all limbs. Sensation seemed entirely normal until pinprick **as pain** was tested. She had total loss of pain sensation over C3–T2 on the right. A diagnosis of syringomyelia was made and an MRI scan showed an extensive syrinx from C3 to T2, a further syrinx extending down to the lower thoracic cord, and an Arnold–Chiari malformation.*

The major clue to the diagnosis in this case was the scoliosis, a common presenting symptom indicating an underlying lesion in the nervous system and always worth a neurological opinion.

The Cervical Spine and Cervical Spondylosis

In the cervical region vertebral disease may affect both the spinal cord and the nerve roots. There are many features of the anatomy of this area that must be appreciated to understand the pathogenesis and neurological syndromes caused by cervical spondylosis (Figs 15.12 and 15.13).

1. In the cervical region the spinal cord is expanded and the canal is relatively narrow. The usual variation in sagittal diameter ranges from 15 to 20 mm. Patients with a sagittal diameter of less than 13 mm may develop cord compression with quite mild degrees of degenerative spondylosis.

2. The C1 root emerges over the top of the first cervical vertebra. Therefore the other roots emerge **above** their respective vertebra, that is, the C6 root emerges in the C5/6 interspace (compare with the lumbar roots).

3. Cervical spondylosis is caused by disc degeneration and protrusion, with bony overgrowth of the adjacent vertebrae. These bony ridges plus the extruded and often calcified disc material constitute the spondylotic bar that may compress the cord.

4. These changes are maximal at C5/6, C6/7 and C4/5 spaces respectively. These are the mobile segments at which most movement occurs. The atlantooccipital joint allows only nodding movements and C7/T1 is immobilized by the thoracic cage.

5. The mobility of the neck makes great demands on the cervical cord. In forward flexion the length of the canal is increased by some 2 cm and the cord must stretch. This probably accounts for the transient cord symptoms known as Lhermitte's sign (known in the

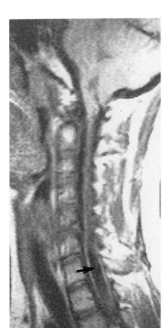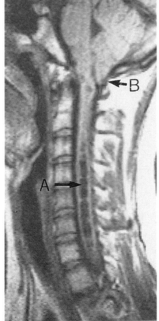

CRIII. *Syringomyelia (A) in cervical and thoracic cord in a 17-year-old with Arnold-Chiari malformation (B)*

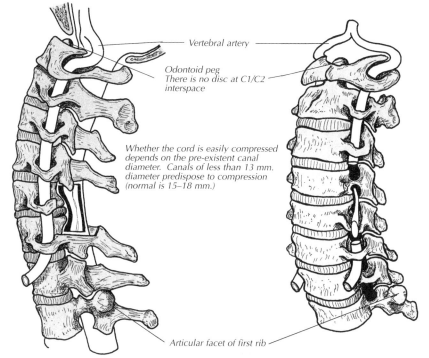

Vertebral arch cut away at C5 and C6 to show the cord being compressed by a spondylotic bar

The transverse process of C4 is cut away to show the emerging C5 root damaged by the osteophytes in the exit foraminae

Vertebral artery

*Odontoid peg
There is no disc at C1/C2 interspace*

Whether the cord is easily compressed depends on the pre-existent canal diameter. Canals of less than 13 mm. diameter predispose to compression (normal is 15–18 mm.)

C5 Nerve root compressed by lateral disc lesion

Cord being compressed by osteophytes and disc fragments (the spondylitic bar)

Articular facet of first rib

15.12   The cervical spine: lateral and left anterior oblique views.

Lateral View of the
Cervical Spine in Forward Flexion

Lateral View of the Cervical
Spine in Hyperextension

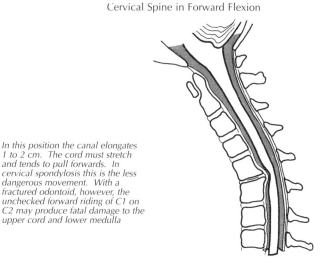

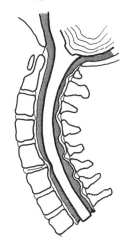

In this movement the cord shortens and would appear to be able to 'flop back' from the bars. But it is by far the most dangerous movement in cervical spondylosis. The roots (see above), the denticulate ligaments, and the forward bulging of the buckled ligamentum flavum all tend to hold the cord forwards. Which of these factors is the most significant in causing damage is much disputed

In this position the canal elongates 1 to 2 cm. The cord must stretch and tends to pull forwards. In cervical spondylosis this is the less dangerous movement. With a fractured odontoid, however, the unchecked forward riding of C1 on C2 may produce fatal damage to the upper cord and lower medulla

15.13   The cervical spine in flexion and extension.

USA as the 'barber's chair sign'). This consists of tingling in all four limbs or electric shock-like feelings down the back on flexing the neck if the cervical cord is damaged by multiple sclerosis, cervical spondylosis or any other condition that distorts or inflames the cervical spinal cord. In hyperextension of the neck the canal shortens and the cord shortens. In this position the spinal cord may be squeezed between the spondylotic bar anteriorly and the buckled ligamentum flavum posteriorly (Fig. 15.13).

6. The cord is not completely free to ride these blows as it is held forward by the anterolaterally directed nerve roots and prevented from riding backwards by the ligamentum denticulatum at each side.

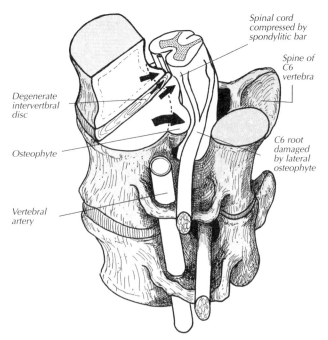

Spinal cord compressed by spondylitic bar

Spine of C6 vertebra

Degenerate intervertbral disc

Osteophyte

C6 root damaged by lateral osteophyte

Vertebral artery

15.14 The effect of cervical spondylosis on the spinal cord and cervical roots.

Clinical Features of Cervical Spondylosis
(Fig. 15.14)

There are two clinical syndromes which may coexist in some patients: these are the root syndromes and compressive cervical myelopathy.

Cervical Root Syndromes

The roots most often affected are, in order, C6, C7 and C5. Roots C3, C4 and T1 are affected so infrequently that other possible causes should be carefully excluded before accepting that damage to any of them is caused by spondylosis. The clinical features of the individual root lesions are fully described in Chapter 16. At this stage it is sufficient to note that the pain in the affected root territory is usually related to neck movement, is generally worse on waking, and is often originally provoked by either known trauma or unusual activity such as painting a ceiling.

Efforts to prevent the damaged root being pulled in and out of the intervertebral foramen should be made. This is best achieved by a soft collar worn at night. This prevents the neck slumping into an abnormal position during the night when the patient is fully relaxed, and acts as a mild physical restraint during the day. Daytime use is less critical as the onset of pain will usually inhibit provocative movement; the use of a collar during the day more often serves as a badge of courage or a symbol of disability than as an aid to treatment. If combined with dark glasses and the use of a stick, a non-organic basis is virtually guaranteed. The

symptoms usually subside in a few weeks and may not recur for years if the provocative activity is avoided.

Compressive Cervical Myelopathy

Fortunately, this condition occurs less frequently than the root syndromes. The patient may be predisposed to compression by a congenitally narrow canal, and will usually present with either an acute or a slowly progressive spastic paraparesis. The acute onset often follows a fall on to the face which sharply extends the neck, or a fall on to the back of the head producing sharp hyperflexion.

Although root symptoms may not be a major feature of the history, quite often the examiner will find that the biceps and supinator reflexes (C5 and C6) are absent, and that the triceps reflex (C7) is brisk. This indicates that the roots and the cord are being compressed at the C5/6 interspace, and this particular combination is almost pathognomonic of cervical spondylosis with cord compression. MRI scanning or myelography is always indicated and surgical efforts to decompress the cord by anterior discectomy is advisable, although carrying some risk and no guarantee of improvement.

A collar is often advised but this rarely seems to have any effect on the myelopathic condition, although it may relieve any coexistent root pain. Unfortunately, so many middle-aged patients have some degree of cervical spondylosis on plain X-ray that its presence cannot be regarded as confirming that their condition is due to spondylosis. This problem is discussed in greater detail as progressive cervical myelopathy in Chapter 14. If MRI scanning shows no evidence of compression, the diagnosis may subsequently prove to be multiple sclerosis or motor neuron disease. On the other hand, an unexpected neurofibroma or meningioma is occasionally discovered. As discussed in Chapter 14, it is wise to keep the diagnosis of cervical spondylosis with neurological complications under continual review.

As an example of the problems of a diagnostic 'near miss' in an elderly patient with degenerative disease in the neck, and indeed other coexistent neurological problems in the arms, the following is a superb example.

CASE REPORT IV

The patient was first seen in 1977, with paraesthesiae down the right inner forearm, aching in the right elbow and similar but less severe symptoms on the left. These developed while he was hunting and he related it to bouncing up and down on his horse. He then developed numbness in a very clear-cut ulnar nerve distribution in the right hand and nerve conduction studies revealed slight slowing through the elbow segment in the right arm. The patient was reluctant to consider surgery and, as he had been in the habit of shuffling around on his elbows, was advised to discontinue doing this

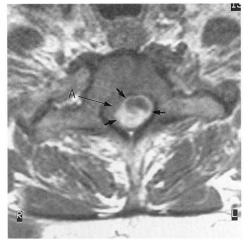

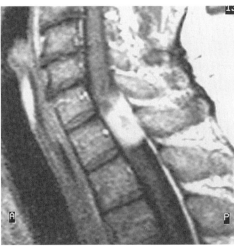

CRIV. *Cord compression by neurofibroma at T1 level. (A) Spinal cord, small arrows indicate tumour.*

in the hope that his symptoms would remit. He was not seen again until 1993, but in the interim had had cancer of the larynx in 1986, which was treated with radiotherapy. He had taken up jogging since his retirement and continued his hunting, and in the year before presentation had become aware of increasing difficulty in using the left leg, which seemed to drag, and he found it difficult to operate the clutch while driving. There were some symptoms in the right leg but he thought that this was due to overuse of that leg. He had had a sensation as if his shoes were too tight, with occasional electric shocks radiating up the left leg. There was no sphincter disturbance. On physical examination there was a marked increase in tone in the left arm, with increased in reflexes in both arms. The right leg was spastic, with a chronic extensor plantar response. The left leg was much less spastic but there was loss of pain and temperature sensation to T3 on the right and posture impairment in both lower limbs, more marked on the left. The picture was typical of the insidious development of a spastic paraparesis with marked sensory deficit and the possibility of radiotherapy damage to the spinal cord had to be considered, although the delay of nearly 8 years since the radiotherapy suggested that this was unlikely. An MRI scan revealed cord compression by an extensive intradural tumour, with marked cord compression.

This was successfully removed and proved to be neurofibroma.

It is interesting to speculate that the original symptoms 16 years previously could have been related to the presence of this neurofibroma, and that what were thought to be symptoms due to ulnar nerve lesions were in fact due to C8 root irritation. Against this diagnosis, however, is the very long delay and the virtual clearance of those symptoms in the interim, but it is also unusual for ulnar nerve compressive lesions to settle, so the possibility that these were the first symptoms of this tumour remains unresolved.

The Lumbar Spine and Lumbar Disc Lesions

The most important anatomical difference between the cervical and the lumbar spine is that the spinal cord ends opposite the lower border of L1 vertebra. Therefore, lumbar disc lesions can **only** cause root syndromes. Any lesion below L1 vertebral level cannot cause spinal cord damage or a spastic paraparesis. It is also important to recognize that as there are eight cervical roots and only seven cervical vertebra, the relationship of the root to the interspace also alters below T1. Therefore, the lumbar roots emerge **below** their respective vertebrae, that is, the L4 root emerges at the L4/5 interspace. It is also less well recognized that a disc lesion may damage a root **anywhere** between its origin from the cord and its exit foramen: the S1 root, for example, could be damaged anywhere along its 6-inch intraspinal course. Fortunately, disc lesions **do** damage the appropriate root in the majority of cases because individual roots are always most vulnerable just above their exit foramen. They are then the most anterior and most lateral root in the canal and lie in the immediate path of a lateral disc prolapse (Figs 15.15 and 15.16).

The root exits very high in its foramen, often above a disc that is prolapsing into its own interspace. Because of this the disc usually damages the root that is passing to the interspace below. Thus, a disc lesion at L4/5 will damage the L5 root and a disc at L5/S1 will damage the S1 root.

These anatomical features all require very careful consideration when one is investigating a patient with lumbar or sacral root lesions. Because of the peculiar anatomy of the cauda equina a neurofibroma on the L2 root could easily present as an apparent S1 root lesion. A serious error is the failure to examine the affected root up to its origin from the cord and only looking for a disc lesion appropriate to the symptoms. The following case report is a superb example of this particular problem.

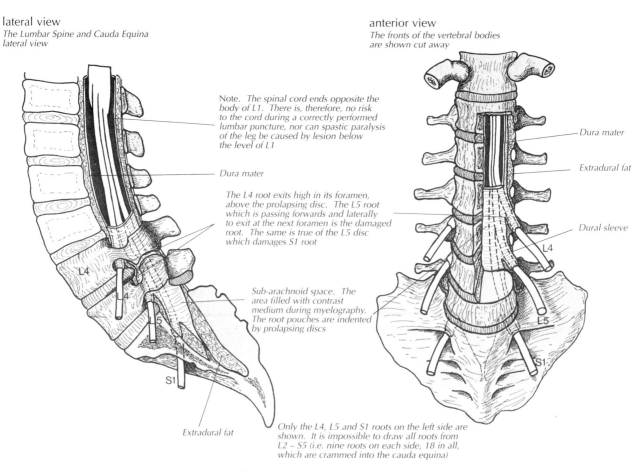

lateral view
*The Lumbar Spine and Cauda Equina
lateral view*

anterior view
*The fronts of the vertebral bodies
are shown cut away*

*Note. The spinal cord ends opposite the
body of L1. There is, therefore, no risk
to the cord during a correctly performed
lumbar puncture, nor can spastic paralysis
of the leg be caused by lesion below
the level of L1*

— *Dura mater*

*The L4 root exits high in its foramen,
above the prolapsing disc. The L5 root
which is passing forwards and laterally
to exit at the next foramen is the damaged
root. The same is true of the L5 disc
which damages S1 root*

*Sub-arachnoid space. The
area filled with contrast
medium during myelography.
The root pouches are indented
by prolapsing discs*

— *Dura mater*

— *Extradural fat*

— *Dural sleeve*

Extradural fat

*Only the L4, L5 and S1 roots on the left side are
shown. It is impossible to draw all roots from
L2 – S5 (i.e. nine roots on each side, 18 in all,
which are crammed into the cauda equina)*

15.15   The lumbar spine and cauda equina.

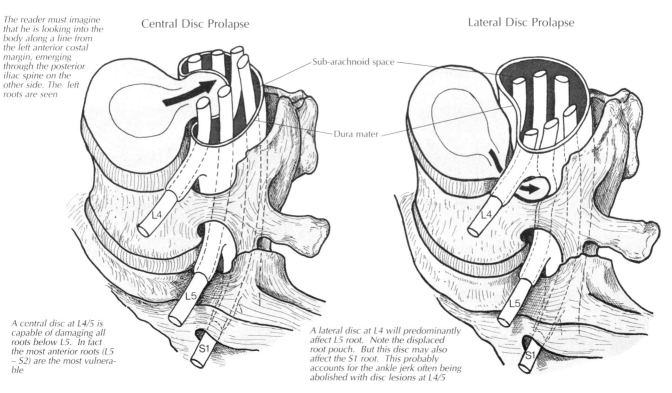

*The reader must imagine
that he is looking into the
body along a line from
the left anterior costal
margin, emerging
through the posterior
iliac spine on the
other side. The left
roots are seen*

Central Disc Prolapse

Lateral Disc Prolapse

Sub-arachnoid space

Dura mater

*A central disc at L4/5 is
capable of damaging all
roots below L5. In fact
the most anterior roots (L5
– S2) are the most vulnerable*

*A lateral disc at L4 will predominantly
affect L5 root. Note the displaced
root pouch. But this disc may also
affect the S1 root. This probably
accounts for the ankle jerk often being
abolished with disc lesions at L4/5*

15.16   Central and lateral disc prolapse.

CASE REPORT V

A 26-year-old man presented with a complete right foot drop that had come on acutely while playing football 6 months previously. He related that he had been dribbling the ball when his foot turned over with a horrifying crack, his ankle blew up like a balloon and since that time he had had a foot drop. He had already had a reportedly negative radiculogram and normal nerve conduction studies elsewhere. There was little wasting and a review in 6 weeks' time was recommended. He failed to attend and was not seen again for 5 years. He returned because not only had the foot drop failed to improve but he had by then developed some weakness in the calf muscles, and had fasciculation in the right thigh and both the right ankle jerk and knee jerk were absent. Electrophysiological studies suggested damage to L4, L5 and S1. A CT can of the L4/5 and L5/S1 interspaces was normal. The myelogram was repeated and a large tumour was demonstrated in the region of the conus at L1/2 level. When the original radiculogram films were reviewed the lesion was clearly present. At operation this

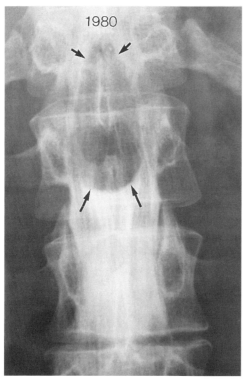
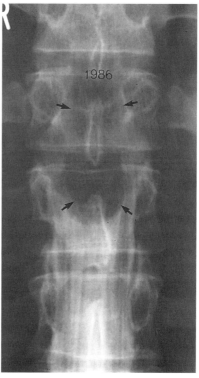

Lesion present but not seen in 1980   *Lesion first identified in 1986*

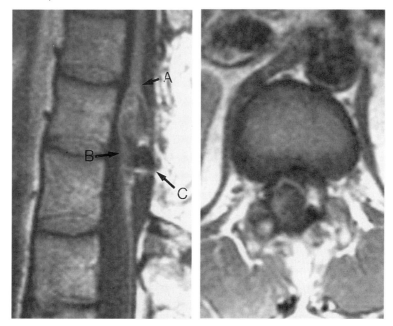

MRI scan 1993. Normal spinal cord (A); expanded spinal cord (B); and dermoid tumour (C)

CRV.   *Dermoid tumour at L1–2 presenting as foot drop.*

proved to be an intradural dermoid tumour arising within the spinal cord, containing epidermoid sebaceous tissue and hair but no bone or teeth. Total removal proved impossible but all his new symptoms rapidly improved, although the foot drop persisted. Five years later his symptoms recurred and an MRI scan revealed recurrent tumour; a further attempt at radical removal was made. He again improved and continues under annual review.

There are many lessons to be learned from this case: how totally misleading the mode of onset can be, the danger of misdiagnosis on radiculography unless the contrast is followed to at least T10 level, and the importance of follow-up, provided the patient complies. Once again, the importance of personally reviewing all previous X-ray films rather than accepting a written report is apparent.

The other major consideration is based on the frequency of disc lesions at various sites. Lesions affecting L5 and S1 roots account for some 95% of disc lesions. Lesions affecting L2, L3 and L4 account for only 5% and the majority of these are at the L4 level. It follows that L2 and L3 root lesions and S2, S3, S4 and S5 root lesions are very unlikely to be the result of uncomplicated disc disease, and urgent investigation is indicated. For more detailed discussion of the clinical features of individual root lesions see also Chapter 17.

There are five syndromes produced by upper lumbar disc lesions.

Anterior Thigh Pain

Pain in the anterior thigh, with wasting of the quadriceps and an absent knee jerk, can be produced by lesions affecting the L3 or L4 roots. Disc lesions are an unusual cause of this picture. Metastatic carcinoma of the prostate gland and diabetic amyotrophy are the main conditions to be excluded. Anterolateral thigh pain without muscle weakness is usually due to meralgia paraesthetica.

Low Back Pain without Radicular Symptoms

So much reliance is placed on radicular symptoms in the leg that if these are absent the question of a disc lesion may not be raised. Occasionally, lesions at the L3/4 level may produce severe local back pain without radicular pain. The most ominous historical feature is rest pain. If the back pain is worse at night or in a lying position, the chance of finding a serious underlying cause is very high.

Sciatic Syndrome

A disc lesion as high as L2/3 interspace may fail to damage the most appropriate root (L3) and present as pain in the L5 or S1 distribution, or even present as bilateral lower root pain syndromes. This adds further emphasis to the need for a complete myelographic or MRI examination of the area, up to and including the lower spinal cord.

Acute Cauda Equina Syndrome

An acute disc prolapse at the L2/3 level may cause bilateral multiple root lesions. The patient will typically complain of severe bilateral leg pain, flaccid paralysis of both legs and retention of urine. This is a surgical emergency, immediately myelography or MRI scan and exploration of the cauda equina is indicated.

Claudication of the Cauda Equina

Severe stenotic lumbar canal disease at any level may cause this syndrome. At lower levels claudication of a single root may occur, but at higher lumbar levels a more general ischaemia of the whole cauda equina may be experienced. This is discussed in greater detail in Chapters 14 and 17.

Cauda Equina Lesions

A lesion in the spinal canal at any level below the T10 vertebra can cause a cauda equina syndrome. There is a dangerous tendency to think of the cauda equina as comprising only the nerve roots lying within the sacrum. The cauda equina includes the terminal spinal cord, all the spinal roots from T12 to S5 and the filum terminale, which is the fibrous band that extends from the tip of the cord to attach to the sacrum (see Fig. 15.15).

Cauda Equina Lesions in Childhood

The embryology of the vertebral column has already been described and the variety of developmental defects that may occur in the lumbosacral region mentioned. It is important to remember that disc lesions are exceedingly rare before 15 years of age.

Symptoms Present Since Birth

Spina Bifida Occulta

Many patients with spina bifida occulta remain asymptomatic throughout life, but associated developmental abnormalities may cause problems. Progressive wasting and weakness affecting particularly muscles supplied by the L4, L5 and S1 roots may be found. Absent ankle jerks and trophic changes in the feet, often first manifest as recurrent chilblains, may occur. The picture may remain static but close follow-up until the teens is necessary to exclude any further progression.

Spina Bifida Cystica

Severe defects in the vertebral column are associated with variable degrees of neural abnormality. These include bulging meninges (meningocoele), a sac containing parts of the terminal cord and nerve roots (myelomeningocoele), and a lump of malformed neural tissue lying free on the surface (myelocoele). Both latter varieties are often associated with aqueduct stenosis and hydrocephalus. The consequences of aggressive surgical treatment of these lesions was discussed earlier.

Symptoms Occurring in Later Childhood

Mild developmental abnormalities of the cauda equina may not produce any disability at birth but the ascent of the spinal cord in the first 5 years of life may cause problems due to cord tethering. Occasionally symptoms or signs may not occur until adulthood.

CASE REPORT VI

A 25-year-old tractor driver presented with pain in his legs. He had been known to have a soft swelling over the lower end of his spine since birth, which had only recently been identified as a meningocoele. Over 5 years he had complained of increasing difficulty with micturition. Surprisingly, he claimed that sexual function was entirely normal. This led to referral to a genitourinary medicine clinic, which occasioned some embarrassment for his wife. He was then referred to the urology clinic, where investigations failed to demonstrate any abnormality of his urinary tract. His problem was sudden painful incontinence of urine if he did not respond instantly. He had noticed that if he worked in a flexed position while sitting on his tractor he developed very severe pain down the back of both legs and perineal numbness. This would improve within minutes of standing up. On physical examination, there was a large soft meningocoele with no cutaneous abnormality. There was saddle anaesthesia from S2 to S5 on the left and from S1 and S5 on the right. Both ankle jerks were absent and there was wasting in both calf muscles. The plantar responses were uncertain owing to numbness in the feet. An MRI scan revealed a torpedo-shaped lesion tethering the spinal cord, which at operation proved to be an intradural lipoma of the filum terminale. His pain cleared but micturition difficulty persists.

The development of weakness, numbness, trophic change or disparity in the size or shape of the feet should prompt careful investigation. Pain is an unusual feature in the developmental cauda equina syndromes of childhood. Pain should prompt an urgent search for evidence of primary malignant disease in the vertebral column or sacrum: retroperitoneal malignancy and the possibility of seeding of the lumbar theca by a medulloblastoma should be considered.

Cauda Equina Lesions in the Adult

There are three main clinical pictures.

Lateral Cauda Equina Syndrome (Fig. 15.17)

The most frequent cause of the lateral cauda equina syndrome is a neurofibroma. Rarely, a high disc lesion may be responsible. The symptoms include anterior thigh pain, quadriceps wasting, weakness of inversion of the foot (L4 root lesion) and an absent knee jerk. If the lesion is very high and lies lateral to the terminal spinal cord there may even be pyramidal signs below the lesion, in which case the ankle jerks may be very brisk with ankle clonus and an extensor plantar

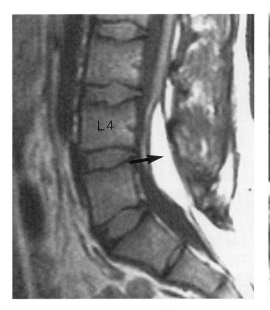
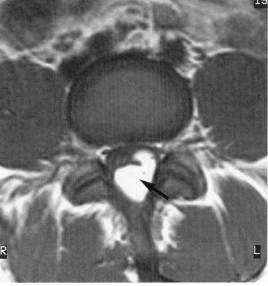

CRVI.   *Intradural lipoma associated with meningocoele and symptoms due to cord tethering (arrows indicates the lipoma)*

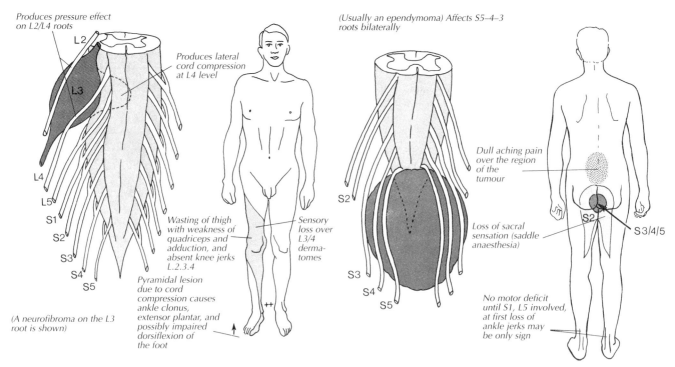

15.17   Lateral cauda equina syndrome.

15.18   Midline cauda equina lesion.

response. With these signs any sphincter disturbance is likely to be due to the cord compression. (See Case Report I in Chapter 17)

Midline Cauda Equina Lesions from Within
(Fig. 15.18)

This is also known as a 'conus lesion'. The usual causes are an ependymoma, a dermoid tumour or a lipoma of the terminal cord. The roots are damaged from the inside, i.e. S5 → S4 → S3 and so on. The initial symptoms include rectal pain, genital pain, micturition disturbances and loss of potency, with no definite physical signs unless the perianal sensation and anal reflex are carefully tested. Later loss of the ankle jerks and weakness of the L5 and S1 muscle groups will occur. In the case of an ependymoma the patient may have a 5-year history of dull backache before any other symptoms or signs appear.

CASE REPORT VII

A 38-year-old man presented with a 5 year history of urinary urgency, constipation, bilateral sciatic pain and impotence. He normally lived in the Orkneys and had only sought advice on the 'off-chance' while in the area on a course. Physical examination revealed marked wasting of the legs below the knee, and generalized impairment of sensation over both L5 and S1 root distributions. A radiculogram revealed a large lesion occupying the sacral sac. At operation this was found to be a myxopapillary ependymoma, which was successfully removed, with remarkable resolution of his long-standing symptoms, before his return home.

In this instance the anticipated sacral sensory loss was not present, although undoubtedly sacral root dysfunction was a major component of his presenting symptoms. It would have been difficult to explain these symptoms on the basis of a disc lesion unless an extremely rare central disc at upper lumbar level were postulated.

Midline Cauda Equina Lesions From Outside

The hallmark of this situation is bilateral lumbar and sacral root lesions. Root pain in unusual dermatomes – L2 or L3 or S2 or S3 – should be regarded with great suspicion. Pain in an L4, L5 or S1 distribution may be readily and not unreasonably attributed to simple disc disease. Severe pain not relieved by appropriate measures and the detection of neurological signs indicates the need for investigation, not just to confirm a disc lesion but to exclude alternative pathology. In the adult the alternatives are extremely unpleasant, and include primary sacral bone tumours (chordomas), metastatic disease (especially prostatic disease), reticulosis, leukaemia or direct seeding from malignant tumours in the CNS, notably medulloblastomas, ependymomas or pinealomas.

CASE REPORT VIII

A 20-year-old woman was admitted as an emergency with severe headaches of 1 month's duration and papilloedema. She gave a 5-year history of left S1 root pain, ascribed by a neurosurgeon to a disc lesion. On physical examination there was papilloedema, neck stiffness, a positive Kernig's test and an absent left ankle jerk. An ependymoma with a spinal sub-arachnoid haemorrhage was suspected but at operation a piloid astrocytoma was found, with evidence of recent haem-orrhage.

This case emphasizes the danger of diagnosing a disc lesion in a 15-year-old and the surprisingly slow clinical course of lesions in this situation. The cause of papilloedema in such cases is uncertain: it has been attributed to very high CSF protein but in this instance CSF from above the tumour was not obtained, and whether this was the cause was not established. The papilloedema was no longer in evidence when the patient was reviewed 10 years later because of instability at the level of her laminectomy.

Proctalgia Fugax

An important benign cause of rectal pain that must be considered here is the benign but excruciating syndrome known as proctalgia fugax. This can occur in either sex at any age, but seems to be more frequent in men. Attacks are mainly nocturnal and may accompany erection or ejaculation. The pain is an intense gripping sensation around the rectum about 2" inside the anal ring. Attacks typically last 15–20 minutes and then subside. Bearing down may relieve the pain slightly. It is thought to be due to cramp in the levator ani muscles.

Depressive Rectal Pain

In recent years an increasing number of men, usually elderly widowers have been seen complaining of a constant burning pain, likened to a red-hot poker in the rectum. It is present 24 hours a day and interferes with all activities. It defies surgical diagnosis and treatment, which is assiduously sought by the patient. The pain has many features in its quality and persistence that are similar to the painful tongue syndrome of elderly ladies who also have an underlying cancer phobia (see Chapter 21). It may well represent a monosymptomatic depression and sometimes responds to amitriptyline.

Although low backache and various aches and pains in the perineum and the legs are one of the most frequent reasons for hospital referral, the importance of detecting unusual features in the history and a careful neurological examination in all cases is mandatory.

Tumours and the Spinal Cord

Now that the anatomy of the spinal cord in relation to the vertebrae has been fully described it is appropriate to consider tumours and the spinal cord. This subject

has been deferred until this stage because from an investigational and pathological point of view the relationship of the tumour to the vertebral column is of great importance. Furthermore, the relationship of the tumour to the cord and its coverings often provides a preoperative clue to the pathology, and to some extent governs the surgical approach.

As so often in neurological disease, we have to consider cord tumours in children and adults separately as there is a dramatic difference in the pathological possibilities in different age groups and, for certain tumours, a marked difference in the sex incidence. As with cerebral tumours, there is also a significant risk of a spinal tumour being due to a metastasis from malignant disease elsewhere.

In stark contrast to cerebral tumours, 50% of spinal tumours in children are metastatic, usually by direct spread from retroperitoneal neuroblastomas, ganglioneuromas or sarcomas.

In adults some 20%–30% of all spinal tumours are metastatic. Metastases from carcinoma of the breast in the female (68%) and the prostate in the male (40%) account for the majority. Tumours in the lung (25%), thyroid (15%), uterus and cervix (10%) and direct spread into the spinal canal of Hodgkin's disease and multiple myeloma are the other major causes. In most instances plain films will often show evidence of either the primary lesion or the bone involvement, and often the site of the primary can be suspected from the nature of the plain film changes.

Tumours in both groups are defined as extradural, intradural/extramedullary and intramedullary if actually within the substance of the cord.

The striking difference between childhood and adulthood is best seen in the classification in Table 15.1.

When a patient presents with symptoms and signs suggesting a cord lesion the initial clinical evaluation should enable a distinction to be made between an intrinsic (intramedullary) lesion of the cord and a compressive (extradural or intradural) lesion. Considering the age, sex and site of the damage the probable nature of the lesion can be deduced but operative diagnosis and histology is always required. The following brief profiles of different tumours may be used as a guide.

1. *Neurofibromas*: Sex incidence equal, 30–50 years age, 60% above L1 causing spastic paraparesis, 30% below L1 causing a lateral cauda equina syndrome.

2. *Meningiomas*: Female/male ratio 9:1 usually at mid-thoracic level (T3–T6). Few in foramen magnum, where the female/male ratio falls to 2:1.

3. *Ependymomas*: Male/female ratio 2:1, average age 30 years, either intrinsic within cord at C6–T2

Table 15.1 Age differences in spinal tumour type

	Childhood			Adulthood	
Extradural	(50 %)	Neuroblastomas Ganglioneuromas Sarcomas		(20 %)	Chordomas Sarcomas
Intradural	(10 %)	Meningiomas Neurofibromas Lipomas Angiomas		(60 %)	Meningiomas Neurofibromas
Intramedullary	(40 %)	Ependymomas Epidermoid tumours		(20 %)	Gliomas Ependymomas

(mimics a syringomyelic cavity) or on the filum terminale (central cauda equina syndrome). Very high incidence of associated syringomyelic cavitation, making the lesion seem much more extensive than its actual size.

4. *Gliomas*: Sex incidence equal, average age 35–45 years, nearly all in cervical cord and quite rare.

5. *Dermoids*: All sacrococcygeal in location, usually associated with spina bifida typically present at 15–20 years of age.

6 *Chordomas*: Slight male predominance, 80% sacrococcygeal, 12% in sphenoid. Considerable bone destruction and pain are major features.

7. *Vascular tumours*: Vascular tumours affecting the cord are discussed in Chapter 14.

Investigation of Spinal Tumours

Routine physical examination and chest X-ray to exclude a primary neoplasm is essential. A rectal examination is particularly important in the male to detect carcinoma of the prostate and a careful examination of the breast in the female is appropriate.

In the absence of any focal signs or symptoms to indicate the level of the tumour the cervical spine, including the foramen magnum and the thoracic spine, including at least the L1 vertebra, should be X-rayed if the clinical picture indicates a spastic paraparesis. If the picture is one of low backache, lumbar root pain and mixed upper and lower motor neuron signs in the legs the region T10–L3 is the most important from a radiological point of view. If there is rectal or genital pain the sacrum should be included in the X-rays but the importance of including the spinal column up to T10 level must be stressed.

MRI scanning of the appropriate level of the spinal canal is now the investigation of choice for all suspected spinal lesions where bony abnormality is not demonstrable on plain X-ray. Where MRI scanning is not available, myelography is still the only alternative investigation. In spite of concern that iodophenylate (myodil) may have caused adhesive arachnoiditis,

there was no other substance available for nearly 30 years. The earliest water-soluble contrast medium, caused considerable problems, epileptic fits during the procedure and bilateral central dislocation of the hips due to muscle spasm being two of the most serious; the successor metrizimide was not entirely innocuous and has now been replaced by methglucimide (Niopam).

The old rules surrounding myelography still apply: a lumbar puncture should not be attempted if it is anticipated that myelography will be needed within the next few days, as subsequently it might be very difficult; a Queckenstedt test should not be done for fear of upsetting the delicate dynamic balance if there is a cord compressing lesion; and finally myelography should not be undertaken unless neurosurgical facilities are readily available if a lesion is demonstrated, as sudden deterioration after the procedure is not uncommon.

Micturition and Neurological Disease
(Fig. 15.19)

Micturition disturbances are a common feature of spinal cord disease and cauda equina lesions and it is therefore appropriate to discuss them at this point.

The normal anatomy and physiology of micturition is not well understood and hence the mechanisms of micturition disturbance in disease remain rather speculative. Males have a very considerable advantage over females in both length of urethra and additional sphincter mechanisms designed to isolate the bladder and contract the urethra during erection and ejaculation. In males the detrusor fibres at the bladder neck form an internal sphincter. In females they do not and the main sphincteric action is derived from the muscle fibres surrounding the urethra.

The angle the bladder makes with the urethra is important and in both sexes collapse of the pelvic floor, allowing the bladder to flop back, or gross faecal impaction, by tilting the bladder forward, may have an effect on bladder function for purely mechanical reasons.

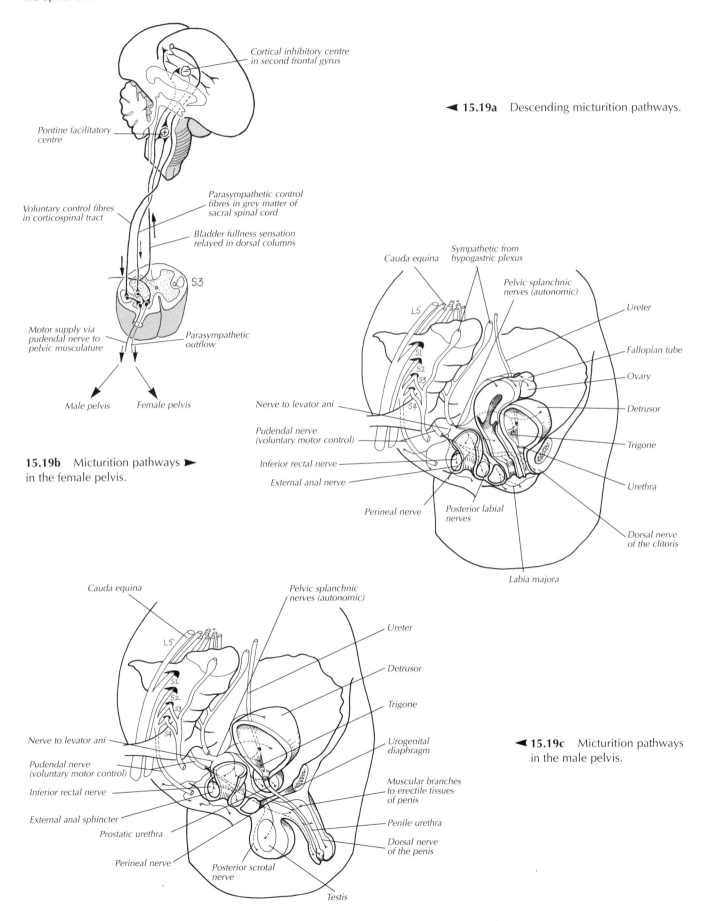

Cortical inhibitory centre
in second frontal gyrus

Pontine facilitatory
centre

Voluntary control fibres
in corticospinal tract

Parasympathetic control
fibres in grey matter of
sacral spinal cord

Bladder fullness sensation
relayed in dorsal columns

S3

Motor supply via
pudendal nerve to
pelvic musculature

Parasympathetic
outflow

Male pelvis

Female pelvis

15.19a Descending micturition pathways.

15.19b Micturition pathways
in the female pelvis.

Cauda equina

Sympathetic from
hypogastric plexus

Pelvic splanchnic
nerves (autonomic)

Ureter

L5

Fallopian tube

S1

Ovary

S2

Detrusor

S3

Nerve to levator ani

S4

Trigone

Pudendal nerve
(voluntary motor control)

Urethra

Inferior rectal nerve

External anal nerve

Dorsal nerve
of the clitoris

Perineal nerve

Posterior labial
nerves

Labia majora

Cauda equina

Pelvic splanchnic
nerves (autonomic)

Ureter

L5

Detrusor

S1

Trigone

S2

S3

Urogenital
diaphragm

Nerve to levator ani

S4

Pudendal nerve
(voluntary motor control)

Muscular branches
to erectile tissues
of penis

Inferior rectal nerve

External anal sphincter

Penile urethra

Prostatic urethra

Dorsal nerve
of the penis

Perineal nerve

Posterior scrotal
nerve

Testis

15.19c Micturition pathways
in the male pelvis.

There is a true external sphincter muscle under voluntary control at the urogenital diaphragm which is only just capable of controlling continence – a fact well known to examination candidates!

The initial assessment of any patient with bladder dysfunction must include details of any drugs that might affect bladder function, exclude the possibility of urinary tract infection, consider prostatic hypertrophy and the possible mechanical effect of severe constipation on the bladder neck.

The anatomy of the bladder and pelvis is shown schematically in Figure 15.19. It is important to notice that part of the urethra lies in the abdomen and is subject to the same external pressure alterations as the bladder itself, so that a high pressure differential is not created by coughing or sneezing.

The neural control of the bladder is extremely complicated. There are three basic reflex mechanisms involved:

1. A vesicosympathetic reflex which relaxes the bladder and tightens the urethra.
2. A vesicoparasympathetic reflex, which contracts the detrusor and relaxes the urethra.
3. A vesicopudendal reflex based on motor cells in the lateral ventral horn at S3 level (Onuf's nucleus), which controls the striated muscle of the pelvic floor and the external sphincter and which is inhibited during micturition.

The following details are fundamental to an understanding of pathological bladder function.

1. The bladder is basically a hollow bag of smooth muscle containing stretch receptors and contracting under the influence of parasympathetic nerves. This constitutes an autonomic stretch reflex which spends 99% of its time accommodating increasing volumes of urine without allowing the intravesical pressure to rise.

2. The parasympathetic reflex is based on the S3 roots and S3 segment of the cord.

3. The stretch receptors fire impulses proportional to the stretch of the bladder wall and the weight of urine in the bladder. Therefore, there is less afferent activity when lying down than when standing: hence the instant desire to pass urine on getting up in the morning. Any infection or inflammation of the bladder wall will heighten the sensitivity of the stretch receptors. Stimulation of the perineum and anal canal inhibits the discharge.

4. The basic sacral reflex arc controls micturition in infancy, senility, unconsciousness and following various lesions to the nervous system.

5. The voluntary mechanisms involve inhibition of the conditioned reflex, some volitional control over the hypothalamic and pontine facilitating centres, and direct physical control over the rather weak external sphincter and pelvic floor. This is all controlled by an area in the second frontal gyrus and the main descending pathways lie in or adjacent to the corticospinal tracts. This accounts for the early disturbance of micturition control in patients with spinal cord compression and the early loss of bladder control associated with parasagittal intracranial lesions (see Chapter 8).

6. The sympathetic outflow from T11 to L2 via the hypogastric plexus descends into the pelvis and has an essentially inhibitory role in micturition. It relaxes the detrusor muscles, inhibits transmission in parasympathetic ganglia, contracts the trigone and the urethra and may have a role in the urethral sphincter mechanism. All these actions oppose the onset of micturition.

Micturition involves complete relaxation of volitional control. The external sphincter and pelvic floor relax and the local reflex is allowed to take over. As the detrusor contracts the bladder neck is pulled open and this combined with inhibition of the weak internal sphincter, allows urine to flow by a combination of rising intravesical pressure and gravity. If there is any mechanical obstruction to flow an additional voluntary increase in intra-abdominal pressure by a combination of the Valsalva manoeuvre and contraction of the abdominal muscles comes into play. This is the cause of the condition known as micturition syncope (see Chapter 22).

Neurological Disorders Affecting Bladder Function

It is important that a low pressure is maintained in the bladder at all times. Large floppy bladders do not have sustained high pressures and although there is an infection risk due to urine stasis, back pressure effects on the kidney are less likely to occur. Small high-pressure bladders, as found in spinal cord disease, are potentially much more hazardous as the high back pressures may rapidly lead to secondary renal damage.

There are four main types of neurological bladder dysfunction.

Uninhibited Bladder

This condition is due to a lesion affecting the second frontal gyrus and the pathways leading from it down to the pontine centre. These include local lesions, such as frontal lobe tumours, parasagittal meningiomas, anterior communicating artery aneurysms, normal pressure hydrocephalus, Parkinson's disease and multisystem atrophy. In the latter incontinence is always associated with impotence. If loss of control of micturition is an early feature of dementia, a focal frontal lesion should be carefully excluded. The features are:

Urgency at low bladder volumes (detrusor hyper-reflexia)

Sudden uncontrollable evacuation.

No residual urine therefore little risk of infection

If severe intellectual deterioration occurs urine may be passed at random, without appropriate concern.

Lesions at pontine level, although theoretically capable of causing a similar picture, are likely to present with rather more dramatic neurological problems than uncontrolled voiding of urine. In 75% of children who have pontine gliomas **retention** of urine is an early feature, often associated with pyramidal features and internuclear ophthalmoplegia. MRI scanning has revealed that the lesions usually lie in the dorsal pons and midbrain. It would seem likely that damage to the pontine facilitatory centre or pathways allow essentially inhibitory mechanisms to operate.

Spinal Bladder

This condition results from damage to the spinal cord by trauma, cord tumour, multiple sclerosis or other spinal lesions. The features are:

1. Bladder fullness is not appreciated and intravesical pressure rises may only be indicated by sweating, pallor, flexor spasms and dramatic rises in the blood pressure. This may be so high that the diagnosis of phaeochromocytoma may be suspected unless this well known reflex response is appreciated.

2. Reflex emptying of the bladder may occur without warning.

3. Evacuation may be incomplete but may improve with practice and sometimes be performed at will, if the bladder is massaged and suprapubic pressure is applied. The basic condition is known as detrusor–sphincter dyssynergia. There will always be evidence of bilateral pyramidal lesions in such patients, such as enhanced reflexes and extensor plantar responses.

The bladder is small and contracted and only capable of holding a maximal volume of 250 ml.

Autonomous Bladder (Subsacral Lesions)

An autonomous bladder results from damage to the motor and sensory components in the cauda equina or pelvis. It is a feature of cauda equina lesions, pelvic surgery, pelvic malignant disease, spina bifida and high lumbar disc lesions. An MRI scan or myelogram to exclude a high disc lesion is obligatory in this situation, which can occur with minimal pain (see Case reports earlier in this chapter). The features are:

Continual dribbling incontinence

Considerable residual urine with high infection risk

No sensation of bladder fullness and a large atonic bladder

It may be associated with perineal numbness and loss of sexual function.

Sensory Bladder

Although the features are similar to an autonomous bladder the anatomical explanation is uncertain. It is an consequence of several rare disorders, such as tabes dorsalis and subacute combined degeneration of the cord it may also occur in multiple sclerosis and diabetes mellitus, conditions that have as a common denominator sensory deafferentation of the bladder and loss of the spinal reflex. This may lead to massive retention of urine. The features are:

Dribbling incontinence of sufficiently large volumes that the patient may claim that they have normal micturition

Residual urine measured in litres, with high infection risk

Voiding possible with considerable straining but evacuation is incomplete.

Retention of urine in the female is rare and is usually due to mechanical obstruction, such as uterine fibroids or an incarcerated pregnancy in the pelvis. Until recently hysteria was regarded as the only other cause, but sphincteric EMG studies have revealed the possibility of a functional disorder of the urethral sphincter mechanism, which is more highly developed in the female, which may be responsible in some cases. The diagnosis of hysterical retention should therefore be attached with some reservations until this possibility has been considered.

During history-taking the main questions to be asked of a patient with possible neurological bladder dysfunction are:

Do they have any sense of bladder filling?

Can they feel the urine passing?

Can they stop urine passing in midstream at will?

Does the bladder leak continually or suddenly pass large volumes?

Is there any associated rectal disorder?

Is there any disorder of potency in the male?

Is there any numbness in the perineum?

Based on the type of dysfunction identified, further history and examination must be directed to the exclusion of neurological disorders potentially responsible for the disorder described.

The methods of investigation now include biochemical investigation of renal function, urine examination and culture, measurement of residual urine after attempted complete evacuation, cystometrography, sphincteric electromyography and MRI of the brain and spinal cord. Further discussion of the specialized techniques is beyond the scope of this present text.

Neurological bladder dysfunction is very difficult to treat. Incontinence may be helped by anticholinergic drugs such as propantheline 15 mg t.d.s., imipramine 10–25 mg t.d.s. or the drug of choice, oxybutynin 5 mg t.d.s. If drugs fail various pelvic nerve sections, intermittent self-catheterization, urinary diversion procedures or the creation of an artificial bladder may have to be considered.

The most obvious solution, permanent catheterization, although effective in many instances, has the serious and potentially fatal risk of infection and has now been replaced in many cases by intermittent self-catheterization. Where the patient is unable to manage this, the use of silastic long-term catheters continues. In females the urethra may become so enlarged that the catheter is ineffective in preventing leakage of urine. The seriousness and misery of bladder dysfunction in neurological disease is a major and often insoluble problem of neurological management.

Disorders of Potency

Although the impact of perineal sensory loss or urinary incontinence is the same in both sexes the associated disorder of potency in the male is a source of great frustration and anxiety, and may lead to divorce in some 50% of patients with chronic neurological disease.

There are four components to sexual function in the male: erection, secretion, emission and ejaculation. All these are basically autonomic reflexes but the importance of psychic influences, intact descending spinal cord pathways and endocrine status greatly complicates the issue and leads to a wide range of possible causes of impotence that is not always easy to explain.

1. Erection requires a suitable psychic state and an intact parasympathetic reflex arc at S2/3. The sympathetic plays a role at this stage in improving blood flow. The initiation and maintenance of the erection requires a strong sensory input from the glans penis and adjacent skin, and this is mainly through the S2 dermatome. Sensory loss in this region is likely to be associated with damage to the reflex arc itself. Malignant infiltration of the S2/3 roots, usually due to malignant lymphomas or leukaemia, may cause a constant painful erection, a condition known as priapism.

2. Glandular secretions from the seminal vesicles, Cowper's gland and the prostate lubricate the urethra under parasympathetic control.

3. Emission of semen into the urethra is mediated via sympathetic activity in the vas deferens and closure of the bladder neck to prevent retrograde ejaculation into the bladder.

4. Ejaculation is partially voluntarily controlled by the rhythmic contraction of bulbocavernosus and ischiocavernosus muscles. This also permits a degree of voluntary inhibition of ejaculation at orgasm.

Causes of Loss of Potency

Psychiatric Disorders

Anxiety states, depression and psychoses may all cause impotence. In recent years it has also been recognized that impotence may be an early symptom of a temporal lobe tumour, and as such tumours may also be associated with personality changes there is a real risk of serious misdiagnosis. It has also been noted that there is a higher incidence of impotence in men with chronic temporal lobe epilepsy. A useful clue to intact reflex mechanisms is a history that the patient still has normal waking erections or that successful intercourse outside the marital situation has been achieved. If doubt still exists a strain gauge device round the penis may be used overnight to monitor erections, combined with EEG recording in a sleep laboratory, as nocturnal erections specifically occur during REM sleep.

Spinal Cord Lesions

Spinal cord compression, transection, multiple sclerosis, tabes dorsalis and subacute combined degeneration of the cord all cause impotence. In many instances the exact cause of the difficulty cannot be identified with certainty. Following spinal cord transection reflex erection occurs easily, even though there is no sensory appreciation at cortical level and no descending influences. Ejaculation rarely occurs in this situation.

Cauda Equina Lesions

Cauda equina lesions tend to affect erection by a combination of penile sensory loss and direct damage to the reflex arc. In this situation dribbling emission of semen may occur. Causes of cauda equina lesions are discussed earlier in this chapter.

Autonomic Nerve Lesions

Autonomic neuropathy occurs in diabetes mellitus, chronic polyneuropathy due to any cause (see Chapter

17) and as an important part of the Shy–Drager syndrome (see Chapter 12). Impotence is often the earliest symptom in these cases and is usually associated with micturition disturbance and postural hypotension. The sympathetic nerve supply itself may be injured by crush fractures of the L1 vertebra, damaging the hypogastric plexus, or by deliberate surgical extirpation for peripheral vascular disease. In both instances normal erections may occur but ejaculation is impossible or incomplete due to retrograde ejaculation into the bladder. Ganglion-blocking agents block both erection and ejaculation, but modern antihypertensive agents, which confine their action to adrenergic nerve endings, may impair ejaculation without affecting erection.

Renal Failure and Alcoholism

Both these medical conditions, owing to their effect on endocrine, vascular and nerve function, commonly cause impotence.

Endocrine Disorders

Potency is affected in many endocrine diseases in which the clinical signs are usually obvious. From a neurological point of view the most important consideration is the possibility of hyperprolactinaemia or panhypopituitarism due to a pituitary tumour. In the male the first symptom is invariably declining sexual function, often occurring several years before field defects or headaches appear (see Chapter 3). The patient himself rarely mentions this symptoms unless specifically asked. Usually the wife refers to the problem colloquially as 'he hasn't been himself'. Body hair, skin texture and testicular size should be assessed, the visual fields examined, plain X-rays of the pituitary fossa taken and, where suspicion is high, an MRI scan of the hypothalamus and pituitary region should be performed.

The ready availability of prolactin assays has transformed the investigation of male impotence, and impotence due to hyperprolactinaemia is now readily identifiable and more common than previously appreciated. Most endocrinological departments can provide full screening to exclude subclinical endocrine dysfunction and this is recommended in those patients who are impotent and are thought not to have psychological problems or neurological disease.

Vascular Disease

The association of erectile impotence with vascular disease, due either to inadequate arterial flow or to venous incompetence, has recently been recognized and investigation using penile blood pressure recordings with a Doppler probe enables the condition to be identified. Intracavernous papaverine can also be used as a diagnostic test: A normal erection will be produced in patients with endocrine and neurogenic impotence but not in those with vascular disease. The use of venous occlusive devices or vacuum devices may provide some help in vascular impotence.

Treatment

A range of surgical procedures have been devised for impotence, involving the insertion of solid plastic rods or inflatable plastic tubes into the dorsum of the penis. The value appears to be cosmetic rather than satisfying for the partners involved. A more successful approach is the use of self-injected intracavernous papaverine, as noted above. With the exception of vascular impotence a satisfactory erection is achieved but may persist longer than is desirable and require medical assistance to achieve detumescence. It does not necessarily permit ejaculation, and where the penis is insensitive the injected party obtains little or no sexual satisfaction. Many patients abandon the technique once its limitations become apparent. Sadly, it rarely prevents marital break-up where sexual dysfunction has become a source of conflict.

Lumbar Puncture

For both anatomical and clinical reasons it is appropriate at this point to discuss lumbar puncture, the procedure that is most often used in the investigation of suspected spinal cord disease and peripheral nerve diseases, which are discussed in Chapter 19.

In spite of repeated pleas from neurologists and neurosurgeons, general physicians in hospitals that lack neurological facilities continue to regard lumbar puncture as an alternative to more precise diagnostic procedures such as CT or MRI scanning. Used in this way the test may be extremely hazardous and, far from helping to clarify the situation, it may result in the neurological unit having to accept a moribund patient requiring life-saving procedures instead of diagnosis.

Many years ago a general medical firm borrowed a bed on the neurological service during their 'take' day. Unknown to the neurologists a lumbar puncture was performed on a teenage girl with a short history of headache, vomiting and ataxia. Not only was a pressure into the bulb of the manometer recorded, but a second manometer was mounted on to the first so that the rise in pressure when the Queckenstedt test was performed could be seen. Fortunately, the patient, who had a cerebellar tumour, survived this potentially lethal investigation and the CSF was quite normal apart from the grossly raised pressure, so that no useful information was gained. Nowadays the failure to do a preliminary CT scan in this situation could be regarded as negligent.

Apparently the reason for embarking on the lumbar puncture was 'because there was no papilloedema'. This is a perennial fallacy. Often a whole series of doctors will take a vote on whether or not a patient has papilloedema and then require a neurologist to give the casting vote. If the history is such that there seems to be a real possibility that the intracranial pressure ought to be raised, **whether or not** there is papilloedema is of no consequence – lumbar puncture should **not** be attempted. It is likely that the risk of coning is greatest in the very acute situation where papilloedema has not had time to develop than where a long slow pressure rise has already led to some compensatory brain shifts and a tenuous equilibrium has been established.

Although these cautionary comments may seem a strange way to introduce a description intended to make lumbar puncture easier to perform, it would be unforgivable not to include these reservations, and whenever a lumbar puncture is contemplated the following questions should be considered:

1. Why am I doing this lumbar puncture? Is it because it is the only test available to me?
2. What positive information will it give me? Just to confirm that it is normal is a dubious indication.
3. Is this a potentially hazardous situation? Is there anything in the history to suggest that the patient may have raised intracranial pressure?

This raises the question of the so-called 'careful' lumbar puncture. Apart from the obvious implication that a majority of lumbar punctures are less than careful, there can be no such thing. Either the sub-arachnoid space is entered by a needle or it is not. Once a hole is made the fluid will continue to leak out after the needle is withdrawn. Although a smaller needle may slow the rate of leakage the risk of coning is still present. In the UK lumbar puncture still enjoys a fearsome reputation among patients, who often refer to it as a 'lumbar punch' – possibly an accurate description in some instances?

Indications for Examination of the CSF

Peripheral Nerve Diseases

Suspected Guillain–Barré syndrome (acute infective polyneuritis)
Diabetic polyneuropathy, especially the proximal variety affecting the leg
Suspected hypertrophic polyneuritis (Dejerine–Sottas disease).

Suspected immunologically based peripheral neuropathy.

Lumbar puncture and CSF examination is a standard investigation in all cases of peripheral neuropathy.

Suspected CNS Infection

In all cases of suspected meningitis or cerebral abscess a CT scan should be performed before lumbar puncture if the facilities are available. Even in uncomplicated meningitis the patient's clinical condition may deteriorate markedly following lumbar puncture if there is significant cerebral oedema. It has even been suggested that in childhood, broad-spectrum antibiotics, without lumbar puncture, may be the management of choice. Suspected viral, bacterial or fungal meningitis and suspected neurosyphilis (primary, secondary or tertiary) are other indications.

As an example of the potential hazards of lumbar puncture in this situation the following case may be cited.

CASE REPORT IX

An 18-year-old girl had been sent into A and E as a possible case of meningitis. Her GP father contacted a neurologist and asked if he would see her. The neurologist arrived in A and E just as a lumbar puncture trolley was being wheeled to the bedside. The girl was extremely drowsy, falling asleep before she could complete a sentence. She was pyrexial and had not only a stiff neck but also slight neck retraction. Although the plantar responses were flexor, the right pupil was slightly dilated and the reaction less brisk that on the left. No CT scanner was available but the lumbar puncture was aborted at the neurologist's insistence; immediate transfer to the neurosurgical unit on a mannitol infusion was arranged. On arrival, a CT scan confirmed that in addition to the meningitis she had blockage of the right foramen of Monro and massive dilatation of the right lateral ventricle, and was about to develop a tentorial pressure cone. Had the lumbar puncture been performed it is almost certain that she would have died immediately.

Suspected Intracranial Bleeding

Preliminary CT scanning may preclude the need for CSF confirmation of subarachnoid or intracerebral haemorrhage, much to the patient's advantage. Many patients deteriorated rapidly after CSF examination when that was the only way of confirming the diagnosis.

Suspected Multiple Sclerosis

For over 50 years CSF examination provided the only indirect confirmation of the clinical diagnosis of multiple sclerosis. Confirmation was based on finding a raised CSF protein, a positive Pandy test which indicates increased globulin content, and a paretic Lange curve, a protein precipitation test which in the absence of positive serology for syphilis was often found in patients with MS. In some acute cases a raised CSF white cell count was found, consisting mainly of lymphocytes. All these findings could indicate other disorders. In the 1970s the advent of immunoelectrophoresis of the CSF permitted the identification of specific proteins that were elevated in patients who had MS, and before MRI scanning became available a combination of raised CSF immunoglobulin, abnormal VERs and the clinical picture constituted a diagnostic triad for MS. MRI scanning has reduced the need for routine CSF examination, but where the scan leaves diagnostic uncertainty, or is not available, CSF examination still has an important role to play in diagnosis.

Contraindications to Lumbar Puncture

Suspected Raised Intracranial Pressure

Any patient with headaches who has definite signs of an intracerebral lesion in the hemisphere or in the posterior fossa should not have a lumbar puncture.

Headache

With the exception of suspected infection or subarachnoid haemorrhage, with their associated signs of meningeal irritation, and subject to the reservations noted above, lumbar puncture is obviously a potentially dangerous way of investigating headache. The only situation where lumbar puncture **to confirm** raised intracranial pressure is permissible is in patients who are thought to have benign intracranial hypertension, suggested by CT scanning. This is because subsequent repeat lumbar punctures are necessary to check the effectiveness of treatment in lowering the pressure.

Unconsciousness

Over 60% of unconscious patients do not have neurological disease, so that the CSF will be normal. The 40% who do have neurological problems are likely to be unconscious because of an intracranial 'catastrophe' and the chances of a lumbar puncture making the situation worse are considerable. Unless infection seems likely, lumbar puncture should await neurological advice and ideally be performed only after precautionary CT scanning.

Local Sepsis

Severe pustular acne on the back, or infected bedsores, greatly increases the risk of CSF examination and may possibly result in iatrogenic meningitis or epidural abscess. This risk is particularly high if a lumbar epidural abscess is already suspected, because traversing the abscess and entering the subarachnoid space will cause meningitis.

Suspected Spinal Cord Compression

In the past, if a lumbar puncture was performed in the investigation of suspected cord compression, the acute alteration of the CSF dynamics, especially during the Queckenstedt test, sometimes led to abrupt worsening of the clinical status. It also made it extremely difficult to perform a myelogram within the next few days because the contrast medium easily entered the subdural space under these circumstances. Therefore, not only was the patient's condition acutely worsened but the necessary subsequent investigation was made more difficult. Fortunately, MRI scanning, when available, has virtually replaced myelography in this acute situation. Where such facilities are not available these problems remain unavoidable and taxing for the neurologist involved. In such instances a myelogram, with the neurosurgeons already alerted, is the correct way to handle any situation in which the patient appears to have rapidly developing cord compression.

Neck Stiffness

This sign is widely recognized as the prime indication that a patient may have a subarachnoid haemorrhage or meningeal infection, but it must also be pointed out that it is also the physical sign that accompanies herniation of the cerebellar tonsils through the foramen magnum. Usually the clinical course in a patient with infection or haemorrhage will be a fairly acute one. If a patient becomes drowsy with a stiff neck after several days or weeks of illness it is as well to consider the possibility of coning, withholding lumbar puncture until a CT scan or urgent neurological advice can be obtained. It is also not unusual for patients with severe headache during viral illness or severe migraine to have both neck stiffness and photophobia, mimicking meningeal infection or haemorrhage.

The vast majority of patients sent to hospital with suspected meningitis have one of these conditions. In such instances the CSF will be normal but many of these patients are coded out as having had 'encephalitis', which is extremely rare in the UK and an unlikely diagnosis in a patient with a normal CSF. Others in the past have given such a convincing history of subarachnoid haemorrhage that it has been argued that even though the CSF was normal, 'the blood had not had time to get down to the lumbar theca' and they were subjected to four-vessel angiography anyway. The following is as good an example as could be devised to demonstrate the fallacy of this suggestion.

CASE REPORT X

A 37-year-old woman who had originally been seen 4 years previously with episodes of left-sided paresthaesiae thought to be due to migraine, was admitted with a history suggestive of a subarachnoid haemorrhage. In view of the previous history migraine was thought more likely, and it was decided to do a lumbar puncture to exclude haemorrhage rather than a CT scan to confirm one. The very experienced house physician achieved an atraumatic tap and slightly pink CSF emerged. It did not clear as the second specimen was taken, and yet did not look sufficiently blood stained to diagnose a subarachnoid haemorrhage. Suddenly the patient shouted 'Oh, my head', and as she did so the fluid instantly emerged at a faster rate and became heavily blood stained. The procedure was abandoned and a CT scan performed which revealed not only subarachnoid blood but also intraventricular blood in the right lateral ventricle. Further investigation and subsequent operation revealed a choroid plexus papilloma that might well have been responsible for her original symptoms, but she subsequently continued to have migraine headaches.

Technique of Lumbar Puncture

Notwithstanding these reservations and contraindications, once the decision to perform a lumbar puncture has been taken, it is worth performing properly. In the past many patients have required extensive investigation for what was an iatrogenic 'subarachnoid haemorrhage' following a traumatic tap. Unfortunately, once there is blood in the CSF from a traumatic tap there is nothing that can be done about it. CT scanning has greatly reduced the risk of this unfortunate sequence of events. Because of this possibility, if a lumbar puncture to exclude subarachnoid haemorrhage is to be performed, it should be done by the most experienced doctor available. The tragic outcome of not following this advice is seen in the following case.

CASE REPORT XI

A 17-year-old girl was referred to hospital on Christmas morning with the acute onset of severe headache and vomiting. There was no previous history of headache. A lumbar puncture was performed by the most junior houseman, who had no previous experience. Heavily bloodstained fluid was obtained after an extremely lengthy and traumatic procedure. All specimens were so heavily bloodstained that there was no demonstrable differential red cell count in the three tubes. The registrar on call decided that this was a bloody tap and, as the parents were keen that the patient should not miss Christmas, they were allowed to take her home. She collapsed and died 3 hours later with a further massive subarachnoid haemorrhage.

The morbidity of lumbar puncture – subsequent backache and headache – is greater in tense individuals, whose worst fears are realized when they experience a really badly performed procedure. This is not to say that these symptoms never occur after technically perfect lumbar punctures. Unfortunately, many doctors qualify without ever having performed a lumbar puncture under supervision. Once qualified, they teach themselves – to the patient's disadvantage. It is wise for all doctors to do their first few lumbar punctures under expert supervision: it is not a 'see one, do one, teach one' procedure!

Positioning the Patient (Figs 15.20–15.22)

The single most important factor in performing an easy, atraumatic tap is the correct positioning of the patient. Very often the most junior nurse is left to put the patient 'on their side' while the doctor scrubs up. If the operator is right-handed the patient should lie on their left side, as shown in the diagrams, even if the bed has to be moved out from a wall. It is surprisingly difficult to perform a lumbar puncture with the patient lying the other way round.

1. The patient should be pulled to the edge of the bed, which will provide firm support and helps to keep the back straight.

2. One or two pillows should be placed between the legs. This provides support for the top leg and prevents the patient rolling forwards. By providing support for the right arm it also prevents the shoulders rolling over.

3. There is no need for a nurse to forcibly flex the neck, or nearly suffocate the patient in the fully flexed position. If the patient is in a comfortable position, cooperation is encouraged. Note in Figure 15.20 the incorrect, rolled-over 'Rokeby Venus' posture and the effect this has on the target area between the laminae of the two vertebrae and compare this with the correct position shown in Figures 15.21 and 15.22. The importance of repeatedly checking that the back is vertical (which keeps the target area directly beneath the palpable spines) must be stressed.

Sterile Procedures

Meningitis after lumbar puncture is exceptionally rare. Nevertheless, sterile precautions should be observed. Although rubber gloves spoil the feel, which is sometimes very important in a difficult lumbar puncture, the advent of AIDS has unfortunately introduced the possibility of the doctor contracting an illness from the patient, rather than the previous concern that they might inadvertently introduce a skin organism into the patient's subarachnoid space, and gloves are now obligatory. It is still important to be sure that the hands are correctly scrubbed and that the shaft of the needle is not touched during the procedure.

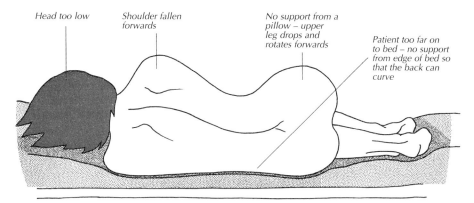

Head too low

Shoulder fallen forwards

No support from a pillow – upper leg drops and rotates forwards

Patient too far on to bed – no support from edge of bed so that the back can curve

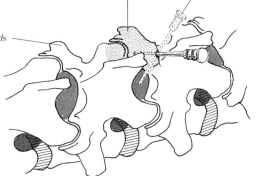

The apophyseal joints now lie directly under the interspinous line if the needle is inserted correctly – hence bone is repeatedly encountered

Direction needle must follow to achieve puncture

Vertebrae rotate forwards

15.20   Incorrect ('Rokeby Venus') position.

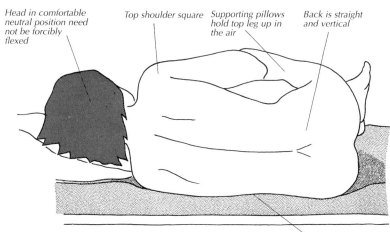

Head in comfortable neutral position need not be forcibly flexed

Top shoulder square

Supporting pillows hold top leg up in the air

Back is straight and vertical

Back right to edge of bed for firm support

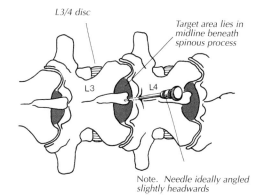

L3/4 disc

Target area lies in midline beneath spinous process

L3

L4

Note. Needle ideally angled slightly headwards

15.21   Correct position.

a   b

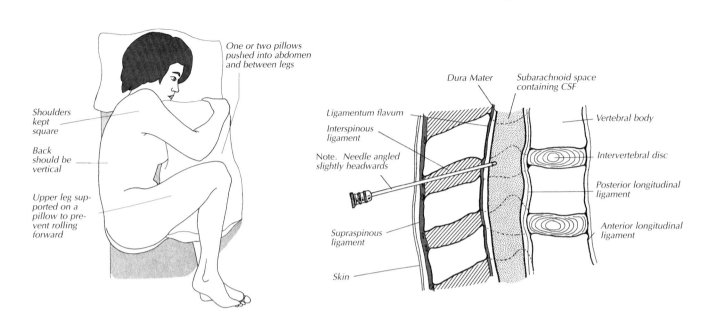

15.22   Correct position seen from above (a) with needle correctly inserted (b).

Equipment

Most hospitals now provide either a standard lumbar puncture pack or single-use equipment as required. The older reusable type of needle, which was often blunt, with an ill-fitting stilette, has fortunately become a thing of the past. The disposable needles do not have an integral stopcock and either a direct connection to the manometer via a flexible tube or a small push-on stopcock adapter should be available if manometry is required. The equipment provided varies so much from hospital to hospital that no specific advice can be given. However, the most important thing is to check that all the needles, stopcocks and manometers fit each other. Always check that the stilette removes freely even if using disposable equipment; check that the stopcock rotates freely and check the flow direction in the different stopcock positions. Finally, make sure that the manometer is not broken inside its pack. Having established that there are not going to be any delays caused by equipment failure, the actual lumbar puncture can begin.

Technique

1. Select a medium-sized $3\frac{1}{2}$ inch (90 mm) needle. Needle sizes are 18, 19, 20 and 21 – the higher the number the smaller the bore. A number 20 is best for general use, a number 21 for children other than infants. Occasionally the more rigid size 18 or 19 needle may have an advantage in the elderly patient

with an osteoarthritic back, although the risk of incapacitating post-lumbar puncture headache increases with needle size.

2. Select the interspace between the spines of L3 and L4. This lies just below the line joining the anterior superior iliac spines. Mark the position of the spines with a ball pen for further reference if needed.

3. Clean the area with whatever skin cleansing agent is available, and finally with alcohol. Allow to dry. Then, finally prepare the skin over an area about 6 inches square, centred on the chosen space, with either mercurochrome or weak iodine solution (Fig. 15.23).

4. Arrange three towels as shown in Figure 15.24. The upper one should not hang down on to the needle, but it is particularly useful for moving the patient about and checking the position of the anterior superior iliac spine, if the landmarks are lost, without jeopardizing sterility. A towel with a window in it is sometimes provided but this makes it difficult to see the necessary landmarks to maintain needle orientation, and tends to fall down on to the needle unless it is of the self-adhesive type. Its use is best avoided.

5. While the skin preparation is drying, draw up 1–2 ml of 2% lignocaine with adrenaline in a 2 ml syringe. There is no need to infiltrate the area widely with 5–10 ml of anaesthetic as this usually causes a lot of bleeding and turns the entry route into a bloody mush that destroys the 'feel'. Warn the patient that the local anaesthetic will 'sting' for about 10 seconds. Raise a skin bleb about 1 cm across, as shown in Figure 15.25,

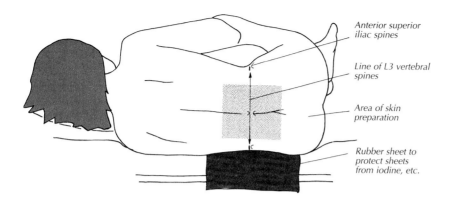

Anterior superior iliac spines

Line of L3 vertebral spines

Area of skin preparation

Rubber sheet to protect sheets from iodine, etc.

15.23 Area to be prepared for lumbar puncture.

15.24 Towelling up for the procedure.

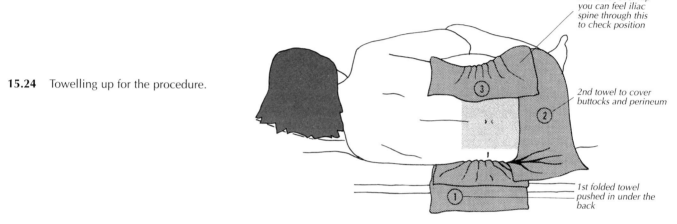

3rd towel over hip – you can feel iliac spine through this to check position

2nd towel to cover buttocks and perineum

1st folded towel pushed in under the back

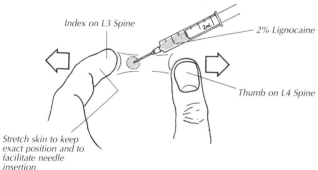

Index on L3 Spine

2% Lignocaine

Thumb on L4 Spine

Stretch skin to keep exact position and to facilitate needle insertion

15.25 Injecting the skin.

and then inject another 0.5 ml just below the skin. Massage it in with a finger. If the skin is not held taut as in the diagram, the area actually anaesthetized may end up some way from the midline.

6. Check that the skin is anaesthetized in the correct interspace, testing with the local anaesthetic needle. Then check that the patient has not altered position and warn them that they will feel a pushing sensation against the back. Ask them to report immediately if they feel any sharp pain. Holding the skin as shown in Figure 15.25, push the needle through the skin. It is generally recommended that the bevel on the needle should face upwards, the theory being that this will make it easier for the needle to slip between the longitudinally arranged fibres of the various ligaments and

the dura and will not cut these fibres transversely, which is what would happen if the bevel were facing up or down the line of the spine. It is thought that this may reduce the risk of post-puncture headache. Insertion through the skin may prove difficult but do not lunge at it or the needle will suddenly plunge in too deeply. As soon as the needle is through the skin check that the position between the spinous processes is still correct and then penetrate the dense supraspinous ligament in its midpoint just below the upper spinous process (Fig. 15.22). Once the needle is through stop, let go of the needle and see that it stays at 90° to the back, which should still be vertical. A correct line through the centre of this ligament is essential. If the needle has been deflected off line start again.

7. Once the needle is correctly aligned push it gently inwards and slightly angled towards the head. Usually the interspinous ligament is quite easily penetrated and little effort is needed at this stage.

8. If the line is correct at about $1\frac{1}{2}''$ depth a slight resistance will be felt. Check the needle line again and, if it is in the correct position, give it a little push, quite firmly but only for about $\frac{1}{8}''$. This should penetrate the ligamentum flavum with a slight 'pop'. As the same push often also penetrates the dura do not advance the needle any further without withdrawing the stilette. If no fluid emerges rotate the needle through 90° as a nerve root may be lying across the end. If this is unsuccess-

ful, replace the stilette (never advance the needle without the stilette in position) and advance the needle another 1/8" and withdraw the stilette again. Continue advancing the needle in this way until fluid emerges, firm resistance is encountered or the patient complains of pain down either leg.

9. If firm resistance is encountered do not force the needle: it may be against the opposite intervertebral disc and this can be damaged. If a nerve root is hit, ask which leg was affected. If the pain was in the right leg, withdraw the needle almost to the skin and then reinsert it angled slightly towards the left side, hopefully nearer to the midline than on the previous needle track. To pull back only half an inch or so is not sufficient as the needle will usually go straight back down the same track and hit the same root again!

10. Do not make more than three attempts in any interspace and do not be afraid to ask someone more senior to try at another interspace (usually L2–3). A failure may occur after 100 or more successful punctures and you will not be thanked for traumatizing three interspaces before seeking advice. Remember that a bloody tap creates more diagnostic problems than it solves.

Never attempt a tap above L2–3 or the spinal cord could be damaged. Never use a syringe to aspirate CSF during a lumbar puncture. The reason for a very low CSF pressure may be a serious one, such as tonsillar impaction or spinal block, and active aspiration may cause a disaster. At a less dangerous level, if the needle is blocked by a root lying across the end severe damage and prolonged sciatica may occur if the root is 'aspirated'.

11. Assuming the subarachnoid space has been entered reinsert the stilette as soon as fluid appears. The pressure cannot be estimated from the rate of flow from the needle and if the pressure needs to be measured it should be checked with the manometer as the next part of the procedure. If the pressure goes very high, above 250 mm H_2O do not panic and pull the needle out and waste the fluid. Collect the fluid from the manometer but do not attempt to remove any more. At 300 mm H_2O the manometer will contain 7–8 ml of fluid, which is more than adequate for all CSF examinations and having run the risk to obtain the fluid it is silly to waste the specimen.

If the pressure is normal, as it should be if the case was properly evaluated, take the manometer contents first and then two further specimens dripping directly from the needle of about 2.5 ml each (about 1/2" of fluid in the standard bottles that are usually provided). A 2 ml specimen should also be taken into a fluoride bottle for glucose estimation.

12. Remove the needle with a gentle pull. There is no need for a dramatic flourish, with a thumb placed immediately on the exit hole: the hole in the dura is the one that needs plugging and that is impossible! Place a sterile gauze square over the hole and fix it, in place with nobecutane spray or a simple plaster, which may be removed a few hours later. If the patient is not told that it can be removed they may arrive at the clinic 2 weeks later with it still in place!

13. Following the puncture the nurses will traditionally confine the patient to bed for 24 hours, with all the minor discomforts that this implies. It is advisable for the patient to lie almost flat with one pillow for 3–4 hours. They may then get up, but if a headache occurs there will be little difficulty persuading them to stay in bed. Post-lumbar puncture headache is quite unmistakable: every time the patient sits or stands they develop a sensation as they had been struck over the nape of the neck with a brick. The pain stops immediately they lie flat. Relatively few patients develop a headache if they have not one so within the first 12 hours. If the headache comes on 12–24 hours later it may take several days to clear and be quite incapacitating.

14. Finally, it is the doctor's responsibility to make sure that the bottles have been labelled 1, 2 and 3 in the sequence collected, especially if the tap was a traumatic one, so that the red cells can be counted in sequential specimens. This is not foolproof. Even with a clean tap a dural vein may be hit while penetrating the dura and continued severe bloodstaining may occur, mimicking a subarachnoid haemorrhage. A clue to this possibility is a tendency for the blood to swirl in the CSF as it emerges from the needle, whereas in subarachnoid haemorrhage the blood is completely admixed. Furthermore, if the fluid is centrifuged immediately, xanthochromia of the supernatant fluid indicates contamination by blood breakdown products prior to the lumbar puncture.

What to do if the Pressure is Abnormally High

A pressure over 200 mm H_2O is technically abnormal. However, in a very tense patient, especially if the procedure was difficult, the pressure may easily exceed this level. Allow the patient to relax for a few minutes and recheck the pressure. If the patient is extremely obese and has been held fully flexed the intra-abdominal pressure will elevate the CSF pressure. Carefully straighten the patient without dislodging the needle and allow them to breathe quietly for a few minutes before rechecking the pressure. If the pressure is genuinely elevated, and especially if it is in excess of 300 mm H_2O take the manometer specimen and pull the needle out.

Examine the patient's pupils immediately and record their size and symmetry. Check the patient's pulse rate and blood pressure and enter them on a head-injury observation chart. Raise the bottom of the bed and lie the patient face down without a pillow. Arrange an immediate CT scan and advise the neurosurgical team of the situation. Start an infusion of 20% mannitol, which should be given 1 g/kg by rapid infusion over 20 minutes. Continue observing the pupils, pulse, and blood pressure, looking for evidence of a developing pressure cone. This will produce pupillary asymmetry, a slowing pulse and a rising blood pressure. Often no specific measures will prove necessary but the lethal potential of this situation should never be underestimated. There is no evidence that attempts to replace the CSF with saline before removing the needle are of value. Raising the pressure may encourage further leaking, and during the unavoidable movements of the needle while fitting the syringe the dura may be torn and this will further increase the rate of CSF leakage.

What to do if the Pressure is Abnormally Low

It is not generally appreciated that a low pressure also carries considerable danger for the patient. A pressure of less than 80 mm H_2O can be regarded as below the normal range. In this situation CSF flow will be poor and the temptation to aspirate it with a syringe must be resisted. When lumbar puncture was the only neurological investigation available, one of the well recognized causes of low CSF pressure in a patient who had a cerebral disturbance was a subdural haematoma. This was due to the outflow of the CSF into the spinal canal being impaired by impaction of the cerebellar tonsils in the foramen magnum, preventing the pressure being transmitted to the spinal theca. Similarly, with a complete spinal block the pressure below the block may fall and the difficulty in obtaining CSF may be further magnified by the increased viscosity of CSF containing increased protein often as high as 2 g/100 ml. This is called the Froin syndrome. Attempts to aspirate this syrupy fluid may cause irreversible cord damage.

CASE REPORT XII

In 1965 a young man was admitted to a neurological hospital with several days' history of headaches, dizziness, unsteady gait, a stiff neck and a slight temperature. His CSF was examined. The pressure was 85 mm. H_2O and the fluid con-

tained 35 lymphocytes. No firm diagnosis was made but the possible significance of the low pressure was not appreciated. He was found dead in his bed 2 hours later. He had a cerebellar abscess with a tonsillar pressure cone.

This example also dramatically emphasizes the risk of mistaking neck stiffness caused by tonsillar coning for meningitis.

The management of low pressure is the same as for raised pressure.

Although details of the technique for performing lumbar puncture have been given, considerable stress has been laid on the importance of carefully assessing the need for the test, and the potential hazards of the procedure. Because occasional well-intentioned and carefully planned lumbar punctures may reveal raised pressure or low pressure the management of these complications has been included. The Queckenstedt test has not been discussed. It is time-honoured part of the ritual of lumbar puncture but has no special or reliable significance. It consists of compressing the jugular vein on each side alternately while recording the pressure. The pressure in the manometer will steadily rise as long as the vein is occluded, as the venous pressure in the head rises. If the patient has a lateral sinus thrombosis the pressure will not rise when the appropriate jugular vein is compressed, and in pre-scanning days this could be helpful. If, however, the patient had a temporal lobe abscess related to middle ear infection, the test could prove lethal. In the presence of spinal cord compression the rise in pressure could not be transmitted to the lumbar subarachnoid space if the block were complete. Unfortunately, in that situation the test could further damage the cord by acutely altering the vascular dynamics within the spinal canal. It was the thoughtless following of this ritual that led to the Queckenstedt test being performed, fortunately without fatal results in the patient quoted in the first paragraph of this section on page 273.

Lumbar puncture is never a life-saving procedure and can only too easily be turned into a life-threatening one, unless great care is exercised in the selection of patients.

16. Diagnosis of Cervical Root and Peripheral Nerve Lesions Affecting the Arm

The neurological anatomy of the arm is very intimidating at undergraduate level and many physicians are consequently reluctant to attempt an accurate anatomical diagnosis. There is also a widely held misconception that plexus lesions are a frequent cause of disease affecting the nerve supply of the arms. The anatomy of the brachial plexus is daunting. Plexus lesions are quite rare in most civilized countries, with a frequency proportional to the deliberate or accidental misuse of firearms and knives. There are few disease processes that primarily affect the brachial plexus other than the difficult differential diagnosis between recurrent carcinoma of the breast and delayed radiation fibrosis, which is discussed in detail later.

The clinical problem usually involves a relatively simple distinction between a peripheral nerve lesion and a root lesion affecting upper limb function. Therefore, in this chapter the anatomical and clinical differences between nerve root and peripheral nerve lesions will be compared and contrasted. A final section on plexus lesions is included containing a specially constructed diagram of the brachial plexus based on a functional approach which should make localizing diagnosis less intimidating.

The clinical problem can usually be reduced to a simple consideration: whether the pain or weakness lies in the territory supplied by a single nerve root or a single peripheral nerve or one of its branches.

Definitive diagnosis usually depends on a very careful evaluation of motor function because in the arm motor findings are much more reliable than sensory findings, for reasons to be discussed later. To facilitate diagnosis these findings are summarized in Tables 16.1 and 16.2, which are based on a simple evaluation of the motor supply of the arm tested by twelve movements, which in all but the most exceptional cases should provide all the information required for accurate diagnosis.

Vulnerable Areas of the Nerve Supply to the Arm

Figure 16.1 shows the entire course of each of the roots and peripheral nerves supplying the arm. Emphasis has been given to those areas where the relationship of the neural structures to bone or muscle may predispose to traumatic damage. Note that the radial nerve is vulnerable at three positions along its course, the ulnar nerve at two positions and the median nerve mainly at the wrist. Damage to the median nerve at the wrist and the ulnar nerve at the elbow are the lesions most often encountered.

When the cervical roots are considered, C5 and C6 are those most often affected by cervical spondylosis and C7 by acute disc lesions or degenerative cervical spine disease. This is related to the fact that these are the mobile segments of the neck. Because of relative immobility, involvement of the roots above and below these levels by acute or degenerative disc disease is quite unusual. If there is evidence of involvement of C2 and C3 or C8 and T1 roots, careful consideration of other diagnostic possibilities is necessary.

T1 root damage is quite a common consequence of altered anatomy in the area of the apical pleura, due to a cervical rib or invasion by neoplastic disease in the upper part of the lung. The older scalene muscle syndromes possibly never existed, but were used to explain what in retrospect were probably cervical root syndromes and carpal tunnel syndrome. Neither of these extremely common neurological conditions was an accepted clinical entity until the mid-1950s.

Clinical Evaluation of Sensory Symptoms and Signs

The unreliability of sensory phenomena in the arms has already been noted. This probably stems from the complex central representation of the limb and considerable overlapping of nerve territories at the periphery. Root pains may range from tingling paresthaesiae in a well localized distribution to very severe pain which the patient cannot localize accurately (Fig. 16.2). Individual root irritation typically causes discomfort and pain in the following distributions:

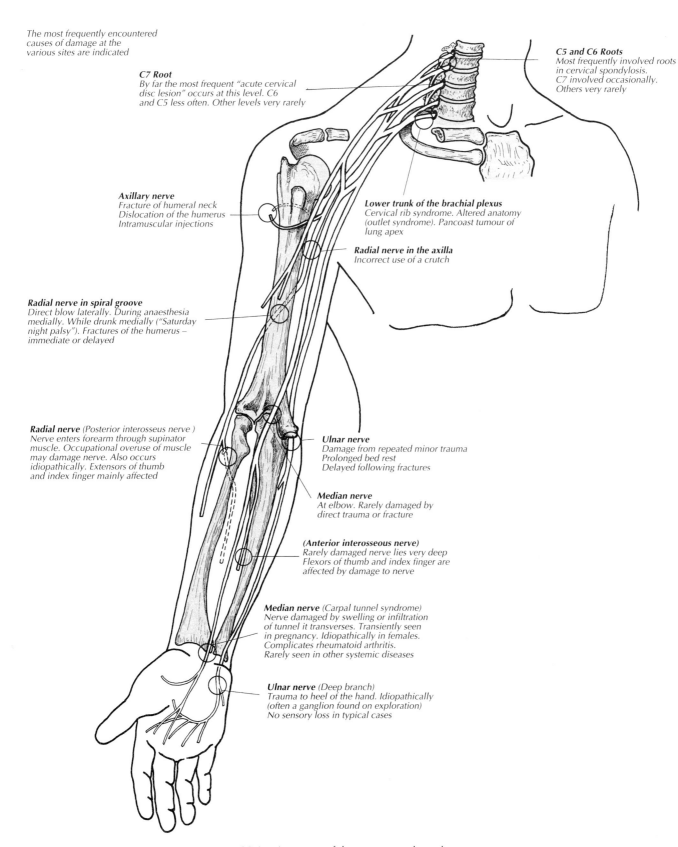

The most frequently encountered causes of damage at the various sites are indicated

C7 Root
By far the most frequent "acute cervical disc lesion" occurs at this level. C6 and C5 less often. Other levels very rarely

C5 and C6 Roots
Most frequently involved roots in cervical spondylosis. C7 involved occasionally. Others very rarely

Axillary nerve
Fracture of humeral neck
Dislocation of the humerus
Intramuscular injections

Lower trunk of the brachial plexus
Cervical rib syndrome. Altered anatomy (outlet syndrome). Pancoast tumour of lung apex

Radial nerve in the axilla
Incorrect use of a crutch

Radial nerve in spiral groove
Direct blow laterally. During anaesthesia medially. While drunk medially ("Saturday night palsy"). Fractures of the humerus – immediate or delayed

Radial nerve (Posterior interosseus nerve)
Nerve enters forearm through supinator muscle. Occupational overuse of muscle may damage nerve. Also occurs idiopathically. Extensors of thumb and index finger mainly affected

Ulnar nerve
Damage from repeated minor trauma
Prolonged bed rest
Delayed following fractures

Median nerve
At elbow. Rarely damaged by direct trauma or fracture

(Anterior interosseous nerve)
Rarely damaged nerve lies very deep
Flexors of thumb and index finger are affected by damage to nerve

Median nerve (Carpal tunnel syndrome)
Nerve damaged by swelling or infiltration of tunnel it transverses. Transiently seen in pregnancy. Idiopathically in females. Complicates rheumatoid arthritis. Rarely seen in other systemic diseases

Ulnar nerve (Deep branch)
Trauma to heel of the hand. Idiopathically (often a ganglion found on exploration) No sensory loss in typical cases

16.1 Anatomy of the nerve supply to the arm.

Table 16.1 Comparative data – root lesions in the arm

Roots	C5	C6	C7	C8	T1
Sensory supply	Lateral border upper arm to elbow	Lateral forearm including thumb & index	Over triceps, mid-forearm & middle finger	Medial forearm to include little finger	Axilla down to the olecranon
Sensory loss (Main location)	As above over deltoid	As above over thumb & radial border of hand	Middle fingers Front & back of hand	Little finger Heel of hand to **above** wrist	In axilla (usually minimal)
Area of pain	As above and medial scapula border	As above, esp. thumb & index finger	As above and medial scapular border	As above (up to elbow)	Deep aching in shoulder & axilla to olecranon
Reflex arc	Biceps jerk	Supinator jerk	Triceps jerk	Finger jerk	None
Motor deficit (muscles most involved and easily tested)	Deltoid Supraspinatus Infraspinatus Rhomboids	Pronators and supinators of forearm Biceps Brachioradialis Brachialis	Triceps Wrist extensors Wrist flexors Latissimus dorsi Pectoralis major	Finger flexors Finger extensors Flexor carpi ulnaris (Thenar muscles in rare patients)	**All** small hand muscles (thenar muscles via C8 in rare patients)
Causative lesions	Brachial neuritis Cervical spondylosis Upper plexus avulsion	Cervical spondylosis Acute disc lesions	Acute disc lesions Cervical spondylosis	Rare in disc lesions or spondylosis (See T1 usually affected by same pathology)	Cervical rib Altered anatomy of first rib Pancoast tumour Metastatic carcinoma in deep cervical nodes Outlet syndromes

1. C5 root pain occurs over the shoulder and into the lateral arm. It does not extend below the elbow. A confirmatory clue is often an aching pain down the medial scapula border. (This scapula pain may also occur with C6 and C7 root irritation).

2. C6 root pain causes deep aching pain in the biceps muscle which spreads down the lateral forearm, involving the thumb and index fingers on both the palmar and dorsal aspects.

3. C7 root pain is inherently diffuse as the C7 root supplies the periosteum of the bones of the arm, with a long cutaneous distribution down the centre of both the front and back of the arm. There is usually deep aching in the triceps muscle and pain down the front and back of the central forearm, radiating mainly into the middle finger and into both the index and ring fingers. When C7 root pain is very severe patients may complain that the entire arm is painful.

4. C8 root pain is relatively uncommon. It radiates from just below the olecranon down into the little and the entire ring finger. This can sometimes be difficult to distinguish from pain due to an ulnar nerve lesion at the elbow (see below).

5. T1 root irritation causes a deep aching sensation in the shoulder joint and axilla, and down the medial side of the upper arm to the olecranon.

When considering the sensory symptoms due to the involvement of peripheral nerves there are three special considerations (Fig. 16.3).

1. The area supplied by the radial nerve is so readily overlapped by other nerves that detectable sensory loss is quite unusual and sensory symptoms may be confined to slight tingling over the dorsal aspect of the thumb and index finger.

2. On purely anatomical grounds compression of the median nerve at the wrist should produce pain only in the lateral palm and the thumb, index, middle and half the ring finger. In practice, many patients with carpal tunnel syndrome complain that the pain radiates up the central forearm to the elbow and occasionally to the shoulder, and others insist that at the height of the pain the fifth finger is also involved. The reasons for this are not clearly understood, but certainly the pain in all the fingers of the hand may well be related to the large number of sympathetic nerve fibres to the blood vessels of the hand, which are almost exclusively carried in the median nerve. This explanation is supported by the fact that most patients who claim that there is pain in all fingers notice that at the height of an attack the fingers blanch and appear to be swollen, rather like Raynaud's phenomenon, and often describe the fingers as feeling 'like a bunch of cold sausages' or 'bananas'.

3. The ulnar nerve is usually damaged at the olecranon or where it enters the cubital tunnel. Its sensory distribution begins at the skin crease at the wrist and includes the front and back of the little finger and the medial half of the ring finger. On anatomical grounds there should be no pain or sensory disturbance above

Table 16.2   Comparative data – nerve lesions in the arm

Nerves	Axillary	Musculo-cutaneous	Radial	Median	Ulnar
Sensory supply	Over deltoid	Lateral forearm to wrist	Lateral dorsal forearm and back of thumb & index finger	Lateral palm Index, middle & lateral half ring finger	Medial palm and fifth & medial half ring finger
Sensory loss	Small area over deltoid	Lateral forearm	Dorsum of thumb & index (if any)	As above from skin crease at wrist	As above but often none detectable
Area of pain	Across shoulder tip	Lateral forearm	Dorsum of thumb & index	Thumb index & middle finger. Often spreads up forearm to elbow (reason unknown)	Ulnar supplied fingers & palm distal to wrist. Occasionally pain along course of nerve up to elbow (can be confusing)
Reflex arc	None	Biceps jerk	Triceps jerk & supinator jerk	Finger jerks (flexor digitorum sublimis)	None
Motor deficit	Deltoid (teres minor cannot be evaluated) usually very obvious	Biceps Brachialis (coracobrachialis weakness not detectable)	Triceps Wrist extensors Finger extensors Brachioradialis & supinator of forearm	Wrist flexors Long finger flexors to thumb index & middle finger Abductor pollicis brevis	All small hand muscles excluding abductor pollicis brevis. Flexor carpi ulnaris. Long flexors of ring & little finger
Causative lesions	Fractured neck of humerus Dislocated shoulder Deep i.m. injections	Very rarely damaged	Crutch palsy Saturday night palsy Fractured humerus In supinator muscle itself	Carpal tunnel syndrome Direct trauma to wrist Suicide attempt Falling on glass Palmar space infection	*Elbow* Local trauma Bed rest (resting on elbow) Fractured olecranon *Wrist* Local trauma Ganglion at wrist joint

the wrist. In practice many patients notice a dull ache down the ulnar border of the forearm along the line of the nerve, which may mimic a C8 root distribution. The mechanism of this is not clear and it is a similar situation to the pain up the medial forearm with median nerve entrapment at the wrist. This could be a diagnostic trap in both circumstances.

In most patients with peripheral involvement of the median or ulnar nerves, appropriate sensory impairment may be found. Two-point discrimination sensation in the fingers is a particularly useful test to detect minimal sensory loss, but it must be realized that in many instances quite severe compression of either the median or the ulnar nerve may occur in the absence of any sensory symptoms or any sensory findings. It is this feature that can make confident diagnosis so difficult on some occasions.

In the case of root involvement, although the pain may be exceptionally severe it is very unusual to be able to document any definite sensory loss and extremely unusual for the sensory loss, if found, to occupy the entire anatomical area supplied by a root. For example, in the case of a C6 root lesion some

numbness over the dorsum of the index finger and thumb may be detected, even though sensation in the area of the forearm supplied by the root may appear normal.

It should be noted that the failure to demonstrate sensory loss in any situation where there is pain in the arm should not be taken as evidence that the patient's symptoms have a functional basis. For this reason the motor findings are very important.

Clinical Evaluation of Motor Function in the Arm

For diagnostic purposes it is important to forget the multiplicity of roots contributing to the formation of individual peripheral nerves, particularly the radial and median nerves. Each movement of the arm is controlled almost exclusively by a single root and it is not necessary to evaluate all the muscles contributing to that movement. The only consideration is then, which nerve carries the root to this particular muscle or group of muscles?

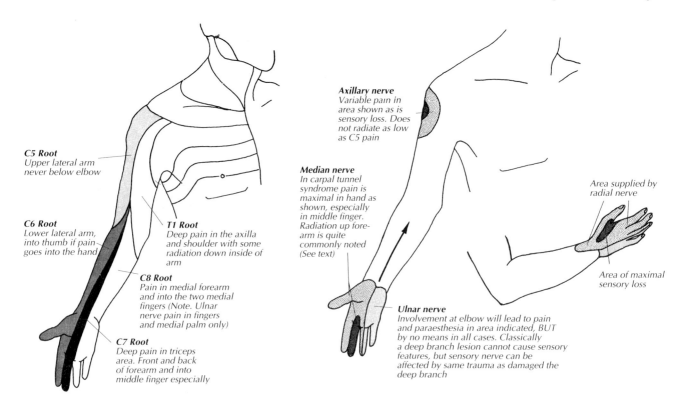

16.2 Distribution of root pain and paraesthesiae.

16.3 Distribution of pain and paraesthesiae in peripheral nerve lesions.

The following reflexes can be elicited in the arm:

1. *Pectoralis jerk*: Elicit by placing the fingers on the belly of the pectoralis major just medial to the deltoid and tap the fingers sharply with the hammer. The shoulder will adduct. This is a C7/C8 reflex conveyed through the lateral and medial anterior thoracic nerves. Its dual innervation reduces its localizing value.

2. *Biceps jerk*: Place the thumb on the bicipital tendon at the elbow, with the patient's arm flexed to 90°, and tap the thumb with the tendon hammer. The elbow will flex. This is an almost pure C5 reflex conveyed in the musculocutaneous nerve.

3. *Supinator jerk*: With the arm flexed at 90°, tap the tendon of the brachioradialis about 4" above the base of the thumb. The muscle will be seen to contract and the arm will flex. This is quite painful for the patient and should not be repeated unnecessarily. It is a C6 reflex conveyed through the radial nerve.

4. *Triceps jerk*: With the patient's arm flexed at 90° and pulled across the chest, tap the triceps tendon about 1" above the olecranon. The tendon is very short and tapping higher up may elicit a direct percussion response from the muscle itself. This is a pure C7 reflex also conveyed in the radial nerve.

5. *Finger jerk*: With the patient's palm upturned and the fingers half-flexed, hold the tops of the fingers with your own half-flexed fingers, which are then tapped. The patient's fingers will be felt to flex and, most strikingly, the free thumb will be seen to flex. This is a C8 reflex conveyed through both the median and ulnar nerves to the long finger flexors.

For each of the basic movements of the arm there is a root value and a peripheral nerve value, indicated in Figures 16.4 and 16.5. It follows that each reflex in the arm also has a root value and a peripheral nerve value, as detailed above. Referring to these figures, it will be noted that the traditional methods used for testing arm function, the grip and opposition of the thumb and fifth finger, are not included. These movements involve several muscle groups, multiple nerves and multiple roots in their performance and their diagnostic value is almost nil in terms of differentiating root and nerve lesions.

Special points that need to be emphasized with regard to testing motor function in the arm are as follows.

1. A C5 root lesion will weaken all 180° of shoulder abduction. An axillary nerve lesion, which affects only the deltoid muscle, will only weaken the second 90° of movement. This should not be confused with the frozen

shoulder syndrome in which severe pain prevents the second 90° of movement. This can be further complicated by the disuse atrophy of the deltoid that rapidly occurs in a patient who has a severe frozen shoulder.

2. A C6 root lesion will produce weakness of elbow flexion in both the fully supine position (achieved by biceps and brachialis) and the half-pronated position (achieved by the brachioradialis muscle). A musculocutaneous nerve lesion (an extremely rare event) would only weaken the biceps and brachialis muscles. A radial nerve lesion will only weaken flexion in the half-pronated position and the strength of the intact biceps and brachialis, even when placed at an anatomical disadvantage, is sufficient to produce near-normal flexion. The absence of the brachioradialis muscle contraction is easily observed.

3. A C7 root lesion causes weakness of shoulder adduction, elbow extension, wrist extension **and** wrist flexion because it makes a major contribution to both the radial and the median nerves. In contrast, a radial nerve lesion cannot affect shoulder adduction or wrist flexion and will also affect the brachioradialis muscle. This clinical distinction between a C7 root lesion and a radial nerve lesion is extremely important as both lesions are common and can occur in clinical situations such as neck and shoulder trauma where either or both could be damaged.

4. A C8 root lesion, which is relatively rare, will cause weakness of the long extensors and flexors of the fingers, and many would add the small hand muscles. This latter feature is extremely controversial and it would appear that in some patients there is some contribution from C8 root to small hand muscles, but in the majority the small hand muscles are almost exclusively innervated by the T1 root.

5. A T1 root lesion will cause wasting and weakness of **all** the intrinsic hand muscles. Anatomical peculiarities abound. An ulnar nerve lesion will also cause striking wasting of the intrinsic muscles but typically spares the abductor pollicis brevis muscle, as this is also supplied by the T1 root but via the median nerve. Confusingly, in some 2%–3% of patients with otherwise normal anatomy, **all** the small hand muscles are innervated by the ulnar nerve. This is known as a an 'all-ulnar hand' and is a considerable diagnostic trap. In such instances an ulnar nerve lesion may result in wasting of all the small hand muscles and the patient may be misdiagnosed as having a T1 root lesion or, even more seriously, motor neuron disease.

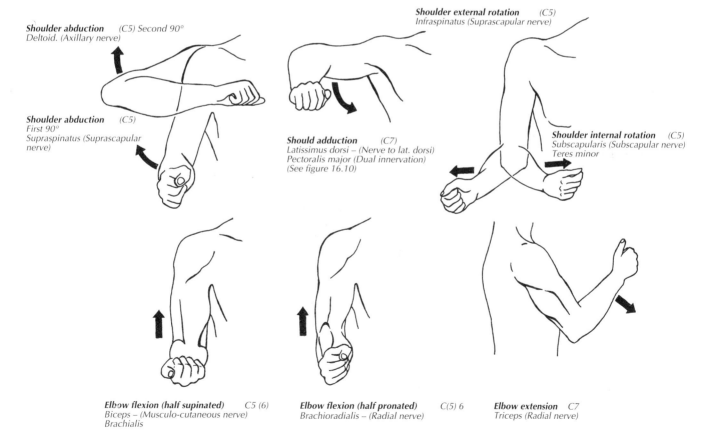

Shoulder abduction (C5) Second 90°
Deltoid. (Axillary nerve)

Shoulder abduction (C5)
First 90°
Supraspinatus (Suprascapular
nerve)

Shoulder external rotation (C5)
Infraspinatus (Suprascapular nerve)

Should adduction (C7)
Latissimus dorsi – (Nerve to lat. dorsi)
Pectoralis major (Dual innervation)
(See figure 16.10)

Shoulder internal rotation (C5)
Subscapularis (Subscapular nerve)
Teres minor

Elbow flexion (half supinated) C5 (6)
Biceps – (Musculo-cutaneous nerve)
Brachialis

Elbow flexion (half pronated) C(5) 6
Brachioradialis – (Radial nerve)

Elbow extension C7
Triceps (Radial nerve)

16.4 Shoulder and upper arm movements.

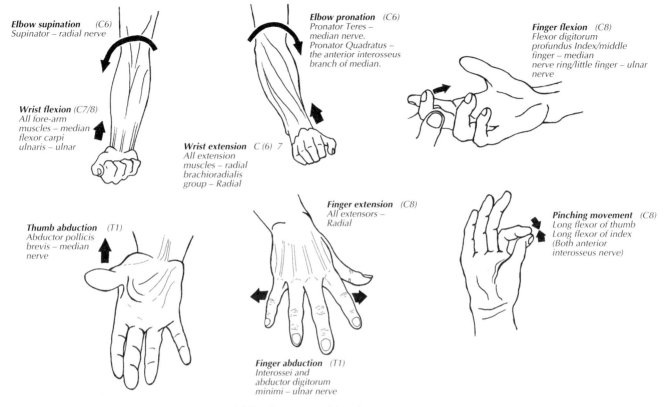

16.5   Forearm and hand movements.

It must be appreciated that this is only a diagnostic guide because several movements have not even been considered. This is solely because their inclusion over-complicates the situation without significantly improving the diagnostic value. In practice, the information gained by testing these movements will enable a confident conclusion to be arrived at in the majority of cases. The value of this approach will be seen when applied to the various clinical conditions that should be considered after an initial history has given some idea as to the possible diagnosis.

The Clinical Syndromes

Root Avulsion Syndromes

These conditions rarely cause differential diagnostic problems as the causative trauma is usually only too obvious. There are two basic syndromes:

1. Erb–Duchenne-type paralysis, which is due to avulsion of the C5 and C6 roots. This is usually the result of trauma to the shoulder tip and occurs following motorcycle accidents, or in infancy during a forceps delivery if the shoulders are stuck and the head is pulled too hard. This causes loss of abduction of the shoulder and loss of flexion at the elbow. This means that the arm hangs limply at the side and cannot be flexed, and therefore the hand cannot be moved to a functional position although hand function itself remains normal.

2. The second type, known as Klumpke paralysis, occurs when the T1 and C8 roots have been avulsed. This tends to occur during falls, when the patient attempts to break the fall by grabbing something and the arm is pulled up while the body continues to move, or when the arm is trapped in a moving machine. In this situation the patient loses the use of all the intrinsic muscles of the hand and the long flexors and extensors of the fingers, so that although the arm can be moved into any position there is no useful function in the hand itself.

In both types severe causalgic pain in the affected areas often complicates root avulsion due to recent trauma and this may result in a lifetime of intractable pain in the affected limb as well as the motor disability.

Root Lesions Due to Cervical Spondylosis

Root lesions due to spondylosis are discussed in detail in Chapter 15. It has already been noted that C5 and C6 are the two roots most likely to be affected. This leads to an almost diagnostic combination of reflex changes. The biceps and supinator jerks being carried by the C5 and C6 roots are usually depressed or absent and the triceps jerk is usually strikingly increased in a typical case. This is due to the local damage to the spinal roots at C5 and C6, blocking the reflex arcs, and the narrowing of the canal at this level, causing some degree of cord compression and enhancing the triceps jerk, which is passing through the C7 reflex arc just below the level of the compression.

In some instances where there is severe cervical spondylosis all three reflexes may be absent in both arms. Root lesions affecting roots other than C5, C6 and C7 are relatively rare and, if roots C2, C3, C4, C8 or T1 are involved, other diagnostic possibilities should be explored.

The presence of cervical spondylosis on cervical spine X-ray is almost universal in the middle aged and elderly as a physiological result of ageing. It is important not to automatically accept that atypical root lesions or rapidly progressive problems in the cervical spine are due to spondylosis, and careful investigation is indicated in unusual cases. The reverse is also true. Surprisingly normal cervical spine X-rays in an elderly patient with clinical evidence of disease affecting the cervical spinal cord or nerve roots, should prompt investigation for other causes.

CASE REPORT I

An 86-year-old woman presented with generalized pain in both arms and surprisingly brisk reflexes and extensor plantar responses. This was in the pre-MRI era and myelography was the only appropriate investigation. The radiologist was reluctant to perform a myelogram in view of the patient's age and frailty, particularly as the changes seen on plain film were minimal. It was successfully argued that the mildness of the plain film changes suggested that cervical spondylosis could not be the cause of this progressive syndrome. Myelography revealed a large meningioma compressing the spinal cord at C2 level, which was successfully removed without incident.

Acute Cervical Disc Lesions

Acute cervical disc lesions are relatively infrequent in comparison with acute lumbar disc lesions. They fall into two main groups:

1. Injuries occurring in an otherwise normal spine. These are typically the result of a sports injury or road traffic accident in a young person and usually produce a unilateral syndrome. The patient develops very severe acute neck pain associated with radicular pain in a specific root distribution, which may be associated with weakness of those muscles innervated by the affected nerve root. The C7 root is the one most often affected by traumatic disc lesions.

CASE REPORT II

A 6'6" tall basketball-playing student was involved in a fracas with gatecrashers at his sister's birthday party and was severely beaten up by six soldiers. He subsequently suffered neck and arm pain and was seen at a hospital on several occasions and told that because his plain neck X-rays were normal there was no traumatic lesion. He presented 2 years later, unable to continue playing basketball because of an insidiously evolving spastic paraparesis and evidence of bilateral C7 root lesions. Myelography revealed a severe traumatic C6/7 disc lesion which required surgery. The root pain was relieved but recovery from the cord damage was incomplete. This case exemplifies, once again, the danger of accepting that normal X-rays indicate that there is no abnormality.

2. Where a neck injury occurs in a patient who already has an abnormal neck due to cervical spondylosis. In such patients sudden flexion or extension of the neck, following a simple trip or in a rear-end collision in a car, may produce acute root symptoms or even acute cord damage. Usually the root symptoms are bilateral, may affect multiple roots, and the accompanying cord damage may cause an acute tetraparesis. The potential seriousness of even minor traumatic events affecting the cervical spine in this way in patients with severe pre-existing spondylosis must be recognised.

CASE REPORT III

A 72-year-old man was given barbiturate sleeping pills and under their influence he fell downstairs and became tetraparetic. He had the typical signs of acute C5/6 root lesions and a mild spastic paraparesis without sensory loss. Plain X-rays showed very gross spondylotic damage and a very narrow canal at C4/5 level. In spite of skilled care he died of bronchopneumonia 6 days following the incident.

CASE REPORT IV

A 73-year-old woman fell in her kitchen, striking her head and forcibly extending her neck. Immediately after the fall both hands had tingled and this rapidly spread up the arms to the shoulders. She did not call a doctor. Increasing weakness in both legs and the left hand and clumsiness over the subsequent month had led to her admission. On examination both arms showed increased tone, more marked on the left, but the arms were areflexic. The left plantar response was extensor but there was no pyramidal weakness in the legs. There was bilateral impairment of pain and temperature sensation over C4–C8 dermatomes. She gave a 20-year history of pins and needles in both hands, unrelieved by previous carpal tunnel decompression. Myelography revealed severe cord compression at C2/3 level but the neurosurgical unit to which she had been transferred made a diagnosis of multiple sclerosis. She was readmitted to the same neurosurgical unit 6 months later, by which time she had pyramidal weakness in both legs and bilateral extensor plantar responses. A diagnosis of peripheral neuropathy due to folate deficiency was sug-

gested. She was seen again by the original neurologist 4 months later, by which time she was tetraplegic with extensive sensory loss to pain and temperature which now extended to include C2 over the back of the head and the entire trunk. Some reservations about the previously suggested diagnoses was expressed and she was referred to an another neurosurgical unit, where she needed an immediate tracheostomy because of rapidly increasing weakness. Water-soluble myelography revealed compression of the spinal cord at C1 but the lesion extended from the body of C2 to the clivus. A transoral cervical decompression was performed which revealed extensive granulomatous tissue, thought to be secondary to previous trauma. Four weeks later atlantoaxial fixation was performed for C1/2 subluxation and within 4 weeks she was walking with a frame, with full recovery of sensation. Six months later, with the exception of areflexic arms and extensor plantars, there were no detectable abnormalities. She died 7 years later of unrelated disease.

In view of the clear relationship to trauma in a patient with a 20-year history and physical evidence of cervical spondylosis, the alternative diagnoses suggested in the face of myodil myelography confirming cord compression remains perplexing. She was saved ultimately by heroic surgery at the eleventh hour. This case is included here because of the critical significance of pre-existing spondylotic change in the pathogenesis of the condition and the likelihood that this would explain the absent reflexes in the arms, which it would seem was regarded as evidence **excluding** cord compression. The diagnostic trap of failing to recognize the inability of pre-existing absent reflexes to enhance in the presence of a cord lesion is referred to in several other chapters.

Several other similar cases have been seen since the advent of MRI scanning, which has revealed that cord compression often seems to occur at C3/4 or C4/5 levels, even though the major degenerative changes are at C5/6 and C6/7. This produces a characteristic clinical picture dominated by numbness in both arms, marked posture sense loss in the legs and a spastic paraparesis or paraplegia. The early symptoms of numbness and tingling in the arms has on several occasions been unsuccessfully treated by carpal tunnel decompression. One patient actually arrived for postoperative review after bilateral carpal tunnel decompression in a wheelchair, having become paraparetic in the 2 weeks following surgery! Discectomy or decompressive surgery is obligatory, even though the end results may be disappointing. Intense burning, tingling paraesthesiae in the hands may persist for many months after surgery and persistent posture sense loss may prevent an elderly patient from mobilizing effectively even if the motor components recover satisfactorily.

Brachial Neuritis (Serum Neuritis, Neuralgic Amyotrophy)

This is a classic neurological condition that was originally recognized as a sequel to immunization procedures involving the injection of serum into the deltoid muscle. The condition is not due to any direct trauma to the peripheral nerves but is believed to be an inflammatory process occurring in the roots. It is very rarely diagnosed correctly at first, because the pain is so severe that more serious pathology is suspected, and later because nobody has examined the patient's back and detected the obvious scapular winging.

In a typical case excruciatingly severe pain over the C5/6/7 dermatomes is followed 2–3 days later, as the pain lessens, by rapid wasting and weakness in some of the C5, C6 and C7-innervated muscles. The involvement may be very patchy. In a particularly severe case there may also be involvement of the sternomastoid and upper trapezius and C7-innervated groups. The most consistent and very striking feature is major involvement of the serratus magnus, with scapular winging. This is one of those physical signs that will not be detected unless specifically sought.

CASE REPORT V

A 35-year-old man was referred because of pain in the left arm and shoulder. The symptoms had started a year previously, after he had been riding his mountain bike and become extremely sweaty on a cold day. Later that day, while leaning forward to wash his hair, he noticed stiffness and aching in his neck. That night he was wakened with such severe pain that it took him 30 minutes to get out of bed to get painkillers, which were ineffectual. The pain radiated across the shoulder and down to the elbow. He also described a sensation as if someone were driving a stake between his shoulder blades. The pain persisted for 7–8 days, by which time he was left with aching in the shoulder and discomfort which had persisted since, in spite of numerous courses of physiotherapy with traction and manipulation and two consultations with a rheumatologist. His main residual symptom was that whenever he used his left arm (he was left-handed) he developed severe aching and stiffness in the shoulder. The history was very suggestive of brachial neuritis and the diagnosis was immediately confirmed when he removed his shirt, by the residual scapula winging.

This explained his ongoing symptoms, which were due to the abnormal posture of the left shoulder joint. It is hard to understand how so many physical therapists had examined this man and diagnosed cervical root lesions without noticing this very strikingly physical finding.

Occasionally the condition may occur bilaterally simultaneously.

CASE REPORT VI

A 32-year-old man presented with a 5 day history of severe bilateral shoulder and arm pain. He had not slept for five days. In the previous 48 hours both arms had become weak and he had already fallen face down on the floor while trying to unplug his T.V. On examination there was profound weakness of all groups supplied by C5–C8 and both arms were areflexic. There were no sensory findings and no long tract signs. A diagnosis of bilateral brachial neuritis was made. Over the following 10 days the pain worsened the weakness arrested but he set fire to his shirt leaning across a candle to get some water in the night. An MRI scan confirmed normality of the cervical cord and roots and CSF examination revealed no cells, a protein level of 107 mg% but no increase in globulins. A 5 day course of immune globulin (Sandoglobulin 24G/24 hours) was given with dramatic improvement in the severity of his pain and also in the weakness which had been established for 3 weeks before the treatment. The motor improvement has continued since that time.

This case suggests that in bilateral cases at least, high dose immunoglobulin infusion at the onset may be very useful in improving the prognosis for quick recovery. Without this treatment cases showing definite evidence of recovery within 5–6 weeks, usually make a full recovery over a period of 3–6 months. Those taking several months before any sign of recovery is apparent may take 18 months to 2 years before maximal recovery is made, and this is often incomplete. In the elderly the affected roots may be predisposed to damage by severe coexisting cervical spondylosis. Many patient cite cold exposure in the hours preceding the onset, although the condition is thought to be related to a viral infection.

CASE REPORT VII

A 45-year-old man and his 15-year-old daughter both presented with brachial neuritis. The right arm was affected in the father and the left in the daughter. Neither had had a virus infection. The day before the onset, both had been involved in strenuous physical activity on a warm autumn afternoon, followed by sudden coldness as the sun went down. Both recollected that their sweat-soaked shirts suddenly felt extremely cold at that time. The father had been chopping wood, right-handed, all the afternoon and the daughter, who was left-handed, had been playing tennis.

These cases are particularly intriguing because of the relationship to activity and cold exposure and show a similarity to acute poliomyelitis, where the first affected limb was often one that had been used strenuously in the hours before the onset, which it is thought may have localized the viral attack.

Cervical Rib Syndrome (Fig. 16.6)

Forty years ago textbooks contained whole chapters devoted to what were known as the 'outlet or scalene

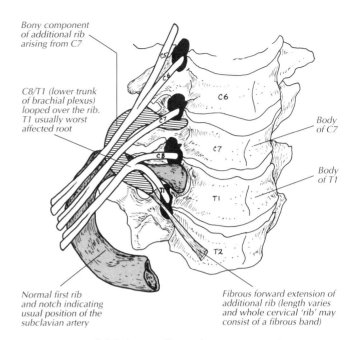

Bony component of additional rib arising from C7

C8/T1 (lower trunk of brachial plexus) looped over the rib. T1 usually worst affected root

Body of C7

Body of T1

Normal first rib and notch indicating usual position of the subclavian artery

Fibrous forward extension of additional rib (length varies and whole cervical 'rib' may consist of a fibrous band)

Subclavian artery lies anterior to roots – stenosis and post-stenotic dilatation at this point may be more significant than root stretching (see text)

16.6   Cervical rib syndrome

syndromes'. At that time, cervical spondylosis and carpal tunnel syndrome were not even recognized entities. With their recognition the outlet syndromes have almost vanished from the diagnostic repertoire. The only unequivocal survivor is the cervical rib syndrome, and to this we may add the situation where a normal first rib is displaced upwards by distortion of the thorax. This may occur in patients with thoracic scoliosis, following artificial pneumothorax or thoracoplasty, and in congenital abnormalities such as Sprengel's deformity, an autosomal recessive disorder with malformation of the shoulder joint and a hypoplastic scapula. The resulting symptoms of cervical rib syndrome may be due to either neural or vascular damage.

Neural Syndrome

The neural syndrome is extremely interesting. The sensory symptoms comprise a deep aching pain in the axilla and down the ulnar border of the arm, often into the hand – in other words, in the territory of both C8 and T1. The motor signs, however, are dominated by damage to the T1 root and in particular to those fibres destined to supply the abductor pollicis brevis muscle, almost to the exclusion of the other small hand muscles. This leads to a situation where the main pain is in the ulnar-innervated fingers, but the main wasting and weakness is in the median-innervated abductor pollicis brevis muscle. Patients have had their median nerve decompressed at the wrist for this syndrome when in fact a careful evaluation of the sensory symptoms should have made the diagnosis of carpal tunnel syndrome untenable.

The situation can be easily confirmed by electromyography and the findings comprise an electromyographic 'syndrome' in which there is evidence of denervation of the abductor pollicis brevis muscle with a normal median nerve action potential, coupled with normal ulnar-innervated muscles in the hand but an absent ulnar action potential at the wrist. On these electromyographic findings alone, even if no cervical rib can be demonstrated on plain X-ray or MRI scan, there is a case for exploring the lower roots of the brachial plexus in the neck, as damage due to abnormal fibrous bands may be found in this situation.

Vascular Syndrome

The vascular syndrome is the result of the abnormally high rib displacing the axillary artery upwards. This causes an area of stenosis with a poststenotic dilatation. Clot may form on the wall of the dilated vessel, small fragments of which then become detached and pass down the brachial artery into the hand. This causes acute embolic episodes resembling Raynaud's phenomenon, ultimately causing ischaemic changes in the fingers. In this situation there may be no abnormal neurological findings, but an incorrect diagnosis of carpal tunnel syndrome may be made when the patient relates the history of repeated attacks of severe pain in the hand associated with blanching and swelling of the fingers.

Further investigation of these patients requires plain X-rays looking for evidence of a cervical rib or an elongated transverse process of the C7 vertebra, MRI scanning of the cervical outlet and, if the vascular syndrome is a feature, angiography to demonstrate the course of the subclavian artery.

It is worth reiterating that the outlet syndromes described in the older books appear to be of dubious validity and it is very doubtful that the so-called scalene syndromes due to abnormal muscle insertions ever existed. A cervical rib or an abnormal fibrous band associated with an unusually elongated transverse process of the C7 vertebra appear to be the only valid causes of the outlet syndrome.

Lesions of the Radial Nerve

The radial nerve in the axilla is often damaged by the incorrect use of a crutch, when the patient takes their whole weight in the axilla. It should be noted, however, that the correct use of the crutch, when the patient takes their weight on the heel of the hand, can damage the deep branch of the ulnar nerve where it enters the palm!

Damage to the radial nerve in the axilla should cause weakness of all the radial nerve-innervated muscles: the triceps, wrist extensors, finger extensors and brachioradialis. Quite often the fibres innervating the triceps seem to be spared by lesions in the axilla, which may mistakenly suggest that the lesion is lower down below the spiral groove. In these cases even the triceps jerk may remain intact. This is an anatomical peculiarity that has to be appreciated.

Damage lower down may be produced in several ways:

1. Trauma to the radial nerve in the spiral groove on the lateral aspect of the upper arm may occur accidentally or be deliberately inflicted by the schoolboy trick in which the outer aspect of the arm is punched hard, causing an acute wrist drop and severe pain down the anterolateral forearm.

2. The nerve may be similarly damaged on the medial aspect of the arm in a so-called 'Saturday night palsy'. This occurs in patients who are inebriated or heavily sedated and go to sleep with their arm hanging over the back of a chair or over the edge of the bed, or following bad positioning during anaesthesia. In recent years sleeping in narrow bunks or berths in caravans or yachts seems to be a common cause of this condition.

3. Fractures of the midshaft of the humerus may involve the nerve either acutely during the actual fracture or during healing if there is overexuberant callus formation. In this situation, although initially the nerve palsy may appear to be progressive it is unusual for permanent damage to result and rarely is surgical exploration of the nerve necessary. Lesions of the nerve at this level usually spare the triceps muscle, the weakness being confined to the wrist extensors, brachioradialis and the finger extensors.

4. Damage to the radial nerve in the axilla or upper arm, although associated with aching, tingling or numbness in the radial nerve cutaneous distribution, very rarely causes detectable sensory loss as the territory is so readily overlapped by the adjacent ulnar and median nerves. If any sensory loss can be detected it is usually over the dorsum of the thumb and index finger.

The radial nerve becomes the posterior interosseus nerve as it enters the forearm, passing between the two heads of the supinator muscle.

Posterior Interosseus Nerve Lesions

Damage to the posterior interosseus nerve causes weakness of the wrist extensors, and in particular the extensors of the index finger and thumb. This lesion may occur idiopathically or following the unaccustomed heavy use of a screwdriver or other twisting movements of the forearm. Cases involving damage to the nerve at this point have also been described following Indian bar wrestling, in which the contestants rest their elbows on the table and try to force one another's hand over backwards, and in an orchestral conductor as a rather unique occupational hazard. The cause in these cases is likely to be the direct entrapment of the nerve by swelling or haemorrhage into the supinator muscle. If the condition is progressive, early exploration of the nerve is advisable.

Lead poisoning, which used to occur in house painters, specifically damaged the posterior interosseus nerve. It is thought that the nerve was predisposed to such damage but it would also seem possible that occupational overuse of the supinator muscle by the painting action predisposes to the localization of the damage to this nerve. Fortunately, with few exceptions, paint no longer contains lead and this condition has become of historical rather than practical significance.

Testing the Intrinsic Hand Muscles in the Presence of a Radial Nerve Palsy

One point of special clinical importance in a patient with a radial nerve palsy is the correct method of excluding coexisting weakness of the intrinsic muscles of the hand. When there is a wrist drop with weakness of the finger extensors, the intrinsic muscles appear to be weak. This can be readily confirmed by attempting to abduct your fingers with the hand fully flexed at the wrist and then with the hand extended at the wrist. There is a striking difference in the observed strength. In the presence of a wrist drop, the patient's hand should be laid flat on a firm surface in a natural position and the intrinsic muscles can then be tested and shown to be unaffected (Fig. 16.7).

Lesions of the Ulnar Nerve

The ease with which the ulnar nerve may be damaged at the elbow is well known from the common experience of hitting the 'funny-bone'. The fact that ulnar nerve palsies may result from repeated and apparently trivial trauma of this sort is less well appreciated. Simple alterations in personal habits, such as using a wooden-armed chair or driving with the arm resting on the door sill are other possible causes of an ulnar nerve lesion at the elbow.

Patients confined to bed often use their elbows to shuffle about in bed and the insidious development of bilateral ulnar nerve palsies is a common sequela. This is a frequent source of neurological referral from the orthopaedic wards, where patients with immobilized legs can only move in this way.

Very gradual damage may occur in women, who normally have a larger carrying angle at the elbow than men, and in whom repeated flexion and extension of

Position 1

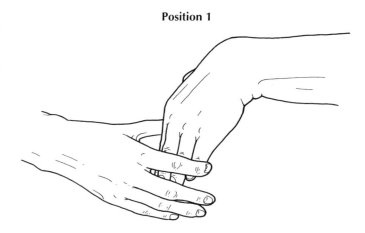

With wrist passively flexed by wrist drop, the dorsal intrinsics can easily be overcome and simulate intrinsic muscle weakness, apparently indicating multiple root or nerve lesions

Position 2

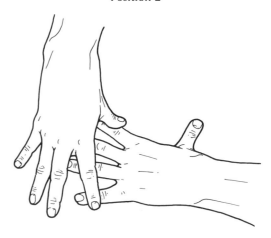

With the hand placed on flat surface the interossei can now use their attachment to the long extensor tendons effectively and normal power will be found (if they are unaffected), thereby excluding additional nerve or root lesions

16.7 Testing intrinsic muscles in the presence of a radial nerve palsy.

the arm is more likely to damage the nerve at the olecranon.

An important variant of this anatomical deformity leads to the condition known as a 'tardy ulnar palsy'. In this situation the patient has suffered a supracondylar fracture of the humerus in childhood, resulting in a developmental deformity of the elbow. As the years pass insidious ulnar nerve damage develops and it may be 20–30 years before its presence is recognized, often with a remarkably acute deterioration at the time of presentation.

CASE REPORT VIII

A 74-year-old man, the proprietor of a nursing home, spent a Boxing Day morning stoking the boiler because of staff sickness. That evening, he noticed aching down the medial forearm and tingling in the little and ring fingers. By the follow-

ing morning he had difficulty using a knife and fork, turning the ignition key in his car and performing any fine tasks with his right hand. When seen the next day he had a severe complete ulnar nerve lesion. He had sustained a fractured elbow at the age of 4 and had developed a markedly increased carrying angle. At surgery the nerve was found to be swollen and trapped in dense fibrous tissue at the olecranon. It was decompressed and transposed, with excellent recovery. This must be one of the tardiest ulnar palsies ever documented!

In many cases where gradual damage to the nerve has occurred the absence of sensory phenomena is quite remarkable. Although tingling and numbness in the ulnar fingers would be anticipated, quite severe and even complete loss of motor function in ulnar-innervated muscles may occur in the total absence of any sensory symptoms. In this situation, unless it is recognized that 2%–3% of the population have an all ulnar-innervated hand, there is a real possibility of the incorrect diagnosis of a T1 root lesion or motor neuron disease because **all** the intrinsic muscles of the hand will be wasted and the clinical distinction between median and ulnar nerve lesions will be lost.

Lesions of the ulnar nerve at the elbow ought to produce weakness of the flexor carpi ulnaris and the medial part of the flexor digitorum profundus. For reasons that are far from clear, it is quite unusual for these muscles to be significantly affected and even more important is the observation that damage to the nerve at the elbow specifically seems to affect those fibres destined to innervate the first dorsal interosseus muscle. Therefore, the patient may present with striking weakness and wasting of the first dorsal interosseus muscle with almost complete sparing of the other interossei and abductor digiti minimi muscles. At first sight this makes it seem unlikely that the nerve is damaged at the elbow and appears to indicate that the lesion is at the wrist.

At the wrist the nerve divides into a superficial sensory part and a deep motor branch.

Deep Branch Lesions of the Ulnar Nerve at the Wrist (Fig. 16.8)

Repeated trauma to the heel of the hand (using the heel of the hand to shut a sticking car door, or the use of a chuck key by a lathe worker etc.) may crush the nerve against the carpal bones. Occasionally the nerve may be affected at the wrist by a ganglion arising from the joint, and if there is no history of trauma to the heel of the hand it is worth exploring the nerve to exclude this possibility. This will only damage the deep branch of the ulnar nerve, which is purely motor. This leads to wasting and weakness of all the ulnar-innervated small hand muscles in the absence of tingling, numbness or other evidence of sensory involvement. This will again raise the clinical suspicion of motor neuron disease,

which may be further compounded if the patient has an all ulnar-innervated hand.

Whenever the intrinsic muscles of the hand are affected by an ulnar nerve lesion, early surgical exploration to decompress the nerve should be performed once the site of damage has been identified. If wasting is allowed to persist, delayed surgery may produce unsatisfactory results and significant intrinsic muscle weakness is extremely disabling.

Lesions of the Median Nerve

The deeply placed median nerve is well protected from trauma in the arm. Rarely, the anterior interosseus nerve, which arises from the median nerve just below the elbow and passes distally on the anterior interosseous membrane, may be damaged in forearm fractures or dislocations of the elbow.

Anterior Interosseus Nerve Lesion

A pure lesion of the anterior interosseus nerve (Kiloh–Nevin syndrome) causes weakness of the long flexors of the thumb and index finger and the pronator quadratus. This impairs the pincer movement of the finger and thumb, which is profoundly disabling. It is usually the result of trauma at the elbow with haemorrhage into the deep musculature. Surgical decompression should be considered.

Carpal Tunnel Syndrome (Fig. 16.8)

In the carpal tunnel the median nerve is extremely vulnerable and damage at this level is the commonest peripheral nerve lesion encountered. Carpal tunnel syndrome is also the commonest neurological complication of pregnancy. It was first described in the mid-1940s but only put on a firm basis with the advent of neurophysiology in the mid-1950s. It is instructive to remember that some eminent physicians denied the existence of this condition for a whole decade after its original description, and insisted that all pain in the hand was due to 'outlet syndromes' and applied the descriptive term 'acroparaesthesiae' to the condition.

The striking feature is that the pain in the hand is particularly severe during the night and may be totally absent during the day. The patient typically wakes with severe pain in the thumb, index and middle fingers and the symptoms are fairly readily relieved by swinging the arm or flexing and extending the wrist. Surprisingly often, the pain extends up the medial forearm and occasionally as high as the shoulder, for reasons that are unclear, and cervical root disease may be suspected. However, the location of the pain in the hand and these relieving movements are diagnostic clues, and however atypical the description of the actual pain

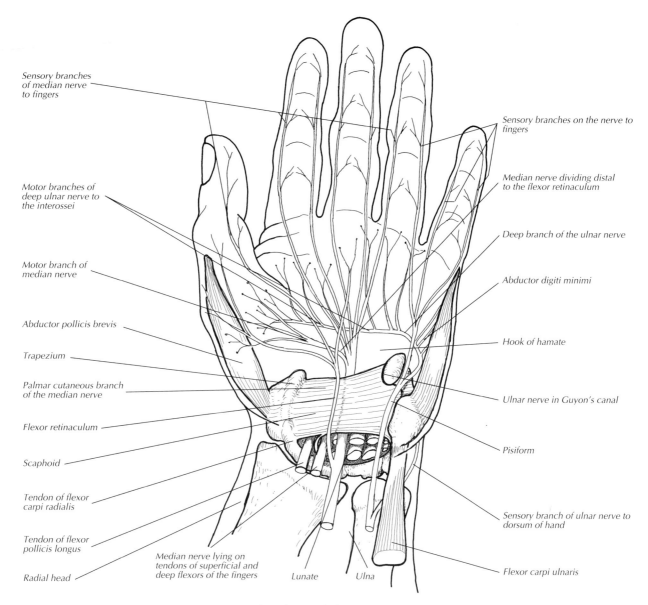

16.8   Anatomy of median and ulnar nerves at wrist and palm.

Sensory branches
of median nerve
to fingers

Motor branches of
deep ulnar nerve to
the interossei

Motor branch of
median nerve

Abductor pollicis brevis

Trapezium

Palmar cutaneous branch
of the median nerve

Flexor retinaculum

Scaphoid

Tendon of flexor
carpi radialis

Tendon of flexor
pollicis longus

Radial head

Median nerve lying on
tendons of superficial and
deep flexors of the fingers

Lunate

Ulna

Sensory branches on the nerve to
fingers

Median nerve dividing distal
to the flexor retinaculum

Deep branch of the ulnar nerve

Abductor digiti minimi

Hook of hamate

Ulnar nerve in Guyon's canal

Pisiform

Sensory branch of ulnar nerve to
dorsum of hand

Flexor carpi ulnaris

may be, night pain in the arm and hand that wakens the patient and is relieved by moving the hand, should be assumed to be due to carpal tunnel syndrome until proved otherwise. Pain that is first noticed on waking in the morning is often due to a cervical root irritation from cervical spondylosis and may be aggravated by neck movement and not relieved by moving the hand.

These peculiarities of the distribution of sensory symptoms in carpal tunnel syndrome have already been pointed out in the introductory part of this chapter. Sensory findings may be quite marked, with total loss of sensation in the median-innervated part of the hand, or sensation may be quite normal in the presence of severe pain.

Motor involvement is usually confined to the abductor pollicis brevis muscle as the other muscles supplied by the median nerve (flexor pollicis brevis and adductor pollicis) either have dual innervation from the ulnar nerve or can be readily compensated for by the long forearm muscles, and it is usually only the wasting and weakness of abductor pollicis brevis that can be easily and convincingly demonstrated. In many cases no wasting or weakness may be apparent. From a clinical point of view it is sufficient to test the abductor pollicis brevis correctly, as shown in Figure 16.5, and then to be certain that the ulnar-innervated muscles are functioning normally.

There are four major presentations of carpal tunnel syndrome:

1. A pure sensory syndrome, which usually occurs in women, in which severe sensory loss in the median nerve distribution develops gradually without significant pain. This variant seems to be related to repeated

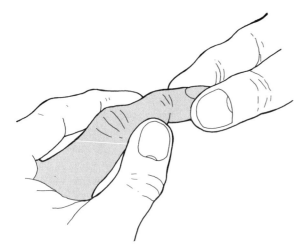

16.9 Correct technique for testing joint position sense in the hand.

movement trauma, such as knitting, sewing or crocheting, particularly in the presence of degenerative arthritic change at the wrist. Making clothing for grandchildren is commonly identified as the cause.

2. A pure motor lesion is usually seen in men who use their hands as tools. Carpenters, plumbers and mechanics are particularly prone to this variant. Sensory symptoms are usually minimal or absent and the patient presents either because of difficulty using the thumb for skilled tasks or because they have noticed the hollowing of the lateral part of the thenar eminence. Considering that the cause is direct trauma to the nerve in the palm of the hand, it is surprising that sensory symptoms are experienced so infrequently.

3. A mainly autonomic presentation with very severe pain is a feature of carpal tunnel syndrome occurring in pregnancy. The patient may be asymptomatic throughout the day but is wakened several times a night by vicious pain which appears to involve the entire hand. It is often described as a feeling that the hand is fat, swollen, cold and clammy, and then as a stinging and burning sensation as recovery occurs, when the arm is either dangled from the bed or swung around. If any attacks occur during the day they are usually provoked by working with the arms elevated, reading a newspaper, or while driving with the hands up on the steering wheel. Each attack recovers surprisingly quickly, and not only is the patient asymptomatic at other times but nerve conduction studies between attacks are usually completely normal. It seems likely that in such cases the autonomic fibres in the median nerve are those preferentially affected.

4. Classic carpal tunnel syndrome includes elements of all the above syndromes and, in a perfect world, the patient would have wasting of abductor pollicis brevis, numbness over the median-innervated part of the hand

and attacks of pain that waken them from sleep. Unfortunately, this classic version seems to be quite rare and therefore this extremely common condition is frequently misdiagnosed or unrecognized for years.

Lesions of the Long Thoracic Nerve of Bell

A classic nerve lesion affecting the arm is due to damage to the long thin nerve that supplies the single but large and important muscle, the serratus magnus. This large sheet of muscle, which inserts to the inner border of the undersurface of the scapula and arises as interdigitations from several ribs, plays a major role in arm movement. It normally holds the scapula flat against the back and rotates the lower scapula laterally during shoulder abduction. When this muscle is paralysed patients notice they cannot hold the affected arm up straight, and when looking in a mirror notice a small hump appearing over their shoulder on the affected side. Relatives may notice the striking protrusion of the shoulder blade, particularly when the patient attempts to put the arm up or push forwards. In many instances the presentation is due to aching and stiffness around the shoulder joint as the spinati and deltoid try to compensate for the lack of rotation of the scapula and become stiff and painful.

There are no specific causes, but involvement of this muscle in brachial neuritis is an almost universal finding and probably the commonest cause. The nerve is vulnerable to maliciously inflicted stab wounds in this area and occasionally to accidental surgical trauma, and is at particular risk during lymph node biopsy in the posterior triangle of the neck, where it lies superficially. Perhaps, due to the length of the nerve, recovery is slow and often incomplete.

Brachial Plexus Lesions

Pathological processes affecting the brachial plexus are rare. Traumatic lesions are certainly the most frequent cause and the only non-traumatic condition presenting a diagnostic problem is damage to the plexus caused by radiation of the axillary area for carcinoma of the breast. A major problem is the difficult decision as to whether the plexus lesion is due to metastatic disease requiring more radiotherapy or to the radiotherapy itself.

There are four main sites of plexus damage producing fairly typical clinical pictures (Fig. 16.10).

Lesions of the Upper Trunk

Damage to this area, which is the most superficial part of the plexus, often occurs with stab or bullet wounds in the neck. C5 and C6 are destroyed, leaving the patient with numbness of the lateral arm, forearm and hand, with loss of abduction, internal and external rotation of

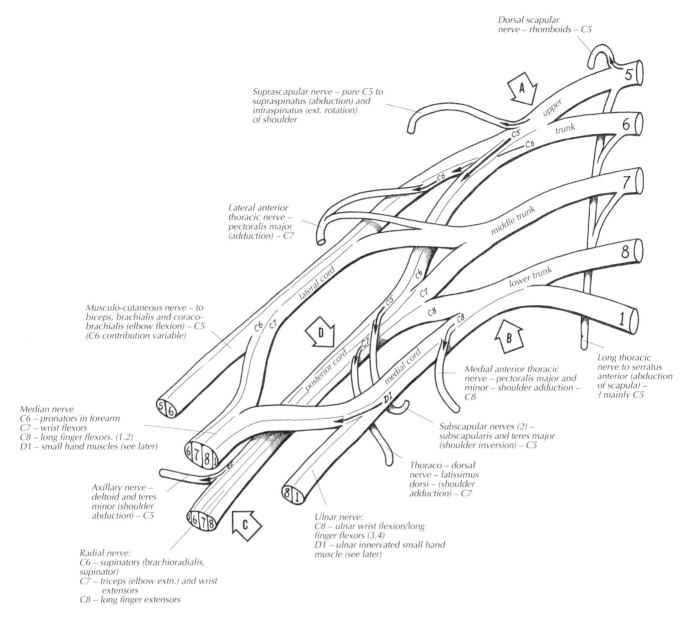

Dorsal scapular nerve – rhomboids – C5

Suprascapular nerve – pure C5 to supraspinatus (abduction) and infraspinatus (ext. rotation) of shoulder

A

upper trunk

C5
C6

C6

middle trunk

Lateral anterior thoracic nerve – pectoralis major (adduction) – C7

C6

C7

C5

lower trunk

Musculo-cutaneous nerve – to biceps, brachialis and coraco-brachialis (elbow flexion) – C5 (C6 contribution variable)

lateral cord

C6 C7

D

C8

C8

B

Long thoracic nerve to serratus anterior (abduction of scapula) – ? mainly C5

posterior cord

C7

medial cord

D1

Median nerve
C6 – pronators in forearm
C7 – wrist flexors
C8 – long finger flexors. (1.2)
D1 – small hand muscles (see later)

5 6

6 7 8 1

Medial anterior thoracic nerve – pectoralis major and minor – shoulder adduction – C8

Subscapular nerves (2) – subscapularis and teres major (shoulder inversion) – C5

Thoraco – dorsal nerve – latissimus dorsi – (shoulder adduction) – C7

Axillary nerve – deltoid and teres minor (shoulder abduction) – C5

6 7 8

C

8 1

Ulnar nerve:
C8 – ulnar wrist flexion/long finger flexors (3.4)
D1 – ulnar innervated small hand muscle (see later)

Radial nerve:
C6 – supinators (brachioradialis, supinator)
C7 – triceps (elbow extn.) and wrist extensors
C8 – long finger extensors

16.10 Anatomy of the brachial plexus, showing the eventual destinations of all root components.

the shoulder, elbow flexion and radial wrist extension owing to weakness in the extensor carpi radialis longus and brevis. The biceps and supinator jerks are absent. Note that as the lesion is distal to the roots it will spare the rhomboid muscles, which are supplied by a branch from the C5 root, and the serratus magnus, which is supplied by branches also arising from the C5, C6 and C7 roots via the long thoracic nerve.

Lesions of the Lower Trunk

Damage to this area has already been described to some extent in connection with cervical rib syndrome.

This is also the area of the plexus that can be damaged by carcinoma of the lung apex extending through the apical pleura (Pancoast's syndrome) and metastatic disease in the axillary glands, from malignant disease in the breast or elsewhere. The clinical picture consists of severe pain in the shoulder, which is particularly severe when lying in bed at night and which may drive the patient to sleep sitting up. This will be accompanied by tingling and numbness down the medial arm and forearm into the little and ring fingers. Weakness of the finger flexors and extensors and the intrinsic muscles of the hand follows.

Radial Nerve Lesion in the Axilla

This has already been discussed under crutch injuries to the nerve in the lower axilla, radial nerve damage may also occur following stab wounds and neoplastic disease in the axillary glands. A complete radial nerve palsy will occur which in this case may well include weakness of the triceps muscle. As noted earlier, the triceps muscle is often spared when external trauma to the axilla is the cause.

Lesions of the Posterior Cord

Lesions of the posterior cord may follow small-calibre low-velocity bullet wounds to the plexus. The bullet traverses the region of the plexus and impacts against the inner surface of the scapula, and the posterior cord seems to be particularly likely to be damaged by this mechanism. The picture is often a transient one, with later recovery. A posterior cord lesion is easy to diagnose as it is essentially a radial nerve palsy combined with an axillary nerve lesion. Therefore, there is inability to extend the elbow, wrist and fingers, and weakness of the second 90° of shoulder abduction owing to paralysis of the deltoid muscle.

Radiation Damage to the Plexus

Patients who have received irradiation to the axillary lymph nodes which surround the brachial plexus, for metastasis from a carcinoma of the breast, may sustain radiation damage particularly to the C7 root, which lies in the centre of the radiation field, with lesser involvement of C8 and T1. The damage does not occur immediately but is typically of fairly sudden onset 12–18 months after radiation is completed. The patient notices progressive numbness and weakness of the forearm and hand, but an important feature is the absence of pain. The numbness and weakness may progress rapidly over a few weeks and then appear to arrest or progress very slowly. Less typically, many years after radiation therapy a very slowly progressive picture may occur. With the long delay before onset there is greater concern that the condition is due to recurrent disease but, as in the more acute condition, the absence of pain is an important and reassuring feature. If the weakness is accompanied by pain, particularly of relentless quality, malignant infiltration is highly likely to be the cause.

MRI scanning, particularly utilizing a stir sequence, may confirm or exclude malignant infiltration in the irradiated area. Previously the absence of pain and the very slow progression of symptoms indicated the more benign pathology. Surgical attempts to explore or decompress the plexus were unhelpful and clearly further irradiation of the area, unless recurrent disease is certain, is wholly inappropriate. Even with MRI scanning this still remains a very difficult diagnostic situation.

The diagnostic problems presented by root and nerve lesions affecting the arm have been outlined. The wide disparity between what actually happens and what ought to happen on purely anatomical grounds has been emphasized. A simplified method of evaluating the arm directly applicable to these circumstances has been outlined. In most instances electrodiagnostic studies can be of considerable value and details of the techniques used and the results to be anticipated are to be found in Chapter 19.

17. Nerve Root and Peripheral Nerve Lesions Affecting the Leg

In the previous chapter dealing with root and nerve lesions affecting the arm three points were emphasized:

1. Anatomical features that place nerves in vulnerable positions in fibrous tunnels against bone or traversing muscles
2. Sensory disturbances that defy anatomical explanation and can make sensory symptoms somewhat misleading
3. The reliability of motor signs utilizing both the reflex responses and muscle weakness in distinguishing between nerve and root injuries.

When root and nerve lesions in the leg are considered, there are some striking differences:

1 The peripheral nerves are much less vulnerable to everyday trauma and, with the exception of the peroneal nerve at the fibula neck, are infrequently damaged compared with the nerves in the arm.
2. Sensory symptoms are extremely reliable in indicating which root is affected. Furthermore, the two commonest peripheral nerve lesions, damage to the lateral cutaneous nerve of the thigh and damage to the peroneal nerve, produce pain and discomfort in anatomically accurate areas, making for relatively easy diagnosis.
3. Motor signs in lumbar and sacral root disease are much less reliable because most muscles have a nerve supply derived from two or more roots, making wasting and weakness sometimes difficult to detect if only one root is damaged.

There are five reflexes that can be elicited in the legs that are of diagnostic value:

1. *Adductor jerk*: With the patient's thigh slightly externally rotated and the knees slightly flexed, place the fingers over the adductor tendon in the lower medial thigh. When the fingers are tapped the muscle will be felt to contract and the thigh will adduct. This is an L3 reflex conveyed through the obturator nerve.

2. *Knee Jerk*: With the patient's knee flexed at 45° and supported by the examiner's left hand, locate and tap the patella ligament just above the tibial tubercle. The quadriceps will be seen to contract. This is an L4 reflex conveyed in the femoral nerve.

3. *Ankle jerk*: Although this is most easily examined and the symmetry compared with the patient lying in a frog-leg position, female patients in particular prefer the leg to be crossed over, so that one leg is resting on the other. In either position the tendon should be tensioned by the examiner pulling slightly upwards on the patient's foot and the Achilles tendon struck with the tendon hammer. The calf muscle will be seen to contract and the foot may be felt to flex. This reflex is conveyed through the S1 root via the tibial branch of the sciatic nerve. This can be quite painful for the patient and attempts to elicit the reflex should be abandoned once it is clear that there is no response.

4, 5. *Medial and lateral hamstring jerks*: With the patient's leg in the same position used to elicit the knee jerk, the fingers are placed on the medial and lateral hamstring tendons respectively. A sharp tap with the tendon hammer should readily elicit these reflexes. They are conveyed through the S1 root but it is of potential clinical importance that the medial reflex is carried in the tibial division of the sciatic nerve and the lateral reflex in the peroneal division.

The Spinal Origins of the Root Supply to the Leg

There are several anatomical features of the origins of the lumbar and sacral roots that require emphasis at this stage. All the nerve roots supplying the leg arise from the spinal cord above L1 vertebra level and each root has to traverse several inches in the spinal canal before reaching its exit foramen. It follows that, even if there is evidence of a single nerve root lesion, it could be damaged anywhere along its intradural course. In practice, the root is most commonly damaged at its exit foramen by a disc lesion. Failure to recognize the possibility that the lesion could be higher in the canal, if no local lesion can be demonstrated, occasionally leads to serious diagnostic errors.

CASE REPORT I

A 48-year-old man, a very keen sportsman, had developed very severe sudden backache while bowling at cricket. This extended down across the right buttock and into the right leg. It was managed conservatively by his GP and cleared over a few weeks. This was 1 year before presentation, and in the interim he had noted an occasional tight feeling in the right leg when bending over but denied any significant pain. Over an 8-week period he developed a marked right food drop. Clinically, this was a pure L5 root lesion with no weakness of inversion or eversion of the foot and an intact ankle jerk. There was no sensory deficit. Nerve conduction studies to exclude a peroneal nerve lesion were normal and a radiculogram showed a very mild disc lesion at L4/5. The CSF protein was markedly elevated at 1.05 g/l. Subsequently a CT scan indicated a central disc at that level and at operation a surprisingly large paracentral disc protrusion was removed. As there was no pain there were no immediately obvious beneficial effects, and over the next 6 years he sought several other opinions, all of whom agreed with the findings and with what had been done, and concurred that the nerve root had been irreversibly damaged. He was referred again 7 years after the operation because of progressive weakness in the leg, which had now spread to involve the thigh. Physical examination revealed wasting and weakness of the right quadriceps and an absent right knee jerk, but the ankle jerk was still intact on the right. All other reflexes were brisk. It was thought unlikely that this was due to progressive scarring from the previous operation. By this time MRI scanning was available and revealed a 2 cm diameter, brightly enhancing lesion at T12 level which was pushing the spinal cord to the left-hand side. At operation this was confirmed as a neurofibroma which was successfully removed. It was thought to be arising on a sensory root but the exact level could not be identified. Unfortunately no recovery had occurred when he was reviewed 3 years later.

This case once again not only demonstrates the advantage of MRI in imaging the lumbar roots but demonstrates that, even with water-soluble radiculography, inadequate demonstration of the lower spinal cord can be a major problem. To make matters worse, the patient undoubtedly did have a very large disc lesion, which seemed to be a more than adequate cause for his symptoms. In retrospect, the absence of pain and the high CSF protein were important clues but perhaps the most important was the intact ankle jerk. A disc lesion dramatic enough to damage the L5 root so severely would in most instances distort the passing S1 root sufficiently to abolish the ankle jerk. On the second occasion the very brisk reflexes were the clue to a lesion high enough to produce cord compression, although the plantar responses remained flexor. The diagnostic problems presented by intradural lesions of the lumbar and sacral roots are fully discussed under cauda equina lesions in Chapter 15.

The clinical term 'sciatica' also requires clarification. Sciatica is a symptom and not a disease and simply means 'pain in the leg'. It does not mean inflammation of the sciatic nerve. It is not inevitably due to disc disease and may be the presenting symptom of other more serious diseases. The cutaneous distribution of the sciatic nerve does not extend up the posterior thigh or on to the buttock.

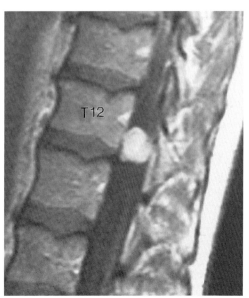 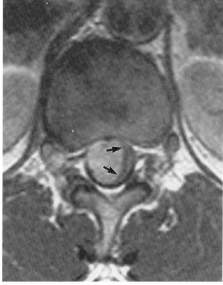

CRI. *Neurofibroma occupying most the canal (arrows indicate extent of tumour)*

Anatomical Features of the Nerve Supply of the Leg

The highest components of the nerve supply to the leg arise from roots L1, L2, L3 and L4, and emerge from the vertebral canal just below the diaphragm to enter the retroperitoneum between the anterior and posterior masses of the origin of the psoas muscle (Fig. 17.1). These four roots form the lumbar plexus and the branches of the plexus have to reach the front of the leg.

The Lumbar Plexus

The L1 root has two named branches, the iliohypogastric and the ilioinguinal nerves, which supply the skin over the pubis and medial inguinal ligament and the upper penis and scrotum or the labia respectively. These nerves are discussed at the end of this chapter.

The L1 and L2 roots combine to form the genitofemoral nerve which, in addition to supplying the skin over the femoral triangle, is motor to the cremaster muscle in the spermatic cord.

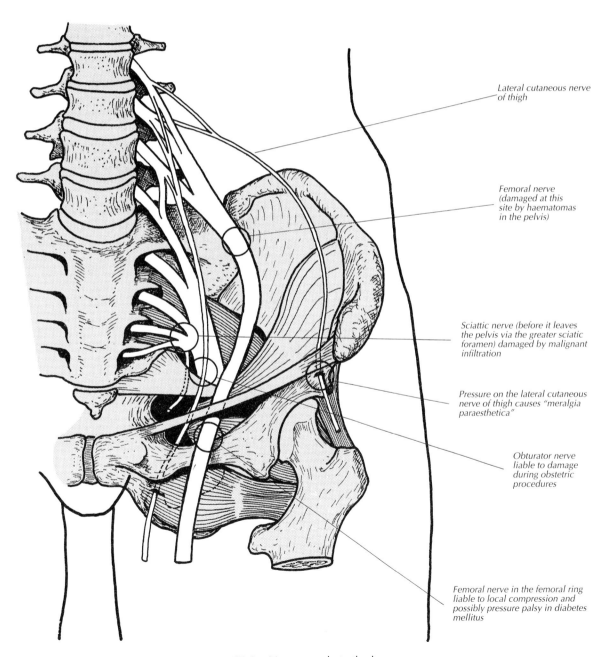

Lateral cutaneous nerve of thigh

Femoral nerve (damaged at this site by haematomas in the pelvis)

Sciattic nerve (before it leaves the pelvis via the greater sciatic foramen) damaged by malignant infiltration

Pressure on the lateral cutaneous nerve of thigh causes "meralgia paraesthetica"

Obturator nerve liable to damage during obstetric procedures

Femoral nerve in the femoral ring liable to local compression and possibly pressure palsy in diabetes mellitus

17.1   Nerve supply to the leg.

The Cremasteric Reflex

For obvious reasons this reflex is only present in the male. Lightly stroking the skin over the inner upper thigh will cause retraction of the testicle on that side. This is mediated through L2 root.

The first clinically important branch, the lateral cutaneous nerve of the thigh (L2 and L3), reaches the thigh by skirting around the pelvic brim and entering the thigh under the lateral part of the inguinal ligament.

The femoral nerve (L2, L3 and L4) passes downwards on the lateral side of the iliopsoas muscle and, with the muscle, emerges under the inguinal ligament into the femoral triangle in the anteromedial thigh.

The obturator nerve (L2, L3 and L4) lies on the medial side of the iliopsoas muscle and comes into close relationship with the uterus in the pelvis before emerging through the obturator foramen into the medial compartment of the thigh. In the pelvis it is vulnerable during obstetric and gynaecological procedures.

The lumbar plexus therefore supplies the hip flexors, thigh adductors, knee extensors and the skin over the medial anterior and lateral thigh, via the obturator, femoral and lateral cutaneous nerves of the thigh

respectively. The sensory continuation of the femoral nerve is the saphenous nerve, which runs across the medial aspect of the knee to supply a long promontory of skin down the medial side of the leg, including the skin over the medial malleolus and occasionally part of the medial aspect of the foot.

The Sacral Plexus

The rest of the leg is supplied by the sacral plexus, which is derived from the combination of the L4, L5, S1 and S2 roots. This plexus forms over the sacroiliac joint and almost immediately leaves the pelvis via the greater sciatic foramen. Its main branches, the gluteal nerves, the sciatic nerve and the posterior femoral cutaneous nerve of the thigh, then lie directly behind the hip joint. It is obvious that fractures of the upper femur, particularly those involving the hip and acetabulum, represent a considerable threat to these nerves but it is surprising how infrequently they sustain damage during such fractures. The sciatic nerve is very vulnerable to damage from a misplaced intramuscular injection in the buttock. The correct position for such injections is shown in Figure 17.2.

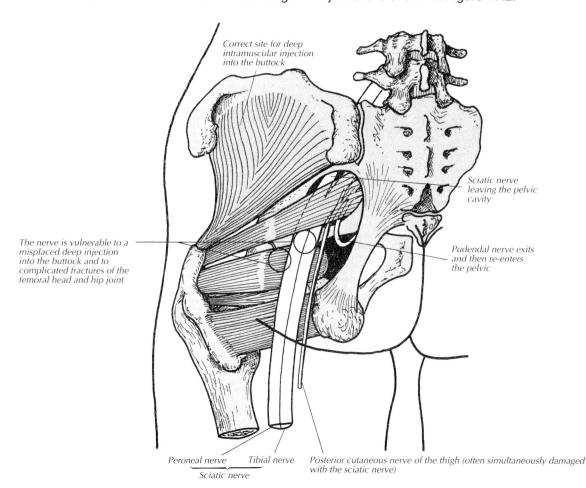

17.2   Nerve supply to the posterior leg.

The sciatic nerve consists of two discrete components invested by the same fascia, the peroneal nerve (formerly called the lateral popliteal nerve) and the tibial nerve (formerly called the medial popliteal nerve). There is an important anatomical peculiarity that even when the whole nerve trunk is traumatized the peroneal component is six times more likely to be damaged than the tibial component. The reason for this is not entirely clear, but this feature has considerable clinical significance and was of critical importance in guiding surgical exploration in the following case in the days before CT scanning.

CASE REPORT II

A 35-year-old women present with a foot drop that had developed gradually over a year. Electromyographic studies revealed severe denervation, confined to the anterior compartment but with no evidence of a peroneal nerve lesion at the fibular neck. Plain X-rays of the pelvis and lumbosacral spine were normal. A myelogram was entirely normal with no evidence of an L5 root lesion. She was observed for a further 6 months with no improvement; indeed, a slight deterioration occurred, and an orthopaedic surgeon was asked to explore the sciatic nerve behind the hip joint based on the known anatomical peculiarity of the peroneal nerve, which indicated that this seemed to be the only possible site of damage. At operation, a hard knob of tumour was found emerging from the greater sciatic notch which was compressing the sciatic nerve trunk. It proved to be chondrosarcoma originating on the inner aspect of the ileum. This was substantially removed through an intra-abdominal approach by a general surgeon and although the peroneal nerve failed to recover, the patient is alive and well, 20 years later. No radiotherapy was given.

This is a superb example of the clinical application of this intriguing anatomical peculiarity, which is equally applicable to blunt trauma and gunshot wounds in the area behind the hip joint.

Following its separation into the two individual nerves in the lower thigh, the tibial nerve remains deeply placed and is very rarely damaged (Fig. 17.3). The peroneal nerve, however, has to gain access to the anterior and lateral compartments of the leg, and in doing so becomes extremely vulnerable as it winds round the fibula neck.

The subsequent division of the peroneal nerve into the deep peroneal nerve, anterior tibial nerve, the superficial peroneal nerve and the musculocutaneous nerve has little practical significance, as damage to the individual nerves below the fibula neck is extremely rare.

The tibial nerve lies deep in the calf and is almost never subject to damage. The terminal digital branches of the tibial nerve are subject to trauma, as they lie under the metatarsal heads, the basis of the condition known as Morton's metatarsalgia.

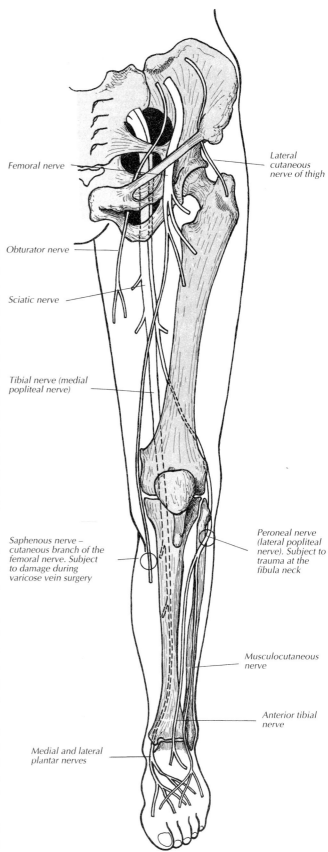

Femoral nerve

Lateral cutaneous nerve of thigh

Obturator nerve

Sciatic nerve

Tibial nerve (medial popliteal nerve)

Saphenous nerve – cutaneous branch of the femoral nerve. Subject to damage during varicose vein surgery

Peroneal nerve (lateral popliteal nerve). Subject to trauma at the fibula neck

Musculocutaneous nerve

Anterior tibial nerve

Medial and lateral plantar nerves

17.3 Bony relationships of the nerve supply to the leg.

Clinically Important Features of the Sensory Nerve Supply to the Leg

Peripheral Nerve Supply

The cutaneous distribution of L1 and L2 through the ilioinguinal, iliohypogastric and genitofemoral nerves is shown in Figure 17.5, 17.8 and 17.9. The area supplied by the lateral cutaneous nerve of the thigh is also indicated. The notable features are that the territory supplied does not cross the midline of the thigh, whereas the area supplied by the L2 and L3 roots (Fig. 17.5) extends to the posterior axial line of the posteromedial thigh.

The long promontory of skin supplied by the saphenous branch of the femoral nerve extends down the medial aspect of the leg. Anatomically this is very important, as sensory loss following a sciatic nerve injury cannot produce complete stocking sensory loss below the knee, as there will always be an area of preserved sensation over the medial side of the leg.

Relative to its size the sciatic nerve supplies a surprisingly small cutaneous area. Unless the posterior cutaneous nerve of the thigh is simultaneously damaged with the sciatic nerve, there will be no numbness over the

back of the thigh and the area of resulting sensory loss will be found over the posteromedial aspect of the leg and the lateral and plantar surfaces of the foot.

A peroneal nerve lesion due to damage at the fibula neck shows some similarities to the effects of a radial nerve lesion in the arm. It causes a foot drop and similarly a remarkable small area of sensory loss, usually a triangular shape over the dorsum of the foot, extending up just across the ankle joint to the lower leg.

Root Supply

The distribution of the nerve roots is shown in Figure 17.5. The L1 root supplies the groin and adjacent genitalia via the iliohypogastric, ilioinguinal and genitofemoral nerves. The cutaneous distribution of lumbar roots L2 and L3 spirals across the front of the thigh and down towards the medial side of the thigh until they reach the posterior axial line. This is in contrast to the distribution of the cutaneous nerves in this area, which run essentially straight down the thigh. The rarity of degenerative disc disease above L4 level makes it immediately apparent that pain in the anterior thigh should not be too readily attributed to disc disease.

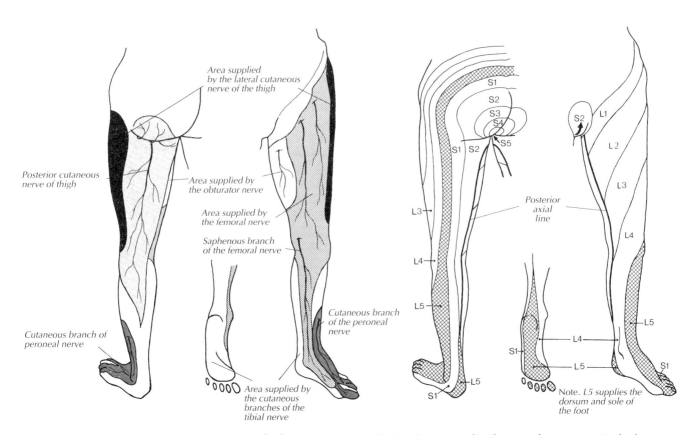

17.4   Cutaneous nerves in the leg.

17.5   Cutaneous distribution of nerve roots in the leg.

This point has been already been stressed in the section on cauda equina lesions in Chapter 15.

The L4 root is the highest root that is commonly affected by disc disease, and even this is relatively unusual. The pain of an L4 root lesion radiates across the front of the knee, on to the medial side of the leg, down to the medial malleolus. It is often described as having a burning quality and seems to be particularly severe across the knee and behind the patella. This quality of sensation is different from that of the other commonly affected roots.

The root most often affected by degenerative disc disease is L5 and the usual radiation of the pain is across the buttock, down the posterolateral thigh, the lateral side of the leg and across the ankle joint on to the dorsum and sole of the foot. Severe pain in the big toe seems to be particularly typical of an L5 root lesion. The pain is usually a dull ache in the buttock becoming a shooting stabbing pain down the posterolateral thigh and anterolateral leg, and ending as a painful tingling on the dorsum of the foot down to the big toe. The pain in the big toe is often likened to the recovering phase after dropping a heavy weight on the toe. This variation in the quality of the pain down the full extent of the root distribution is very important in evaluating pain of dubious authenticity.

The pain of S1 root irritation runs across the inner buttock down the posterior thigh and the lateral side of the leg and extends on to the lateral aspect of the foot. Its quality is similar to that described above for L5. In both L5 and S1 root lesions it is unusual to find definite sensory loss, although slightly altered perception of cutaneous sensation may be found over the dorsum of the foot in an L5 root lesion or over the lateral aspect of the foot in an S1 root lesion.

The lower sacral roots S2–S5 supply the skin of the inner posterior thigh, the inner buttocks and the genitalia. Sensation over these areas should be carefully checked in all patients complaining of pain in the posterior thigh or genitalia, and in patients with sphincter disturbances.

CASE REPORT III

A 14-year-old girl presented with an 8-month history of pain in the back following a fall downstairs. This cleared until she fell again 3 months later while roller skating, and had further pain which again cleared spontaneously. A month later, while sitting on a radiator, she noticed that her right buttock did not feel warm and when she touched the area she found that she was numb over the central part of the right buttock. The pain became worse and was very severe at night, so that she was forced to get up and walk around for relief. Over the next 6 weeks the numbness spread down the inner posterior aspect of the right thigh. In the 2 weeks prior to neurological consulta-

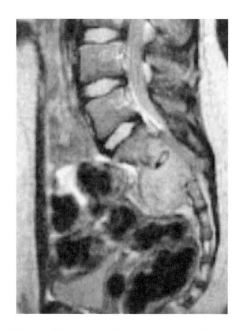

CRIII. *Giant-cell tumour of sacrum presenting as atypical sciatica in a 14-year-old girl.*

tion she had severe pain in the entire right foot and the numbness had spread to involve the back of the right calf and the outer border of the right foot. She had been seen by an orthopaedic surgeon 3 months previously who had requested an A/P and a lateral lumbar spine X-ray, which was reportedly normal, as was a subsequent CT scan through the lumbar discs, although the films were not available when she was seen. She was only referred for a neurological opinion because the rheumatologist to whom she had been referred for an epidural was on holiday. Physical examination revealed sensory deficit over the right L5, S1 and S2 dermatomes and absence of both ankle jerks. It seemed possible that a conus lesion had been missed by not X-raying high enough to detect it. However, an MRI scan of the lumbar sacral spine revealed a large soft tissue mass arising anteriorly in the second sacral segment and expanding the sacrum in all directions. Subsequently review of the original X-rays and CT scan clearly revealed the presence of this tumour. Biopsy revealed a giant-cell tumour of bone and she subsequently underwent a course of radiotherapy, with considerable resolution of her symptoms but little or no resolution of the mass lesion. She died 6 years later in spite of numerous further opinions and total resection of the sacrum towards the end of her illness.

This case exemplifies many critical features: the importance of recognizing the sinister significance of night pain, the recognition of atypical nerve root involvement, that degenerative disc disease does not occur in children and the lesson that any available X-rays should always be examined personally and carefully studied and not just looked at to exclude one diagnosis. These considerations also apply to adults, as exemplified in the following case.

CASE REPORT IV

A 65-year-old woman was referred by an orthopaedic surgeon with a 2-month history of a nagging unpleasant pain in the region of the left hip and down the posterior inner thigh. This was so severe that she could not sit down and was better standing than lying, particularly if she kept her hip slightly flexed. It had consistently wakened her at night and had failed to respond to analgesics. The ESR had been persistently elevated to between 50 and 80 mm/h but had briefly been 120 mm/h 4 years previously, which remained unexplained. All biochemical and haematological studies were normal. On physical examination both ankle jerks were absent and there was a band of sensory deficit very accurately localized to the S2 dermatome. A CT scan and bone scan were arranged and revealed a mass arising in the region of the left sacroiliac joint. Biopsy revealed a malignant fibrous histiocytoma. After an initial response to radiotherapy, the patient deteriorated and died some 6 months after presentation.

Clinically Important Features of the Motor Nerve Supply to the Leg

The correct methods of testing leg movements and their root and nerve values are shown in Figures 17.6 and 17.7

Peripheral Nerve Supply

The nerve supply of the psoas arises from L1, L2 and L3 in the posterior abdominal wall. The femoral nerve (L2 and L3) is responsible for hip flexion, as it innervates the iliacus muscle, and for knee extension as it innervates the quadriceps muscle. A lesion of the femoral nerve within the pelvis will affect both hip flexion and knee extension. This may be complicated when there is an intrapelvic lesion such as haematoma or psoas abscess directly interfering with hip flexion. If iliopsoas is actually weak, or attempts to use it cause such severe pain that contraction is inhibited, it is a clear indication that there is an intra-abdominal lesion causing the problem. From a strictly practical point of view no distinction as to the cause of the hip flexor weakness need be made. The knee jerk is conveyed in the femoral nerve and will always be abolished by a femoral nerve lesion. Although the femoral nerve contains components from L2, L3 and L4, the reflex arc is conveyed purely in L4 and loss of the knee jerk can occur with an L4 root lesion in the absence of significant wasting or weakness of the thigh.

The obturator nerve supplies obturator externus (lateral rotation of the thigh) and all the adductor

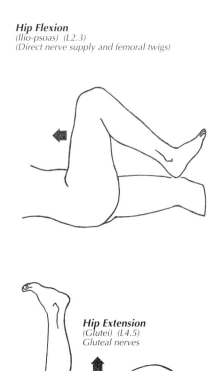

Hip Flexion
(Ilio-psoas) (L2.3)
(Direct nerve supply and femoral twigs)

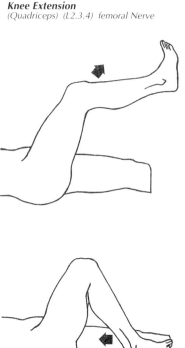

Knee Extension
(Quadriceps) (L2.3.4) femoral Nerve

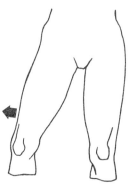

Hip Abduction
(Glutei and tensor fascia lata) (L.4.5)

Hip Extension
(Glutei) (L4.5)
Gluteal nerves

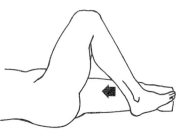

Knee Flexion
(Hamstrings) (L5, S1)
Tibial nerve. Peroneal nerve
(Lateral head of biceps femoris only)

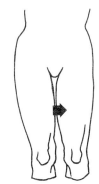

Hip Adduction
(Adductor group) (L2.3.4)
Obturator nerve

17.6   Movements of the leg.

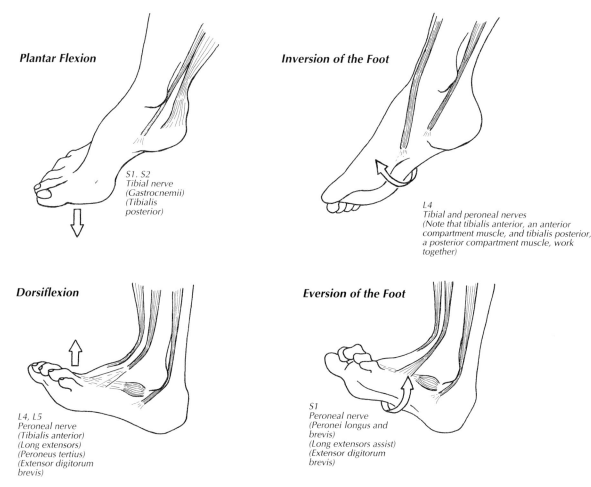

Plantar Flexion

*S1, S2
Tibial nerve
(Gastrocnemii)
(Tibialis
posterior)*

Inversion of the Foot

*L4
Tibial and peroneal nerves
(Note that tibialis anterior, an anterior
compartment muscle, and tibialis posterior,
a posterior compartment muscle, work
together)*

Dorsiflexion

*L4, L5
Peroneal nerve
(Tibialis anterior)
(Long extensors)
(Peroneus tertius)
(Extensor digitorum
brevis)*

Eversion of the Foot

*S1
Peroneal nerve
(Peronei longus and
brevis)
(Long extensors assist)
(Extensor digitorum
brevis)*

17.7   Movements of the foot.

muscles of the thigh. Its integrity can be tested simply by the patient's ability to hold the legs together against resistance. The obturator nerve conveys the obturator reflex, which will be abolished by an obturator nerve lesion, but abolition is also a useful sign of damage to the L2 or L3 roots and this is the highest reflex that can be elicited in the leg.

The peroneal nerve supplies the short head of the biceps femoris (the lateral hamstring muscle), the muscles of the anterior compartment (dorsiflexors of the foot and toes and a major contribution to inversion), the lateral compartment of the leg, the peronei (evertors of the foot) and the extensor digitorum brevis on the dorsum of the foot which contributes to dorsiflexion of the toes. This is the small muscle that can be palpated just below and anterior to the lateral malleolus when the toes are dorsiflexed. The supply to the lateral hamstrings conveys the lateral hamstring reflex through the S1 root. This may be of value in establishing the level of a peroneal nerve lesion and will be preserved if the lesion is at or below the knee, which is usually the case.

The tibial nerve supplies the long head of the biceps femoris and the medial hamstring muscles (knee flexion), the posterior compartment of the leg (plantar flexion and

inversion of the foot) and all the intrinsic muscles of the foot, with the exception of the extensor digitorum brevis, which is the only muscle belly on the dorsum of the foot. The ankle and medial hamstring jerks are conveyed in the tibial nerve through the S1 root.

The Root Supply

The L2 root is predominantly responsible for hip flexion and makes a major contribution to thigh adduction. Knee extension is minimally affected, even though the quadriceps receives contributions from L2, L3 and L4. The contribution of the L2 root to the cremasteric reflex is described earlier.

The L3 root makes a major contribution to both knee extension and thigh adduction, and it would appear on clinical grounds that the main motor innervation of the adductor and quadriceps muscles derives from the L3 root.

The L4 root conveys the knee jerk but seems to make a minor contribution to the motor supply of the quadriceps muscle. Patients who have an L4 root lesion often have minimal wasting and weakness of the quadriceps, with an absent knee jerk. Below the knee the L4 is the almost exclusive supply to the invertors of the foot (tibialis anterior in the anterior compartment of the leg and tibialis posterior in the posterior compartment of the leg). The L4 contribution to these muscles reaches them via the peroneal and tibial nerves respectively. With an L4 root lesion minimal weakness of dorsiflexion and plantar flexion of the foot may be found but there will be marked weakness of inversion of the foot. A patient with a bilateral L4 root lesion walks in a most peculiar way, with the feet flapping on the ground as if extremely flat-footed. Some gluteal weakness and wasting may also be detected in L4, L5 and S1 lesions. This is best seen by direct inspection of the buttocks and observing the muscle when the buttocks are clenched.

In L5 root lesions, if weakness is detectable it is usually maximal in the toe extensors, particularly of the great toe. Because of major contributions from L4 and S1 to the innervation of the muscles responsible for plantar and dorsiflexion of the foot, it is unusual to detect any weakness of these movements. Both L4 and L5 roots contribute to the nerve supply of the gluteal muscles, and wasting and weakness of these very large and powerful muscles is sometimes difficult to detect. No reflex is carried in the L5 root.

An S1 root lesion abolishes the ankle jerk and both hamstring reflexes will also be depressed or absent. Unless the root is totally destroyed weakness may be extremely difficult to detect. Eversion of the foot is the best movement to test when looking for evidence of an S1 root lesion. There may be some detectable weakness of plantar flexion and of the hamstring muscles. The hamstrings present the same problems on examination as the glutei, in that they are very large powerful muscles with a multiple root supply. Weakness and wasting may therefore be extremely difficult to detect in the presence of a single root lesion.

When examining power in the legs in any patient who has either back or abdominal pain, it is necessary to make considerable allowances for inhibition caused by the pain. If the patient is encouraged to make on maximal effort, however severe the pain, it is usually possible to establish whether or not strength is normal, and most patients will make this effort if they understand how important it is. It is not permissible in patients with leg pain to dismiss the motor examination as 'impossible due to pain', as vital localizing diagnostic evidence may be missed if the examination is incomplete.

Specific Clinical Conditions Affecting the Nerves and Nerve Roots of the Leg

Meralgia Paraesthetica

This common condition (entrapment of the lateral cutaneous nerve of the thigh) produces a peculiar numb, tingling, burning hypersensitivity over the middle lateral thigh. In a male patient it may be most noticeable when the hand is placed in the pocket because of the peculiar sensation that is provoked. The condition is most often encountered in obese patients of either sex who have lost a lot of weight, or conversely is sometimes seen in late pregnancy or in the weeks after delivery (it is possible that the sagging anterior abdominal wall pulls on the nerve) or it may occur idiopathically. Occasionally, obvious local trauma from tight jeans and examples due to a young lady sitting on the lap have been seen in young men. The condition usually remits spontaneously and surgical decompression should be avoided, or irreversible entrapment in scar tissue may well cause permanent problems and the pain may then assume a more severe, causalgic quality. It has been suggested that some cases are due to lumbar radicular lesions. If strict anatomical criteria are applied, it is difficult to see how this could be possible.

Femoral Nerve Lesions

The femoral nerve may be damaged in the upper abdomen by primary or secondary neoplasms or psoas abscesses and in the pelvis by an intrapelvic haematoma, a surprisingly common complication of poorly controlled anticoagulant therapy. Direct trauma to the nerve may occur during arterial catheterization or from a femoral artery aneurysm.

Diabetic Amyotrophy

An extremely important and frequently misdiagnosed complication of diabetes which affects either the femoral nerve itself or the three roots contributing to it. This is known as neuralgic amyotrophy or diabetic amyotrophy of Garland. It typically occurs in non-insulin-dependent diabetes mellitus and is more common in males. It is characterized by the onset of excruciating pain down the front of the thigh, often radiating down the medial border of the leg to the medial malleolus. There is usually a history of rapid weight loss and general ill-health in the weeks prior to the onset, which is probably the reason that malignant disease is often misdiagnosed. Within a few days of onset the pain, which may require narcotics for its control, abates and the patient suddenly develops rapid wasting and weakness of the quadriceps, which makes walking impossible.

The condition eventually improves although it may take 18–24 months for full recovery and 6 months may elapse before any recovery begins. In some cases the clinical evidence indicates that it is the L2, L3 and L4 roots that are damaged and not the femoral nerve itself. This produces more widespread weakness and wasting, including the hip flexors and adductor muscles. It is important to establish tight diabetic control, usually with insulin, to guarantee that this very disabling condition will recover.

Pelvic Haematoma

Pelvic haematoma is often due to poor anticoagulant control but may also occur in any haemorrhagic disorder. The onset is similar to diabetic amyotrophy, with severe thigh pain and an acute femoral nerve lesion. Full recovery takes 9–12 months.

CASE REPORT V

An 84-year-old lady had a revision operation for a total right hip replacement. One month later she developed severe groin pain on the same side. She had had prophylactic heparin to cover the original surgery in view of a previous pulmonary embolism. In spite of this a venogram revealed a deep vein thrombosis and she was given more heparin and started on Warfarin. The pain worsened and she developed weakness of the right leg. An MRI of the lumbar spine showed no significant lesion in the spinal canal. She was referred for a neurological opinion. On examination, she had pain in the R hip worse on hip flexion which was weak, and total paralysis of the right quadriceps. A CT scan was recommended to confirm the clinical diagnosis of a psoas haematoma. The CT scan showed marked enlargement of the psoas shadow. The appearances were consistent with a haematoma of some duration. There was no fresh blood and it is probable that the symptoms were due to a haemorrhage into the muscle perhaps at the time of the original surgery.

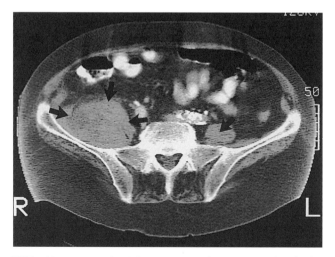

CRV Haematoma in right psoas muscle (arrows). The shadow is almost isodense and probably present several weeks. Note the normal psoas shadow on the left.

CASE REPORT VI

A domiciliary visit was requested on a 17-year-old boy with a 'slipped disc'. He had come back from a Scout camp with a flu-like illness, with fever and coughing. He had been unwell for only 3 weeks when seen. During that time he had increasingly severe backache radiating down into the left thigh, which was particularly severe at night. On examination he was clearly very anaemic, had lost weight and was in severe pain. There was no lymphadenopathy and no organs were palpable. There was marked wasting and weakness of the left quadriceps and the knee jerk was absent. He was barely able to stand. He was admitted to hospital where acute myeloid leukaemia was confirmed. This case was seen before CT scanning was available but the clinical diagnosis, which seems likely to have been correct, was a pelvic haematoma secondary to leukaemia.

Once again, the importance of recognizing the sinister significance of night pain, an atypical distribution and the rarity of disc lesions in young patients is demonstrated.

With the exception of these two classic conditions femoral nerve lesions are extremely unusual.

Sciatic Nerve Lesions

The sciatic nerve may be damaged in the pelvis by the direct spread of neoplasms from the rectum or genitourinary tract. Although sciatica is very common in late pregnancy, it is unlikely that this is due to direct compression of the sciatic nerve.

In the buttock, misplaced deep intramuscular injections, complicated hip fractures or penetrating trauma, especially due to gunshot or knife wounds, are the most frequent causes of sciatic nerve damage.

An unusual feature of damage at this site, mentioned earlier, is that the peroneal division is six times as likely to be damaged as the tibial division in spite of nonselective trauma to the whole nerve trunk. A common diagnostic problem that emphasizes the practical value of this knowledge is as follows. A patient with severe traumatic damage to the hip may not have been examined adequately prior to open joint surgery. Subsequently it is discovered that the patient has developed a foot drop. The question then arises as to whether this is simply due to pressure on the peroneal nerve at the fibula neck due to positioning during the surgery, or whether the nerve was damaged in the buttock by the fracture or during the surgery. The marked difference in prognosis, both in time and the potential for full recovery, is extremely important. A useful clinical sign may be the detection of wasting and weakness in the biceps femoris, the part of the hamstring muscle supplied by the peroneal nerve, as this would be unaffected by a peroneal nerve lesion at the fibula neck. If the lateral hamstring appears wasted the lateral hamstring reflex should be abolished. Electrophysiological studies should readily confirm whether or not the lesion is at the fibula neck, which carries an infinitely better prognosis.

Misplaced injections which damage the sciatic nerve are especially disastrous, as not only is there disabling weakness of both dorsiflexion and plantar flexion of the foot, but such mishaps often result in very severe causalgic pain over the leg and foot, sparing only the medial border of the leg supplied by the femoral nerve. This pain makes it almost impossible for the patient to tolerate the leg splints necessary to compensate for the weakness.

Peroneal Nerve Lesion

This is the nerve in the leg most often damaged by compression at the fibula neck, where the nerve winds round the bone protected only by skin and fascia, the fascia itself holding the nerve tightly against the bone. The nerve is therefore extremely vulnerable to modest compression at this point and compressive damage may occur in healthy patients following a sharp blow to the nerve or after to sitting for prolonged periods with the legs crossed.

In all cases care should be taken to exclude any general medical condition as a possible cause of increased vulnerability due to impaired nutrition of the nerve. Diabetes is probably the commonest cause, but polyarteritis nodosa and other collagen vascular diseases should be excluded. Where it is endemic leprosy is the commonest cause of this situation. In all these conditions other peripheral nerves may be vulnerable to damage by compression, particularly the ulnar nerve, and when multiple compression by palsies occur in this setting the condition is known as mononeuritis multiplex.

The normal peroneal nerve may also be more vulnerable in patients who have lost a lot of weight, when the protective effect of fat and muscle is lost, especially if they are confined to bed. Similarly, below-knee plasters may damage the nerve.

Whatever the cause the patient will develop a foot drop and, if the nerve lesion is complete, there will be weakness of inversion, dorsiflexion and eversion of the foot. These movements are controlled by nerve roots L4, L5 and S1 respectively. The distinction from an L5 root lesion should be simple but some difficulty may be experienced in demonstrating that inversion and eversion are intact when there is severe weakness of dorsiflexion due to an L5 root lesion. Testing can be facilitated by deliberately holding the foot in the neutral position while testing these movements. This is similar to the difficulty experienced when testing the intrinsic muscles of the hand in the presence of a severe wrist drop (see Chapter 16). Electromyography and nerve

conduction studies are invaluable in confirming the clinical diagnosis.

The cutaneous distribution of the peroneal nerve to the lower leg and foot is conveyed mainly in the superficial peroneal (musculocutaneous) nerve and supplies the lower anterolateral leg and on to the dorsum of the foot in a triangular area. A small twig from the deep peroneal nerve supplies the first interspace between the big and second toes. In most cases of peroneal nerve damage there is surprisingly little or no sensory loss. In practice it is unusual to find more than a small area of slightly altered sensation over the dorsum of the foot.

CASE REPORT VII

A 50-year-old hypertensive diabetic man tripped in a rabbit hole while playing golf. The next day he awakened with a severe foot drop. He did not immediately seek advice and was seen 3 weeks later when, if anything, the condition had worsened, with both motor and sensory deficit. The clinical evidence clearly indicated a peroneal nerve lesion at the fibula neck and this was confirmed by nerve conduction studies the same day. There was marked slowing through the affected segment of nerve. The immediately obvious cause was a diabetic compressive peroneal nerve lesion, but the antecedent trauma and the completeness of the deficit suggested that exploration would be wise. A fusiform enlargement of the nerve was found which, when incised, proved to be due to a haematoma in the nerve. A full recovery occurred over the next 6 weeks. It is likely that had exploration been delayed, more permanent damage would have occurred.

This case emphasizes the importance of taking every single aspect of the history into consideration and shows that the most obvious diagnosis is not necessarily the correct one.

Tibial Nerve Lesions

The tibial nerve, unlike the peroneal nerve, is rarely damaged. As already noted, it is much less likely to be damaged by trauma in the region of the hip joint, and throughout the thigh it lies in a deeply protected position. Behind the knee the tibial nerve is deeply placed and well protected from knee trauma, but may be damaged by fracture dislocations through the knee or by a popliteal artery aneurysm. In the calf, the nerve lies deep to the muscles and only becomes superficial where it divides at the flexor retinaculum into the medial and lateral plantar nerves. At this point a syndrome analogous to the carpal tunnel syndrome has been described which is known as the tarsal tunnel syndrome. It is quite rare.

Tarsal Tunnel Syndrome

Both the medial and lateral plantar nerves are affected and pain occurs over the medial aspect of the foot and sole, which has a burning quality similar to that described in carpal tunnel syndrome. There may be weakness and wasting of the intrinsic muscles of the foot and a positive Tinel's sign on tapping the nerve below the medial malleolus. The causes are not obvious. Patients are much more likely to have swollen oedematous feet than swollen oedematous hands, and yet the syndrome is very rarely associated with such obvious pathology. Occasionally decompressive surgery may find a ganglion arising from the ankle joint, which may prove to be the cause if entrapment is confirmed by electrophysiological studies.

The final branches of the tibial nerve are the medial and lateral plantar nerves. These are analogous to the median and ulnar nerves respectively. The medial plantar nerve supplies the skin of the medial sole with a limited muscular supply and the lateral plantar nerve the skin of the lateral sole and makes a very major contribution to the intrinsic muscles of the foot. There is no practical value in attempting to identify the actions of individual foot muscles.

The digital nerves run distally between the heads of the metatarsals and lie superficial to the deep transverse metatarsal ligament. They are therefore subject to both external compression and pinching between the metatarsal heads. The interdigital nerve between the third and fourth metatarsals is particularly vulnerable. Severe pain radiating into the web and adjacent sides of the toes on standing or walking may become quite disabling. Occasionally a neuroma will form on the nerve which is very tender to pressure and may be palpable. Treatment is by resection of the nerve. This condition is known as Morton's metatarsalgia.

Nerve lesions in the legs are relatively rare compared to the arm. Root lesions occur with greater frequency and may be related to serious intrapelvic or abdominal disease, and it is extremely incautious to assume that all leg pain is due to a disc lesion. It is essential to have a clear grasp of the intraspinal and intrapelvic anatomy of the lumbar and sacral nerve roots and to be aware of the clinical clues that suggest more ominous pathological possibilities.

The single most ominous symptom in a patient with back pain radiating into the leg is that the pain is not in an L5 or S1 distribution, is worse at rest and is particularly severe at night. This is in marked contrast to disc disease, in which rest is the main relieving factor.

As an example of the validity of this statement the following case is instructive.

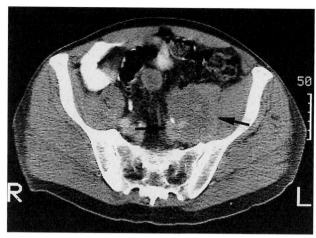

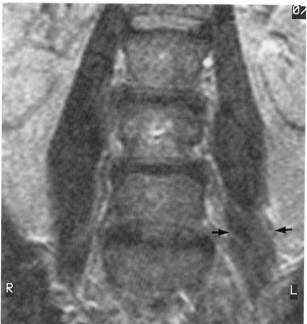

CRVIII. *Metastatic carcinoma in left psoas muscle.*

CASE REPORT VIII

A 58-year-old GP presented with pain in the left thigh. This had been presented for 8 weeks when he was first seen. One year previously he had a carcinoma of the bladder detected following the development of haematuria. This had been treated by radiotherapy and subsequent follow-up had been satisfactory. After a long drive he developed a sensation of burning and soreness in the left inguinal region and down the left lateral upper thigh. He thought that he was developing shingles, and by the first evening was in quite severe pain. The pain had a deep gnawing, burning quality to it and kept him awake. Over the subsequent 8 weeks the pain had become progressively more severe, with an increasing tendency to waken him at night, and could only be relieved by sitting up or walking round. It was not aggravated by movement, coughing or sneezing. He had not slept for several days because of pain. On physical examination there were no motor findings in the legs, the knee jerks and ankle jerks were intact and there was no impairment of hip flexion or adduction. There was impaired sensation over the distribution of the lateral cutaneous nerve of the thigh and over the distribution of the femoral branch of the genitofemoral nerve and the ilioinguinal nerve. Bearing in mind the lymphatic drainage of the bladder and the possibility of an extradural lesion, an MRI scan of the posterior abdominal wall and lumbar spine was obtained looking for evidence of lymph nodes, enlargement of the lower part of the psoas or extradural metastases. The scan was normal. Everyone except the neurologist and the patient was reassured by this finding, but the pain persisted and was unresponsive to narcotics and 6 weeks later, with no change in the physical findings but intractable pain, a CT scan was done with a view to proceeding to another MRI scan if this were also normal. On this occasion the lower part of the psoas was demonstrated to be greatly enlarged and fine-needle aspiration of the area revealed an anaplastic metastatic carcinoma. Radiotherapy was given, with some modest relief of the pain. The patient succumbed six months later.

Problems relating to the lower sacral roots were dealt with extensively under the heading Cauda equina lesions in Chapter 15.

In view of the lessons presented by the case above, it is appropriate at this point to consider the cutaneous nerve supply of the inguinal region, the perineum and the external genitalia in both sexes. This is very rarely discussed in textbooks and the anatomy of the nerve supply to the area is difficult to glean, even from the most detailed anatomical books, and yet it is an area of great clinical importance (Figs. 17.8 and 17.9).

The nerves supplying this area are interesting in that they are derived from the lumbar and sacral plexuses and are bilaterally vulnerable within the spinal canal itself, and therefore patients with bilateral impairment of sensation within the perineal area or genitalia will almost always be found to have lesions within the canal.

Once the nerves exit the canal, however, the situation becomes very different, as the nerves diverge from one another as they skirt round the pelvis and strictly unilateral presentations are then the rule. The iliohypogastric, ilioinguinal and subcostal nerves, which supply the medial and lateral inguinal regions respectively, and the lateral cutaneous nerve of the thigh (see Fig. 17.1) are therefore vulnerable posteriorly to retroperitoneal malignancy and involvement in the retroperitoneal lymphatic tissue, and anteriorly to abdominal incisions. The central part of the inguinal region is supplied by the femoral branch of the genitofemoral nerve, which takes a more direct route into the leg along the lateral border of the psoas, giving off a branch which accompanies the spermatic cord in the male and the round ligament of the uterus in the female, down into and supplying the same areas as are supplied by the ilioinguinal nerve as far as the genitalia are concerned, but do not contribute to the supply of the skin over the thigh.

Due to the descent of the testicle into the region from above, we also have the situation that the anterior

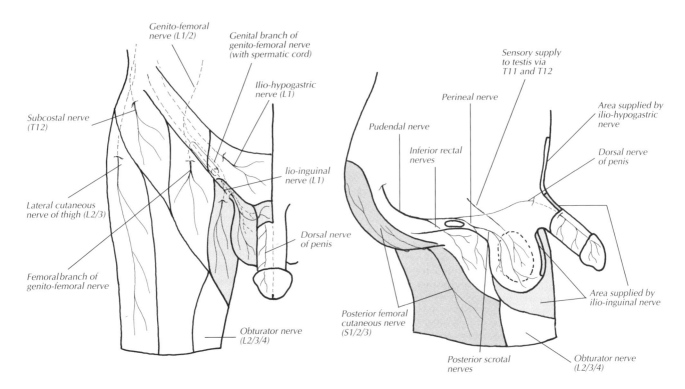

17.8 Cutaneous nerve supply to the inguinal region, perineum and external genitalia in the male.

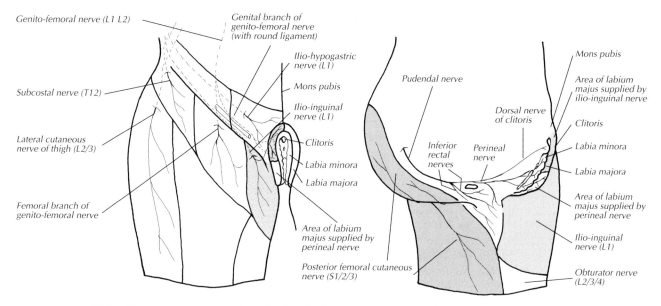

17.9   Cutaneous nerve supply to the inguinal region, perineum and external genitalia in the female.

scrotum is supplied by the ilioinguinal nerve derived from L1, the posterior scrotum by the posterior scrotal nerves derived form S2 and S3, and the contained testis a nerve supply derived from T11 and T12 and carried down into the scrotal sac via the spermatic cord. Similarly, in the female the mons pubis and upper labia majora are supplied by the L1 root via the ilioinguinal nerve, whereas the lower and posterior labium major is supplied by the posterior labial nerves derived from S2 and S3, as are the clitoris and labia minora. There is nowhere else in the body where adjacent skin areas are derived from such distant radicular origins, and this knowledge can be turned to advantage when evaluating localized pain or numbness in the genitalia in either sex.

The lower inner buttock and posterior inner thigh are supplied mainly by the posterior femoral cutaneous nerve of the thigh, but the area around the anal margin and the adjacent upper inner thigh are supplied by the inferior rectal nerves in both sexes, with considerable overlap with the posterior cutaneous nerve of the thigh. The perineal nerve supplies the more anterior perineum in front of the anal margin forward to the area supplied by the ilioinguinal nerve, on the anterior inner thigh. In the male the posterior scrotal nerves supply the posterior part of the scrotum. In the female the posterior labial nerves supply the skin over the posterior inferior labia majora and the skin of the labia minora and the lower third of the vagina. The clitoris is supplied by the dorsal nerve of the clitoris. The male equivalent, the dorsal nerve of the penis, has a much more extensive nerve supply over the dorsal aspect of the penis anterior to the area supplied by the ilioinguinal nerve and the entire glans and prepuce. Thus the root

of the penis is supplied by nerve elements derived from L1, as is the anterior scrotum and the whole penis anterior to this, and the posterior aspect of the scrotum and perineum is supplied by S2 and S3. All the areas of sensation in the male and female ultimately carried in the pudendal nerve are vulnerable to lesions of the rectum, vagina and prostate and the pararectal tissues, and are vulnerable to surgical procedures performed through the perineum. It is worth emphasizing that pain in these areas has a very unpleasant nagging quality and is often worse nocturnally. There is a high likelihood of underlying malevolent disease in all patients presenting with pain in these areas.

Finally a comment on straight leg raising is necessary as this is hard to evaluate. If the history includes typical radicular pain on coughing or sneezing, lifting the leg on the affected side may well prove painful after only 20°–30° of elevation and if it has been tested several times, the patient will tense up as soon as the leg is held preparatory to lifting it. The best test is to flex the leg at the hip with the knee flexed as the leg comes up. Then the examiner straightens the leg at the knee. Often hip flexion of 45° or more will be tolerated when only 10° was achieved when lifting the leg held straight, suggesting a strong emotional component. Side to side comparison is also important. This modification is called Lasegue's sign. Severe totally extravasated disc lesions can be accompanied by completely normal straight leg raising whereas a small disc protrusion in the root canal may cause dramatic loss of straight leg raising. Like all signs in neurology, it must be interpreted in the light of the history and the other physical signs and must not be given undue weight.

Table 17.1   Comparative data – root lesions in the leg

Roots	L2	L3	L4	L5	S1
Sensory supply	Across upper thigh to posterior axial line	Across lower thigh to posterior axial line	Across knee to medial malleolus	Lateral leg to dorsum and sole of foot and great toe	Behind lateral malleolus to lateral foot and little toe
Sensory loss	Often none Lateral area if any	Often none Lateral area if any	Medial leg below knee to medial malleolus	Dorsum of foot to great toe	Behind lateral malleolus and lateral border of foot
Area of pain	Across thigh diagonally	Across thigh diagonally	Down to medial malleolus. Often severe at knee round patella	Back of thigh lateral calf, dorsum of foot and great toe	Back of thigh back of calf lateral foot to little toe
Reflex arc	None	Adductor reflex	Knee jerk	None	Ankle jerk and hamstring jerks
Motor deficit (most readily demonstrated)	Hip flexion Thigh adduction	Knee extension Thigh adduction	Inversion of the foot	Dorsiflexion of toes and foot (latter L4 also)	Plantar flexion & eversion of foot
Causative lesions (in order of frequency)	L2 / L3 / L4	Neurofibroma Meningioma Neoplastic disease Disc lesions very rare (except L4 < 5% all)		L5 / S1	Disc lesions Metastatic malignancy Neurofibromas Meningiomas Congenital lesions affecting cauda equina

Table 17.2   Comparative data – nerve lesions in the leg

Nerves	Obturator	Femoral	Sciatic nerve	
			Peroneal division	Tibial division
Sensory supply	Medial surface of thigh to posterior axial line	Anteromedial surface of thigh and leg down to medial malleolus	Anterior leg, dorsum of ankle and foot	Posterior leg, sole and lateral border of foot
Sensory loss	Often none	Usually anatomical as above	Often only detectable dorsum of foot	Sole and lateral border of foot
Area of pain	Medial thigh	Anterior thigh and medial leg to ankle	Often painless dull ache Anterolateral leg & foot	Often painless Very uncommon
Reflex arc	Adductor jerk	Knee jerk	Lateral hamstring jerk	Ankle jerk Medial hamstring jerk
Motor deficit	Adduction of thigh	Extension of knee	Dorsiflexion, inversion (tibialis anterior) & eversion of the foot Lateral hamstrings	Plantar flexion and inversion of foot (tibialis posterior) Medial hamstrings
Causative lesions	Pelvic neoplasm Pregnancy Pelvic surgery	Diabetes Femoral hernia Retroperitoneal haematoma (anticoagulants) Femoral artery aneurysm Posterior abdominal neoplasm Psoas abscess	Pressure palsy at fibula neck Hip fracture/dislocation Penetrating trauma to buttock Misplaced injection in buttock	Very rarely injured even in buttock Peroneal division more sensitive to damage (reason unknown)

18. Diseases of Muscle and the Muscle End-Plate

Muscles are subject to a wide range of inherited, degenerative, metabolic and toxic disorders. There is a marked similarity to peripheral nerve disease in that a wide range of disorders produce a limited group of symptoms and signs. Differential diagnosis depends on a careful family history, careful documentation of the extent and distribution of the muscle abnormalities and an awareness of all the diagnostic possibilities.

Muscular Dystrophy

Muscular dystrophy is characterized by an inherited degeneration of various muscle groups that begins after a period of apparently normal muscle development and function. In some varieties the onset is delayed until adulthood. Although it is still regarded as a primary muscle disorder, clinical and electrophysiological evidence has suggested a neurogenic component. A full discussion of these controversial views is beyond the scope of the present text. Although clinical features often allow a confident diagnosis to be made it is essential that full confirmatory studies, including electrophysiological tests and muscle biopsy, are performed. The diagnosis must be certain for prognostic purposes and to allow genetic counselling to be firmly based. Occasionally, patients are seen who have been given a lethal prognosis and who are later shown to have a restricted form of myopathy or a neuropathic disease such as Kugelberg–Welander syndrome. The main conditions to be considered are:

Duchenne muscular dystrophy
Becker's muscular dystrophy
Limb-girdle dystrophy (pelvifemoral type, Leyden–Mobius variety and scapulohumeral type)
Facioscapulohumeral dystrophy (Landouzy–Dejerine)

Dystrophia myotonica (Steinert's disease)
Myotonia congenita (Thomsen's disease)
Ocular dystrophies (oculopharyngeal muscular dystrophy).

The muscular dystrophies are identified and classified as a result of the sequence and distribution of weakness in the various types. This distribution, and the ancillary clinical features relevant to each condition, are illustrated in Figures 18.1–18.6

General Clinical Features of Muscular Dystrophy

1. There is often a positive family history. It is always worth remembering that family histories can be unreliable or impossible to obtain. Only a positive family history has any significance.
2. The distribution and sequence of muscle damage will vary widely depending on the type of dystrophy. Indeed, these features form the basis of the classification of muscular dystrophy.
3. In muscular dystrophy the muscles become weak before significant wasting is apparent. This is because the degenerating fibres are often replaced by fat, and the muscles may even appear hypertrophied. Such muscles have a stodgy, doughy feel. This is quite the reverse of neural disease, in which the atrophy often proceeds faster than weakness develops.
4. Reflexes are often depressed or absent very early in the course of muscular dystrophy and long before the muscle is significantly wasted. This is one of several features that has led to the suggestion that there is a neurogenic component in some cases.
5. In the terminal stages of muscular dystrophy it may be impossible to make a clinical diagnosis as the widespread muscle wasting, weakness and loss of reflexes could equally well indicate a diffuse neurogenic disorder.

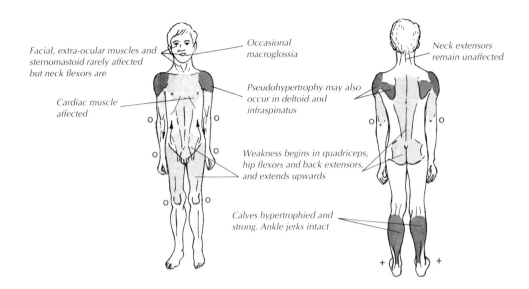

Facial, extra-ocular muscles and
sternomastoid rarely affected
but neck flexors are

Cardiac muscle
affected

Occasional
macroglossia

Pseudohypertrophy may also
occur in deltoid and
infraspinatus

Weakness begins in quadriceps,
hip flexors and back extensors,
and extends upwards

Calves hypertrophied and
strong. Ankle jerks intact

Neck extensors
remain unaffected

Duchenne muscular dystrophy

1. Males, inherited as a sex-linked recessive due to a defect in the short arm of the X chromosome leading to absence of a specific cytoskeletal muscle protein dystrophin. (Rare female cases reported. Nearly all XO, Turner's syndrome.) 30% of all cases are new mutations

2. Onset between 3 and 10 years of age. 30 cases per 100 000

3. No abortive cases, most die within 6 years of onset, usually by age 20

4. Onset in proximal muscles of leg, especially quadriceps and lower trunk muscles: later shoulder girdle and then extends peripherally. Contractures occur early and are severe. Early neck flexor involvement may be detected by careful examination

5. Important early signs include loss of reflexes, except the ankle jerk, which usually remains intact and excludes a neuropathy, as does the striking preservation of strength in the foot flexors and invertors

6. Diaphragm, extraocular and facial muscles very rarely involved

7. Other features include macroglossia, pseudohypertrophy of calves, deltoids and infraspinatus. ECG shows tall R waves and deep Q waves in 90% of cases

8. Bone thinning, scoliosis, pathological fractures, fatty infiltration of the heart and respiratory infections are important complications that may lead to death

9. 30% of affected patients have an IQ of less than 75

10. The carrier state may be detected by serum enzyme studies and EMG. Early on in affected children enzymes are very high, with a later fall into normal range when atrophy is severe. Gut muscle involvement may cause bowel obstruction

11. Although steroids may improve strength in early cases it has no effect on prognosis.

18.1   Duchenne muscular dystrophy.

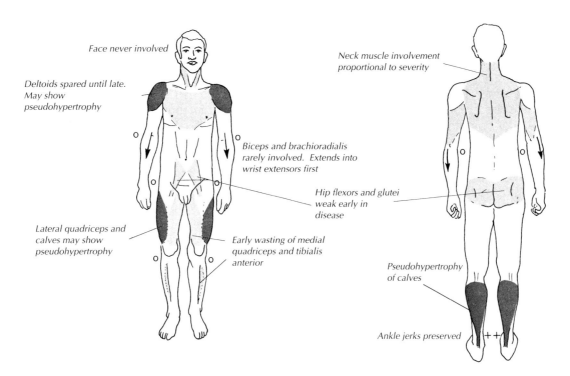

Face never involved

Deltoids spared until late. May show pseudohypertrophy

Biceps and brachioradialis rarely involved. Extends into wrist extensors first

Lateral quadriceps and calves may show pseudohypertrophy

Early wasting of medial quadriceps and tibialis anterior

Neck muscle involvement proportional to severity

Hip flexors and glutei weak early in disease

Pseudohypertrophy of calves

Ankle jerks preserved

Limb girdle dystrophy (This group remains controversial and the diagnosis should only be made after extensive investigation to exclude other diagnoses)

1. Males/females equally affected, autosomal recessive but occasionally dominant or sporadic

2. Onset between 10 and 30 years of age

3. Abortive cases with incomplete picture occur with mainly pelvic (pelvifemoral form) or shoulder girdle (scapulohumeral form) involvement. Usually causes disability over 10–20 years after onset

4. Onset may be either pelvic or shoulder girdle and may remain confined to these areas and apparently static for years. Eventually considerable peripheral wasting and weakness may occur. Contractures are unusual

5. Proximal reflexes are often impaired and, as in Duchenne dystrophy, the ankle jerks are usually preserved until late in the disease

6. Cardiac involvement is extremely rare and facial muscles are only slightly affected if at all

7. Pseudohypertrophy may occur in the calves and deltoids and strikingly in the lateral quadriceps, often associated with early and gross wasting of the medial thigh

8. There are no special complications and lifespan is unaffected

9. Intelligence is normal

10. The serum enzymes are slightly elevated or normal

11. The differential diagnosis should include polymyositis, late-onset congenital myopathies, lipid and mitochondrial myopathy and Kugelberg–Welander syndrome

18.2   Limb girdle dystrophies.

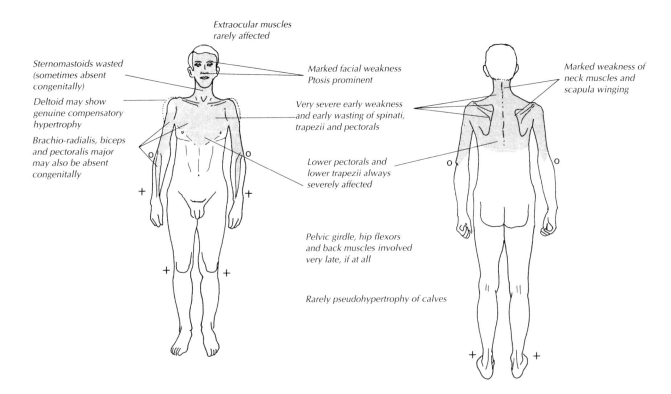

*Extraocular muscles
rarely affected*

*Sternomastoids wasted
(sometimes absent
congenitally)*

*Deltoid may show
genuine compensatory
hypertrophy*

*Brachio-radialis, biceps
and pectoralis major
may also be absent
congenitally*

*Marked facial weakness
Ptosis prominent*

*Very severe early weakness
and early wasting of spinati,
trapezii and pectorals*

*Lower pectorals and
lower trapezii always
severely affected*

*Marked weakness of
neck muscles and
scapula winging*

*Pelvic girdle, hip flexors
and back muscles involved
very late, if at all*

Rarely pseudohypertrophy of calves

Facioscapulohumeral dystrophy (Landouzy–Dejerine)

1. Males/females equally affected, autosomal dominant, occasionally recessive

2. Onset at any age between 10 and 40 years of age. 3–10 cases per 100 000

3. Mild abortive cases common. Siblings or parents of a patient often have only facial weakness

4. Weakness begins in the face then involves the shoulder girdle, particularly the lower trapezil and pectoralis, triceps and biceps. Forearm muscles may show striking true compensatory hypertrophy. Pelvic girdle is rarely significantly involved and very late if at all. Contractures very rare

5. Reflexes only impaired at biceps and triceps. Progression extremely slow. Disability is relatively minor

6. Pseudohypertrophy is rare, the deltoids are often enlarged by true hypertrophy to compensate for other weak muscles

7. Special features include congenital absence of pectoralis, biceps or brachioradialis. Occasionally tibialis anterior may be the only muscle involved below the shoulder girdle

8. Normal lifespan

9. Normal intelligence

10. Serum enzyme studies show slight increase in 50% of cases

18.3   Facioscapulohumeral dystrophy.

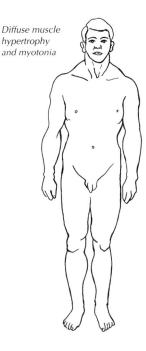

Diffuse muscle hypertrophy and myotonia

Myotonia congenita (Thomsen's disease)

1. Both sexes affected. Inherited as an autosomal dominant. 2 cases per 100 000

2. Myotonia is present from birth and first noticed as a peculiar cry, difficult in feeding or inability to reopen the eyes while having face washed

3. Muscle hypertrophy becomes apparent in the second decade but athletic ability is poor due to slowness and stiffness of movement. Once warmed up the stiffness eases and some patients can compete in long-distance events. The myotonia is much worse in the cold and this makes winter games such as football virtually impossible

4. The muscle hypertrophy is the result of almost continual involuntary isometric exercise

5. The myotonia becomes less severe with age and often responds well to procaineamide, phenytoin or quinidine. Patients are well advised to pursue an indoor occupation. One patient, a glazier, was unable to work in winter because whenever he offered up a piece of glass to a window frame he was unable to let go, much to the consternation of his helper!

6. There are no associated abnormalities and the condition has no effect on life expectancy

7. Thought to be due to a defect in chloride conductance in muscle membrane

8. An autosomal recessive form exists which is associated with progressive weakness

18.4   Myotonia congenita.

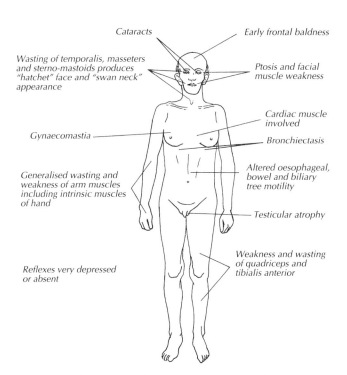

Cataracts

Early frontal baldness

Wasting of temporalis, masseters and sterno-mastoids produces "hatchet" face and "swan neck" appearance

Ptosis and facial muscle weakness

Gynaecomastia

Cardiac muscle involved

Bronchiectasis

Generalised wasting and weakness of arm muscles including intrinsic muscles of hand

Altered oesophageal, bowel and biliary tree motility

Testicular atrophy

Weakness and wasting of quadriceps and tibialis anterior

Reflexes very depressed or absent

1. Males/females both affected. Inherited as an autosomal dominant in most cases. 3–5 cases per 100 000

2. Onset at any age is possible, including congenital, but in most cases disease develops between 20 and 30 years of age. Where the mother is the carrier the age of onset is earlier, even in infancy, and apparent improvement in childhood is then followed by rapid deterioration at the more usual age of onset

3. There is a general impression that the disease shows incomplete penetrance and it has been claimed that cataracts in a previous generation are minimal evidence of the disease. It is also possible that the disease appears earlier in successive generations, but this may merely reflect earlier recognition. These points are all subject to considerable controversy

4. The onset may be either dominated by weakness or myotonia or a combination of both. Difficulty in releasing the grip may present problems if delicate skills are required or pure weakness if manual work is involved. In some patients with leg weakness, difficulty in kicking a ball or "pseudo" drop attacks due to quadriceps weakness may be the presenting symptoms. In most cases the flexor muscles of the arms are myotonic and the extensors muscles weak

5. Important additional clues to the diagnosis are numerous. These include frontal baldness (in females this may be disguised by a wig), loss of facial expression and ptosis, marked wasting of masseters and temporalis giving a haggard, wasted appearance to the face. Posterior capsular cataracts always ultimately occur. There may be dysarthria due to myotonia of the tongue. Wasting of the sternomastoids to the point of disappearance is a prominent early feature and patients may have difficulty in lifting the head from a pillow. The neck is thinned, producing a 'swan neck'. If the tongue is percussed on a tongue depressor or the thenar eminence percussed, a slow myotonic contraction of the muscles is seen

6. Numerous other abnormalities occur, including gynaecomastia, gonadal atrophy with impotence, cardiac abnormalities with syncopal attacks and motility disorders of the entire bowel and biliary tree. Respiratory infections are common due to bronchial muscular difficulties and occasionally abnormalities in immunoglobulins. Many patients have a low IQ and dementia may occur in the course of the disease

7. The diagnosis is usually unmistakable on clinical grounds alone and the EMG changes of myotonia are easily detectable in almost any muscle

8. Premature death is the rule and is usually due to cardiac failure or overwhelming chest infection

18.5   Dystrophia myotonica (Steinert's disease).

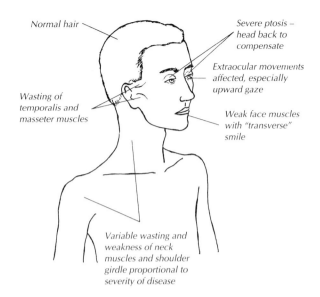

Normal hair

*Severe ptosis –
head back to
compensate*

*Extraocular movements
affected, especially
upward gaze*

*Wasting of
temporalis and
masseter muscles*

*Weak face muscles
with "transverse"
smile*

*Variable wasting and
weakness of neck
muscles and shoulder
girdle proportional to
severity of disease*

Progressive ocular myopathy (including
oculopharyngeal muscular dystrophy)

1. Both sexes affected. Dominant or sporadic inheritance

2. Clinical features range from ptosis alone to ptosis with eye
    movement disorder and facial weakness, and in some 25% of
    cases shoulder girdle involvement

3. 50% have dysphagia; in some families this is the major feature and
    the other clinical signs are only found on careful examination. The
    term oculopharyngeal muscular dystrophy has been proposed for
    this group. These cases may be dramatically helped by
    cricopharyngeal myotomy. One emaciated patient put on 40 lb in
    6 weeks postoperatively

4. Some families have retinitis pigmentosa, visual difficulties,
    endocrine abnormalities, cardiac involvement and cerebellar
    abnormalities. Electrical and histological studies suggest a
    neuropathic rather than a myopathic basis in some patients

5. The disorder may lie somewhere between the muscular
    dystrophies and metabolic neuropathies such as Refsum's disease,
    and clinically must be distinguished from dystrophia myotonica

18.6   Progressive ocular myopathy.

Congenital Myopathies

For many years the term 'floppy infant' was used to
describe a group of muscular disorders, present from
birth, in which the child was hypotonic and showed
delayed motor activity and development. The disabilities may be sufficiently severe to threaten the childs'
survival. A wide range of disorders may be responsible.

In some cases the condition is merely evidence of
severe cerebral damage, as spasticity and choreoathetoid movements cannot develop until 1–2 years of
age. Werdnig–Hoffman disease may be so severe at
birth that floppy paralysis is already present. This is
fully discussed in Chapter 19. Dystrophia myotonica is
another possible cause of the 'floppy infant' syndrome,

although the usual onset is in the second or third
decade.

This leaves several other disorders that appear to be
due to a myopathic process, ranging from a benign
variety with delayed but normal motor development, to
a progressive myopathy. The routine use of muscle
biopsy, including electron microscopy and histochem-
istry, has revealed several different pathologies.
Currently four varieties of congenital myopathy have
been identified. On muscle biopsy all show an increase
in the number of type 1 fibres and the additional pathological changes are confined to this fibre type.

Central Core Disease

In this condition the muscle fibre demonstrates abnormal
structure and absence of muscle enzymes in the central
areas of the muscle fibre. It is inherited as an autosomal
dominant. The abnormal core is only found in type
1 fibres and a higher number than usual of type 1 fibres
are present. It is still unclear whether this is myopathic
degeneration or secondary to a neurogenic disorder.

Nemaline-Rod Myopathy

In this condition thread like structures are found in the
type 1 muscle fibres. Inheritance is usually autosomal
dominant but may also be recessive or sporadic. It is
characterized by a thin dysmorphic facies and is associated with kyphoscoliosis and pes cavus.

Myotubular Myopathy

In this condition the type 1 muscle fibres have a tubular
structure similar to foetal muscle. It is inherited as an
autosomal recessive. In childhood there is marked
weakness of the extraocular and facial muscles. Some
rare cases of adult onset with limb-girdle dystrophy
have now been described.

Congenital Fibre-Type Disproportion

The muscle demonstrates a markedly abnormal ratio of
muscle fibre type, with an excess of type 1 fibres which
are smaller than usual. Fifty per cent of cases are
associated with congenital dislocation of the hip, foot
deformities, arched palate and kyphoscoliosis. Mild
muscle biopsy changes similar to this occur in the three
other types and it is still not clear whether this is a discrete entity, but infants with this condition have very
severe floppy weakness and are readily misdiagnosed
as having Werdnig–Hoffman disease. Some degree of
improvement beginning at 2 years excludes the latter
diagnosis.

Most patients with these disorders survive into adulthood, with various degrees of disability due to proximal myopathy.

Metabolic Myopathy

A complete discussion of muscle metabolism is beyond the immediate scope of this book. For brevity, discussion will be confined to generalizations which given an idea of the biochemical function of muscles upon which discussion of the different types of metabolic myopathy can be based.

There are three main metabolic considerations:

1. Protein metabolism must be normal to maintain the integrity of the contractile proteins. In some endocrine myopathies contractile protein abnormalities may contribute to muscle weakness.

2. The metabolism of energy production in the muscle must be intact. This basically means that glucose availability and the glycogen breakdown pathways must be normal. Several muscles disorder are based on either glucose assimilation disorders or enzyme deficiencies in the glycogen breakdown pathway.

3. Normal sodium, potassium and calcium metabolism is of importance in maintaining normal resting membrane potentials, and is critical in the induction and cessation of contraction.

The metabolic pathways and interrelationships of these metabolic activities are summarized in Figure 18.7. The metabolic myopathies tend to cause chronic progressive muscle weakness, but in the initial stages episodes of sudden severe weakness during or following exertion are the most typical feature. The distinction can often be made on a typical history of the acute episodes.

Muscle Disease due to Abnormal Glycogen Metabolism

Although there are seven glycogen storage disorders only four are associated with clinically significant muscle disease.

Pompe's Disease (Type II Glycogenosis)

This is usually a disease of infancy and invariably fatal. It is inherited as an autosomal recessive disorder and the gene is located on the long arm of chromosome 17. In recent years, a few cases of a mild form of this disorder have been recognized in adults. In the infantile form

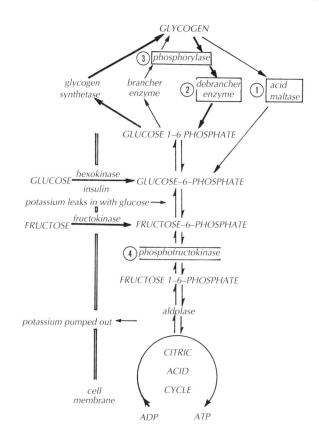

The following glycogen storage disorders produce muscle disease. The enzyme block is indicated on the figure
1. Pompé's disease (Type II glycogenosis)
2. Cori's disease (Type III glycogenosis)
3. McCardle's Syndrome (Type V glycogenosis)
4. Tarui's disease (Type VII glycogenosis)
Note also the leak of potassium into the cell during glucose uptake and the active pump mechanism which keeps the intracellular potassium down (see the periodic paralyses)

18.7   Glucose–glycogen metabolism in muscle

the heart, liver, kidneys and the CNS itself are also affected, and either cardiac failure or muscle weakness may be the first evidence of the disease. The condition is very difficult to distinguish from Werdnig–Hoffman disease, including the fact that EMG shows profuse fibrillation – an indication of ventral horn cell disease or denervation. This is thought to be due to ventral horn cell infiltration by glycogen. The clinical diagnostic clues lie in the finding of cardiac damage and often a very large tongue, which may suggest the alternative diagnosis of cretinism with a proximal myopathy. Neither of these features occurs in Werdnig–Hoffman disease.

In the adult form a slowly progressive proximal myopathy occurs. The very patchy involvement may simulate polymyositis, emphasizing the vital importance of muscle biopsy as the EMG findings may be similarly confusing, with evidence of both myopathic and neurogenic change. Muscle biopsy will reveal glycogen-filled vacuoles throughout the muscle cells.

Debranching Enzyme Disease (Limit Dextrinosis or Type III Glycogenosis)

This condition is inherited as an autosomal recessive and the main feature is infiltration of the liver, causing hepatomegaly, stunted growth and hypoglycaemia. A mild proximal myopathy with hypotonia is present in infancy and a few adult cases have been reported, with a clinical picture easily mistaken for motor neuron disease.

Myophosphorylase Deficiency (McArdle's Syndrome or Type V Glycogenosis)

This condition is usually inherited as an autosomal recessive but dominant transmission has now been reported. It is three times as common in males. The abnormality in this condition is confined to the skeletal muscles. The abnormality is only apparent on exertion, as the defect blocks the glycogen – glucose conversion. Because the enzyme has no role in glycogen synthesis there is only a minimal excess of glycogen in the muscle. The disorder causes easy fatiguability and severe muscle cramping on exercise, with breakdown of muscle proteins leading to myoglobinuria and eventually renal failure in 8% of patients. As in all metabolic muscle disorders there is a tendency for patients to develop permanent limb-girdle muscle weakness later in life, and this occurs in 20% of cases of McArdle's syndrome.

The classic investigation is to exercise the forearm muscles with a cuff on the arm so that the muscle is ischaemic. This increases the need for anaerobic glycolysis and the muscle promptly goes into severe cramp. If a venous sample of blood is taken from the exercised arm there is no rise in the blood lactate level and EMG sampling of the muscles in cramp will reveal electrical silence. This is quite the reverse of normal muscle cramp. The disorder is extremely rare. Avoidance of sudden or prolonged exertion is the only useful advice to give the patient as there is no specific treatment.

Phosphofructokinase Deficiency (Tarui's Disease or Type VII Glycogenosis)

The clinical details of this disease are virtually identical to McArdle's syndrome but in this case the block in the glycogen–glucose breakdown pathway is several stages further on (see Fig. 18.7).

Muscle Disease due to Abnormal Potassium Metabolism

These conditions are known as the periodic paralyses and are associated with alterations in serum and tissue potassium levels. The defect probably lies in muscle membrane permeability, the serum potassium levels merely reflecting massive uptake or loss of potassium from the muscles. Although the serum potassium levels are diagnostic, recent studies suggest that alterations in sodium conductance across muscle membranes may also play a critical role. There are three types.

Familial Hypokalaemic Periodic Paralysis

This is inherited as an autosomal dominant affecting males more than females in a ratio of 4:1. In females the gene shows reduced penetrance, which accounts for this difference. The condition becomes evident between 10 and 20 years of age and tends to remit after 35 years of age. Attacks typically occur after rest, usually on waking in the morning. They particularly occur if a heavy carbohydrate meal or excessive exercise were taken on the previous evening. Stress, cold exposure or excess alcohol may also be provocative.

An excess of potassium enters the muscles fibre during the high rate of glucose uptake, following a meal or after exercise. The serum potassium falls weakness becoming apparent at a level of 3.5 mmol/l and maximal at 2.5mmol/l, suggesting that it is the high intracellular potassium that causes the weakness rather than the serum level, as much lower levels of potassium are necessary to induce weakness in normal people.

An attack is rarely fatal as the diaphragm, respiratory muscles and eye muscles are unaffected. This is because the continual activity of these muscles even during sleep keeps pumping potassium out of the cells: further evidence that it is the rising intracellular potassium that is critical in causing weakness.

Attacks usually last 8–24 hours and tend to become less frequent and severe with age. An attack may be relieved by 10 g of potassium chloride in water taken orally. Acetazolamide 150 mg daily will provide some protection in patients having frequent attacks by preventing potassium entering the muscle cells. The condition is much more common in patients of Asian origin, in whom a very high association with thyrotoxicosis is also seen.

CASE REPORT I

A 28-year-old waiter from a Chinese restaurant was referred with attacks of weakness. These tended to occur on Sunday mornings. On Saturday nights when the restaurant closed, he and his colleagues ate all the leftover food and played mahjong until 6 a.m. He then went to bed. On many occasions, when he wakened in the morning he was totally paralysed and took several hours to recover fully. He was admitted to hospital and on a standard NHS diet over 4 days his serum potassium level remained obstinately normal. Thyroid tests proved that he was thyrotoxic. On the Saturday evening he was sent back to work in the restaurant and asked to behave as usual, and was readmitted to the ward at 6 a.m. At 8.30 a.m. his serum potassium was 1.8 mmol/l and he was again paralysed. Treatment of his thyrotoxicosis and avoidance of the provocative activities proved highly successful. Three years later he produced a fellow waiter from another Chinese restaurant with the same condition!

Genetic exploration via the family history can sometimes produce unanticipated problems. While questioning an 18-year-old boy with the condition in the presence of his mother, it emerged that the only person he was aware of with the condition was his father's best friend. The expression on his mother's face at that moment suggested that further discussion along these lines might prove embarrassing.

Adynamia Episodica Hereditaria (Gamstorp's Disease or Hyperkalaemic Periodic Paralysis)

This version of potassium-related weakness is characterized by the sudden onset of weakness some 30 minutes after exercise. If the patient senses the stiffness and weakness coming on further exercise may delay the onset but the subsequent attack is then more severe. Unlike the hypokalaemic condition, fasting may provoke this type of attack.

The proximal muscles are particularly affected and become stiff and myotonic. Individual attacks last 30 minutes to 2 hours. Attacks usually start between 5 and 15 years of age and tend to remit after 20 years of age. Unfortunately, a chronic proximal myopathy tends to develop after the condition has apparently burnt out.

The weakness is probably due to the sudden release of potassium from the muscles as it occurs when the serum level is only just over 5 mmol/l. In patients with potassium retention weakness does not occur until a serum level of 7 mmol/l is reached.

Attacks may be provoked by oral potassium and prevented by the use of acetazolamide 50–100 mg daily and an acute attack may be terminated by 1–2 g of calcium gluconate intravenously or 100 g glucose given as dextrose saline with 10 units of soluble insulin. The rapid uptake of glucose facilitated by the insulin transports potassium back into the muscles cells.

Normokalaemic Periodic Paralysis

It is very uncertain whether this condition exists: It is thought that many reported cases are examples of Gamstorp's disease. An unusual feature is that the condition occurs in infancy, between 2 and 10 years of age. The attacks consist of sudden episodes of flaccid quadriplegia that may last from 1 to 3 weeks. They may respond to sodium chloride and can be prevented by the use of salt-retaining steroids such as fludrocorti-

sone. The relationship of this disorder to potassium metabolism is obscure.

Secondary Metabolic and Endocrine Myopathies

Some features of endocrine myopathy are due to coexisting electrolyte disturbances so that some degree of overlap is inevitable in discussing these problems.

Electrolyte Disturbance

Sodium Metabolism

Several disorders of sodium metabolism cause cerebral symptoms and these dominate the clinical features. Milder disorders of sodium metabolism may contribute to muscle weakness in adrenal disease.

Hypokalaemia

Hypokalaemia of less than 2.5 mmol/l causes severe flaccid tetraparesis. The most frequent causes are:

   Conn's syndrome (aldosterone-secreting adrenal tumour)
   Renal disease (Fanconi syndrome, renal tubular acidosis)
   Potassium-losing enteritis and severe diarrhoea
   Excessive diuretic therapy (thiazide diuretics)
   Carbenoxolone therapy (liquorice extract used in peptic ulcer disease)
   Bartter's syndrome
   Amphoteracin B toxicity
   Alcoholism – both acute and chronic myopathies
   Lithium poisoning
   Mineralocorticoids (especially fludrocortisone)
   Thyrotoxicosis.

An immediate serum potassium determination is indicated in **any** patient with acute or subacute flaccid paraparesis. One patient with Conn's syndrome was only diagnosed when a third attack of acute paralytic poliomyelitis was thought to be an unlikely diagnosis!

Hyperkalaemia

Hyperkalaemia greater than 7 mmol/l causes a severe ascending quadriplegia that may mimic Guillain–Barre syndrome. It is extremely rare for the extra ocular muscles to be affected. The most frequent causes are:

Renal failure

Adrenal insufficiency

Rhabdomyolysis

Excessive administration of potassium salts in i.v. infusions

Aldosterone antagonists (spironolactone).

There is a much greater risk that the cardiotoxic effect of hyperkalaemia will kill the patient before the onset of paralysis. However, this is not always the case.

CASE REPORT II

A 81-year-old man was referred because of sudden falls when his legs seemed to buckle under him. This occurred after two cataract operations and an episode of congestive heart failure treated with diuretics. He had noticed an ongoing but variable difficulty getting in and out of chairs, which he attributed to increased weight. When he fell it was as if his legs had suddenly collapsed under him. On examination, apart from slight thinning of both thighs, there was no neurological abnormality. The neurophysiologist who was asked to do EMG and nerve conduction studies wrote, 'I think I shall have to give up EMG if I continue to get results like this, which do not make much sense with the clinical picture'! The EMGs were quite normal but he had motor velocities of 21 and 24 M/s in the legs and 34 M/s in the ulnar nerves. There were no sensory action potentials. While waiting for these studies he had resumed taking salt with his meals and thought that he had improved. He was therefore admitted for metabolic studies. On examination the normality of the nervous system was confirmed. In particular the reflexes remained normal and there was no sensory deficit. He was dyspnoeic with slight ankle oedema and a raised JVP. Routine biochemistry revealed a serum potassium of 8.2 mmol/l. All other electrolytes were normal except for a slightly reduced magnesium level. His creatinine was 250 mmol/l. Thyroid function was normal. He was treated immediately with 10 ml of 10% calcium gluconate and calcium resonium suppositaries and a glucose and insulin infusion was started. Twenty-four hours later the potassium had fallen to 6.7 mmol/l and, without further intravenous therapy, continued to fall into the normal range and threatened to go even lower because of severe constipation, preventing him passing the ion exchange resin. As the potassium reached 5.5 mmol/l he became asymptomatic. The exact mechanism of the illness remained mysterious and the nerve conduction studies cannot be explained. Unfortunately he was lost to follow-up, as after discharge he moved out of the area.

Hypocalcaemia

Chronic hypocalcaemia causes attacks of tetany and muscle weakness. In infancy hypocalcaemia may cause convulsions, papilloedema and calcification of the basal ganglia. Hypocalcaemia should be carefully excluded in any young person who develops cataracts. Causes include primary or secondary hypoparathy-roidism, renal disease or bladder diversion procedures, deficient diet or lack of vitamin D. Rarely, for reasons that are obscure, it may be related to osseous metastases.

CASE REPORT III

A 66-year-old man with known carcinoma of the prostate, with widespread osteosclerotic and osteolytic metastases resulting in pathological fractures of both thighs, was referred for advice on proximal muscle weakness that had been diagnosed elsewhere as carcinoma-associated polymyositis. He had profound proximal weakness and considerable wasting of both thighs, partly related to his fractures. It was thought unlikely that a prostatic carcinoma would be complicated by polymyositis and EMGs, particularly in the shoulder girdle, were suggestive of denervation rather than a myopathy. Muscle biopsy showed only atrophic changes. The initial serum calcium was 1.46 mmol/l and the phosphate 0.26 mmol/l. All other electrolytes were normal, including the serum magnesium at 0.6 mmol/l. The biochemical team was totally unable to explain this. Large doses of oral calcium gluconate, 12 g daily, and high-potency vitamin D 1.25 mg t.d.s. were given but the serum calcium dropped to 1.36 mmol/l before rising over 4 weeks to 2.1 mmol/l, at which point there was a dramatic improvement in the proximal weakness. The serum level continued to fluctuate between 1.8 and 2.2 mmol/l while he continued on this large intake of calcium and vitamin D, and he was able to mobilize on sticks. He subsequently became anaemic following further radiotherapy and blind in the left eye due to an orbital metastasis. He died 3 years after the hypocalcaemic myopathy was diagnosed but remained mobile until 2 weeks before his death.

Although the mechanism in this case remains unexplained, both the dramatic proximal weakness produced by hypocalcaemia and the need to consider metabolic disturbance in any patient with proximal weakness are again emphasized.

Hypercalcaemia

Sudden hypercalcaemia causes severe cerebral dysfunction or acute psychosis. A slower onset causes quite severe but variable proximal muscle weakness. This is usually combined with very brisk reflexes, which may raise the possibility of motor neuron disease. The most frequent cause is primary hyperparathyroidism due to a parathyroid adenoma. It may also occur in patients with metastatic malignancy who have osteolytic metastases or as a complication of oat-cell carcinoma with ectopic secretion of parathormone. Multiple myeloma may cause diffuse bone destruction and hypercalcaemia. Sarcoidosis, excessive intake of vitamin D, milk–alkali syndrome and idiopathic hypercalcaemia of infancy are other possible causes.

Endocrine Disease

Thyroid Disease

There are several ways in which the thyroid gland may be associated with muscular disorders.

1. Myasthenia gravis is often associated with thyrotoxicosis (in 10% of cases) and routine thyroid investigations are indicated in any patient with myasthenia gravis.

2. Hypokalaemic periodic paralysis occurs in association with thyrotoxicosis, particularly in Asian patients but also in other ethnic groups.

3. The most frequent muscular complication is thyrotoxic myopathy, which particularly affects the shoulder girdle (spinati, deltoid and triceps) or pelvic girdle (hip flexors and quadriceps). It can be the only overt manifestation of the disease and occurs particularly in males, even though thyrotoxicosis occurs three times as commonly in females. An important clue to this diagnosis is the presence of very brisk reflexes. The picture is similar to hypercalcaemic myopathy and could also be misdiagnosed as motor neurone disease.

4. Extraocular muscle disease in thyrotoxicosis was described in Chapter 5.

5. Myxoedema causes proximal muscle weakness which may be mistakenly regarded as part of the general slowing down. In some 25% of patients a full-blown proximal myopathy occurs and is known as Hoffman's syndrome. The more dramatic neurological complication of myxoedema is cerebellar degeneration (see Chapter 11). Proximal muscle weakness also occurs in cretinism. This is known as the Kocher–Debre–Semelgaine syndrome.

Adrenal Disease

In Cushing's syndrome due to hyperadrenalism, very striking wasting and weakness of the pelvic girdle and thigh muscles occurs with wasting of the buttocks and upper legs. When accompanied by excessive fatty tissue over the upper trunk and lower cervical spine, the combination produces the clinical appearance known as a 'buffalo hump'. The similarity of body shape to a buffalo in affected patients is very striking. The diagnosis is usually clinically very obvious but the following case presented considerable diagnostic difficulties, not the least being that the Cushing's syndrome developed in parallel with the onset of Parkinson's disease.

CASE REPORT IV

A 63-year-old man, a former international sprinter, was referred following bilateral hip replacements, with bilateral ulnar nerve lesions and the beginnings of the right-sided tremulous Parkinson's disease. Both ulnar nerves were trans-

posed with improvement and antiparkinsonian medication was introduced. The response was difficult to gauge: although the more overt features, tremor and rigidity, seemed to improve, his general mobility did not and he suddenly reported a series of falls because his thighs felt weak. When he was first seen he had a rather flushed face and thin arms and legs and a large trunk. The limb signs were thought to be due to his various orthopaedic difficulties. He continued to complain of generalized weakness and the thinning of the limbs progressed and the redness of the face increased, but he denied drinking. This was after 2 years of treatment. His physical shape and the history suggested the possibility of Cushing's syndrome. Midnight cortisols on 4 consecutive nights were raised with minimal dexamethazone suppression. A 24-hour urinary cortisol was 345 nmol/l and ACTH level was 49 ng/l. The tests were repeated with all his antiparkinsonian medication stopped, with similar results. CT scans of the pituitary and adrenal glands were normal. After much discussion the endocrinological and biochemical teams recommended bilateral adrenalectomy followed by full replacement therapy. The increasing weakness that had made management of his Parkinson's disease increasingly difficult improved markedly and all the features of Cushing's syndrome cleared. Eight years later his Parkinson's disease has progressed sufficiently to produce major disability.

An identical picture can be produced by exogenous steroid treatment, including the redistribution of body fat and a severe proximal myopathy of rapid onset. In the neurological field, this is particularly common in patients on high-dose dexamethasone for control of the symptoms of raised intracranial pressure, and can occur within a matter of weeks. The weakness recovers surprisingly quickly if the steroids can be safety withdrawn.

In Addison's disease due to adrenal failure, general lethargy, muscle cramps and weakness are an integral part of the disease. This is usually due to the hyponatraemia.

Conn's syndrome (hyperaldosteronism) with hypokalaemic muscle weakness was mentioned earlier.

Parathyroid Disease

The effects of parathyroid disease on muscle have already been described in the section on disordered calcium metabolism.

Inflammatory Muscle Disease

Muscles are remarkably resistant to infection, with the exception of gas gangrene caused by *Clostridium Welchii*, bacterial infection is rare. Some 80% of patients suffering from sarcoidosis develop a mild to severe proximal myopathy. This is particularly common in female patients over 50 years of age and may respond to the use of steroids.

Muscle inflammation in viral disease is exemplified by Bornholm disease (epidemic pleurodynia) and the general myalgia and listlessness of influenza which may mimic the onset of acute poliomyelitis,

Parasitic involvement is very rare in the UK. *Trichinella spiralis* particularly affects the extraocular muscles and is a rare cause of pain and weakness in these muscles. Cysticercosis is usually an asymptomatic collection of calcified cysts in the trunk muscles of a patient who has become the accidental intermediate host in the lifecycle of the pork tapeworm. This usually causes epilepsy due to cerebral cysts, but plain X-rays of the trunk muscles to show the calcified cysts are important in establishing the diagnosis. It is important to stress that the cerebral cysticerci do **not** calcify and are not visible on skull X-ray, but are readily seen on CT scanning.

Idiopathic Inflammatory Myopathies

The most important inflammatory muscle diseases are the idiopathic inflammatory myopathies. There are three main conditions that fall into this category: inclusion body myositis, dermatomyositis and polymyositis.

Inclusion Body Myositis

This polymyositis-like condition, which has been relatively recently delineated, occurs in an older age group and tends to show a slower progression and a very poor response to the use of steroids. It is only diagnosable by muscle biopsy. The clinical features are otherwise very similar to polymyositis.

Dermatomyositis

The proximal myopathy of polymyositis may be associated with skin changes and the significance of this depends on the patient's age. The combination is known as dermatomyositis. The skin rash consists of a lilac-coloured rash over the cheeks, nose and eyelids and thickened, reddened skin over the interphalangeal joints, elbows and knees. The nailfold may be reddened and telangiectatic.

CASE REPORT V

A 56-year-old woman presented with rapidly increasing generalized weakness over several weeks. There were widespread skin changes diagnostic of dermatomyositis. The response to steroids was dramatic. She had had a carcinoma of the breast removed 10 years previously and all subsequent follow-ups had failed to reveal any evidence of residual or metastatic disease. Initial reinvestigation for recurrent disease still showed no abnormality. The good response to steroids was maintained for several months but sudden deterioration prompted a further screening for malignancy, and widespread metastatic disease was then identified. She died a few months later of metastatic carcinoma of the breast.

In this case, even though the index of suspicion of carcinoma was overwhelming, screening tests failed to demonstrate any abnormality. There is some controversy as to how far attempts to eliminate underlying disease should be taken in such patients and uncertainty as to whether the discovery of the underlying lesion, alters the prognosis in any way. This case emphasizes the difficulties encountered in such cases, even when the likelihood of underlying disease is known to be virtually certain.

Dermatomyositis is the **usual** pattern of the disease in childhood but is **never** associated with underlying malignant disease in this age group. Systemic symptoms, however, are very common in childhood and the disorder may be associated with bowel perforation, intestinal obstruction and the deposition of calcium in the skin and subcutaneous tissues, which may erode out through the skin as calcified lumps.

Children with dermatomyositis should be treated with steroids in the expectation of a good response. A myasthenic syndrome may occur in association with dermatomyositis in childhood, and if the child's clinical status worsens or fluctuates an edrophonium test is indicated to exclude this possibility.

In adulthood less than 50% of patients show skin changes but the risk of underlying malignant disease is virtually confined to this group. There is also a marked sex difference. Over the age of 50, up to 70% of males with dermatomyositis are eventually found to have underlying malignant disease. In females the risk is only 25%. The underlying malignant disease is usually found in the breast in females and in the lower bowel in males. In patients over 50 years of age with dermatomyositis, if no tumour in the breast or lung can be demonstrated investigation for an underlying bowel tumour is justified, although whether its discovery will alter the outcome is uncertain.

Polymyositis

The importance of this disorder lies not only in the muscle problem, which may be considerable, but also in the association with serious underlying disease. There is underlying collagen vascular disease in some 20% of cases; rheumatoid arthritis, scleroderma, systemic lupus erythematosus and Sjogren's syndrome and some carcinoma-associated cases do not have the skin changes discussed above.

As so often in neurological disorders, the beginner's problem is less one of classification than of recognizing the condition in the first place. Polymyositis shares with porphyria and Guillain–Barré syndrome the distinction of being easily misdiagnosed as a functional disorder or hysteria. Some of the difficulty stems from the name and the usual descriptions, which suggest that muscle tenderness is a prominent feature and that the weakness is proximal and symmetrical, making the diagnosis very obvious. This is unfortunately quite inaccurate, as less than half the patients have demonstrable muscle tenderness and the weakness may be no greater than enough to make the patient feel rather listless. It may be remarkably localized, affecting only the glutei or one shoulder or the neck extensors, and show a tendency to easy fatigue, a symptom suggesting myasthenia gravis or too readily dismissed as being due to depression or anxiety.

General Clinical Features

1. Females are affected twice as often as males and the typical age range is 50–70 years.

2. Muscle weakness is the usual presenting symptom and usually affects the pelvic girdle first. This causes difficulty climbing stairs or getting up from a chair.

3. This is followed by shoulder girdle weakness, with difficulty reaching objects on shelves, washing the face or brushing the hair. Weakness of the neck muscles and dysphagia are very common at this stage but facial weakness and extraocular muscle weakness are extremely rare which is an important distinguishing feature from myasthenia gravis; however, as emphasized later, myasthenia gravis without ocular involvement can readily mimic polymyositis.

4. Pain and tenderness of the affected muscles occurs in less than half the patients and is usually most obvious in the shoulder girdle muscles.

5. Systemic symptoms such as weight loss, anorexia, fever and lassitude occur more frequently in childhood polymyositis.

6. Atrophy of the affected muscles is late and mild and it is always difficult to detect atrophy in the plump pelvic area or in the fleshy upper arms and shoulders of females. It is usually more readily detected in the relatively defined musculature of elderly males.

7. Evidence of collagen vascular disease such as Raynaud's phenomenon, arthralgia, pneumonitis and renal damage is found in 20% of cases.

8. Tendon reflexes are usually preserved until very late in the course of the disease.

CASE REPORT VI

A 58-year-old man returned from abroad to live with his family. He related that he had been slowing down physically for 2 years. This had been ascribed to depression following his wife's death and he had been on antidepressants. On his arrival he showed marked physical inertia and had a persistent cough with profuse watery sputum. On examination he clearly had parkinsonism but the most dramatic finding was gross weakness and wasting of the proximal muscles. A chest X-ray revealed a cavitating carcinoma of the right upper lobe and EMG studies showed findings consistent with polymyositis.

He responded well to levodopa and prednisone but died a few weeks later while receiving palliative radiotherapy.

This is an example of malignancy associated polymyositis and the good response to steroids is not unusual. Surprisingly often, patients who are subsequently shown to have underlying malignant disease show the most dramatic response to steroids, and this may be an ominous indicator of the need for continual monitoring for underlying disease.

Polymyalgia Rheumatica

Muscle tenderness, severe aching and very severe deep burning, tearing pains in the muscles, often described by the patient 'as if the flesh were being torn from the bone' are the main symptoms of a peculiar disease known as polymyalgia rheumatica. Apparent weakness is usually secondary to pain in the muscle and the EMG changes are mild and non-specific. The ESR is usually elevated and an almost immediate response to indomethacin or steroids provides strong support for the diagnosis. The relationship of the disease to other collagen vascular diseases is uncertain, but a special feature is that some 40% of patients later develop temporal (cranial) arteritis. If the patient is being discharged from the clinic they should be advised to report immediately any headache they may develop in the future.

An inflammatory proximal myopathy has been identified in association with HIV infection and shows some response to steroids. Its relationship to polymyositis is as yet uncertain. Furthermore, zidovudine used in the treatment of the condition may also cause a myopathy.

Myasthenia Gravis and Myasthenic Syndromes

Myasthenia gravis was the first neurological disease to be clearly identified as being due to an autoimmune disorder. The association with underlying thymomas had been long recognized and thymectomy had been performed since the early 1940s, with clear benefit in some cases, and by the 1950s thymectomy in the absence of a thymic tumour had been shown to benefit young females with rapidly progressive disease of short duration. In the 1960s steroids were shown to be of benefit and then the demonstration of end-plate antibodies, now an important diagnostic test, led to treatment with full-scale immunosuppression.

To understand the illness the normal anatomy and physiology of the neuromuscular junction (NMJ) must be understood and this is detailed in Figure 18.8. The

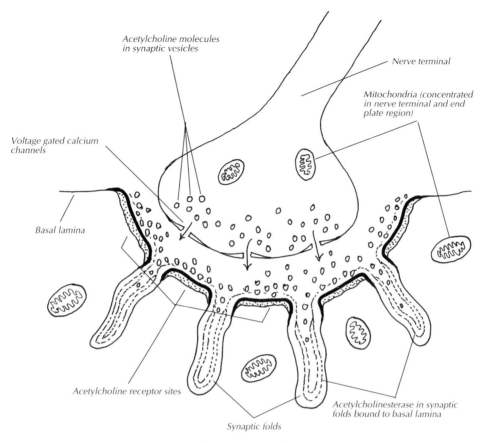

*Acetylcholine molecules
in synaptic vesicles*

Nerve terminal

*Mitochondria (concentrated
in nerve terminal and end
plate region)*

*Voltage gated calcium
channels*

Basal lamina

Acetylcholine receptor sites

*Acetylcholinesterase in synaptic
folds bound to basal lamina*

Synaptic folds

18.8   The neuromuscular junction.

antibodies in myasthenia gravis are directed against the acetylcholine receptor site and in Lambert–Eaton myasthenic syndrome (LEMS) against the voltage gated calcium channels of the presynaptic terminal. The end result in both cases is partial failure of neuromuscular transmission. The site of antibody production is uncertain. Patients who have hypertrophied thymocytes or thymic tumours do well after thymectomy and in some patients little or no benefit is seen, suggesting antibody production elsewhere. Relatively few patients are able to completely discontinue steroids and immunosuppressants after thymectomy.

It is important to recognize the striking age and sex differences of this condition. There are two distinct groups in whom the condition typically occurs, but it can also occur in elderly women and young men, although much less often.

Young women (20–35 years) tend to have an acute onset of typical severely fluctuating myasthenia gravis involving the eye muscles, with generalized weakness.

Elderly men (60–75) present with oculobulbar myasthenia gravis in an age range where cerebral vascular disease and motor neuron disease are other possible diagnoses, and where the LEMS syndrome is more likely to occur owing to underlying disease.

The difficulty with myasthenia gravis is in considering the diagnosis in the first place. Any patient with muscle weakness, even if there is no variability and even if there are no eye symptoms or signs should be regarded as a possible case of myasthenia gravis until an edrophonium test and muscle end-plate antibodies prove otherwise. Even these tests are not infallible, as well be evident in a later case report.

Like many diseases, classic myasthenia gravis presenting as a droopy eyelid with variable diplopia is easy to diagnose, but atypical presentations are extremely common and the first symptoms can be very difficult to recognize, and other disorders more readily suspected. This is usually because the diagnostic features of variability and fatiguability may not be obvious and the patient may present with an apparently permanent mild ptosis or a fixed deficit of eye movement that may be misdiagnosed as an incomplete extraocular nerve palsy. If the bulbar muscles are affected by a nonvariable weakness, motor neuron disease or a brainstem vascular accident may be suspected.

In contrast, extremely brief attacks of diplopia or dysarthria may occur and mimic a breaking-down squint or a transient brainstem ischaemic attack. Because both stress and fatigue may provoke myasthenic episodes, non-organic mechanisms are readily suspected.

Even if the diagnosis is correctly made attempts to confirm it with the edrophonium test are fraught with difficulty in interpretation. The basic requirement for the test is an observable and measurable degree of weakness in a specific muscle. In the early stages of the disorder myasthenic muscles may show an uncertain response to Tensilon, or even to a trial of longer-acting anticholinesterase drugs given orally.

The Edrophonium (Tensilon) Test

This test should ideally be performed in hospital with the patient resting on a couch and equipment available in case of collapse. It should not be done with the patient sitting in a chair in the outpatient clinic.

The patient should be warned that when the edrophonium is injected they may notice that their heart races, they may feel faint, their throat may feel tight, the facial muscles may twitch, they will notice stinging and watering of the eyes and many report a peculiar taste. A dummy run using saline is sometimes recommended as a control, but in a positive test the result is so dramatic and unanticipated by the patient that this is probably an unnecessary sophistication.

Ten milligrams of edrophonium are drawn up and 2 mg injected intravenously and flushed in with saline. The patient will notice most of the side-effects and even this small dose may be sufficient to cause syncope. It may also provide an immediately obvious positive response, with a dramatic improvement in the strength of the test muscle that has been selected for observation. This might be the patient's ability to speak without slurring – usually tested by counting – or the ability to swallow water without choking and, where appropriate, the elevation of a droopy eyelid or the disappearance of diplopia.

If no response is seen to the first injection after 2 minutes and the if patient has no distressing side-effects, 3 mg are then injected and the same observations made. Most positive responses will be apparent at this dose. If this also fails and the patient is not distressed, the final 5 mg should be injected as a bolus and the observations repeated.

A strongly positive response typically disappears in several minutes, but occasionally persists for 10–15 minutes. A positive response to edrophonium is perhaps the most dramatic event in neurological practice and is quite unmistakable. Unfortunately, a negative response does not necessarily disprove the diagnosis.

CASE REPORT VII

A 29-year-old woman was referred because of intermittent drooping of the left eyelid, which had come to light when she had a security-pass photograph taken and saw for the first time that her eye was almost closed. There was no response to an edrophonium test on two separate occasions over the next 3 months and autoimmune studies were normal. She then developed diplopia and within 6 months had developed generalized weakness with bulbar difficulties, culminating in a thymectomy when the situation was not contained by high-dose steroids and immunosuppression. The histology showed an involuted thymus without lymphoid hyperplasia. Unfortunately, the thymectomy, after an initial improvement, did not produce the anticipated long-term benefit and 8 years later she remains fully immunosuppressed on steroids and anticholinergics but is unable to follow her employment and can barely cope with housework.

As already indicated variable ptosis of one or other eyelid and variable diplopia are the most frequent presenting symptoms, closely followed by weakness of chewing, dysarthria or difficulty in swallowing.

Limb symptoms in such cases are a late and relatively minor symptom in the majority of myasthenics. It is unusual for the reflexes to be altered: in fact, they are often brisker than normal.

Myasthenia may occur transiently in 10% of children born to myasthenic mothers. If the mother has needed large doses of anticholinesterases during labour the child may born with cholinergic blockade. This is unusual, as in general myasthenia tends to improve during pregnancy and the mother's medication may have been reduced.

In childhood myasthenia is quite rare, but is invariably associated with severe generalized weakness, quite unlike the adult form. Otherwise the clinical features are similar to the adult. In childhood myasthenia there is a good possibility that a spontaneous remission will occur. As noted earlier, the condition may complicate dermatomyositis in this age group.

In adults with long-standing disease a proximal 'myasthenic myopathy' may supervene, and in most cases progressive atrophy of the maximally affected muscles with diminishing responsiveness to anticholinergic drugs occurs. It is hoped that modern management with steroids and immunosuppression will prevent proximal myopathy developing. So far this hope seems justified.

In all cases thyrotoxicosis should be excluded. This occurs in 10% cent of males and 20% of females with myasthenia gravis. Routine thoracic CT scanning to exclude a thymic tumour is always indicated.

Treatment of Mysthenia

The original treatment of myasthenia gravis with anticholinergic drugs dates back to 1934, when an inspired guess proved correct and it still has a definite but diminishing role in management. The mainstay of current management is to consider thymectomy early, particularly in young females and in any age range in the presence of a thymic tumour.

Anticholinergic Drugs

These drugs tend to cause abdominal cramping, sweating, tachycardia, muscle fasciculation and blurred vision, and should be used with caution. Neostigmine 15–30 mg 4-hourly is relatively quick acting and of short duration; it can be used to establish the effectiveness of anticholinergic treatment and also as a quick-acting interventional drug at any stage of the illness. Pyridostigmine 30–120 mg 6–8 -hourly is longer lasting and slower acting and is best used as a background drug supplemented by 'as necessary' doses of prostigmine. Prior to the 1960s this was the only treatment available and many patients managed quite well. Unfortunately, this treatment has no effect on the underlying pathology and many patients became unresponsive to medication and progressed to a proximal myopathy.

Steroids

The use of oral prednisolone is now standard and elderly men may respond to extremely small doses, 2.5–5 mg t.d.s. Younger female patients may require doses as high as 60–120 mg (1– 1.5 mg/kg) on alternate days to be effective. On these very high doses the possibility of steroid myopathy has to be considered as a possible complication.

Immunosuppression

Azathioprine has become the standard immunosuppressant in a dose range of 25–50 mg t.d.s., (2.5 mg/kg/day): the dose that produces an increase in red cell diameter to between 105 and 110 μm is a useful guide, provided the white cell count is satisfactory. The benefits are not immediately obvious and some patients may take 6 months to respond. Haematological parameters must be monitored monthly.

With modern treatment myasthenic crises are now rare, but the use of plasmapheresis or intravenous immunoglobulin has proved successful in acute life-threatening relapses. Although the risks of very long-term steroids and immunosuppression in these quite young patients are a source of concern it must not be forgotten why the condition was called myasthenia 'gravis', it was lethal in many cases prior to modern management.

Myasthenic Syndrome (LEMS)

This condition is also known as the Lambert–Eaton myasthenic syndrome and usually occurs in association with an oat-cell carcinoma of the lung. The weakness is found mainly in the proximal muscles of the pelvic and shoulder girdles. The neck and trunk muscles are affected but involvement of the bulbar or extraocular muscles is unusual. The initial presentation can be similar to myasthenia gravis, including both obvious and very atypical features. Unlike myasthenia gravis, repetitive activity of the muscle leads to increasing strength rather than weakness, although the patients rarely notice this. Only half the patients have a detectable malignancy at diagnosis, but close follow-up is necessary as the syndrome may precede the identification of the underlying malignant disease by several years. The treatment is basically the same as for myasthenia gravis, except that acetylcholine release can be improved by the use of 3, 4 -diaminopyridine 10–20 mg q.d.s. This will produce immediate improvement, but in most patients combination with steroids and azathioprine is necessary for long-term management.

Muscle Disease due to Drugs

In the past 20 years the number of drugs, toxins and chemicals identified as causing weakness and paralysis by affecting the neuromuscular junction and the muscle itself, has increased enormously and has become of considerable clinical significance. In view of the importance of severe muscle weakness as a presenting symptom, an extensive review of these agents is justified, and for completeness even rare causes have been mentioned.

Drugs Affecting the Neuromuscular Junction (NMJ)

Drugs may temporarily affect the normal NMJ, produce a myasthenia-like syndrome, unmask pre-existing NMJ abnormality or delay recovery after the use of NMJ blocking agents during anaesthesia.

Antibiotics

All aminoglycosides may damage the NMJ. Neomycin and tobramycin are the worst offenders. Gentamicin, kanamycin, neomycin, tobramycin and streptomycin may all temporarily block the normal NMJ. Erythromycin, penicillin, sulphonamides, tetracycline and fluoroquinolones may unmask latent myasthenia gravis. Polymyxin and colomycin may cause problems, even in topical use, in the presence of renal failure.

Anticonvulsants

Phenytoin may affect the NMJ by a membrane-stabilizing effect, which finds clinical use in myotonic conditions in which membrane instability is a pathological feature.

β-blockers and Calcium Channel Blocking Agents

β-blockers may affect the NMJ by blocking ion pump mechanisms in the muscle membrane. Timolol eye-drops may cause diplopia by directly affecting the extraocular muscles. Calcium channel blocking agents often cause muscle cramping as a side-effect, which may be severe. The mechanism of this effect is uncertain.

Steroids

All steroids may affect the NMJ. When used in a myasthenic patient the weakness may at first be aggravated. Long-term steroids also produce a myopathy by damaging type 2b muscle fibres. The fluorinated steroids dexamethasone and betamethasone, under occlusive dressings, may cause localized effects on underlying muscles.

Lithium

Lithium affects NMJ function by depleting sodium from the nerve terminals and interfering with ion pump mechanisms at presynaptic level.

D-Penicillamine

This agent, used to treat rheumatoid arthritis, Wilson's disease and cystinuria, causes very complex muscle weakness. It provokes the production of antiacetylcholine receptor antibodies, simulating myasthenia gravis, and can also produce an inflammatory myopathy showing all the features of polymyositis.

Organo phosphates

These agents, particularly malathion and diazanon, which are used as insecticides, block the NMJ by irreversible inactivation of acetylcholinesterase, producing a depolarizing blockade. Similar chemicals have potential use as nerve gases in warfare.

Botulinum Toxin

Botulinum toxin binds to the voltage gated calcium channels of the presynaptic membrane, causing progressive fatal paralysis if not identified and treated. The recent therapeutic use of botulinum in the treatment of hemifacial spasm, blepharospasm and torticollis is discussed in Chapters 6 and 12. The nerve ending recovers by making new presynaptic terminals, a process that takes 7–12 weeks. Botulism occurs in infants following wound infection with *Clostridium botulinum*, can occur for no detectable reason and classically is the result of ingestion of the toxin produced by the bacterium in inadequately preserved foods. The most recent cases in the UK followed contamination of a hazelnut purée used in yoghurt.

Tick Bite

The paralytic toxin involved in tick bite paralysis and its mode of action have not been identified. The identification and removal of the responsible tick is curative.

Snake Venoms

There are two types of venom-related NMJ blockade, affecting the presynaptic and postsynaptic terminals respectively. The presynaptic-acting toxins are phospholipases and are lethal. They are as follows and the snake responsible is named in brackets. β-bungarotoxin (the Krait); notoxin (Tiger snake); taipotoxin (Taipan); crotoxin (Brazilian rattlesnake); and myxotoxin (sea snakes). The postsynaptic-acting toxins are polypeptides and are much less lethal. They are α-bungarotoxins and act by binding irreversibly to the acetylcholine receptor site. This property has made them an important experimental tool. They are produced by all species of pit vipers (the rattlesnake in the USA and the common viper in the UK).

Myopathy due to Drugs

Necrotizing myopathy

Muscle damage due to drugs produces rapidly worsening proximal muscle weakness, muscles that for some reason are specifically vulnerable in metabolic disorders, as discussed earlier. A feature of the acute condition is severe muscle pain and tenderness which may mimic polymyositis. In some instances the rapid breakdown may lead to myoglobinuria (see below). In some cases the onset may much more insidious, producing a chronic myopathy, and the possible role of drugs is less readily suspected.

Laevostatin

This agent, used in familial hypercholesterolaemia and following renal transplantation, has an interestingly variable tendency to cause problems. If used alone the risk of myopathy is 1%; if used with gemfibrozil the risk rises to 5%; and if used in combination with cyclosporin in a renal transplant patient the risk of myopathy increases to 30%.

Clofibrate

This branched-chain fatty acid ester, another cholesterol-lowering agent, is particularly prone to cause myopathy in patients with renal failure due to nephrotic syndrome, as the drug is albumin bound and excreted by the kidney.

Epsilon-Amino Caproic Acid

This agent, used to prevent rebleeding in subarachnoid haemorrhage by blocking fibrinolysis, may cause myopathy if used for longer than 14 days.

Other Agents

Etretinate, which is used to treat psoriasis, may cause a myopathy after 3–7 months, use, as can procaineamide, especially in renal failure. A cytotoxic drug, 5-azacytidine, especially if used in a patient with liver failure, may cause myopathy. Zidovudine, used in AIDS, may cause muscle weakness after 6–17 months of use and ipecac (Emetine) can produce a reversible proximal myopathy in prolonged use.

Myoglobinuria

The dramatic release of myofibrillar components in acute necrotizing myopathy may block the renal tubules, causing myoglobinuric renal failure with anuria. This may occur with all the agents mentioned above, but specifically complicates muscle crush injury, snake envenomation and is secondary to the dramatically increased muscle activity produced by phencyclidine (angel dust) intoxication.

Amphiphilic Myopathy

This type of myopathy is caused by a large group of drugs with a wide range of therapeutic indications. They have in common large cationic amphiphilic molecules with a hydrophobic region and a hydrophilic region, the latter with a substituted amine group with a net positive charge permitting interaction with both cell membranes and cell organelles. The hydrophobic regions react with plasma membrane and cause acute necrotizing myopathy or chronic low-grade myopathy with loss of microtubules. The hydrophobic group includes chlorpheniramine, chlorcyclizine, triparanol and iprindol.

The hydrophilic region reacts with liposomes, causing lipid-containing vacuolation of the muscle fibre described as 'lipoidoses'. The hydrophilic group includes choloroquine, hydroxychloroquine, doxorubicin and amiodarone.

The following drugs have a very similar chemical structure but have **not** yet been shown to cause an amphiphilic myopathy: popranolol, amantadine, tocamide, tamoxifen, clomiprimine, desiprimine, nortriptyline, fenfluaramine and haloperidol. Clearly, the use of any of these agents in a patient developing muscle weakness should be viewed with suspicion.

Antimicrotubular Agents

There are two drugs in common use which may cause myopathy by affecting the lysosomes and interfering with the microtubular system of muscle. These are vincristine, which more commonly causes a peripheral neuropathy, and colchicine, particularly in patients in renal failure when used for the treatment of gout, Mediterranean fever, amyloidosis, primary biliary cirrhosis and proliferative vitreo-retinopathy.

Muscle Damage Secondary to Drug-Induced Hypokalaemia

Prior to the advent of the H_2 antagonists, carbenoxolone (liquorice extract) was widely used in the treatment of peptic ulceration and many cases of acute muscle weakness and paralysis due to severe hypokalaemia were reported. Similarly, thiazide diuretics can cause loss of potassium, resulting in very acute severe muscle weakness, although this risk is now better recognized than in the early days of oral diuretic therapy.

From this extensive list of medications in relatively common use, it is apparent that the history of current and past medication is a very important facet of history-taking in any patient presenting with muscle weakness. Although the first thought of students when asked about their knowledge of muscle disease is to think of the muscular dystrophies, these actually represent a relatively small part of the field of muscle disease. Of much greater importance are the inherited biochemical disorders, the autoimmune-based inflammatory disorders, the ubiquitous myasthenic syndromes and the increasingly significant problem of drug-induced myopathy.

19. Peripheral Neuropathy and Diseases of the Lower Motor Neuron

The classic signs of a lower motor neuron lesion are wasting and weakness of the supplied muscles and loss of local reflexes. These signs may be associated with other phenomena such as muscle cramps, muscle pain on exercise, easy fatigue and fasciculation. These additional features may indicate specific entities such as motor neuron disease or myasthenia gravis. Unfortunately, any or all of these symptoms and signs can be found in any condition that affects the lower motor neuron anywhere on its course from the ventral horn cell to the muscle end-plate.

The symptoms and signs of a neuropathy vary widely depending on the disease responsible. Sometimes sensory symptoms dominate the picture, varying from mild paraesthesiae to severe pain. Actual sensory impairment may range from slight numbness with hypersensitivity to painful stimuli to gross loss of pain perception. In others the picture is essentially a motor one, almost to the exclusion of sensory phenomena.

The only constant physical finding is depression or absence of reflexes, even in those patients with pure sensory symptomatology. As a broad generalization, if a patient has normal reflexes it is unlikely that they are suffering from a peripheral neuropathy. These symptoms and signs must be very critically evaluated in every case, and it is essential to remember that it may be quite impossible to distinguish between nerve and muscle disease on clinical grounds alone.

The Phenomena of Peripheral Nervous System Disease

Muscle Wasting

Muscle atrophy is a feature of all lower motor neuron disorders and many muscle diseases. The exceptions are pseudohypertrophy, hypertrophy secondary to myotonia and compensatory hypertrophy in unaffected muscles in some of the localized myopathies (see Chapter 18).

Muscles normally thin with age and as part of any generalized weight loss. In both situations muscle stamina may decrease but strength is not affected. Even very frail patients should be able to produce one full-strength effort in each muscle. If they can do so it is unlikely that they have peripheral nerve or muscle disease. If called upon to make repeated efforts with the same muscle, fatigue may rapidly occur and raise the suspicion of myasthenia gravis, but the absence of ocular or bulbar muscle weakness will exclude this diagnosis in many – but certainly not all cases. In Lambert–Eaton myasthenic syndrome (LEMS) repeated activity may **improve** strength and reflexes may reappear. Generalized weakness without ocular involvement often occurs in myasthenia gravis and in such cases, particularly if the weakness is stable, the diagnosis may not even be considered. It is a useful rule to regard any patient with recent-onset weakness, even if striking variability is not a feature, as a potential case of myasthenia gravis and an edrophonium test can produce many surprises.

CASE REPORT I

A 49-year-old man complained of progressive weakness for 6 months. This followed a domestic incident which he initially thought was the cause. However, over 6 months he had deteriorated from playing daily squash and being captain of his golf club to being able to play only two holes and unable to walk upstairs. He felt that the main weakness was in his shoulders, and washing his hair had become almost impossible. On examination the cranial nerves were entirely normal and the neck muscles were strong. There was marked wasting and weakness of the shoulder girdles and some weakness of the distal arms and hand muscles. The leg muscles remained well developed, with modest proximal weakness. The reflexes were intact, the plantars were flexor and there was no sensory deficit. Myasthenia seemed unlikely because of the lack of variability, absent eye signs and marked wasting. Nerve conduction and EMG studies were entirely normal but repetitive stimulation was not attempted. CSF examination was performed and revealed an increase in the IgG, raising the unlikely possibility of demyelinating disease. He was admitted to hospital, the diagnosis still uncertain. On the morning of the second day in hospital he was for the first time unable to get out of the bath unassisted. A few hours later, physical examination was much as previously and he was able to get in and out of the bath without assistance. With this first evidence of fatiguability appearing in the history, an edrophonium test was done. Within 30 seconds he was able to walk normally and run up the stairs. A diagnosis of myasthenia gravis was made. He required increasing doses of anticholinergics and steroids. Although the control was excellent, he insisted on a second opinion because he did not like the high doses. He was referred to a colleague with a special interest in the condition who, following an intercostal muscle biopsy, was able to demonstrate that this was Lambert–Eaton syndrome. The patient remains well 13 years later but on very much higher doses of steroids and immunosuppressants than prompted him to ask for a second opinion!

Certain muscles waste rapidly with disuse, the best example being the quadriceps, which may show appreciable wasting within days of the patient being confined to bed. In this situation the muscle is not weak. The important point is that wasting is not necessarily associated with weakness, and disuse atrophy affects stamina and not strength.

Muscle Weakness

Patients in pain have difficulty in cooperating with muscle testing. It is essential that they do so, and the majority of patients are prepared to bear the pain for one maximal effort. Patients who absolutely refuse to make the effort tend to be suffering from a non-organic pain syndrome. Indeed, 'grunting and groaning' while being apparently completely unable to contract a muscle is almost diagnostic of non-organicity, especially if it happens behind the curtains within earshot of the examiner as the patient undresses!

Weakness in the legs secondary to unbearable back pain is a common feature in depressive low back pain syndromes. The weakness affects **all** muscle groups. In patients with organic disc disease, if weakness is present it should be confined to muscles innervated by one root and typically in the distribution of either L5 or S1.

Non-organic weakness is usually described as 'give-way' weakness. This is a bad term, as all weakness eventually leads to the muscle giving way, but in non-organic weakness there is a typical variable weakness proportional to the amount of resistance offered by the examiner. If the examiner suddenly exerts less effort after a brief lag the patient stops trying and 'gives way'. Often the patient's performance on testing is grossly at variance with their ability to walk into the clinic, undress and climb on to a couch. Occasionally, when total weakness of a muscle is present on a non-organic basis, if the antagonist muscles are palpated at the same time they will be felt to contract every time the patient tries to use the 'weak' muscle. There is an enormous amount of grunting and groaning, facial grimacing and stiffening of the entire body in such cases, quite different from the quiet but ineffectual efforts made by the organically paralysed patient. It is surprising how often patients who have global weakness of a leg when examined on the couch actually walk with the 'paralysed' leg held **stiffly**, when they first come in to the consulting room. They also characteristically tend to lean on their walking stick with both hands and, if using a crutch, can often be seen swinging the crutch forward while bearing their full weight on the 'affected' leg.

Loss of Reflexes (Areflexia)

Many otherwise normal people have depressed or absent reflexes. Such patients may recollect being asked to perform the reflex reinforcement manoeuvres at previous physical examinations, or actually being told that their reflexes were absent. Recent loss of previously intact reflexes is a very important physical sign, and if previous medical examinations have been performed some effort to obtain the old notes for confirmation of the presence of the reflexes is worthwhile. Often the notes will only state 'CNS $\sqrt{}$'. This emphasizes the importance of accurate documentation of physical findings at all examinations and the importance of documenting if a system was specifically **not** examined. It is perfectly permissible not to examine an area if any findings would be irrelevant to the case, but unless this is clearly stated subsequent review of the notes may be misinterpreted as indicating that all was well at that time.

Total loss of reflexes is a feature of peripheral neuropathy and often occurs in patients with muscle disease. Loss of individual reflexes should indicate disease affecting the nerve root or peripheral nerve conveying that particular reflex. Elderly patients may have very depressed or absent ankle reflexes of uncertain significance, but in children in particular an absent ankle jerk should never be dismissed as a chance or insignificant finding. As a broad generalization, brisk reflexes may indicate no more than an anxious patient but **an absent reflex should always be explained**.

Muscle Cramps

Muscle cramps are a common experience. They usually occur when a muscle contracts when already shortened, notably the small foot muscles when the foot is already flexed by the weight of bedclothes. Salt depletion or a low serum calcium may predispose to cramping, but usually in obvious climatic situations or associated with disease. The majority of patients with cramps do **not** have an electrolyte disturbance or any physical disease: it is a common physiological phenomenon. Although muscle cramps are a frequent symptom in motor neuron disease, unless other definite signs are present there is no need to entertain this diagnosis.

Muscle Pain on Exercise

Muscle pain during or following exercise is frequently the result of unusual activity. The whole basis of training for any form of sport or activity is to reduce muscle pain or delay its onset. Probably the commonest type is known as 'shin splints'. This consists of severe pain in the tibialis anterior muscle following unaccustomed activity. Occasionally, the swelling of the muscle within its confined compartment may lead to ischaemic damage and surgical decompression may be required. This is called the 'anterior compartment syndrome' and is a surgical emergency. Muscle pain and cramping following exercise is common in inflammatory myopathy, polymyalgia rheumatica and glycogen storage diseases. It may also occur in even more surprising situations.

CASE REPORT II

A 38-year-old woman presented with the complaint of severe generalized muscle pain following the slightest exertion. She was embarrassed by her inability to do housework and shopping, and even collecting the children from school by car was an ordeal. She felt that there was some weakness but pain limited her activity so much that fatiguability had not been noticed. There were no ocular or cranial nerve symptoms. On physical examination there was marked proximal weakness and exquisite tenderness of the proximal muscles, particularly around the shoulder. A diagnosis of polymyositis seemed certain. An ESR was 6, an emergency CPK (creative phosphokinase) estimation was 35 iu/ml, and an EMG showed no evidence of inflammatory muscle disease. A Tensilon test produced a dramatic and immediate restoration of strength, and within 24 hours of starting prednisolone 10 mg t.d.s. and pyridostigmine 60 mg t.d.s. the patient was totally asymptomatic with no weakness and no pain. It would appear that the pain was a dramatic complication of profound weakness that had been scarcely noted by the patient because pain prevented sufficient activity to bring this feature into prominence.

This is another excellent example of an atypical presentation of myasthenia gravis.

Fasciculation

Visible spontaneous contraction of groups of muscle fibres is known as fasciculation. It is a physiological phenomenon that usually follows exertion. It is particularly common in previously athletic patients who have reduced their participation in sports and is most striking in relaxed dependent muscles such as the calves. Although it does occur in motor neuron disease it is not specific for this condition and may occur in any disease of the lower motor neuron. In the absence of any other signs, such as wasting or weakness of the fasciculating muscle, it is unlikely to be of sinister significance. It is one of the most common causes of self-referral of doctors to their neurological colleagues. Doctors who notice fasciculation in their own muscles usually require very considerable reassurance before they will accept that they do not have motor neuron disease. It is also surprising how frequently patients who actually have motor neuron disease are totally oblivious of widespread fasciculation in their trunk and limb muscles. It is almost never the reason for the consultation.

Sensory Symptoms

When considering peripheral nervous system disease we are concerned with symmetrical sensory symptoms or symptoms within the territory of a sensory dermatome or the cutaneous distribution of a peripheral nerve (see Chapters 16 and 17).

Generalized sensory symptoms usually begin in the legs and rarely affect the hands until the symptoms in the leg reach knee level. They consist of non-stop fine tingling paraesthesiae coupled with subjective numbness, although it is often difficult to detect any actual sensory loss. These sensations may be more severe in a warm bed or while standing, but do not remit completely. Patients with **intermittent** peripheral paraesthesiae are almost invariably suffering from an anxiety state, with hyperventilation (see Chapter 22). Similar but **non-stop** symptoms occur in multiple sclerosis and the distinction from neuropathy is best made by the state of the reflexes. If the reflexes are present or brisk multiple sclerosis is the likely diagnosis; if absent or depressed a peripheral neuropathy may be the cause.

In peripheral neuropathy, as tingling extends centrally numbness follows in its wake in a 'glove and stocking' distribution. This is another pejorative expression, like 'give-way' weakness, which is subject to serious misinterpretation as it is usually used to describe non-organic sensory deficits, ignoring the fact that organic sensory loss produces similar findings. In organic sensory loss sensation gradually becomes normal over a few inches, with an intermediate zone of altered sensation. The distinguishing feature of non-organic loss is that there is usually a sharp transition from total sensory loss to intact sensation. Furthermore, in organic sensory loss it is unusual for all modalities to be equally affected and there is often relative preservation of some modalities. In non-organic situations complete sensory loss to all modalities is claimed; even vibration sense may be perceived an inch higher up on the ankle or an inch across the midline of the sternum, than where it is apparently completely absent. Overshoot of pinprick loss across the midline is **not** a common non-organic finding. Such patients do claim sensory loss to the midline very precisely, hence the stress placed on the use of vibration sense as a more useful test for non-organic sensory loss (Fig. 19.1).

Further discussion will be divided into two major groups of diseases, those affecting the ventral horn cells and those affecting both the motor and sensory peripheral nerve fibres.

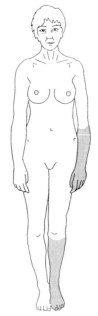 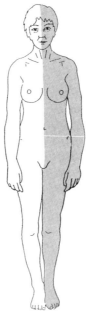 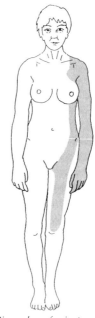

'Glove-and-stocking' anaesthesia Complete loss of all modalities with sharp upper edges would never be found in organic disease

Complete loss of all modalities down one side is virtually impossible. Patients will often claim loss of vibration sense across sternum or skull. Claimed loss is usually strictly midline and rarely overshoots or undershoots the midline as some texts claim

Bizarre loss of pain, temperature and touch in localised areas is not consistent with a root or nerve lesion. Claimed loss halfway across the shoulder or only the lateral aspect of the trunk is quite common and could not be explained on any organic basis

19.1   Examples of non-organic sensory loss distribution.

Ventral Horn Cell Disease

This is a group of disorders due to a variety of genetic, infective or toxic causes, many of which have a lethal prognosis. It is most appropriate to include them with diseases of the peripheral nerves and muscles, as the overlap in the clinical presentations may make for serious misdiagnosis. In particular, the incorrect diagnosis of motor neuron disease may have devastating consequences for the patient and such a diagnosis should only be made after all other possibilities have been completely excluded, unless the clinical picture is absolutely diagnostic.

Inherited Ventral Horn Cell Disease

This category includes three or possibly four conditions, if we include the fact that 5% of patients with motor neuron disease have a family history of this disorder.

Werdnig–Hoffman Disease (Infantile Spinal Muscular Atrophy)

This lethal disease is inherited as an autosomal recessive. The disease begins in utero and the mother may be aware of poor fetal movements in late pregnancy, particularly if she has had a previously affected child.

At birth the child may be a 'floppy' infant with difficulty breathing and feeding, and when supine the arms and legs flop out in a frog-like posture. They may be areflexic. Frank fasciculation may not be seen because of subcutaneous fat, but little jerks of the fingers and toes may indicate fasciculation in the underlying muscles. The facial and tongue muscles are often spared but respiratory muscle paralysis occurs early and is responsible for death in most instances. This is often detectable as indrawing of the intercostal spaces as the child breathes. In its most severe form the child may die within weeks, but death within the first year of life is the usual outcome.

Intermediate Form

A less severe form of the condition may occur in which the child appears to develop normally in the first year of life but weakness of the legs becomes apparent when they should start walking. The arms may be mildly affected and, unlike the lethal disease, tongue wasting and fasciculation are prominent. The disease appears to arrest and if respiratory involvement does not occur the child may survive. Whether this represents variable expression of the Werdnig–Hoffman gene or is a separate entity is unknown.

Wohlfart–Kugelberg–Welander Syndrome (Juvenile Spinal Muscular Atrophy)

This rare disorder occurs in both autosomal recessive and dominant forms. Onset is usually in late childhood or early teens and is dominated by weakness of the proximal muscles, with clear-cut fasciculation but relatively modest wasting. The long tracts are spared, the reflexes are not enhanced and the plantar responses are flexor. It is the mildest of the inherited motor neuron diseases. The weakness is most pronounced in the pelvic girdle and the disease is often misdiagnosed as a limb-girdle myopathy or Becker's muscular dystrophy. The prognosis is relatively good, with some gait disability and later some shoulder girdle weakness but rarely any bulbar muscle involvement. Most patients eventually need a wheelchair and it is likely that many cases of apparent long survival with motor neuron disease are due to this condition. Whether this is a separate genetic disorder or a benign form of Werdnig–Hoffman disease is uncertain.

CASE REPORT III

A 27-year-old accountant was referred for advice on his proximal muscular dystrophy as he had applied to join his company's pension plan. A prognosis was required. The history was unusual. He had not started walking until 3 years of age but then walked reasonably normally until 10 years of age. He then deteriorated rapidly, so that he was using a wheelchair by the age of 14 and totally unable to walk by 15 years of age. He had had investigations done under anaesthesia but was not sure of the results. There was no family history of any similar illness. On examination the cranial nerves were entirely normal. There was global weakness down to grade 2 or 3 in all limbs, but more marked distally than proximally. There was marked wasting of the intrinsic muscles of the hands and feet. He was areflexic with bilateral flexor plantar responses. There was a fixed flexion deformity of both knees. All routine studies, including CPK, were normal. EMGs revealed severe chronic partial denervation of proximal and distal groups in all four limbs. There was no fasciculation and minimal fibrillation. Motor and sensory conduction was normal. These findings were entirely consistent with the clinical diagnosis of Kugelberg–Welander syndrome and his company pension plan doctors were advised accordingly.

This particular patient was certain that there had been no progression since the age of 15, although the rapidity with which this severe degree of disability had developed is unusual.

Motor Neuron Disease

Some 5% of patients with motor neuron disease have a positive family history and the pattern of inheritance indicates an autosomal dominant gene. Gene analysis has indicated a defect in the enzyme superoxide dismutase in 40% of familial cases. This defect has not been demonstrated in sporadic cases, and as yet this has not led to any advance in our knowledge of the mechanism or led to treatment for this condition. The clinical features are discussed in greater detail in the following section.

Amyotrophic Lateral Sclerosis

The variant of motor neuron disease most relevant to the present discussion is progressive muscle atrophy, in which the brunt of the damage falls on the ventral horn cells and, by definition, there is no evidence of corticospinal or corticobulbar pathway disease. This means that the reflexes are not enhanced, the plantar reflexes are flexor and the weakness is in a myotomal pattern rather than a pyramidal distribution.

If signs of upper motor neuron involvement appear, the condition is then called amyotrophic lateral sclerosis and this is the most common pattern of the disease.

A pure upper motor neuron version is thought to exist and is known as primary lateral sclerosis. This produces a very severe progressive spastic paraparesis and may mimic cord compression or multiple sclerosis. The prognosis for survival in this form is good and many patients live for 20 years or more after the onset of the disease. Considerable disuse atrophy of the muscles may appear but nerve conduction and EMG studies show no evidence of lower motor neuron damage and no sensory disturbance or bladder disturbance occurs to indicate other relatively benign pathologies as alternative causes (see Chapter 14). All the possible patterns of motor neuron disease involvement are shown in Fig. 19.2.

Sporadic Progressive Muscle Atrophy

This variant of motor neuron disease starts with distal wasting and weakness, which may affect either arms or legs. It may therefore mimic an ulnar nerve lesion when it affects the hand or a peroneal nerve lesion when it affects the leg, producing a foot drop. However localized the damage, the failure to demonstrate any evidence of peripheral nerve damage in the presence of clear-cut denervation of the affected muscles on EMG studies should always indicate this diagnostic possibility. With time it usually becomes symmetrical and the diagnosis is then more obvious.

CASE REPORT IV

A 38-year-old nursing sister was referred with a progressive left foot drop. She gave a history of very severe night cramps in the left leg and a gradual progression to a foot drop. She had seen a neurologist 8 years previously with some back

A   Classical amyotrophic lateral sclerosis   **B   Single limb presentation**   **C   Severe generalized disease** (may mimic polymyositis or cachexia of occult disease)

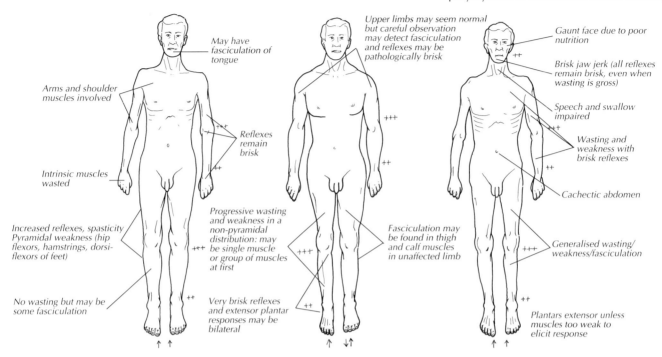

19.2   Motor neuron disease (major presentations).

pain and had had a myelogram at that time on the suspicion of a spinal tumour. Unfortunately no physical signs had been documented and the myelogram had been destroyed. She was told that she had a disc that had 'popped in and out'. On examination she had global weakness, a severe foot drop and widespread fasciculation in the left leg, brisk reflexes and a left extensor plantar response. There seemed to be some sensory deficit over the L5/S1 dermatomes. EMGs showed evidence of denervation in the L4/5 myotomes bilaterally. A myelogram and CSF examination were normal. The initial fear that this was motor neuron disease seemed to be further excluded by increasing sensory loss on subsequent examination, but a repeat EMG evaluation showed bilateral evidence of denervation and again the diagnosis of motor neuron disease seemed likely. A senior colleague agreed, although he was also surprised at what seemed to be an unequivocal sensory deficit. Unfortunately, the disease then evolved very rapidly, became generalized and led to her death 4 years after the diagnosis was finally made.

Although in retrospect the diagnosis of motor neuron disease seems obvious, a reluctance to make this diagnosis and the confusing and still unexplained sensory deficit seemed to offer a diagnostic escape route, until the evidence became overwhelming. The simple rule regarding increased reflexes in the presence of wasting and the extensor plantar response should perhaps have led to greater diagnostic confidence.

In the elderly, the bulbar ventral horn cells seem particularly vulnerable and a rapidly progressive bulbar palsy is probably the most common presentation of the disease in the over-60 age group. The first symptom is usually slurring of speech, and on the telephone the patient may sound as if they have been drinking. Difficulty is then experienced with chewing and forming a food bolus, and the patient becomes aware of having to make a conscious effort to swallow. Choking on fluids is the next new symptom. When first seen, wasting, weakness and fasciculation of the tongue are the most striking signs and poor or absent palatal movements may be detected. It is unusual to find any other signs and the jaw jerk should not be enhanced. In many instances widespread fasciculation in the trunk muscles may have passed unnoticed by the patient and clearly confirms the diagnosis.

CASE REPORT V

A 75-year-old man was referred because of difficulty swallowing saliva for about 6 months. He was otherwise well and still playing golf with one arm, having lost his left arm in 1942. He complained that the symptoms had become much worse since he had been put on quinine for very severe cramp in his legs. This combination of symptoms was suggestive of motor neuron disease, a suspicion increased by the fact that his 36-year-old daughter was dying of the condition. On examination he had a slightly brisk jaw jerk and sparse fasciculation in the tongue, but speech and swallowing appeared normal. However, there was widespread fasciculation throughout the trunk and all limbs, particularly prominent in the thighs and shoulders. All reflexes were brisk and both plantars were extensor. EMG studies were diagnostic. He died one year after diagnosis.

The initial findings suggested that the bulbar involvement was of the upper motor neuron type, with a relatively good prognosis, but within 6 months his speech was incoherent and he required a feeding enterostomy, which he declined. He had not noticed the generalized fasciculation. Severe muscle cramping is a common early symptom in motor neuron disease and the physical findings, when bulbar symptoms begin, can be misleadingly minimal. Of further interest here is the familial pattern of the disease, which is quite the reverse of the normal familial situation where the children develop the disease 40 years after their parents have died of it. This case is being investigated genetically.

Aspiration pneumonia may rapidly overwhelm the elderly patient and death within 6 months of the onset is not uncommon. The differential diagnosis lies between motor neuron disease of this type and bulbar myasthenia gravis or pseudobulbar palsy due to cerebrovascular disease. There may be considerable variability in the slurred speech and swallowing difficulty in the early stages, and even an apparent response to Tensilon may further confuse the diagnosis.

Pseudobulbar palsy due to vascular disease is relatively easy to distinguish because the onset is always acute and the jaw jerk is enhanced. It is also often accompanied by marked emotional lability, which is not a feature of the other two conditions.

Infective Ventral Horn Cell Disease (Acute Anterior Poliomyelitis; Infantile Paralysis)

As a consequence of effective vaccination programmes this is now a rare disease in developed countries but previously yearly epidemics occurred. Rare cases still occur following vaccination and occasional cases appear in the non-immune relatives of children who have recently had the oral vaccine. The illness remains a major risk to non-immune travellers in the tropics and less sanitary areas of the world, as the virus is transmitted by faecal soiling of drinking water.

The commonest manifestation is aseptic meningitis, which in only 1% of cases goes on to become potentially fatal paralytic poliomyelitis. The disease is also known as 'infantile paralysis', an expression which belies the fact that adults are 15 times more likely to become paralysed and are more likely to die.

Some 3 weeks after an acute viral upper respiratory tract infection, severe myalgia, painful paraesthesiae and a mild meningitic picture with headache and photophobia develop. Four or five days later weakness rapidly developed, with severe cramp and fasciculation in the affected muscles. These were usually groups of

muscles supplied by the same motor neuron pools in the lumbar or cervicothoracic enlargement. Sometimes the weakness localized to an actively used limb, for example the tennis player's arm or the runner's legs. Death was usually the result of bulbar and respiratory muscle paralysis. All modern developments in respiratory care owe their origins to the equipment originally designed for the management of acute poliomyelitis. Many patients survived and some muscle groups that were originally paralysed recovered, but most survivors were left with considerable but sometimes remarkably localized disability.

There is a distinct impression that in the past any form of paralysis in childhood was likely to be called 'polio'. Many patients are still seen with conditions ranging from cerebral palsy and spina bifida to Friedreich's ataxia, whose families had been told they had had 'polio' when young. It would seem a wise precaution to carefully review the physical signs in any patient who gives such a history.

'Old polio' typically produces a group of severely atrophied and weak muscles with loss of local reflexes. Vasomotor changes in the affected limb produce a violaceous swollen clammy extremity. If there is ataxia, sensory loss, or if the reflexes are intact the diagnosis cannot be 'old polio'.

The Post-Polio Syndrome

It has long been suspected that there is a higher risk of a motor neuron disease-like illness developing in survivors of poliomyelitis, although this concept has always been disputed. Motor neuron disease occurring in polio survivors was said to run a more benign course. This condition is now called the post-polio syndrome and is thought to represent ventral horn cell death in cells that have previously 'recovered' from the acute attack by the polio virus. This typically occurs 30–40 years after the original infection and therefore in the 60–75-year old age group, where the chance coincidental occurrence of motor neuron disease is more than possible. To make the distinction it is important to be able to correctly identify the changes of previous poliomyelitis.

In the upper limb, polio particularly affected the shoulder muscles and relatively infrequently involved the intrinsic muscles of the hand. The biceps and triceps jerks would have been abolished in the original attack. The finding of brisk arm reflexes and marked involvement of the intrinsic muscles of the hand would point to new pathology.

In the lower limb a striking difference is the very marked autonomic change. As in the arm, the paralysis may be proximal and patchy but the limb is usually cold, puffy, purple in colour and oedematous. This is usually associated with a flail foot. It is thought that these changes are not just secondary to paralysis and dependent oedema, but that the polio virus also damaged autonomic cells in the spinal cord.

The main clues to the development of motor neuron disease affecting the leg would be brisk reflexes and an extensor plantar response, but if the reflexes were already abolished they could not become brisk, and if the anterior compartment muscles were weak an extensor plantar response could not occur. This leaves only a distribution of weakness more typical of pyramidal disease than the patient's pre-existing weakness as the clue to the new development of an upper motor neuron lesion.

Trunk muscle weakness may produce mixtures of kyphoscoliosis, lordosis and segmental loss of the intercostal or abdominal musculature. With increasing age, secondary degenerative change in the spinal column may produce increasing pain and disability.

In post-polio syndrome the new muscle involvement tends to occur in muscles that the patient recalls were involved in the original attack which subsequently recovered. This provides strong support for the view that these are damaged neurons undergoing premature degeneration, rather than a new disease process. Six-monthly review over 1 or 2 years will usually exclude the more explosive development of true motor neuron disease in this setting. Unfortunately, electromyographic studies do not provide definitive evidence for or against either diagnosis.

CASE REPORT VI

A 63-year-old retired professor was referred with 6 months' progressive clumsiness and weakness of the left arm that he had been told was due to cervical spondylosis, although the development had been quite painless. He had had poliomyelitis 30 years previously, which had left him with some residual weakness in the legs, and although it had affected the arms acutely they appeared to have recovered completely. On examination he had marked weakness of the intrinsic hand muscles on the left, with wasting of the forearm and brisk reflexes throughout the left arm. The right arm was neurologically normal. Both legs showed clear-cut evidence of old poliomyelitis. They were areflexic, with generalized thinning and modest vasomotor changes, but the left plantar response was extensor. The clinical picture was clearly inconsistent with cervical spondylosis and the distal wasting, brisk reflexes in the arm and the extensor plantar response suggested that this was indeed motor neuron disease. This was more than adequately confirmed by the clinical course over the next 6 months. It was motor neuron disease developing in a patient with previous polio.

CASE REPORT VII

A 58-year-old woman was referred because of increasing weakness in the legs. At the age of 24, when she was a PE teacher, she developed polio which at its height resulted in

generalized paralysis, although she did not need respiratory support. She was in hospital for 2 years and was able to walk with sticks, with quite severe residual weakness in both legs. She had always been aware of weakness in the quadriceps muscles but they now seemed to be getting weaker. She had recently put on 20 lb in weight. On examination she had typical vascular changes of old polio in both legs. The main weakness was in the hip flexors, quadriceps and evertors and dorsiflexors of the feet, which were areflexic. There were no plantar responses due to weakness. EMG revealed bizarre prolonged repetitive giant units in a greatly reduced interference pattern, with no fasciculation or fibrillation. These findings were suggestive of very chronic changes with no evidence of new disease and muscles that were functioning on relatively few surviving units. Six-monthly follow-up over 3 years has confirmed this view, with no further deterioration, helped by some weight loss.

CASE REPORT VIII

A 46-year-old man was referred because of weakness while chewing, particularly affecting the right side. He had been born in India and at 6 years of age contracted an illness while swimming in stagnant water. He had little recollection of the illness and was told that he had been in coma for 2 weeks. During the recovery phase he recalled that he could only eat by using his hands to push his lower jaw up and down to chew. The illness had also left him with a complete right lower motor neuron facial palsy. His mother came over from India to give further details and said that a diagnosis of poliomyelitis was never suggested. She confirmed that he took nearly a year to recover the ability to speak and chew normally. On examination he had marked weakness of the right pterygoids and a dense right facial nerve palsy. There were no other physical findings and the bulbar musculature was entirely normal. EMGs in the right pterygoids revealed a remarkably similar picture to the patient above, with a very reduced number of identical repeating giant units but no evidence of fibrillation or fasciculation. There has been no progression during 12 months of follow-up.

It seems very likely that this was an example of bulbar poliomyelitis. A persistent facial palsy was reportedly the commonest residual of the condition. There is historical evidence of involvement of the muscles of mastication during the acute attack and now, 40 years later, he is developing weakness in the same muscles. It is tentatively suggested that this is a perhaps unique example of post-polio syndrome. Certainly it would be an even more atypical presentation of motor neuron disease.

Toxic Ventral Horn Cell Disease

Fortunately, there are no drugs that are known to damage the ventral horn cell but at least one chemical, tri-ortho-cresyl phosphate, does and this has twice caused tragic outbreaks of disease in the last 50 years. The first was its use as 'Jamaica ginger', a component of illicit liquor during prohibition in the USA. The second occurred fairly recently, when aviation oil containing the chemical was sold as cooking oil in Morocco. An epidemic of poisoning occurred leaving many survivors severely disabled. An epidemic of peripheral neuropathy with similar features occurred in Spain, and although cooking oil has been suspected the exact cause has not yet been established.

The third 'toxic' cause of ventral horn cell damage, or at least a polio-like illness, is tick paralysis. This is due to a toxin released from a tick embedded in the skin, usually in the scalp or neck. The particular species involved are found in the Rocky Mountains of Canada and the USA, and also occur in South Africa, Australia and southeast Europe, including the Balkan states. Within days of the entry of the tick, fever, delusions, facial paraesthesiae and difficulty in swallowing occur. This is rapidly followed by ascending paralysis, which may prove fatal if the tick is not found removed.

Electric Shock and Ventral Horn Cell Disease

In recent years it has been recognized that survivors of severe electric shock may develop acute spinal cord damage in the affected area. As the shock often enters through the arm and goes to earth through the opposite arm or leg, the cord at C5, C6 or C7 is maximally affected. Within months progressive wasting and weakness in these motor units occurs, producing symptoms and signs indistinguishable from motor neuron disease. The condition usually arrests but the damage is permanent.

Peripheral Neuropathy

Lesions affecting individual nerve roots and peripheral nerves are discussed in Chapters 16 and 17. In this chapter we are concerned with inherited, infective, metabolic, toxic and obscure disorders in which the peripheral nerves are diffusely damaged.

In infancy and childhood peripheral neuropathy may cause failure to achieve normal motor milestones, clumsiness or abnormal gait. Rarely does the child complain of peripheral paraesthesiae, the classic symptom of a neuropathy. Because of the absence of subjective symptoms children with peripheral nerve damage are often thought to have muscular dystrophy, and electrophysiological studies in children are essential in differential diagnosis.

In the adult the typical symptoms of peripheral paraesthesiae, sensory loss and clumsiness, usually due to a mixture of slight loss of dexterity and sensory impairment, make the diagnosis more obvious even though the aetiology often remains obscure.

In all age groups a very detailed family history is vital. Sometimes several members of a family are found to have the same disease masquerading under several different diagnostic labels. If there is any doubt

it is worth considerable effort to examine other family members to establish whether or not an inherited disorder is present. A detailed history of all drugs previously used and any possible chemical exposure is important. Dietary habits, previous abdominal surgical procedures and details of alcohol intake should be taken into consideration as nutritional deficiency is an important cause of neuropathy.

Inherited Peripheral Neuropathies

The inherited peripheral neuropathies have been extensively reclassified in the last 15 years and the new classification is used in further discussion, but the original names of the conditions have been included for both historical and practical reasons, as many patients still carry the old appellation in their clinical records. They are now called the hereditary motor sensory neuropathies (HMSN I–III) and hereditary sensory neuropathies (HSN I–IV).

Hereditary Motor Sensory Neuropathies

HMSN I (Peroneal Muscular Atrophy, Charcot–Marie–Tooth Disease, Roussy–Levy Syndrome)

This condition is inherited as either an autosomal dominant or recessive gene defect on chromosome 1. The gene shows variable penetrance, so that a spectrum of conditions, ranging from an abnormal foot to a full-blown neuropathy, can occur.

Physical signs may be found at any age. Kyphoscoliosis or pes cavus may be noted in infancy and orthopaedic advice sought. Often the significance of these findings is not appreciated at that stage, although examination of the parent's feet will often reveal similar deformity. The type of foot deformity is best remembered if the deformity of the foot that would be produced by kicking a concrete football is imagined, the foot is foreshortened, the arch is high and the lateral border of the foot does not touch the ground, the toes are bunched up and appear to arise from the upper surface of the metatarsals rather than at their ends. This type of deformity may be found in association with any of the inherited neurological disorders and intraspinal diseases and is a key neurological sign known as a Friedreich's foot (Fig. 19.3). Typically the condition becomes more obvious between 10 and 20 years of age. It starts with wasting and weakness of the peroneal muscles, producing a foot drop, and progressive worsening of the pre-existing pes cavus. Later the calf muscles and the distal third of the thigh atrophy, resulting in a leg shaped like a 'stork leg' or a

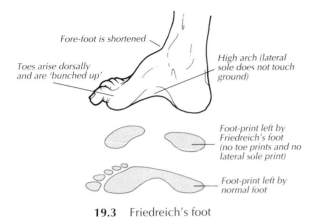

19.3   Friedreich's foot

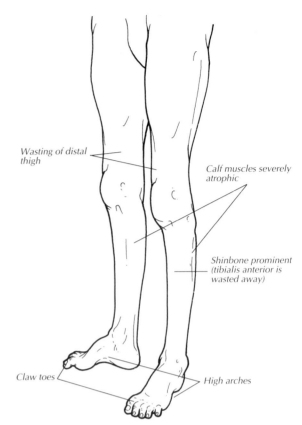

19.4   Charcot–Marie–Tooth disease (HMSN I or II): 'champagne glass leg' or 'stork leg'.

'champagne glass'. Vibration sense is impaired early and later some joint position sense loss may occur. The motor disabilities are always much more in evidence than sensory deficit, although in some kindreds sensory loss may be an important feature (Fig. 19.4).

In a severe long-standing case the distal forearms and small hand muscles may also waste. The reflexes are lost and some thickening of the peripheral nerves is detectable in about 50% of cases. In some families the condition is associated with coexisting benign essential tremor. This is the variant that used to be called Roussy–Levy syndrome.

The hallmark of HMSN I is profound slowing of peripheral nerve conduction, with velocities reduced to 10–20 m/s and loss of sensory action potentials. Clinically unaffected family members may also have nerve conduction abnormalities. Pathologically, peripheral segmental demyelination and dorsal column degeneration are found. The prognosis for survival is good and relatively few patients become wheelchair-bound.

HMSN II

This condition is inherited as an autosomal dominant and is virtually identical to HMSN I except that the onset is later, at about 20–30 years of age. The condition is milder, affecting only the legs, and less progressive. The distinguishing feature is that nerve conduction velocities and nerve action potentials are minimally reduced. The pathology in this condition appears to be in the neuron or axon and the condition has been described as the 'neuronal form' of peroneal muscular atrophy.

HMSN III (Hypertrophic Peripheral Neuropathy, Dejerine–Sottas Disease)

This condition is inherited as an autosomal recessive and symptoms begin in early childhood or adolescence. The affected patients are usually of short stature, kyphoscoliotic, and may have deformities of

the hands and feet. Motor milestones may be delayed. The reflexes are absent and the peripheral nerves are enlarged and easily palpable, and sometimes even visible, particularly the supraclavicular nerves and the cutaneous nerves on the dorsum of the foot.

Weakness starts in the legs but becomes generalized and, unlike HMSN I and HMSN II, severe sensory deficit occurs. This particularly affects posture sense and may result in pseudoataxia and pseudoathetosis. Hearing is frequently impaired. Nerve conduction studies reveal extreme slowing down to 10 m/s or less and sensory action potentials are absent. The pathological changes are surprising, given the thickening of the nerves. The normally myelinated nerve fibres are hypomyelinated or non-myelinated and there is evidence of segmental demyelination. The nerve fibres are encased in concentric layers of basal lamina. The thickened nerves are very vulnerable to extrinsic compression and a mononeuritis multiplex type of neuropathy may occur. The illness is severely disabling and most patients become wheelchair bound in their 20s.

Neuropathy in Friedreich's Ataxia

Although this is not classified as one of the hereditary motor sensory neuropathies it is appropriate to mention it here, as a mild sensorimotor neuropathy characterized by slow conduction down to the 20–30 m/s range is a characteristic feature of the condition. The identical foot deformity is also a feature and any patient with a neuropathy and foot deformity should be very carefully examined for evidence of ataxia or dysarthria (see also Chapter 14).

Hereditary Sensory Neuropathies

HSN I (Hereditary Sensory Neuropathy of Denny–Brown)

This rare familial disorder of autosomal dominant inheritance specifically affects pain pathways and, to a lesser extent, other modalities, particularly in the legs. Clinical symptoms begin between 10 and 20 years of age. The underlying pathology is a slowly progressive sensory distal axonal degeneration affecting non-myelinated and small myelinated fibres, hence the severe loss of pain and temperature sensation. The main problems are due to recurrent painless trauma and ulceration of the feet, which may later progress to a severe destructive arthropathy of the ankle joints (Charcot's joint). Autonomic function is unaffected, and provided the condition is recognized and care taken of the feet, the prognosis is good.

HSN II (Morvan's Syndrome, Infantile Syringomyelia or Congenital Sensory Neuropathy)

This is very rare autosomal recessive disorder producing distal sensory deficit leading to painless deformity and ulceration of the hands and feet. It is similar to HSN I except for its onset in infancy.

HSN III (Riley–Day Syndrome, Familial Dysautonomia)

This is very rare autosomal recessive disorder most often seen in Jewish families. It is due to the congenital absence of autonomic and dorsal root ganglia sensory neurons. The clinical picture is dominated by severe autonomic neuropathy, with fluctuating body temperature, no tears, a dry mouth, postural hypotension, impaired taste sensation with a strikingly smooth tongue, and generalized loss of pain and temperature sensation. All reflexes are absent. Most children die by the age of 15 due to autonomic dysfunction.

HSN IV (Congenital Sensory Neuropathy With Loss of Sweating)

An extremely rare autosomal recessive disorder presenting in infancy with episodes of high fever due to the absence of sweating mechanisms. Mental retardation and short stature are common. Congenital insensitivity to pain is a notable feature. The prognosis is poor.

Metabolic Neuropathies

These conditions are also inherited, but in each the biochemical defect causing the neuropathy has been identified and they are therefore classified separately.

Amyloid Neuropathy

The peripheral nerves may be damaged in amyloidosis by direct deposition of amyloid around the nerve fibres, deposition of amyloid in the coverings of the nerve fibres and by microvascular deposition of amyloid leading to a 'vasculitic' type of neuropathy. The clinical picture is dominated by damage to the small-diameter fibres producing pain and temperature loss and autonomic neuropathy, which is a constant feature.

There are four varieties of inherited amyloid neuropathy. The first type to be reported was initially detected in patients of Portuguese extraction, but Japanese and Swedish origins have now been established. This produces a very unpleasant, relentlessly progressive and ultimately fatal neuropathy that starts in the legs in the third decade and runs its course over some 10 years. The second variety has been reported in families of Swiss and German origin and is a milder disorder, usually starting in the arms with a carpal tunnel-like syndrome. Vitreous opacities are common in this variety. The third variety is a generalized neuropathy starting between 30 and 40 years of age with minimal autonomic involvement. This was first recognized in Iowa in a family of British origin. The fourth type has only been reported in Finland and produces multiple cranial nerve lesions and corneal dystrophy.

Systemic amyloidosis of non-familial origin may be complicated by peripheral neuropathy. Primary amyloidosis, including that occurring in patients with multiple myeloma, produces a generalized symmetrical sensorimotor neuropathy with later serious autonomic involvement. The diagnosis is made by biopsy of the sural nerve, rectum or gum. Death is usually due to cardiac or renal involvement by amyloid.

Lipoprotein Disorders and Peripheral Neuropathy

This is a group of very rare disorders where the other components of the condition may be of greater significance than the neuropathy, but they are best included at this stage for clarity.

Cerebral Lipoidoses

The cerebral degenerative diseases associated with the deposition of abnormal lipids in the brain, although dominated by cerebral problems, include a peripheral neuropathy as part of the picture. Nerve conduction studies and nerve biopsies will often confirm the diagnosis without resort to cerebral biopsy. The two conditions are metachromatic leukodystrophy and Krabbe's disease. Both are inherited as autosomal recessive conditions.

Metachromatic Leukodystrophy

This condition is due to a deficiency of arylsulfatase A, leading to the deposition of sulfatides in the tissues. Widespread demyelination of the brain produces intellectual impairment and a progressive picture not unlike multiple sclerosis, unless the peripheral neuropathic features are identified. There are infantile, juvenile and adult forms but all are fatal within a few years of onset.

Krabbe's Disease

This condition is due to a deficiency of galactosylceramide beta-galactosidase. Galactocerebroside accumulates in the brain and peripheral nerves. Progressive cerebral degeneration and evidence of neuropathy dominate the picture, which is fatal within 1–2 years of the onset, which is usually within the first year of life.

Neuropathy due to Glycoprotein Deficiency

Two conditions have been identified associated with glycoprotein deficiency. These are Bassen–Kornzweig syndrome and Tangier disease.

Bassen–Kornzweig Syndrome (A–betalipo proteinaemia)

This is an autosomal recessive condition in which triglycerides accumulate in the intestinal mucosa and impair the absorption of fat-soluble vitamins. Serum cholesterol levels are extremely low. The clinical picture is dominated by malabsorption with developmental delay and progressive ataxia, dysarthria and peripheral neuropathy, with marked impairment of posture sense due to large fibre involvement. It may be associated with retinitis pigmentosa. Patients may live to middle age. The laboratory feature other than the extremely low cholesterol is the presence of acanthocytes in the blood film. These are red cells with spiny projections. It is thought that the use of high doses of fat-soluble vitamins and dietary fat restriction may modify the progression of the neurological signs.

Tangier Disease (High-Density Lipoprotein Deficiency)

This fascinating autosomal recessive condition may present as a peripheral neuropathy. The most striking clinical feature is the deposition of cholesterol into the tonsils, producing swollen yellow tonsils that may cause difficulty in swallowing and breathing. The biochemical basis of the condition is uncertain, but high-density lipoproteins are virtually absent in the serum and the cholesterol level in the blood is extremely low. The small myelinated and unmyelinated fibres are affected, which tends to produce severe impairment of pain and temperature sensation mimicking syringomyelia. The neuropathy progresses extremely slowly.

Refsum's Disease (Hereditary Ataxic Neuropathy, Phytanic Acid Storage Disease)

This very rare condition is due to the inability to break down phytanic acid, which is found mainly in dairy products, fish oils and beef. The condition usually starts in the late teens and is dominated by retinitis pigmentosa, with night blindness, deafness, ataxia and progressive peripheral neuropathy. Ichthyosis may be an early feature. Early identification and treatment by a low phytol diet may modify the disease, which is otherwise fatal due to later cardiac involvement.

Fabry's Disease (Angiokeratoma Corporis Diffusum, α-Galactosidase A Deficiency)

This condition is inherited as an X-linked recessive and starts in childhood. The skin lesion is a telangiectatic rash of the lower trunk and upper legs. An abnormal lipid is deposited in all tissues and present in body fluids. Renal failure is the commonest cause of death. The feature of the peripheral neuropathy is very severe pain of excruciating burning type. This may be constant and occasionally severe in so-called 'crises'.

All the inherited neuropathic conditions produce signs of a peripheral neuropathy: basically, loss of all reflexes and sensory impairment, which may preferentially affect pain or temperature sensation if small fibres are affected and loss of proprioception with consequent ataxia if large fibres are involved. This differential sensory loss can sometimes mimic cord disease unless it is appreciated that dissociated sensory loss can sometimes be due to peripheral nerve disease. The routine evaluation of all patients with suspected peripheral neuropathy should include a careful family history, palpation of the peripheral nerves, examination of the eyes for vitreous opacities and retinitis pigmentosa and examination of the tonsils. A routine blood film, serum cholesterol and lipoprotein determination, and blood phytanic acid level should be included in the screening investigations if the clinical picture is appropriate. In genetically determined and metabolic neuropathies a frequent finding is marked slowing of nerve conduction, which may be in the 10–20 m/s range (normal 38 m/s and higher). In other types of neuropathy slowing to the lower range of normal occurs, but with the exception of Guillain–Barré syndrome this extreme degree of slowing is rarely found, and extreme slowing is the hallmark of inherited neuropathies.

Metabolically Triggered Neuropathy (Acute Intermittent Porphyria)

Three of the six variants of abnormal porphyrin metabolism are associated with damage to the brain and peripheral nerves. The classic condition is acute intermittent porphyria due to a defect in uroporphyrinogen-1 synthetase. The mechanism of damage to the nervous system is uncertain but toxicity of abnormal metabolites is that most favoured. Attacks are most often triggered by certain drugs, but again the mechanism is unknown.

The condition is inherited as an autosomal dominant and the incidence is 1.5/100 000. Many of the most provocative drugs are no longer in general use, which may explain the rarity of acute attacks. The most notable were sulphonamides and barbiturates (see Table 19.1). Many other less frequently used drugs have also been implicated. Attacks may also be precipitated by fasting and fever.

The clinical picture is remarkable for its ability to simulate other conditions, conditions sometimes requiring the use of further provocative agents such as sulphonamides, if the picture indicates urinary tract infection, or general anaesthesia with barbiturates if an acute abdomen is suspected.

Severe colicky abdominal pain with vomiting and constipation may mimic bowel obstruction. Acute emotional upset with abnormal behaviour, often psychotic in degree, may require acute psychiatric intervention.

The rapid onset of a severe ascending neuropathy resembles Guillain–Barré syndrome but the association with a peculiar piecemeal onset and unusually severe pain in a mentally disturbed patient might easily suggest a diagnosis of hysteria. In a typical case severe painful paraesthesiae, often without sensory loss, is a major feature. If sensory loss occurs it may start proximally in a so-called 'swimming trunks' distribution. A rapidly ascending flaccid areflexic paralysis with cranial nerve involvement is the usual motor picture. Autonomic involvement may occur and be responsible for the gastrointestinal symptoms. Attacks of severe abdominal pain (visceral crises) and tachycardia with postural hypotension are the usual clues to the autonomic involvement.

Previously the diagnosis was made by the detection of excess porphobilinogen and δ-amino-laevulinic acid in the urine, but now direct determination of erythrocyte urobilinogen-1 synthetase is the diagnostic test. The deep red colour of the urine, which occurs during an attack, only develops if the urine is left standing in the light and allowed to oxidize.

Secondary metabolic dysfunction is common and there may be evidence of inappropriate secretion of ADH (antidiuretic hormone), salt-losing nephropathy and liver damage.

The mortality rate is high, at 25%–50%, and is due to paralysis and cerebral dysfunction. Survivors begin recovering at 6–8 weeks, but recovery is slow and

Table 19.1 Drugs precipitating attacks of porphyria

Alcohol
Barbiturates
Carbamazepine
Chloramphenicol
Chlordiazepoxide
Dichloralphenazone
Ergotamine derivatives
Glutethimide
Griseofulvin
Imiprimine
Levodopa
Meprobamate
Methsuximide
Methyldopa
Oestrogens (including contraceptive pill)
Pentazocine
Phenytoin
Sulphonamides
Tolbutamide

often incomplete. Attacks should be treated with intravenous glucose at the rate of 10–20 g/h and haematin 4 mg/kg per 12 hours, which reverses the metabolic defect. Phenothiazines may be used for sedation: chlorpromazine seems particularly useful. Other metabolic disorders are treated as appropriate.

CASE REPORT IX

A 26-year-old woman developed a urinary tract infection which was treated with sulphonamides. The back pain changed to abdominal pain with vomiting but no surgical cause was found and she continued on sulphonamides. Increasing distress and emotional lability led to admission to a general hospital and subsequent transfer to a mental hospital. Increasing neurological disability, with pain, numbness and weakness, was thought to indicate hysteria. Arrangements were made for neurological assessment and on the day of transfer she was made to crawl along the corridor to the ambulance because 'she had to do it to hasten her recovery'. On arrival at the neurological unit, she was dyspnoeic and slightly cyanosed, with severe generalized weakness, bilateral facial weakness, areflexia and difficulty in swallowing and speaking. She clearly had a severe fulminant neuropathy. A urine specimen turned deep red after 2 hours on the ward window-sill and biochemical analysis confirmed the diagnosis of acute intermittent porphyria. Chlorpromazine 25 mg t.d.s. was used to control her symptoms and she narrowly avoided respiratory support and made a good recovery.

This sequence of referrals – surgical–psychiatric–neurological – is almost diagnostic of the condition in itself, but acute intermittent porphyria is so rare and the presentation so variable and atypical that failure to identify it immediately is almost the rule. Like all rare conditions, anyone can make the diagnosis once it has been thought of, the problem is to think of it in the first place.

Once again, the importance of a complete history of all drugs taken by the patient within previous months is highlighted. There may be no family history until the first case is detected. Full family screening may then reveal other members who have yet to have an attack, and who may even have taken provocative drugs in the past without developing symptoms.

There are six neuropathies related to infective organisms: leprosy and herpes zoster, which are due to direct infection of the nerves; diphtheria, due to a toxin produced by the bacterium in the body; sarcoidosis, an infection-related chronic granulomatous condition; and immunologically triggered neuropathies, Guillain–Barré syndrome and the chronic relapsing inflammatory neuropathies. Botulinum poisoning due to an ingested toxin is discussed in Chapter 18, as it is the nerve end-plate and not the nerve that is damaged.

Leprosy (Hansen's Disease)

Leprosy is probably the single most important cause of peripheral neuropathy on a worldwide scale. There are 13 million sufferers in the world. There are two main types, lepromatous leprosy with generalized skin involvement and generalized nerve damage due to Schwann cell infection by *Mycobacterium leprae*, and the localized tuberculoid form with patchy skin lesions affecting the cutaneous nerves, producing depigmented and anaesthetic patches. The difference in type is due to the immune response. This is poor in the generalized form and very dramatic in the localized form. The organism infects via the skin in the cooler areas of the body, the face, hands, feet and male genitalia. The small fibre cutaneous nerves are first affected, leading to striking pain and temperature loss mimicking syringomyelia. The thickened nerve trunks later become vulnerable to compression palsies. Prolonged treatment may arrest the disease but the recovery of the nerve lesions is poor and incomplete.

CASE REPORT X

A 50-year-old man who had worked in North Africa for several years slammed the door of his Land Rover and tried to walk away. He found that he was caught and thought that his jacket sleeve was in the door, but was surprised to find that it was actually his fingers, which were severely mangled although quite painless. Later that day he demonstrated to his colleagues that he could hold his damaged hand over an open fire without flinching, with fairly devastating results. Biopsy revealed tuberculoid leprosy.

Fortunately, leprosy is now rare in Europe but is endemic throughout Africa and the Middle East. It is not very infective and travellers are unlikely to contract the disease, but contract workers who live in these areas for prolonged periods are at some risk. As noted above, the main nerve trunks are thickened and become pressure sensitive so that sudden pressure palsies of particularly vulnerable nerves (i.e. the ulnar and peroneal nerves) punctuate the slow development of a diffuse neuropathy. The patient may therefore develop a 'mononeuritis multiplex'. The other main causes of this condition are diabetes and polyarteritis nodosa.

Herpes Zoster

Herpes zoster classically affects individual nerve trunks or nerve roots, producing pain and sensory loss. What is not generally appreciated is that motor involvement is common. This is most readily detected when cervical or lumbar roots are involved. The segmental motor weakness of thoracic root involvement is less readily detected unless specifically sought. Attacks of herpes zoster are probably due to a localized breakdown of the immunological mechanism that prevents replication of the herpes virus, which has been present in the sensory root ganglia since the patient had chicken pox many years previously. The virus travels down the nerve to the skin, erupting as vesicles in the affected dermatome, a process normally taking 4–5 days after the onset of very severe localized pain. The severe scarring of the nerve roots produced by the attack may cause postherpetic neuralgia, one of the most unpleasant and painful conditions known. Herpes zoster can occur in a generalized form in immunosuppressed and immunocompromised patients.

Diphtheritic Neuropathy

In most civilized countries this disease has become a rarity due to mass immunization programmes, but occasional outbreaks still occur and reveal that the disease remains a very serious and often lethal infection of childhood. Neural involvement occurs in 20% of infected patients. The toxin produced by the bacterium inhibits myelin synthesis by Schwann cells. The generalized neuropathy typically occurs 4–8 weeks after the acute infection and, like Guillain–Barré syndrome, produces a rapidly ascending paralysis which may be fatal due to respiratory muscle involvement. Death is usually due to diphtheritic myocarditis. Survivors make a complete recovery. During the acute infection paralysis of accommodation causes blurred vision and palatal weakness causes nasal speech. This is thought to be due to a direct local toxin effect and occurs in the first 2 weeks of the illness. Similar localized paralysis may occur with diphtheritic infection in tropical ulcers on the legs.

Sarcoidosis

This complex and ill-understood disorder, which usually causes pulmonary problems, is complicated by peripheral nerve lesions in 5% of cases. It is a chronic granulomatous disorder with no identified pathogen. The commonest nerve lesion is a Bell's palsy and the condition should always be considered in patients with bilateral or recurrent attacks of Bell's palsy. Single thoracic or lumbar root lesions have been described and rarely sensorimotor neuropathy may occur. Sarcoidosis is one of those conditions that can enter into the differential diagnosis of almost any neurological disease, but all these manifestations are extremely rare.

Guillain–Barré Syndrome

The incidence of Guillain–Barré syndrome is 9.5 cases per million. Most cases present in A and E departments. They are a source of considerable diagnostic difficulty as there is a wide range of clinical presentations and only the classic progressive ascending type is likely to be immediately recognized. Serious diagnostic errors are common.

CASE REPORT XI

A very anxious 28-year-old man presented at an A and E department in the early evening complaining of generalized paraesthesiae and difficulty in breathing. He was thought to be suffering from an anxiety state with hyperventilation and was sent home. His condition deteriorated but he was reluctant to return to the original hospital as it had been made clear to him that he was wasting the department's time. Four hours later he was admitted to another hospital in cardiopulmonary arrest. By then he had lost all his reflexes and was totally paralysed. He did not survive.

CASE REPORT XII

A 32-year-old woman, a known alcoholic under psychiatric care, complained of difficulty speaking and swallowing and generalized weakness. Her psychiatrist was called to the house and diagnosed an acute anxiety state. Two hours later increasing difficulty with breathing prompted her husband to call for an ambulance. She collapsed in the ambulance and in spite of cardiopulmonary resuscitation arrived at the hospital with fixed dilated pupils, generalized hypotonia and areflexia. Guillain–Barré syndrome was confirmed by CSF examination and nerve conduction studies. She was ventilated and survived for 2 years in an intensive care unit, during which time her reflexes returned and power recovered, enabling the limbs to become spastic and to demonstrate decerebrate posturing for the first time. She had cortical blindness. She died following a chest infection.

These cases exemplify the relatively non-specific onset and show how easily this may be misdiagnosed as anxiety, and also illustrate the potentially fulminant nature of the illness. Immediate admission to a unit with full facilities for assisted respiration is vital, and early

tracheostomy is advised once it is clear that respiratory function is compromised and respiratory support is going to be required.

CASE REPORT XIII

A 20-year-old student was travelling in the Far East and Australia. During a somewhat adventurous period in Thailand, where he got tattooed and used illicit substances, he developed painful paraesthesiae in both feet. This had already been present for a week when he flew to Australia, by which time the tingling had extended to the lower abdomen, the legs had become numb and tingling and numbness was developing in the hands. He was finding it increasingly difficult to walk and carry his bags. He sought medical advice in Australia. No diagnosis was offered but it was suggested that he returned to the UK as soon as possible. On admission to hospital he had generalized weakness which by then involved the facial musculature and there was marked sensory deficit to the mid-thigh and mid-upper arm. He was areflexic. He was immediately infused with 24 g immunoglobulin (Sandoglobulin), repeated daily for 4 days. Within 3 days the sensory loss had improved to wrist and ankle level and power had improved sufficiently that he could stand with help. Within 6 weeks his only residual difficulty was some numbness of the feet and weakness of dorsiflexion of the feet and toes.

This case is a more classic example of the condition, with perhaps a more insidious onset and more extensive sensory deficit than is usually seen.

This condition is thought to be a single response of the nerve roots to a variety of infective processes. It often follows acute upper respiratory tract or gut infections and specifically complicates glandular fever in 1% of cases. It may also occur in association with a remote carcinoma. It can occur at any age, and the clinical findings may be very variable and hysteria is often suspected.

The first symptoms are usually painful peripheral paraesthesiae but often unaccompanied by definite sensory findings. Weakness may come on quite explosively and a patient may become extremely weak in 30 minutes, although more typically the period of advancing weakness in an acute case is some 12–48 hours. The weakness is often most marked in the proximal muscles, so that the patient may be unable to sit or stand at a time when peripheral strength is quite normal. It is this combination that may lead to the diagnosis of hysteria, as most doctors tend to examine the distal strength, hand grips and feet movements and often fail to test the much more important proximal muscles if peripheral strength is normal.

In most cases the main clue, and almost diagnostic finding, is the total abolition of reflexes, even at the stage when the weakness has not yet become severe. It is very important to ask the patient whether their reflexes have previously been present. Many will remember eliciting their knee jerks as a schooldays exercise and anyone who has been in the services is usually aware that their reflexes were elicited at their induction medical. Unfortunately, there are many patients who have never been examined and it is worth remembering that some 5% of the general population have very depressed or absent reflexes. Only the loss of previously detected reflexes is significant. It may be possible, if the patient is seen early in the course of the illness, to document reflexes disappearing under observation and this really is diagnostic!

Atypical presentations are very common indeed and include bilateral facial weakness, which is easily missed unless eye closure, cheek blowing and lip pouting are routinely tested. If present this is another virtually diagnostic sign of Guillain–Barré syndrome. It is extremely rare in other forms of neuropathy.

A descending version of the disorder, starting with facial weakness and then involving the upper limbs, can occur and anyone with bilateral facial weakness with areflexic arms should be regarded with suspicion.

Ascending paralysis may be associated with cord inflammation, producing a coincidental transverse myelitis, and this may mimic spinal cord compression.

In some patients profound loss of posture sense may produce such severe deafferentation of the limbs that static tremor and ataxia may occur. This is particularly likely in those cases with cranial nerve involvement, and this has been subclassified as the Fisher syndrome.

Some 25% of patients have significant respiratory problems and the 10% mortality rate is a measure of the potential danger of this disease. Great emphasis is always placed on the typical CSF protein elevation but this may take several days to occur, and in the very acute stages of a severe attack some lymphocytes may be found in the CSF, raising other diagnostic possibilities such as poliomyelitis.

Suspected Guillain–Barré syndrome is one of the few conditions that should be regarded as an acute neurological emergency, yet it is often casually treated and regarded as a benign condition by those who see the occasional case that runs a mild course with recovery over a few weeks.

CIDP and CRIP Syndromes

Chronic inflammatory demyelinating polyradiculoneuronopathy (CIDP) and chronic relapsing inflammatory neuropathy (CRIP) are two Guillain–Barré-related syndromes. They are perhaps best characterized as Guillain–Barré syndrome that keeps going (CIDP) or keeps coming back (CRIP). Both conditions clearly have an immunological basis and respond to steroids, immunosuppressants and, in the acutely worsening situation, to IgG infusions.

Toxic Neuropathies

There are a wide range of chemicals that can cause peripheral nerve damage and a full history of possible chemical exposure should be part of the routine questioning in patients with peripheral neuropathy. Some of the toxins are of mainly historical interest.

Arsenic has been widely used as a poison in the past, was the first effective treatment for syphilis (neo-arsphenamine), and in the not too distant past was used by one neurologist in the UK as a treatment for multiple sclerosis, resulting in several cases of arsenical neuropathy.

Lead is still a potentially 'hidden' toxin. Its removal from paint has solved the problem as far as painters are concerned and protected children from the consequences of chewing lead-painted toys, but isolated examples resulting from burning batteries to retrieve the lead, lead glazes on pottery, make-up from the Indian subcontinent and tetraethyl lead poisoning from petrol sniffing, still occur.

Thallium, widely used as a cockroach poison in the USA, has caused cases of peripheral neuropathy and a famous case in the UK, where a man now in Broadmoor poisoned three workmates with thallium, producing an illness which defied diagnosis until later confirmation, when the bodies were exhumed when a third workmate became unwell and poisoning was first suspected.

Tri-ortho-cresyl phosphate caused a motor neuropathy when used as a flavouring agent in illicit alcohol during prohibition, and more recently in industrial oil sold as cooking oil in Morocco, producing an epidemic of severe motor neuropathy. The actual agent involved in the recent Spanish 'toxic' cooking oil epidemic has not been identified.

Organic solvents have been implicated in nerve damage in survivors of repeated glue-sniffing. Cases have been identified in the shoemaking industry due to the solvents n-hexane and α-methyl-hexane used in industrial glues. Acrylamide, an industrial polymer, was one of the first identified neurotoxins of the modern era.

Clearly, a history of all occupations past and present and any chemicals used in hobbies should be an essential part of any diagnostic work-up for neuropathy, and in the younger generation the illicit use of a variety of possible toxins has unfortunately to be considered.

Drug-Induced Neuropathy

Drug-induced neuropathy has long been recognized and it is interesting to recall that a peripheral neuropathy due to thalidomide had already been identified prior to the discovery of the teratogenic effect of this drug. Some of the heavy metals discussed in the section above were used as therapeutic agents for several centuries and might be considered as 'drugs', and the continuing use of gold in the treatment of rheumatic conditions, with a risk of neuropathy among other hazards, is worthy of mention.

There are two major groupings of drugs that are particularly prone to cause neuropathy, the antibiotics and the antineoplastic agents.

Among antibiotics, metronidazole in long-term use for fungal disorders, nitrofurantoin, especially in chronic renal disease, dapsone in leprosy and *Pneumocystis carinii* infections in AIDS, and the use of isoniazid and ethionamide in the treatment of tuberculosis, are particularly notable. Chloramphenicol has caused neuropathy but this is rare as it is never used long term.

Antineoplastic drugs are a special problem because they are used in conditions that may lead to direct or remote peripheral neuropathy as a complication of the disease being treated. This is a particular problem in the treatment of malignant lymphomas with vinca alkaloids. These agents tend to produce a painful peripheral neuropathy with striking wasting and weakness of the intrinsic hand muscles, and most patients on vinca alkaloids quickly become areflexic. The use of cisplatin in ovarian carcinoma is also important because ovarian carcinoma has also been associated with peripheral neuropathy as a remote complication.

Among other drugs that have been reported to cause neuropathy are several in common use. They include phenytoin, disulfiram, hydrallazine, penicillin, perhexilitine, cliquinol, sodium cyanate and pyridoxine, which paradoxically is used to prevent neuropathy in patients on isoniazid.

Miscellaneous Neuropathies

This category includes several important general medical conditions, including diabetes, alcoholism, renal disease and malignancy, in which the exact relationship to the underlying disease or concurrent drugs is uncertain. Each will be discussed as a separate entity.

Alcoholic Peripheral Neuropathy

Worldwide alcohol is a common cause of peripheral neuropathy, but in the UK it is not a common disorder. It is still uncertain whether the neuropathy is due to a direct toxic effect of alcohol or secondary to accompanying vitamin B$_1$ deficiency. Although severe vitamin B$_1$ deficiency causes a neuropathy similar clinically to that of alcoholism, vitamin B$_1$ replacement alone is not successful treatment unless alcohol is also withdrawn. Well-fed heavy drinkers seem less likely to develop neuropathy than nutritionally deprived alcoholics. The neuropathy is characterized by severe pain in the feet, with very marked hypersensitivity to light touch or painful stimuli. The patient cannot bear the bedclothes to touch their feet or put their feet to the ground. The onset may be remarkably acute and because of pain most patients present early, before significant motor damage can occur. Occasionally a relatively painless

motor neuropathy can occur with very slow and incomplete recovery. With the acute painful onset, however, alcohol withdrawal and high-dose vitamin B$_1$ therapy will rapidly reduce the discomfort and a good recovery will ensue provided the patient abstains.

Heavy drinkers are also prone to compression palsies caused by lying on nerves while inebriated. The classic condition is a so-called 'Saturday night palsy' due to radial nerve compression. A peroneal nerve palsy due to compression at the fibula neck may also occur, especially if the leg is thinned by poor nutrition.

Diabetic Peripheral Neuropathy

Diabetes in all its forms is the commonest cause of neuropathy in the developed world. Its occurrence is often related to the duration and severity of the disease, and is more prevalent in males. Some 50% of diabetics who have had the condition for over 20 years have some degree of neuropathy. In maturity-onset diabetes, however, neuropathy is a common **presenting** symptom.

All fibre types are affected – motor, sensory and autonomic – producing a wide range of clinical manifestations. Even the basic pathology is complicated. Primary axonal degeneration with secondary demyelination may be further modified by proximal vascular lesions of the nerve and compression palsies, to which the nerves are vulnerable because of poor vascularity. These additional features may lead to almost static or slowly progressive peripheral nerve problems, punctuated by dramatically sudden but potentially recoverable acute nerve lesions, some of which are unique to the diabetic state.

Diabetic neuropathy may occur in the following forms:

1. *Mild peripheral sensory neuropathy*: Slight numbness of the feet and loss of ankle reflexes, it is found eventually in nearly all diabetics.

2. *Sensorimotor neuropathy*: Definite distal sensory loss to all modalities, affecting both feet and hands, and generalized areflexia. This may be relentlessly progressive and lead to significant disability. A major feature is pain which is refractory to all treatment. Amitriptyline, phenytoin and carbamazepine may sometimes be of benefit. The recent introduction of capsaicin ointment 0.075% is of uncertain value and many patients find its application too uncomfortable to bear. Severe loss of deep pain perception may lead to Charcot joints at the knee and ankle. This is a painless destructive arthropathy now almost exclusively found in diabetic neuropathy.

3. *Autonomic neuropathy*: This may cause impotence, diarrhoea, postural hypotension, tachycardia, gastrointestinal stasis, pupillary constriction and potentially hazardous impairment of the autonomic response

to hypoglycaemia, which many patients rely on to indicate the onset of a hypoglycaemic attacks. The advent of autonomic neuropathy is a very bad prognostic feature in diabetes.

4. Nerve compression palsies: Carpal tunnel syndrome, ulnar nerve compression at the elbow and peroneal nerve compression at the fibula neck are common and may occur in sequence and produce a mononeuritis multiplex syndrome. These nerve palsies are recoverable with appropriate decompression and pressure avoidance.

5. Vascular nerve lesions: Recurrent and multiple extraocular nerve palsies are discussed in Chapter 5. Some patients, particularly those with unstable diabetes, may develop sudden pain and numbness in thoracic dermatomes, with paralysis of the intercostal muscle. It would seem likely that these are vascular lesions of the intercostal nerve. They are all recoverable.

6. Diabetic amyotrophy: This is a very important and often misdiagnosed condition, sometimes referred to incorrectly as a femoral neuropathy. It is fully discussed in Chapter 17 but is worth detailing again here. The features are:

1. Maturity-onset diabetes, particularly in males.
2. Onset characterized by sudden dramatic weight loss without obvious deterioration in the diabetic state.
3. Excruciating pain in the front of the thigh down to the medial malleolus. This is in both the femoral nerve distribution and the L4 root distribution. The pain is severe for 5–10 days.
4. As the pain peaks the patient will start to stumble and fall, with rapidly progressive weakness of the quadriceps, and the knee jerk disappears. Rapid wasting of the thigh muscles ensues.
5. Careful motor evaluation will often reveal weakness in the hip flexors and thigh adductors, indicating that this is a lumbar plexopathy affecting L2, L3 and L4 rather than a femoral nerve lesion or an L4 root lesion, which is a common misdiagnosis.
6. Recovery usually occurs over a period of 6–18 months, depending on the severity and exact location of the presumed vascular lesion of the nerve roots or nerve trunks in the pelvis.

This condition may be the presenting symptom of diabetes, and unless it is considered pelvic malignancy or extradural malignancy will usually be suspected. An elevated blood sugar is a much less expensive way of making the diagnosis than negative MRI and CT scans of the pelvis and lower back.

Diabetes should be excluded in any patient presenting with any form of peripheral neuropathy before any other investigations are considered.

Ischaemic Peripheral Neuropathy

The probable role of nerve ischaemia in diabetic neuropathy has been mentioned above. Many 70–80-year-old patients complain of tingling paraesthesiae in the feet, particularly in a warm bed or on standing. This may be accompanied by definite blunting of cutaneous sensation over the feet. This is almost certainly due to poor skin nutrition affecting the cutaneous nerve filaments and the nerve endings in the skin. Nerve conduction studies rarely show evidence of neuropathy. No treatment is of any benefit.

Of more sinister importance is the neuropathy complicating collagen vascular disease and, notably, neuropathy in association with polyarteritis nodosa. This condition may not only produce individual ischaemic cranial nerve lesions but can also cause a widespread diffuse sensorimotor neuropathy due to severe vasculitis, and it is one of classic causes of mononeuritis multiplex. Over several days a patient may develop compression palsies of all the vulnerable peripheral nerves, resulting in an acute 'generalized' neuropathy. This can recover provided further compression is avoided and the underlying condition controlled with appropriate treatment.

Rheumatoid arthritis may be complicated by carpal tunnel syndrome due to local arthritic changes at the wrist joint, and more diffuse damage may occur as a result of local trauma around inflamed joints. It is still uncertain whether a true neuropathy due to the disease itself can occur.

Systemic lupus erythematosus may produce an acute Guillain–Barré like picture, a diffuse sensorimotor neuropathy or mononeuritis multiplex. In this complex disease this may be partially vascular and partially immunologically based.

Neuropathy of Chronic Renal Failure

Chronic renal failure causes peripheral neuropathy. In the past some cases may have been due to the use of nitrofurantoin but it was always suspected that some of the nerve damage was due to the uraemia. This has now been more than adequately confirmed with the advent of renal dialysis, and in the early days of dialysis serial nerve conduction studies were used as one of the indicators as to its efficacy. A generalized mild painful sensorimotor neuropathy is the usual picture.

Neuropathy Associated With Malignant Disease

Neuropathy associated with malignant conditions is accorded much greater importance in most discussions than is justified by its rarity. Neuropathy due to chemotherapy is more prevalent. The main interest lies in the widely different mechanisms of damage, involving all the potential ways in which peripheral nerves can be damaged.

Carcinoma-Associated Neuropathy

A progressive mild generalized sensory neuropathy with minor motor features should raise the possibility of an underlying disease if diabetes and alcohol have been excluded as possible causes.

The more classic neuropathy is a pure peripheral sensory neuropathy which is pathologically due to damage to the dorsal root ganglion cells. Painful paraesthesiae and ataxia due to severe posture loss are the prominent features. It is rapidly disabling and then stabilizes. It is most often found in female patients.

Both types of neuropathy are associated with oat-cell carcinoma of the lung. Other underlying carcinomas are extremely rare, with the exception of carcinoma of the ovary. There is a problem of differential diagnosis when cisplatin is used in therapy for this condition and a neuropathy develops.

Lymphoma-Associated Neuropathy

Lymphomas may cause sensorimotor neuropathy with the important additional feature that the neuropathy is more likely to improve with effective treatment of the underlying disease than is carcinoma-associated neuropathy. Unfortunately, the use of vinca alkaloids may cause a neuropathy which recovers very slowly, but only if the agent can be withdrawn without jeopardizing the patient's survival.

Myelomatosis

In addition to the major neurological complication of multiple myeloma, which is spinal cord compression due to extradural deposits, there are a variety of ways in which the peripheral nerves may be damaged. Myeloma protein may be deposited particularly in the carpal tunnel. Secondary amyloid deposition may damage the peripheral nerves and abnormal immunoglobulins may produce an immune-based peripheral neuropathy. All three types may associated with severe pain.

In some cases an axonal neuropathy which is thought not to be due to any of the above mechanisms produces a much more insidious neuropathy. The immune-based demyelinating type causes a mainly motor neuropathy. Successful treatment of the underlying myeloma may permit some improvement.

Neuropathy due to Other Paraproteinaemias

All disorders that produce abnormal immune proteins may affect the peripheral nerves. The benign monoclonal IgG or IgM gammopathies, which may be precursors of malignant plasma-cell dyscrasia, may present as a sensorimotor neuropathy. Waldenstrom's macroglobulinaemia may cause either a low-grade sensorimotor neuropathy or present as an acute

Guillain–Barré-like syndrome. Cryoglobulins usually cause peripheral vascular difficulties, which may lead to acute mononeuritis multiplex but can also cause a low-grade sensorimotor neuropathy.

From the above it is clear that in any patient with a sensorimotor neuropathy and no obvious cause, careful exclusion of a lung tumour, breast carcinoma or ovarian cancer is fully justified. Serum protein electrophoresis will usually identify the dysproteinaemic disorders. More extensive searches for underlying carcinoma are usually unrewarding and harder to justify. Repeat screening 6-month intervals for the common underlying conditions is justified because occasionally the neuropathy can antedate clinical evidence of the tumour by several years.

CASE REPORT XIV

A 62-year-old retired bank messenger gave a 1-year history of severe lower back pain and numbness extending from the back to involve the entire right leg and the anterior aspect of the left leg. Two months before admission he had developed paraesthesiae with weakness in the left hand, and 5 weeks later in the right hand. He had lost 8 lb in weight. On admission there was weakness and wasting of the intrinsic hand muscles, more marked on the right than the left. Both quadriceps were wasted and weak. There was minimal distal weakness. Both ankle jerks were absent. All arm reflexes except the right triceps jerk were present. There was a glove-and-stocking sensory loss and a band of loss of pinprick sensation on the trunk between T7 and T10. A myelogram was normal but the post-myelogram CT scan suggested lower dorsal cord expansion; an MRI scan was negative. The CSF was normal and EMG and nerve conduction studies were consistent with a peripheral neuropathy with minimal slowing, suggesting an axonal basis. A second opinion was obtained and the diagnosis of neuropathy of unusual distribution was confirmed; further extensive general investigations were normal. The patient remained in very severe pain. Two months later, after a further 8 lb weight loss and increasing weakness and peripheral numbness, he was readmitted for review. There was severe weakness of all limbs and generalized loss of vibration and joint position sense. He was unable to stand without support. All investigations were again normal, including bronchoscopy. Four months later he had increasingly severe painful paraesthesiae and was by now barely able to walk with support. There was no further weight loss. Further progression of both weakness and sensory findings was confirmed and the liver edge was palpable. Complete rescreening was performed and was again completely normal. Five months later he was admitted after collapsing with dehydration and weakness. There was no further neurological change but the serum sodium was 114 mmol/l. He was treated with intravenous hydrocortisone and further biochemical investigations confirmed Addison's disease and inappropriate ADH secretion. He was treated with hydrocortisone and carbamazepine and continued on high doses of morphine to control the painful paraesthesiae. One month later he developed a scaly skin eruption thought to be carcinoma related, and some small lumps within the skin under the right arm. Biopsy confirmed metastatic oat-cell carcinoma. The chest X-ray was still normal but 3 weeks later he suddenly became jaundiced and a few days later died, 30 months after the onset of his symptoms.

In this case a very atypical onset at first more suggestive of cord disease was quickly shown to be a painful axonal neuropathy, two features strongly indicative of underlying carcinoma. In spite of repeated investigations and conviction that an oat-cell carcinoma was the likely cause, which was apparently confirmed when he developed the SIADH syndrome, it was not until weeks before his death, 2 years after the onset of his neuropathy, that the diagnosis was confirmed, and then only because of cutaneous metastasis. It is doubtful whether early discovery of the lesion would have made any difference, and to some extent this case confirms that such searches are often futile.

Electromyography and Nerve Conduction Studies

The study of the electrical activity of resting and contracting skeletal muscle and conduction of the nerve impulse has become one of the most useful diagnostic tools in neurology. At experimental level the technique has been responsible for a complete reappraisal of neuromuscular diseases, and clinically EMG studies may completely alter the diagnosis and prevent a serious diagnostic error. EMG and nerve conduction studies have become indispensable in the diagnosis and management of peripheral nerve and muscle disease. It is really only possible to learn these techniques by practical experience, but it is worth understanding the terms used descriptively in EMG reporting and these are described below. The general principles of nerve conduction studies are described and their application to specific situations is shown Figures 19.6 and 19.7.

Electromyography

Electromyography is carried out by the insertion of a twin-core needle electrode into the muscle. The electrical potentials in the muscle are observed on an oscilloscope during insertion of the needle, with the muscle at rest and during full muscle contraction. The muscle to be sampled is selected depending on the clinical diagnosis. A mildly affected muscle is preferred to a severely affected muscle as in the latter case there may be so few surviving muscle fibres that the EMG findings are confusing (Fig. 19.5).

Denervation (Fig. 19.5a)

If the nerve supply to a muscle is damaged by disease of the ventral horn cell, nerve root or peripheral nerve the muscle is 'denervated' and the EMG findings are known as 'chronic partial denervation'. Each ventral horn cell

and its axon supplies a group of muscle fibres, the whole being known as a 'motor unit'. This means that if a ventral horn cell or its neuron is damaged a discrete and limited group of muscle fibres ceases to function. It has been shown that surviving neurons are capable of branching and taking over adjacent denervated muscle fibres, enlarging the size of the surviving units. These basic changes lead to the following EMG findings in a denervated muscle. Denervated muscle fibres are very irritable and show spontaneous electrical activity. On needle insertion the normal brief injury potentials are greatly prolonged (increased insertional activity) and occasionally continue in a burst of decreasing frequency and amplitude (a pseudomyotonic run).

With the needle held still in the resting muscle transient alterations in the muscle membrane potential of 50–200 μV size and of extremely brief duration occur. These are fibrillation potentials. They may occasionally be of longer duration and monophasic, and are then known as a positive sharp wave. Contractions of entire motor units produce fasciculation potentials. These are the contractions visible to the naked eye and sometimes incorrectly referred to clinically as 'fibrillation'. They are not necessarily pathological.

When the resting activity has been observed the patient is asked to contract the muscle gently while the examiner steadies the needle. Individual units are studied. The normal motor unit produces a bi- or triphasic potential of up to 2 mV size in a proximal muscle and 5 mV in the small hand or foot muscles. When a unit has been enlarged by the branching of its nerve fibre to incorporate adjacent muscle fibres two things happen: the duration of contraction of the unit is increased, producing a polyphasic potential, and the amplitude of the units is greatly increased, often reaching 5–10 mV in foot muscles and up to 15 mV in the small hand muscles. These are known as giant units.

The patient then contracts the muscle as hard as possible against resistance. In a normal muscle the activity is continuous, as units contract and rest as others take over. The baseline sweep is completely obliterated. This is known as the interference pattern. In a denervated muscle gaps appear in the pattern, marking the former position of a damaged unit in the sequence and the surviving units are typically large and polyphasic. From their identical appearance it is often clear that it is the same giant unit repeating at regular intervals. This is known as a reduction in the interference pattern. These findings may be patchy, and in some diseases the fastest-conducting fibres seem to be affected first, so that the most striking findings of denervation are in the periphery of the muscle. This is a particular feature of motor neuron disease. It must be stressed that these findings only indicate damage to the nerve fibres or ventral horn cell; the level at which the damage has occurred must be deduced from the clinical features and nerve conduction studies. Chronic partial

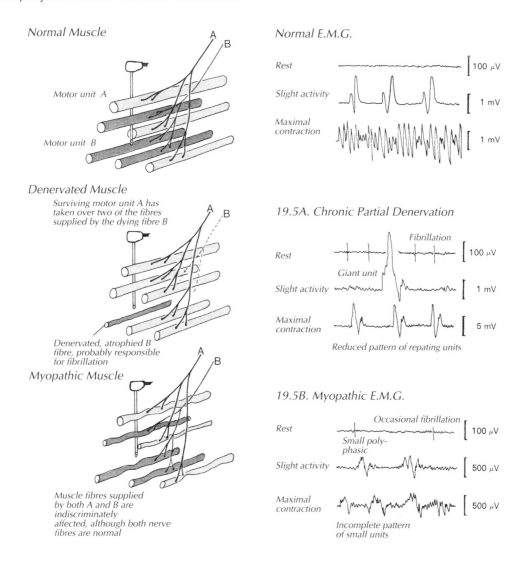

19.5 EMG appearances.

denervation does not automatically indicate ventral horn cell disease.

Myopathic Changes (Fig. 19.5b)

In muscle disease the situation is quite different. The disease process affects all or some muscle fibres in an entirely random way without regard to motor units. The only exception to this is in polymyositis, in which the changes may be extremely patchy and full-depth sampling in several areas of a muscle may be necessary before an area of typical damage is detected. Furthermore, the damaged muscle fibres in polymyositis may be very irritable and if the region of the nerve end-plate is affected changes similar to denervation may be found.

The following features are typically found in muscle disease:

1. Damaged muscle fibres, particularly in inflammatory myopathies such as polymyositis and in Pompe's disease (see Chapter 17), in which glycogen storage disease affects both the muscle fibre and the ventral horn cell, may be irritable and demonstrate fibrillation, which may lead to an incorrect diagnosis of denervation.

2. As the process is often patchy in individual fibres there is delayed or blocked conduction along the fibre, both dispersing the unit and reducing its size. The end result is a small – 200–500 μV – polyphasic action potential. The interference pattern is usually full as part of all units survive, but the small polyphasic potentials produce a very characteristic 'crackling' noise on the EMG amplifier, rather like rustling greaseproof paper.

3. In muscle disease associated with myotonia, the prolonged discharges that produce the typical stiffness of the muscles are audible as decrementing bursts of potentials that were formerly likened to 'dive-bomber' noises, but a more accurate contemporary description would be the sound of a highly tuned motorcycle engine. The bursts often superimpose on one another, quite unlike the

single pseudomyotonic burst provoked by needle movement in irritable, partially denervated muscles.

4. EMG techniques have a limited place in the diagnosis of myasthenia gravis as the muscles typically affected are often inaccessible to EMG techniques. If a suitable muscle can be found, a burst of stimuli at 20 Hz may produce a clearly decrementing response in myasthenia gravis or an incrementing response in Lambert–Eaton syndrome. This technique is quite painful for the patient but can produce unequivocally diagnostic results.

Nerve Conduction Studies

The basic requirements for motor nerve conduction studies are that a suitable muscle is available and that its nerve supply can be stimulated at two points along its course. The time taken from the stimulus nearest the muscle is known as the distal latency and includes not only the time taken for the impulse to travel down the nerve but also the delay at the end-plate and initiation of contraction. If the nerve is then stimulated higher up a second latency can be obtained, the difference in the time taken being an accurate measurement of the time taken for the impulse to traverse a measured length of nerve. From this the conduction velocity in metres per second is easily calculated. Very carefully documented velocity ranges for all the nerves that can be studied in this way have been reported. Most commonly these are the median and ulnar nerves in the arm and the peroneal and tibial nerves in the leg. Nerves such as the radial and femoral can only be readily stimulated at one point, and a latency to an appropriate muscle is all that can be measured.

In general, if a muscle is denervated and it can be shown that the lesion responsible is above the proximal stimulus, it is probably affecting the nerve root or ventral horn cell. The positions of electrodes and velocities for the standard conduction studies in the arm and legs are shown in Figures 19.6 and 19.7.

Nerve action potentials can be measured in two ways, orthodromically or antidromically. Here the main requirement is a nerve near enough to the surface to be picked up by a surface electrode or anatomically constant in position, allowing needle electrodes to be inserted adjacent to it. Both the median and ulnar nerve action potentials can be detected at the wrist by stimulating the interdigital nerves of the appropriate fingers. Nerve action potentials in the leg present more of a problem. The techniques are shown in the figures.

In the case of ulnar nerve lesions at the elbow or peroneal nerve lesions at the fibula neck due to compression some patients may not demonstrate slowed conduction through the damaged area. A very useful ancillary test is to study the quantitative muscle action potentials. Using maximal shocks the full muscle potential produced from stimulation at the wrist or ankle is measured. The nerve is then stimulated just below the elbow or fibula neck as appropriate. A slight reduction on potential size of some 10% is normal. The nerve is then stimulated above the elbow or in the popliteal fossa, respectively. A dramatic drop in the potential is often seen and a reduction of 40% or greater in potential size in this second stimulation position is diagnostic of nerve damage below the upper stimulus, even though the velocity in the surviving fibres may be normal. Usually a combination of slowing and reduced fibres is found. Using this technique the actual point of damage may be detected at a position where the nerve is almost inexcitable. This technique is known as 'inching' as the stimulus is moved only slightly up or down the nerve.

More Advanced Techniques

In recent years improvements in electrophysiological apparatus, particularly digital averaging, have greatly extended the scope of nerve conduction studies. Very small action potentials in almost any cutaneous nerve can now be detected above background activity, using antidromic or orthodromic excitation and standardised variations for size of potential and latency have been established for most peripheral nerves.

There are few situations however, where such information is critical to clinical diagnosis. In the motor field one of the major disadvantages was the inability to study conduction in the proximal part of the nerve.

In the upper arm conduction velocities can be obtained by stimulating in the axilla or the supraclavicular fossa over Erb's point, although the depth of the nervous structures at these levels requires rather painful shocks. Useful information, particularly in suspected cervical outlet syndromes or brachial plexus leisons can be obtained using these techniques. Clearly this is more readily applicable to damage in the upper roots of the brachial plexus. The lower cervical roots often implicated in these pathological processes are harder to stimulate. Techniques were developed using nerve stimulating electrodes inserted close to individual nerve roots adjacent to the spinal column.

The use of needle recording electrodes enables evoked potentials in deeper nervous structures to be studied and surface electrodes over the nape of the neck and head, extend this information further centrally as somatosensory evoked potentials (SSEPs).

All these techniques require considerable technical skill and are not generally available. At a simpler level, some information can be gained by studying the F wave response when performing simple peripheral nerve conduction studies. This makes use of the fact that when the nerve being studied is stimulated distally, the immediate contraction of the muscle is followed some 30 seconds later by a second, much smaller contraction of the muscle. The impulse also passes

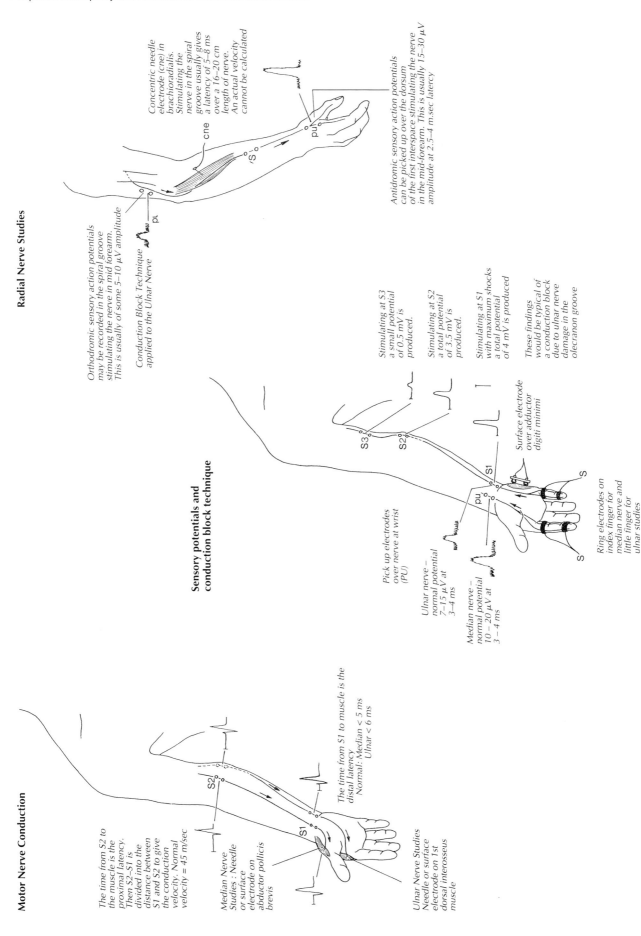

Radial Nerve Studies

Concentric needle electrode (cne) in brachioradialis. Stimulating the nerve in the spiral groove usually gives a latency of 5–8 ms over a 16–20 cm length of nerve. An actual velocity cannot be calculated

cne

Orthodromic sensory action potentials may be recorded in the spiral groove stimulating the nerve in mid forearm. This is usually of some 5–10 μV amplitude

Conduction Block Technique applied to the Ulnar Nerve

Antidromic sensory action potentials can be picked up over the dorsum of the first interspace stimulating the nerve in the mid-forearm. This is usually 15–30 μV amplitude at 2.5–4 m.sec latency

Sensory potentials and conduction block technique

Stimulating at S3 a small potential of 0.5 mV is produced.

Stimulating at S2 a total potential of 3.5 mV is produced.

Stimulating at S1 with maximum shocks a total potential of 4 mV is produced

These findings would be typical of a conduction block due to ulnar nerve damage in the olecranon groove

Surface electrode over adductor digiti minimi

Pick up electrodes over nerve at wrist (PU)

Ulnar nerve – normal potential 7–15 μV at 3–4 ms

Median nerve – normal potential 10 – 20 μV at 3 – 4 ms

Ring electrodes on index finger for median nerve and little finger for ulnar studies

Motor Nerve Conduction

The time from S2 to the muscle is the proximal latency. Then S2–S1 is divided into the distance between S1 and S2 to give the conduction velocity. Normal velocity = 45 m/sec

Median Nerve Studies : Needle or surface electrode on abductor pollicis brevis

The time from S1 to muscle is the distal latency. Normal: Median < 5 ms Ulnar < 6 ms

Ulnar Nerve Studies Needle or surface electrode on 1st dorsal interosseus muscle

19.6 Nerve conduction studies in the arm.

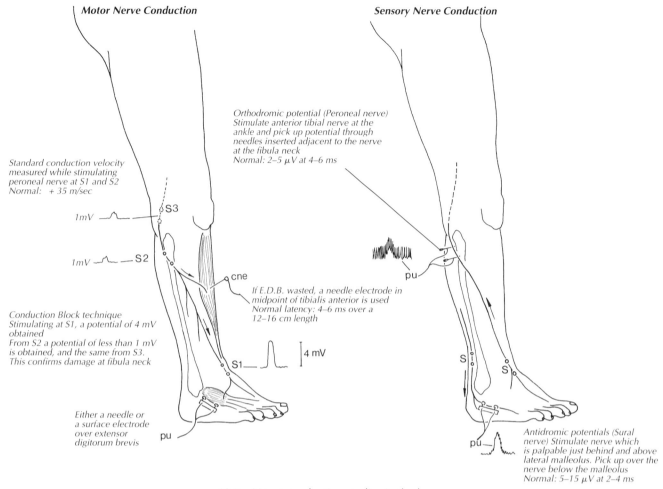

Motor Nerve Conduction

Standard conduction velocity measured while stimulating peroneal nerve at S1 and S2 Normal: + 35 m/sec

1mV S3

1mV S2

Conduction Block technique Stimulating at S1, a potential of 4 mV obtained From S2 a potential of less than 1 mV is obtained, and the same from S3. This confirms damage at fibula neck

Either a needle or a surface electrode over extensor digitorum brevis pu

Sensory Nerve Conduction

Orthodromic potential (Peroneal nerve) Stimulate anterior tibial nerve at the ankle and pick up potential through needles inserted adjacent to the nerve at the fibula neck Normal: 2–5 μV at 4–6 ms

cne

If E.D.B. wasted, a needle electrode in midpoint of tibialis anterior is used Normal latency: 4–6 ms over a 12–16 cm length

S1   4 mV

pu

S   S

pu *Antidromic potentials (Sural nerve) Stimulate nerve which is palpable just behind and above lateral malleolus. Pick up over the nerve below the malleolus Normal: 5–15 μV at 2–4 ms*

19.7   Nerve conduction studies in the leg.

antidromically up to the ventral horn cells and causes a second discharge back down the nerve. An increased latency between the normal muscle response (M wave) and the delayed response (F wave) indicates proximal damage to the nerve or nerve root.

These techniques were established to try to enhance the clinical information in the days when the main imaging modalities for spinal cord, spinal canal and radicular lesions were myelography or radiculography, with all their imperfections. The advent of MRI scanning has to some extent made many of these techiques obsolete, as a confident clinical diagnosis can usually be readily confirmed by MRI scanning without resorting to these technically complex techniques which can also be difficult to interpret.

Similarly, the use of electromyography in the paravertebral musculature, to try to demonstrate denervation in territories supplied by individual cervical or lumbar nerve roots has lost much of its limited value,

now that the underlying lesion can be so readily demonstrated anatomically.

Single fibre electromyography (SFEMG) is another very specialised technique which can study electrical activity in single muscle fibres. The phenomenon known as 'jitter' is a variation in the voltage and firing rate of the individual fibres at rest and this is modified in many peripheral nerve conditions but has particular value in the early diagnosis of myasthenia gravis. Considerable experience and skill is needed in interpreting these findings.

There is no standard examination for any patient referred for EMG and nerve conduction studies. The clinical problem is considered and a combination of muscle sampling and nerve studies is performed appropriate to the situation. All neurologists should have a detailed working knowledge of electrophysiological techniques and their interpretation.

20. Headache

Headache is the most common symptom in medicine and may account for up to 40% of all consultations. At a conservative estimate 10% of the population suffers from migraine, the commonest cause of severe recurrent headache.

Many texts contain long classifications of multiple causes of headache that seem to indicate that the differential diagnosis of headache is a mere formality. With the exception of all but the most classic cases of migraine, this implication is certainly unjustified. The degree of overlap between both the aetiological factors and some of the features of the headache may make differential diagnosis extremely difficult. For example, most patients with headache who are referred as 'diagnostic problems' are suffering from migraine headaches, the diagnostic difficulty usually having arisen because the headache was not frontal, strictly unilateral or throbbing in nature. All these features are obligatory for a diagnosis of classic migraine, but none of them need to be present for a diagnosis of migraine headache to be made.

When aetiological factors are considered, a major problem is the role played by tension in an individual case. Just because the patient is tense it does not automatically follow that they have tension headache. Migraine is often precipitated by tension, and any patient who has had a series of bad migraine headaches soon becomes tense. Failure to appreciate the cardinal importance of the nature and particularly the patterning of the headache may lead to prolonged ineffectual therapy with tranquillizers and sedatives, and deny the patient possible symptomatic relief.

There are considerable similarities in the diagnostic approach and aetiological factors in patients with headache and face pain, and it is advisable to read this and the subsequent chapter in sequence.

General Considerations Concerning Headaches

There is a widely held misconception, not confined to the general public, that the most common causes of headache are eye strain and sinus disease and that all bad headaches are due to brain tumours. Very few patients are referred who have not already had their eyes tested and many have also had their sinuses X-rayed, and even had multiple ineffectual ENT procedures.

Refractive errors may cause pain in and around the eye when the eyes are used for unusually long periods or in poor light. Refractive errors cannot cause intermittent severe headache which is not linked to the use of the eyes for close work or reading, and it is clearly absurd to attribute headaches, present on waking in the morning, to eye strain. Considerable delays are caused by referral to opticians, as it takes some time for the patient to obtain new glasses and discover that they do not relieve the headache.

Many patients complain of lifelong 'sinus headache' often abbreviated to the more colloquial 'sinus'. Close questioning usually reveals a typical history of migraine. Sinus disease causes pain in the affected sinus which may be referred to other areas of the face and head, but the underlying pain in the affected sinus is identifiable. The suggestion that chronic subclinical sinus infection can cause recurrent severe headaches over decades is no longer acceptable. The absence of nasal blocking or nasal discharge should exclude sinusitis, but unilateral nasal discharge and blocking may be a feature of neuralgic migraine. In these cases the blockage and discharge stop immediately the headache stops and as attacks only last 1–2 hours there should be no diagnostic difficulty in excluding sinusitis as the cause.

The term 'ordinary headaches' is often used by patients and this term seems to mean that the headaches have been sufficiently infrequent, so short-lived or responsive to simple analgesics that the patient has not previously sought advice. It is essential to try to establish the exact nature of any such previous headaches and not to accept the patient's own diagnosis or allow them to dismiss them as 'normal'. Patients with recent-onset severe headaches become quite cross when they are extensively questioned as to the nature of previous headaches, and yet in many instances this is the single most important part of the history. The patient feels that such questioning is unnecessarily delaying the brain scan that they and all their friends know is immediately required because the headache is so bad.

The possibility that a headache is due to something serious does not increase in proportion to the severity of the headache. In fact, the most severe recurrent headaches are usually due to migraine. Patients who are harbouring cerebral tumours may complain of a 'dull' or 'muzzy' headache, only on direct questioning. It is rarely the headache itself that prompts the patient to seek medical advice.

In the past X-rays of the skull were demanded by patients but rarely gave useful information. Now patients demand a brain scan, which is certainly capable of giving more helpful information, but with the likelihood that there is only a 1:2000 chance of a headache being due to a cause demonstrable by a brain scan it is clearly not appropriate to accede to the patient's wish in every instance. Surprisingly often, the reason advanced by the patient for demanding a scan is that the headaches have been so bad **for so long**, a situation that has already virtually excluded the possibility of a sinister cause. Unfortunately, the increasing availability of CT scanning has led to the absurd diagnostic label of 'scan-negative headache', a diagnosis that rarely seems to cure the headache, reassure the patient, or immediately indicate an effective method of treatment.

The most important investigation in the evaluation of headache is the history.

Migraine Headache

In the introductory paragraphs the emphasis placed on the recognition of migraine headache will be apparent. This is because migraine or migraine variants are responsible for the headache in a majority of patients referred to hospital, and particularly those with severe headache.

The difficulty in making the diagnosis may be due to atypical features of the headache, which is not unusual. However, it is often due to the uncritical acceptance of the patient's history that they have only had 'sinus' or 'ordinary' headache previously. Headache apparently starting at the age of 55 years may indicate a serious problem, but when seen in the setting of lifelong migraine (hitherto called 'sinus') the diagnosis becomes less challenging.

Attributing a causal role to tension, when the tension is secondary to the headache itself, is another problem. Although the tension component may well require appropriate therapy with suitable medication, it is unlikely that this will succeed if the underlying headache is due to migraine, as the concomitantly prescribed simple analgesics will not relieve a migraine headache. This is because in the majority of migraine

sufferers simple proprietary analgesics and even narcotics do not significantly alleviate the pain. At the very best analgesic combinations may achieve some 10%–20% relief from the headache, however administered. Genuine migraine sufferers are not impressed that sufficient aspirin, taken at the right moment, is effective.

The pattern of occurrence of migraine is of critical importance in making the diagnosis and this is not sufficiently emphasized. Many patients notice that their attacks are seasonal and that specific weather patterns are provocative; the critical role of weather has become increasingly appreciated in recent years and such weather may lead to occasional 'epidemics' of migraine. The classic thunderstorm-associated headache is perhaps the most readily appreciated example, but prolonged periods of low atmospheric pressure with high humidity in warm or cold weather seems equally provocative. The mechanism of this association is not clear.

Nearly all sufferers eventually realize that their attacks come on at the end of periods of stress, and this is seen in its simplest form in the tendency for attacks to be present on waking in the morning, especially at weekends. This may sometimes be aborted by following a normal working-day routine at weekends. The ultimate expression of these relaxation-provoked migraine attacks is found in some patients who only have headaches during their holidays! Severe serial migraine, when the patient has attacks on a daily basis, frequently follows prolonged periods of stress such as the terminal illness of a relative, a house move or a marital break-up. In such situations, if the patient's life has been in a turmoil they seem even more likely to develop a firm conviction that they now have a fatal brain tumour, which can be extremely hard to dispel, and this is probably the most difficult group of patients to manage.

In female patients the relationship to periods, pregnancy and the menopause have been appreciated for centuries, but again the mechanism defies explanation. Young girls will often have cyclical headache in the 2 years prior to the onset of periods, and once the periods begin will notice a tendency to develop the headache in the few days before and on the first day of the period. In the late teens attempts to take the contraceptive pill may lead to uncontrolled headaches whatever the type and however low the dose of the pill. In the majority of patients pregnancy produces a dramatic improvement in migraine and many female migraineurs cite their pregnancies as the most headache-free time of their life. Unfortunately, they typically suffer a very severe migraine 6–12 weeks following delivery, and the previous pattern of headaches then resumes.

At the menopause migraine often becomes less predictable, as do the periods, and quite often assumes more neuralgic quality where the pain becomes localized in the eye or face, and the patient is often fearful that this is a sinister new development. The use of hormone replacement therapy, if anything, appears to make this situation worse, especially if there is a previous history of severe headaches when the patient attempted to take the contraceptive pill.

There is also a group of female patients who develop migraine for the first time at the menopause. Unfortunately these patients tend to continue having migraine for the rest of their lives, whereas those who have had migraine since their menarche often notice a considerable reduction in the severity and frequency of attacks after the menopause.

There are several other factors that may operate in the provocation of migraine that are less generally applicable than those discussed above.

1. It is not uncommon for migraine to follow relatively trivial blows to the head, and in some men heading footballs may provoke migraine sufficiently predictably to prevent continued participation in the sport. In children such post-traumatic vascular headaches are a source of great anxiety to parents, who regard headache following head trauma as obviously indicative of a major intracerebral catastrophe, however trivial the injury. It is a source of surprise to neurologists involved in medicolegal work that following really serious head trauma headache is an unusual symptom, but is such a major problem following minor blows to the head.

2. Migraine sufferers often note that intercurrent infections, particularly upper respiratory tract infections with fever, will produce a very severe headache indistinguishable from their usual migraine. If there is no known history of migraine a patient who is febrile, with photophobia, nausea, severe headache and occasionally even a stiff neck, presents a clinical picture mimicking meningitis or a subarachnoid haemorrhage. A majority of patients referred to hospital as possible meningitis cases fall into this group, with a negative CFS examination and an unfortunate tendency to develop particularly severe post-lumbar puncture headache, which often keeps them in hospital for several days longer than the presenting illness would have justified.

3. Bright light and noise are well recognized as being unpleasant during an episode but are less well known as provocative agents in their own right. Many sufferers will report that driving into a setting sun, winter sunlight through trees and sun reflected off a wet road after a summer shower, will actually provoke a headache. Very loud noise may have a similar effect, and older patients often recollect having migraine following visits to the cinema when they were children, after the noise and flickering light of the film itself and coming out into the bright light. Other patients may cite sunlight reflected off snow while skiing, or looking out of the cabin windows in aeroplanes, having a similar effect.

4. The role of dietary factors in migraine has gradually become relegated to a very minor position in the provocation of migraine, although enjoying continuing popularity in women's magazines. At one time the concept held such sway that patients announced that their headaches could not be due to migraine because they had stopped eating chocolate, cheese and oranges and the headaches were still occurring. The data that at first sight provide some support for the concept is probably derived from the association of hunger with migraine.

Many patients know that one certain way to provoke an attack is to allow themselves to become very hungry. Others relate that one of their warning symptoms of a pending migraine is sudden ravenous hunger, often for very sweet foods. Under both these circumstances the patient is likely to eat a readily available food: if they are away from home a bar of chocolate will suffice, and if at home cheese is probably the most readily available food in the refrigerator. Nearly all patients comment that they are surprised how often they can eat the foods they have been told will cause migraine, **without** having an attack, even those who are convinced that their attacks **are** due to such foods.

Perhaps the best example of the variability of vulnerability to an attack is seen with alcohol. Migraine sufferers find that they can drink wine or spirits of any variety on many occasions without trouble, and at other times a minute quantity will provoke an instant migraine. This is not the way an 'allergy' to any other substances in any other condition behaves. It is clearly sensible, if the patient has any clear evidence that anything they do or eat provokes attacks, that they should avoid them if possible, but what is not acceptable is that blanket restrictions on foodstuffs should be recommended on the basis of a discredited theory.

Site of the Headache

Classic migraine is frontotemporal in site and is unilateral. There should be little difficulty in suspecting the diagnosis when the headache is located in that area (Fig. 20.1).

The location shown in Fig. 20.2 causes more difficulty. Such stress is laid on tension in the neck muscles as being responsible for tension headache that it is assumed that any occipital headache is bound to be due to tension. Many cases of otherwise typical migraine start in the occipital area and radiate forward to the 'classic' frontotemporal site. Patients will often comment that headaches showing this pattern of onset occur when they have been under a lot of stress, and

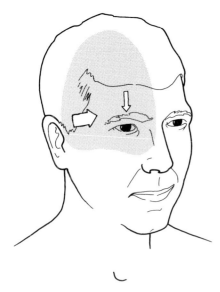

The headache starts in the temple on one side and spreads to involve the whole side of the head. It is a pulsatile headache and any or all of the common migraine concomitants may occur. It usually remains strictly unilateral but may occur on either side on subsequent occasions. Usually self-limiting, lasting from 30 minutes to several hours

20.1 Classical migraine (hemicrania).

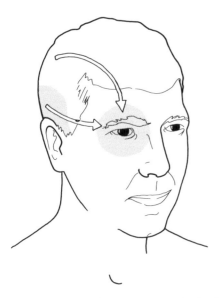

This is the type of headache most often requiring hospital referral. The onset is less dramatic, often a dull ache in the occipital area, which extends forwards around the temple or deep into the area behind the eye. A dull bursting ache behind the eye is an important diagnostic clue. The pain may also be bilateral in this type, although the pain on one side is usually worse than the other. Other migraine concomitants may not be present and the headache may last several days, usually regenerating overnight on each successive day

20.2 Occipital–orbital migraine.

indeed as a direct response to stress, rather than the overnight delayed response which is more typical. The pain starts suboccipitally and radiates forward into the temple or deep behind the eye. It is often bilateral, although one side is usually more severely affected than the other.

The third variety (Fig. 20.3) is the one most often attributed to sinus disease. The pain is essentially

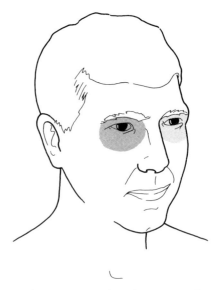

This is a variant of migrainous neuralgia. The pain is predominantly a deep nagging ache behind one or both eyes with occasional stabs of pain 'like a needle in the back of the eye'. Photophobia is common and bright light or sudden movement provokes the pain. This variety is seen as a common variant of the vascular headache produced by oral contraceptives and HRT

20.3 Orbital migraine

confined to a position deep behind the eye. It may be bilateral and particularly aggravated by bright light. It is more or less continual over days or weeks, with periodic exacerbations, and is usually referred to as migrainous neuralgia. It often occurs in patients who have a previous history of isolated attacks of migraine and its unusual ongoing nature is the main reason for referral. It is more common in females, unlike cluster headache, which is almost confined to males. This pattern of headache seems particularly likely to be provoked by the contraceptive pill or hormone replacement therapy.

Type of Pain

Although throbbing is always emphasized as a typical feature of migraine, the headache does not have to be of this character for the diagnosis to be entertained. Even with pain in the classic location, throbbing may only occur as the headache develops, the eventual pain being more or less constant. At the height of the headache throbbing can usually be provoked by sudden movement, such as sitting up in bed, suddenly standing or particularly bending over or running upstairs.

In the locations other than frontal, described above, it is unusual for throbbing to be a prominent feature. The deep bursting or pressing pain in the eye or back of the orbit must be emphasized, as not only is it the main diagnostic feature in these cases but it also often provides the diagnostic clue in the facial migraine syndromes to be discussed in the next chapter. Intense prickling sensations, likened by patients to a bunch of stinging nettles, may intrude into this severe orbital pain. Occasionally the patient may experience a sensation like a red-hot dagger through the eye, which is virtually diagnostic of migraine. These dagger-like sensations may occur in any other part of the head, particularly the orbit and ear, and often shoot diagonally through the head and are so sudden and vicious that they frighten the patient more than almost any other feature of the migraine syndrome. Other sensations of similar sort may be described, such as the eye 'smarting' or as if 'a little bunch of red-hot needles' were being jabbed into the back of the orbit.

It is not uncommon for the head to become extremely tender in the area of maximum headache and an incorrect diagnosis of cranial arteritis may be entertained, even in 20-year-old patients! Even when the headache has subsided, the whole area may feel bruised and tender for several days.

Associated Symptoms

In descriptions of classic migraine great emphasis is always placed on dramatic prodromal symptoms such as fortification spectra. These are said to resemble the plan view of castle battlements. More often the patient describes zig-zag lines or little incomplete jagged circles, like a letter C back to front when drawn by the patient. These phenomena are particularly typical when only one eye is affected. When both eyes are affected the visual phenomena are usually hemianopic and are described as the vision to one side becoming 'watery'; this appearance slowly extends across to the midline, by which time only half a face or a clock is seen. These visual phenomena usually precede the headache: they typically evolve slowly over 5–10 minutes and clear quickly at about 20–30 minutes as the headache develops. They are not a universal feature of migraine and many patients with migraine have never experienced any of them, although most have experienced photophobia and slight blurring of vision.

The majority of patients feel extremely nauseated during an attack but severe vomiting is relatively unusual. Indeed, it is a useful rule that if vomiting is a new feature of the attacks the possibility of more serious disease should be seriously considered. If there is no previous history of migraine the recent onset of headache associated with vomiting should always be regarded as due to a posterior fossa tumour until proved otherwise. More dramatic neurological accompaniments of migraine are discussed below in the section on vasospastic migraine.

Mood changes before, during and after migraine are frequently under-recognized, and may sometimes provide an important clue to a pending episode or a pointer to the correct diagnosis. Many patients feel irritable, edgy and incompetent in the 24 hours prior to a

migraine, and may find that they are making mistakes in their normal day-to-day activities. Sometimes these symptoms will not culminate in a headache, and this state has been graphically described by one patient as her 'slug' day. Others find that these symptoms occur during the headache and persist for several days afterwards.

A more enjoyable mood change may be accurately described as a 'super day'. The patient feels exhilarated, full of energy and 'on a high'. They may also be remarkably productive and efficient at this time: housewives will often spring-clean the entire house in one day and when they collapse with the headache the next day are accused of 'bringing it on themselves', and even the patient sometimes fails to recognize that this mood change is part of a migraine that has already started and that the subsequent headache is inevitable unless specific measures are taken. This is easier to suggest than implement, as patients feel so well that the last thing on their mind is that they might get a headache, until it happens – usually on wakening the next day!

Other Important Migraine Variants

Childhood Migraine

Migraine in childhood is perhaps best characterized as short, sharp and vicious. The onset is usually very sudden and often characterized by pallor, nausea and vomiting, with occasional complaints of blurred vision. In some instances giddiness with true vertigo may dominate the picture, and in others the abdominal pain may be so severe and the complaint of headache so mild that intra-abdominal conditions such as appendicitis are suspected. This so-called 'abdominal migraine' can be very dramatic in childhood. It is unusual for headache to become the main symptom until the child is about 10 years of age.

Occasionally, exceptional 5-year-olds are able to give remarkably accurate descriptions of their attacks, if allowed to do so by their parents. One little boy called his attacks 'headaches with colours'; others call them 'giddy heads' or 'a pain above the eye'. The parents' description of a pale, listless and sleepy child leaves little doubt as to the diagnosis.

As in the adult attacks may be precipitated by exertion, and some athletically inclined children fond of games and physical education find these classes ruined by the onset of their attacks. Unlike adults, however, the attacks may be extremely brief, often as short as 15–20 minutes, with sudden and complete recovery. In the early teens the variant that has been called 'basilar migraine' occurs in which attacks of brainstem ischaemia dominate the picture.

CASE REPORT I

A 13-year-old boy was referred because of five episodes of teichopsia (flashing lights) followed by hemianopia and tetraplegia, each episode lasting nearly 30 minutes. All had occurred over the previous 2 years and all had been followed by a typical migraine headache. Between attacks typical migraine had occurred without the ischaemic symptoms.

Where there is a positive family history of migraine the affected parent will often suspect the correct diagnosis, but when such attacks occur for the first time in a family considerable parental alarm and often extensive overinvestigation follows. The typical time relationships and the full recovery of the child, usually after a brief sleep, should indicate the correct diagnosis.

Vasospastic Migraine

This all-embracing term has been used in preference to 'hemiplegic migraine', which is a very inaccurate name for the condition. Actual paralysis is rare and involvement of the entire side uncommon. The term 'vasospastic migraine' may be criticized on the grounds that there is still controversy as to whether the neurological accompaniments are due to vascular spasm or to a primary disturbance of cortical function. That the clinical phenomena occur in clearly identifiable vascular territories, and in rare cases infarction occurs in the affected area, seems very persuasive in support of a vascular aetiology but it is important to draw attention to the controversy. As a strongly supportive example the following case may be cited.

CASE REPORT II

A 56-year-old woman was admitted with a left hemiplegia and complete left hemianopia. Since her early 20s she had suffered episodes several times a year, when she would develop a left-sided visual disturbance followed by left-sided numbness and weakness, lasting 30–40 minutes, and a severe headache. She usually tried to avoid the headache by going to sleep. On this occasion she had gone to bed in the early evening with an attack under way, had gone to sleep and wakened in the morning headache free but hemiplegic and hemianopic. On admission she was still conscious and talking, and said that she had always been frightened that one day she would wake up and it would not have cleared. A CT scan revealed infarction in the entire right middle cerebral artery distribution, and over 5 days she developed severe uncontrolled cerebral oedema, slipped into coma and died.

It is very difficult to draw any other conclusion than that all her attacks, including the fatal episode, were on the basis of intense vasospasm in the right middle cerebral territory. There seems to be some reluctance by doctors to make a definitive diagnosis of cere-

brovascular accident due to migraine, but this serious complication of the condition is now increasingly recognized.

The most frequent vasospastic features are the visual disturbances discussed in Chapter 3, and their presence is required for a diagnosis of classic migraine. In Chapter 5, ophthalmoplegic migraine, a transient third nerve palsy associated with severe orbital headache, was discussed. Pupillary abnormalities in migraine – either a dilated pupil or a Horner's syndrome – are described in Chapter 2.

Brainstem symptoms, nausea, vomiting and vertigo may be prodromal symptoms of a migraine or an integral part of the actual attack. In children severe brainstem symptoms during 'basilar migraine' were detailed in the previous section. In adults ischaemia in the basilar territory leading to poor perfusion in the distribution of both posterior cerebral arteries may be responsible for the syndrome of transient global amnesia. This is described in detail in Chapter 22.

The most frequent migrainous event mistaken for a transient ischaemic attack has been referred to as 'cheiro-oral' migraine, a name emphasizing that it is only the arm, face and mouth, on the same side, that are affected. Typically the patient will develop tingling in the fingers of one or other hand, and tingling in the lips and tongue on the same side. Over several minutes the tingling advances up the arm and outwards on to the face, leaving a sensation of numbness in its wake. If the right arm and face are affected and the patient is left hemisphere dominant, speech difficulties may occur. This may consist purely of 'word salading', a tendency to jumble up the correct words, or more dramatically involve frank dysphasic difficulty. The affected upper limb will feel both heavy and dead during the attack but demonstrable paralysis and objective sensory loss may be hard to detect. The standard time course is important. The whole picture evolves slowly over 5–10 minutes, persists for 15–30 minutes and subsides relatively suddenly. Headache may occur in parallel, but more often comes on after a delay of 15–30 minutes or may not appear at all, a condition known as 'migraine without a headache'. This latter situation causes much alarm and misdiagnosis, but the slow evolution and time course should make the diagnosis obvious on the history alone.

The risks of such attacks proceeding to infarction may be increased by age alone, or the use of oral contraceptives or hormone replacement therapy. There has also always been concern that the use of ergotamine in such patients may cause vasospasm and the same applies to sumatriptan, which has a similar mode of action. There are, however, no recorded instances of this occurrence, but caution in the use of these drugs in patients with vasospastic phenomena is clearly advisable.

There have been reports of cerebral damage demonstrable by scanning in patients who have had repeated identical episodes of migrainous vasospasm. The following case supports the view that such events are not always benign, and efforts to prevent attacks with vasodilator migraine prophylactic drugs such as propranolol or nifedipine are justified.

CASE REPORT III

A 32-year-old woman presented in 1974 with repeated episodes of right-sided numbness, weakness and speech disturbance over the previous 10 years. The episodes behaved entirely typically of migraine, although the accompanying headaches had been modest and atypical. Extensive haematological, biochemical and cardiological investigations were normal, as was cerebral angiography. In spite of the use of propranolol the attacks continued, culminating in a fatal cerebral vascular accident at the age of 35 years. At post mortem there was evidence of multiple areas of infarction of differing ages throughout the left hemisphere, but no evidence of underlying vascular disease and no source of emboli could be identified. Repeated attacks of migrainous vasospasm remains the likely diagnosis.

Migraine is often seen as a socially convenient disorder. The above discussion and case reports may redress the balance and increase the seriousness with which this very disabling and sometimes lethal disorder is regarded and treated.

Cluster Headache (Fig. 20.4)

This condition ought to be the most readily identifiable form of migraine encountered, yet it is hardly ever correctly diagnosed. The reason for this is almost certainly that the pain is so severe that a cause as simple as migraine is rarely considered, and the patient is always suspected of having acute sinusitis, a ruptured aneurysm, a cerebral tumour or any other 'very serious' diagnosis that springs to mind. When eventually diagnosed, patients have often had annual attacks for many years and many have undergone several ENT procedures and numerous courses of antibiotics for 'sinusitis'. Because of the natural history of the condition, the last thing done has always been credited with success, until the next attack proves otherwise. The American name for this condition, 'alarm-clock headache', has more to commend it than any of the other names, such as cluster headache, Horton's cephalgia or migrainous neuralgia, which give no indication of the cardinal and virtually diagnostic feature. The condition occurs almost exclusively at night in middle-aged men and it is very unusual for there to be a previous history of migraine of other types.

The headache is of very rapid onset and starts as a prickling or tingling sensation in the orbit and nostril on one side. Within minutes, a sensation as if a red-hot

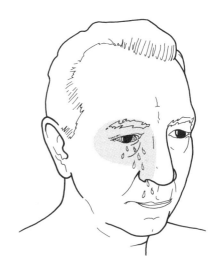

Almost exclusively a disease of middle-aged males. Usually occurs without a prior history of migraine. Attacks last 30 minutes to two hours and are mainly nocturnal. Pain is excruciating in and around the eye. Eye may become bloodshot and nose 'stuffed up'. Lacrimation and nasal watering occur. Especially likely to be provoked by alcohol. Bout lasts 6–12 weeks and may recur at the same time each year. Excellent response to methysergide and lithium

20.4   Cluster headache.

poker were being poked up the nose or acid being poured into the orbit is experienced. The pain in the eye is particularly severe and may reduce strong men to tears. The affected eye rapidly becomes bloodshot and waters, and the nose becomes congested and watery nasal discharge continues throughout the attack. The most characteristic feature is that the initial attacks are strictly nocturnal, and wake the patient from sleep. This may occur two to three times during the night, each attack lasting from 30 minutes to 2 hours. The patient will quickly realize that the attacks occur at the same times every night, with 1 a.m., 4 a.m. and 7 a.m. being the times usually cited.

Daytime attacks are less frequent, the attack ratio usually being three attacks at night to one in the day. Even in the day the same clockwork pattern exists, with attacks 1 hour after lunch and around 6 p.m. being particularly common. During the day many patients notice specific provocation by alcohol. When present, this is another diagnostic feature of the condition. Following each attack the eye and cheek feel bruised and tender, there may be slight ptosis and the pupil may be dilated. This tenderness may persist until the next attack occurs. Because of the 'attack-like' nature of the condition, trigeminal neuralgia is frequently suspected and many patients are put on carbamazepine, which is not only ineffective but may increase their problems, adding nausea and giddiness to the syndrome. It should be stressed that the nocturnal nature of the attack and the pain in the eye and forehead are in stark contrast to the patterning and location of the pain in trigeminal neuralgia, although there is no doubt that the pain approaches the same intensity (see Chapter 21).

Attacks usually occur on a daily basis for 6–12 weeks, and this 'cluster' of episodes gives the condition its name. It may occur at the same time each year for several years, and in the UK the months of December, January and February seem to be particularly provocative. Occasionally attacks are prolonged, and patients are seen who have had daily attacks over several years in spite of a variety of surgical and pharmacological assaults on the condition, which have been unavailing because of incorrect diagnosis.

The most effective treatment for cluster headache is a combination of methysergide maleate and lithium carbonate. Quite small doses may be very effective and methsergide maleate 1 mg at 8 a.m., 2 p.m. and 10 p.m., each dose accompanied by lithium carbonate 125 mg, is effective in the majority of cases and the benefit is apparent within 48 hours. If this fails, doubling the dose of both drugs for 7–10 days may be necessary. Although both ergotamine tartrate 2 mg or sumatriptan 6 mg are effective in the attack, the natural history of an attack with spontaneous recovery in less than 1 hour in the majority of cases does not justify the use of these drugs, unless difficulty controlling the attacks with prophylactic medication is experienced. When attacks have been completely controlled for 10 days, a phased withdrawal of the methysergide maleate will usually indicate whether the cluster is over and the lithium can then be discontinued. The patient should be given a starter supply of medication for immediate treatment of future episodes, although medical supervision is advisable until the cluster is over.

Cluster headache satisfying all the diagnostic criteria is very uncommon in females. Atypical female versions of the condition are perhaps more accurately described as migrainous neuralgia or Sluder's lower-half headache, which is discussed in greater detail in Chapter 21. This emphasizes the major differences, which are that the pain is more generalized in the face and often extends into the mastoid and jaw as well as the orbit and nose, the attacks tend to be longer lasting, and although frequently nocturnal often continue into the day. Attacks during the day are of slower onset and offset than the explosively sudden attacks in males. The treatment is the same as discussed above for cluster headache, but may need continuing for many months as the duration of a female cluster may extend to 6 months or more.

Status Migrainosus

The concept of low-grade ongoing migraine has become controversial, with the demand of headache classifications which were initially intended for research purposes requiring that ongoing headache is regarded as **not** being due to migraine. Such headaches are regarded as chronic tension headaches on the basis of their chronicity rather than on the nature of the headache. Efforts continue to demonstrate anatomical, physiological and pharmacological differences to confirm that tension headache is a distinct entity and not a continuum of the migraine syndrome. Unfortunately, patients with recurrent headaches become extremely tense, which leads to the conclusion that the headache is therefore due to tension. Patients are not really concerned as to the accuracy of the distinction: they are looking for relief from their headache and prophylactic treatment for migraine is often surprisingly successful in those patients thought to be suffering from chronic tension headache. Many long-term migraine sufferers are able to make a clear distinction between an ordinary migraine and one that has been provoked by a stressful situation, but the basic features of the headache remain identical.

This condition is best described as chronic mild migraine. The distribution of the headache is similar to that shown in Fig. 20.3. The episode may have been initiated by a stressful situation but by the time the patient is seen the initial stress is often no longer operative. However, the headache itself has become the stress, owing to the patient, their relatives and almost anyone they meet (except their neurologist) having decided that they must have a cerebral tumour. The importance of treating the headache with antimigraine drugs, as well as treating the tension, is worth reiterating.

In this group reassurance that the patient does not have a cerebral tumour is a vital part of management. Sometimes patients are frightened to voice this fear, but this is such a constant worry in this group that it is worth specifically telling them that the possibility has been considered and excluded on clinical grounds, although it is increasingly likely that a scan will be demanded to back up this view. In former times patients were very happy with a skull X-ray for the same purpose, but now the public perception is that scanning reveals all.

The treatment of this situation can be very taxing: an instant response to any medication is unlikely and it may be difficult to persuade the patient that at least a 4-week trial of any medication is necessary before firm conclusions can be drawn. Provided there are no contraindications, propranolol with its combination of antianxiety and antimigraine effects may be helpful in modest doses. As little as 10 mg t.d.s. is more readily tolerated and can be as effective as 80–160 mg of long-acting propranolol per day. Amitriptyline in a dose of 10–50 mg nocte can be surprisingly effective within days, suggesting that the antidepressant effect is not the mode of action. Pizotifen in a dose of 0.5–1.5 mg at night is less effective in this group, and in males severe drowsiness and in females unacceptable weight gain represent considerable disadvantages if long-term treatment is necessary. The same stricture applies to methysergide maleate, which can be effective in a low dose of 1 mg at night. This permits longer-term use than the recommended dose of 2 mg t.d.s., which few can tolerate, but the patient should be subject to continuing review while they remain on the medication.

Any of these medications has to be preferred to self-medication with large doses of 'over-the-counter' analgesic combinations taken ineffectually for years on end. The majority of cases of fatal analgesic nephropathy have been reported in patients with migraine, using proprietary analgesics in this way. This risk alone justifies the somewhat soul-destroying task of attempting to treat these extremely difficult patients.

Exertional Migraine

This is an under-recognized but quite frequent variant of migraine of some importance which is invariably misdiagnosed as subarachnoid haemorrhage. It may occur during any exertion, but is most frequently reported during sexual intercourse and is now recognized as 'intercourse migraine' or 'benign coital cephalgia'. The increasing enthusiasm for strenuous workouts in gymnasia, particularly weight training, is producing another clearly identifiable group of similarly afflicted patients.

The headache is of explosive onset at climax during intercourse or at the height of exertion in other situations, and it is described as a sensation as if the patient had been hit over the back of the head with a brick. It may be pulsatile but subsides quite rapidly over 10–15 minutes. If the patient attends hospital he is likely to be subjected to an immediate lumbar puncture to exclude subarachnoid haemorrhage. One unfortunate patient had a lumbar puncture on no less than three occasions in 6 months at the same hospital, for intercourse migraine! It is intriguing that this seems to be a self-limiting condition and patients may have a series of attacks over a few months without subsequent recurrence.

Problems arise if the patient is seen some time after such an episode. The condition is sufficiently characteristic for confident reassurance to be given that this had not been due to a 'small bleed', **if** the headache had cleared *completely* within 1–2 hours and was not followed by a stiff neck, nausea, vomiting or low back pain the next day. If the patient is seen in the middle of a series of attacks occurring close together, the use of propranolol 20 mg 1 hour before the intended exertion is extremely effective at preventing the onset of the headache.

Two other headache variants which probably fall into the same category are cough headache and so-called 'thunderclap' headache. Both headaches are of explosive suddenness, and migraine sufferers are well aware that any protracted bout of coughing can provoke the sudden onset of otherwise typical migraine. Sudden-onset vicious headache for no clear reason has been called 'thunderclap' headache, and the benign nature of this condition has been repeatedly demonstrated. Because the headache that accompanies the onset of subarachnoid haemorrhage is of similar suddenness and severity, neurosurgeons who only see patients who **have** had such headaches in association with a proven subarachnoid haemorrhage, have a different perception and claim that all such headaches should be regarded as being due to subarachnoid haemorrhage until proved otherwise. They do not realize that they would be overwhelmed if all such headaches were automatically referred for full neurosurgical evaluation. If a headache of this type builds quickly, is not associated with nausea or vomiting, does not produce confusion or impaired consciousness, and no stiff neck or backache occurs in the next few hours, a subarachnoid haemorrhage is extremely unlikely (see Chapter 11).

Migraine With Vertigo

Migraine is frequently associated with vertigo in all its forms. Benign positional vertigo occurs much more frequently in migraine sufferers than in the general population, and even Menière's disease shows an association with migraine. These conditions are discussed in greater detail in Chapter 7. The importance of recognizing the potential seriousness of headache in association with vomiting which is related to positional change, and accompanied by acute vertigo, must be recognized. Even a patient with long-standing migraine and headaches that seem to be the same as before, should be regarded with great suspicion if the headaches are suddenly accompanied by nausea and vomiting, particularly on change of position. Most will prove to be benign positional vertigo, but this is the group that **does** require further investigation.

CASE REPORT IV

A 31-year-old male coach driver presented with a 10-week history of daily headaches. These were totally different from his lifelong but infrequent typical migraine. The pain was occipital in location and described as being like a nail hammered into the skull. Seven days before admission he turned all the passengers off his coach and drove back to the bus station because he was frightened to continue. Five days prior to admission he had started vomiting on change of position, and commented that he had noticed that he became slightly giddy on change of position over the previous 8 weeks. On examination, with the exception of papilloedema there were no other physical findings. A CT scan revealed a cystic cerebellar tumour with gross hydrocephalus. This proved to be a haemangioblastoma, which was totally resected without incident, and he was allowed to resume coach driving 1 year later.

As discussed earlier, the recurrent vertiginous syndrome which occurs in childhood as a migraine variant also requires careful investigation until a posterior fossa lesion has been excluded. (See Case Report V)

Treatment of the giddy syndromes associated with migraine is very difficult. A combination of prophylactic doses of propranolol 10 mg t.d.s., supplemented with cinnarizine hydrochloride 15 mg t.d.s., is particularly effective for benign positional vertigo, Menière's disease in association with migraine is more difficult to treat, as betahistidine hydrochloride 8–16 mg t.d.s. tends to aggravate the headache and higher doses of propranolol with cinnarizine or prochlorperazine 5 mg t.d.s., may be more effective. Unfortunately, the long-term use of prochlorperazine or cinnarizine may produce an extrapyramidal syndrome or drug-induced parkinsonism, and it is important not to leave patients on this regimen indefinitely. Prochlorperazine seems to be responsible for more cases of drug-induced parkinsonism in the non-psychiatric community than any other agent.

Treatment of the Acute Migraine Attack

In previous discussion the use of various prophylactic drugs and regimens in chronic migraine and in the specific migraine syndromes, has been considered. Prevention of attacks, rather than effective treatment when they occur, is the aim of migraine management and the ambition of migraine patients.

Any appropriate variation in activities or avoidance of provocative factors is desirable, but unfortunately rarely produces a dramatic improvement in the situation because so many of the factors are unavoidable and dietary exclusion is so ineffective in genuine migraine sufferers. The end result is that however much effort is put into management, patients will still suffer acute attacks.

Many adult patients and most children obtain considerable relief if they can get off to sleep, and it is likely that the success of antivomiting sedatives such as prochlorperazine owes as much to the sedation as to the relief of vomiting. The severity of the headache often prevents sleep, and patients find that sitting or even walking around is preferable unless the headache is so severe that they cannot move. The traditional remedy for nearly 100 years has been ergotamine or dihydroergotamine, and both formulations are still available. The actual success rate is hard to gauge and many patients find that the coincidental migrainous bowel upset, nausea, vomiting or diarrhoea is aggravated by the use of ergot. It may be taken orally as a 2 mg tablet, 1 mg subcutaneously or rectally as a 2 mg suppository. An inhaled form is available but a patient at the height of a severe attack cannot be trusted to adhere to the prescribed dose, and an extra puff could be hazardous. Migraine sufferers are notorious abusers of analgesics and other medication, driven by the severity of the headache, drug ineffectiveness and peer pressure to 'do something about it'.

The recent introduction of sumatriptan has improved the management of acute attacks for a higher proportion of patients. Its mode of action is stimulatory on the same receptors as ergotamine and the two drugs should not be used together. It enjoys greater specificity for the cranial circulation than ergotamine and is thought to be less likely to produce coronary artery and peripheral vessel vasoconstriction. It is available as either a 50 mg or 100 mg tablet or a 6 mg self-administered subcutaneous injection. Many patients find that the injection takes 15–20 minutes to take effect and the tablets 60–90 minutes. Many peculiar sensations, including tightness in the chest, tightness in the occipital region and tingling or numbness in the face, may occur and many patients are reluctant to use the drug if these symptoms are particularly prominent.

There is no doubt that one of the major problems with ergotamine was overuse by severe migraine sufferers, resulting in ergot rebound headaches where further headaches were being generated by the previous dose of ergotamine. There is now evidence that in spite of the expense of sumatriptan, some desperate patients are getting into the same situation and sumatriptan rebound headache is a real entity. For this reason, further efforts to reduce the frequency of acute migraine attacks by any and all prophylactic measures should remain the mainstay of management.

It would be extremely helpful diagnostically if the failure of a headache to respond to either ergotamine or sumatriptan indicated that the diagnosis of migraine was incorrect, but unfortunately this is not the case. Attempts at prophylaxis and effective treatment of the acute attack often fail, and the increasingly desperate patient slips into the diagnostic category of chronic tension headache – hardly surprising, because their lives are increasingly disrupted by the condition. It is this group of patients who seem to be so badly served by attempts to make all headaches fit into a contrived grouping, rather than treating each patient as an individual with an individual problem. Less dogmatic and unhelpful reclassification of the patient's headache type may lead to more effective treatment. Too often the patient is told that their headache does not fill all the diagnostic criteria for migraine and therefore no treatment is available. If it is considered that there are as many types of migraine as there are patients who have it, this therapeutic nihilism may be avoided.

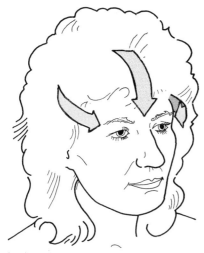

Pain is said to be due to spasm on the scalp and sub-occipital muscles. The muscles are said to be tender and knotted but this is extremely difficult to evaluate. In general the description of 'tightness' like a 'band' or 'scalp too tight' is a frequent clue (this is in contrast to the 'bursting feeling' described by migraine sufferers). These patients are usually overtly anxious and respond to minor tranquillisers and the headache to simple analgesics.

20.5   Tension (muscle contraction) headache.

Tension Headache (Fig. 20.5)

Tension headache is now classified as acute or chronic in type. The basic headache in both types is the same: it is the frequency or persistence of headache that makes the distinction. A typical acute tension headache starts as a tight feeling in the suboccipital muscles and then spreads over the top of the head as a 'tight' feeling. When this follows immediately in the wake of a stressful situation and responds to simple analgesics, or clears overnight without specific medication, the diagnosis seems certain. Similar headaches occurring towards the end of each day, at a time when the patient is aware that they are under stress, allows a similar conclusion. If, however, the stressful situation results in the patient waking with the headache, the alternative possibility that they are migrainously based has to be considered, and further evaluation of the quality of the headache is more important than the fact that it is stress associated.

During the acute tension headache, tightness of the neck muscles and over the scalp, poor concentration, slight dizziness and even difficulty focusing may occur as further evidence of anxiety and distress. Severe photophobia, drowsiness, nausea, vomiting and incapacitation are very unusual in tension headache. A feature that seems to permit a distinction between acute tension-based migraine and tension headache is the localization of severe aching pain in and behind the eye, and specific enquiry for this symptom is worthwhile. It is a striking feature in migraine of all varieties.

If the headaches continue to occur on a daily basis and even persist overnight, or are continuing beyond any definable stressful situation, they are classified as chronic tension headaches. Such headaches become self-generating because of the disruption of the patient's life and work, and are further fuelled by the insistence of workmates and friends that the chronicity of the headaches has to indicate serious disease. Referral of these patients for further investigation constitutes a major part of the work in most neurological outpatients.

Exploring the past history of headache in such patients can be very revealing. There is often a previous history of very typical migrainous-type headache initially dismissed by the patient as 'only ordinary headaches' or due to 'sinus' disease. Occasionally a history of previous prolonged bouts of headaches of a similar sort emerges, and sometimes this is documented in the patient's records and may even be denied by the patient. A long history of recurrent headache of this type may be another indication that this is a low-grade ongoing migraine, and appropriate treatment may be successful where months of sedative drugs and analgesics have failed. The controversy as to whether tension headache, tension migraine or chronic migraine are separate entities or whether they are all the same thing continues, to the disadvantage of the patient.

The most effective prophylactic drug in this group of patients is amitriptyline in a dose of 10–50 mg nocte. Its success in the past suggested that an essentially psychological diagnosis was correct, but the clear identification of similar success in patients with typical migraine no longer allows such a simple conclusion. The speed and effectiveness of doses too small to treat significant depression provides support for the concept that there is a condition of chronic low-grade migrainous headache.

Psychotic Headache (Fig. 20.6)

This is an unfortunate term as the patients are not 'psychotic' in the usual sense of the word. Their symptoms are remarkably constant. There is a pain in the head localized to a discrete area, often able to be covered by a penny piece and usually indicated by the patient with one finger. The quality of sensation described is the feature that has delusional overtones: expressions such as 'I can feel the lump just inside the skull'; 'there are worms crawling about inside the head'; or 'the bone is going rotten', are voiced by the patient. Reassurance is always greeted by 'Well, I know you cannot find anything but I know there is something there!' Such patients regularly invite the examiner to feel the lump overlying the painful area, and the patient, and often the spouse, will confirm that some evenings a lump as big as a hen's egg appears transiently in that position.

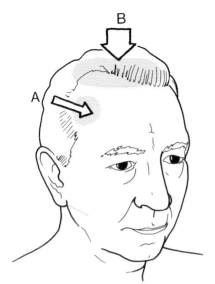

(A)   A specific spot on the head is singled out and bizarre complaints such as 'bone is going bad' or 'worms crawling under the skin' are quickly followed by an invitation to feel the increasingly large lump. Usually nothing other than a normal bulge on the skull is palpable

(B)   A relentless pressure feeling over the vertex is typical of simple depressive headache. Like 'the weight of the world' on the head present 24 hours a day

20.6   Psychotic headache.

These patients willingly undergo and indeed demand repeat investigations and are never reassured by negative tests. Occasionally patients are seen who have had the same symptom for 30 years or more, and it would appear that none are ever cured.

Pressure Headache

The typical description that is said to represent a headache indicating raised intracranial pressure is a headache that occurs on waking, is aggravated by bending or coughing, produces a 'bursting' sensation in the head and does not respond well to analgesics. Unfortunately, as discussed in earlier sections, all these features commonly occur in migraine, so that the diagnosis is far from straightforward. Many patients with such headaches are extensively investigated and no abnormality is found. Headaches that occur only on coughing fulfil some of the criteria, and the decision to embark on full investigation of this symptom requires careful clinical judgement.

What is impressive in neurology clinics and specialist headache clinics is the fact that very few patients with headache actually have serious disease. Conversely, patients who do have cerebral tumours may only reveal on direct questioning that they have had 'muzzy heads' in the mornings for several weeks. It is usually more dramatic neurological symptoms that prompted their seeking medical advice. It is generally accepted that fewer than 1 in 2000 patients is likely to have a serious cause for their headache. The skill in evaluating

patients with headache lies in singling out those who are at particular risk. Two examples of patients that were immediately identified with serious intracranial disease are to be found in Chapter 8. (Case Report XXV and XXVI)

These two examples were included to illustrate rather than alarm, and to emphasize something that has proved to be an important pointer to serious problems. Very short-lived headaches of pounding type related to change of position or straining, with no headache at other times, may indicate a ball-valve type of obstruction in the ventricular system. What is surprising is how rapidly this occurs, and indeed how rapidly it subsides. This is in contrast to cough headache and thunderclap headache discussed earlier, where more protracted provocation is required, or no provocation at all. As discussed in Chapter 8, patients with recent-onset headache associated with positional vertigo and accompanied by very sudden vomiting are the other group of patients in whom investigation is mandatory. It really is not a practical proposition to scan everyone with headache.

In spite of this structure, the following case emphasizes that however classical the history, and even with a previous negative scan in a child with classical migraine, careful physical examination still has a major role to play in management.

CASE REPORT V

*A 13-year-old girl was referred with a recrudescence of migraine first suspected when she was 2 years old. Her GP was concerned that her fundal appearances were abnormal, although he admitted that he had not seen papilloedema for 15 years. At the age of 2 she would cry for 2–3 hour periods and every 15 minutes by the clock she would vomit. She remembers that, at the age of 6, these episodes recurred and were associated with a bad headache and occurred once a week. A CT scan with contrast was reportedly negative (she was living in the USA at that time). The attack rate reduced to once per month on propranolol. By 1991 when she returned to GB, the headaches ceased, the propranolol was stopped and she was well for four years. Three months before consultation she developed similar headaches but in a pattern where the attacks lasted for 2–3 days at 5–10 day intervals. They were still dominated by vomiting and were even more typical of migraine. She developed speckling of vision in the right eye, then blurring of central vision in the one eye, always followed immediately by the headache which started on the left side as a banging sensation in the forehead and 30 minutes later she would start vomiting. This occurred at 10 minute intervals for 2–3 hours (almost identical to the childhood attacks). At the end she slept and the headache cleared. It had become apparent that the attacks often happened on Tuesdays and were not modified by propranolol or pizotifen. From the sequence of symptoms and the intermittency, the diagnosis of migraine seemed ever more certain **but** she did have papilloedema. CT scanning revealed a cerebellar tumour with mild hydro-*

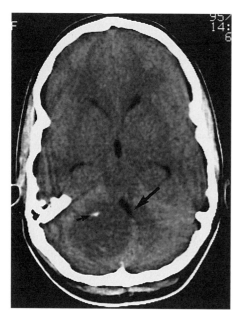

CRV Cerebellar Astrocytoma (non-cystic). Fourth ventricle distorted and displaced (large arrow), small fleck of calcification within the tumour (small arrow).

cephalus. *This showed areas of calcification suggesting a long standing lesion. At operation this proved to be a Grade 1 juvenile astrocytoma.*

It will be interesting to see whether the headaches abate completely (operation May 1995)

Temporal (Cranial) Arteritis (Fig. 20.7)

The original name of this syndrome is unfortunate as it gives the impression that the temporal artery is the only vessel involved. Perhaps the term cranial arteritis should be more generally adopted, and the fact that any artery in the body except the renal arteries may be involved should be emphasized. The classic situation is that an elderly patient (very rarely under 60 years of age) develops pain and tenderness over an obviously swollen temporal artery on one or both sides. The other superficial arteries of the head may also be involved, and occipital pain with local tenderness may easily be misdiagnosed as 'tension' headache.

Although the condition is relatively rare it is safest to assume that all headache starting after the age of 60 years is temporal arteritis until proved otherwise.

For practical purposes this can be readily achieved by performing an immediate ESR. If this is elevated, immediate treatment with high-dose steroids is indicated and arrangements made for the biopsy of the temporal or any other tender artery. The response to steroids alone is usually diagnostic, with dramatic relief of the headache within hours. Further questioning will

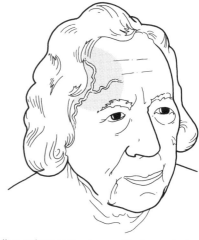

Although swelling, redness and tenderness of the temporal artery and a headache in the distribution of the artery are the hallmarks of the disease this is only in a classical case. A diffuse headache can occur. The occipital artery may be involved and tenderness and swelling in the occipital region occurs. The age of the patient, most often over 60, years of age should help exclude migrainous neuralgia or facial migraine syndromes. General malaise and high ESR or C-reactive protein are diagnostic.

20.7 Temporal arteritis.

usually reveal that the patient has been generally unwell for some time, with generalized muscle aching, sometimes amounting to full-blown polymyalgia rheumatica, loss of appetite with consequent weight loss, and even low-grade pyrexia. All these symptoms remit within days of starting treatment. Sometimes the ESR may be misleadingly normal and occasionally patients with a high ESR may have a normal biopsy, and in such instances the response to steroids may be the mainstay of correct diagnosis.

The important features of the headache are that it is often generalized and the scalp may be very tender. This, combined with the tendency for the headache to be much worse at night, will often result in loss of sleep and the complaint that the patient cannot bear their head touching the pillow. There may be attacks of transient loss of vision or transient ischaemic attacks in vertebrobasilar or other vascular territories. Involvement of the external carotid vessels may lead to claudication of the jaw while chewing or talking, and ischaemic necrosis of the tip of the tongue. Patients may present with unilateral blindness and minimal headache, and only months later when the other eye goes blind does an ESR reveal the diagnosis.

The reason for immediate treatment with steroids is the high risk of blindness due to the involvement of the retinal blood vessels which may occur in some 50% of untreated patients. This risk is rapidly reduced over the first 7 days of treatment. Enteric-coated prednisolone 20 mg t.d.s. should be used for the first 5–7 days, and can then be tailed down in 5 mg steps to 5 mg t.d.s. over 3–6 weeks, using either the headache or the ESR as a guide to the reduction. Many patients remit completely after 1–2 years' treatment but some repeatedly relapse and may need treatment with low doses of prednisolone 2.5–5 mg t.d.s. indefinitely. This may cause problems with osteoporosis, particularly in elderly women, but this risk has to be accepted.

Post-Traumatic Headache

This condition has been left until last as its features underline many of the problems already discussed. Headaches are surprisingly rare in patients who have had serious trauma requiring surgical intervention. If there are headaches in this situation they usually respond to simple analgesics and rarely seem to cause significant difficulty.

Following minor head trauma there is often local tenderness at the site of injury, especially those patients where a small lump has been left, either by a local laceration or as a result of a subgaleal haematoma. These patients often become preoccupied with the idea that their headaches are due to a much bigger lump on the inside of the skull and the belief that headache means that they 'must have been concussed' and that they 'must have been brain damaged'. These concerns guarantee the chronicity of the headaches and lead to demands for repeated investigation to reassure the patient that there are no new developments, because all their friends keep reminding them that clots occur in heads after head injuries, even 10 years later. These symptoms are the commonest cause of medicolegal referral for a neurological opinion.

The post-traumatic anxiety-perpetuated headache consists of a tightness in the head, with localized tenderness at the site of original trauma, and is usually accompanied by poor concentration, memory disturbance, visual difficulties and dizziness. It has many of the features of tension headache and the complexity of that diagnosis has already been discussed.

To further compound the difficulty, post-traumatic vascular headache (migraine-like) is quite common and seems to be a particular complication of trauma to the forehead, orbit and facial area. The usual features of migraine – a pulsatile pain, associated nausea, giddiness, drowsiness and irritability – are present and sometimes sufficiently severe to incapacitate the patient.

As an example of the complexity of post-traumatic headache, and to reiterate the importance of assessing the type of headache before any judgement as to the aetiology is made, the following case is of interest.

CASE REPORT VI

A 32-year-old truck driver suffered a serious injury as the result of a well known hazard of changing the wheels on a 40-ton truck: the wrong bolts were removed and the outer wheel rim flew into the patient's face and chest. This pushed his face back to the extent that the maxillae were under the skull base. His chest was 'stove in', as the surgeons' report so aptly described it. Extensive maxillofacial surgery restored the anatomy of his face to some extent but he was seen 9 months later because of an excruciating headache. Not surprisingly, the headache was bifrontal, continual and not responding to 4-hourly demerol (a synthetic narcotic). The striking part of the history was the dull aching in the backs of the eyes and photophobia. In spite of the obvious severity of the known facial trauma a diagnosis of post-traumatic headache of migrainous type was made. He had been previously suspected of malingering or suffering from tension, owing to the fact that as the original injury was his fault he would not get compensation, and already owed several thousand dollars in medical bills. In spite of all these additional factors he was pain-free within 24 hours of starting treatment with ergotamine, and remained so for 3 months until he was lost to follow-up.

These problems are further discussed in Chapter 23.

Drugs Precipitating Headache

Oral contraceptives and HRT may precipitate migraine or exacerbate pre-existing migraine headache. Less well recognised are migraine-like headaches provoked by NSAIDs especially indomethacin and acematacin. Phenyl acetic acid, propionic acid and similar agents can all cause headache. Sulphasalazine and its derivatives, olsalazine and mesalazine used in the treatment of ulcerative colitis frequently cause low grade headache.

As all these drugs are used long-term, sometimes the association with headache is not immediately obvious.

In conclusion, the **history** is the most important if not the only thing that matters in assessing a patient with headache. It would be extremely unusual for there to be any physical signs **even** in those patients who prove to have serious underlying causes, and the absence of papilloedema on physical examination is of little reassurance to the experienced neurologist. Nevertheless a complete and careful physical examination must be performed in every patient, however certain the diagnosis may seem to be. The severity of the headache is not proportional to the seriousness of the underlying cause, and probably the most frightened and disabled patients will be suffering from one of the migraine variants. Headache due to serious causes is usually an innocuous and minor part of the patient's history. A systematic approach to establishing the history should be followed for every patient if important details are not to be overlooked, and to facilitate this a suggested questionnaire which will identify all the salient features is included in Table 20.1.

Table 20.1 Questionnaire approach to headache diagnosis

Headache	Classic migraine	Common migraine	Cluster headache	Tension headache	Psychotic headache	Pressure headache	Cranial arteritis
Age & sex pattern	Any age M & F	Middle age F > M	30–50 yrs F < M ++	Any age M & F	Middle age M & F	More likely in children	Over 60 M & F
Site	Frontal Unilateral may change sides	Fronto temporal, occipital or orbital Often bilateral	Strictly frontal and in eye, nostril and cheek	Around whole head or pressure on vertex	Local pain in one spot Pressure on vertex	Dull bursting ache over whole head	Superficial usually/often unilateral and over temple
Nature	Throbbing Pulsating Pounding	Dull ache Stabbing pain in eye 'like a bunch of of needles'	Severe stabbing pain in eye	Tight band around head	Weight on top of head	Low-grade ache, no specific quality	Burning, sore quality
Special features	Classically pulsatile	Bilateral but pain maximum behind one or both eyes	Bloodshot eye Lacrimation & rhinorrhoea Pupil dilated Ptosis of lid	Worse when clearly under stress	Present continually, preventing any activity	Brief surges	Tenderness in scalp or temple over affected vessels
Diurnal pattern	During night or on waking or at weekends	Waking or later in day when stressed	Most often nocturnal Like clockwork	Worse at end of day	**All** the time Never remits, according to patient	Mainly waking clearing by mid-day	Usually worse in the night
Aggravating factors	Often none Alcohol Stress off Weather	Bright light Noise Tension Weather	Alcohol Seasonal (may occur same time every year)	Stress Anxiety Fear of tumour	None, often after very stressful event but then self-generating	Bending Coughing Sneezing	Touching or brushing hair or face in affected area
Relieving factors	Rest Dark room Ergotamine Sumatriptan Sleeping	Rest Dark room Prophylactic medication	Attacks short (20 min–2 h) Sumatriptan if attacks last >30 min	Tranquillizer Holidays Change of employment	Anti depressants	Better if standing up Steroids (dexamethasone) Operation	Dramatic response to prednisolone
Associated features	Visual phenomena Nausea Vomiting Diarrhoea Confusion	Dull pain Relentless V. disabling Mood change secondary to headache	May develop partial third nerve palsy or Horner's syndrome in attacks	Other features of anxiety, not least about headache	Weight loss Crying Inability to sleep Poor con-centration	Vomiting Visual blurring Associated features due to underlying lesion Papilloedema	Weight loss Lassitude Aching muscles Visual blurring Jaw/tongue pain when eating or talking

21. Facial Pain

In the discussion of headache (Chapter 20) special emphasis was given to the importance of the history in the differential diagnosis. The same applies to the symptom of pain in the face but, unlike headache, several of the facial pain syndromes are always 'typical' in their historical features. This is particularly true of trigeminal neuralgia, which is the face pain against which all other conditions are judged and which is probably the most severe pain known.

There are several popular misconceptions about facial pain. Prominent among these is the feeling that any pain that is not immediately identifiable as trigeminal neuralgia is automatically due to the condition called 'atypical facial pain'. In reality 'atypical facial pain' is just as 'typical', historically, as trigeminal neuralgia. This underlines the importance of the history. In the case of headache no anatomically discrete areas of involvement are demanded, as the pain may originate in neural, vascular or muscular tissues. The pain is therefore allowed to spread bilaterally, down on to the neck or well on to the face, without concern as to the anatomical substrate.

For the accurate diagnosis of facial pain, a detailed knowledge of the anatomy of the fifth cranial nerve is essential. This information is provided in full detail in Chapter 6 and the sensory distribution of the nerve relevant to this chapter is summarized in Fig. 21.1.

A brief mention of the role of disease of the teeth and the sinuses in the context of face and head pain is necessary. A diseased tooth in the upper jaw can cause headache on the same side, that is, not in direct continuity with the pain in the tooth, which may radiate into the orbit and face. A diseased tooth in the lower jaw may cause considerable pain in the distribution of the mandibular division of the nerve, including pain deep in the ear. In both cases the pain in the involved tooth dominates the picture: there should be no difficulty in recognizing that the pain is coming from a diseased tooth.

Sinus disease is similar. Experimental work has shown that the lining of the sinuses is relatively pain insensitive, and that most pain in sinus disease is due to pressure in the sinus secondary to congestion of the nasal mucosa and the turbinates. As this produces symptoms of nasal congestion and nasal discharge the diagnosis should be obvious. This also means that in the absence of these symptoms the time-honoured search for evidence of chronic subclinical sinus infection or nasal polyps as the explanation for repeated attacks of pain in the face is unnecessary. The common finding of some thickening of the mucosa in the antrum is of dubious significance.

On the premise that there was such a thing as chronic subclinical sinus infection causing facial pain, various aetiological hypotheses were suggested. The most popular of these held that various autonomic nerves and ganglia were irritated by sinus infection and caused pain. Entities such as vidian neuralgia, ciliary neuralgia, sphenopalatine neuralgia and petrosal neuralgia were described and a variety of surgical procedures were designed to ablate the offending nerves and ganglia. These conditions are now recognized as facial migraine syndromes, and include cluster headache and Sluder's lower-half headache. A major feature of these syndromes is a tendency to serial attacks with long remissions, sometimes lasting years, which explains the apparent success of the surgical procedures – fortuitously performed when a natural remission was about to occur. Critical evaluation of these treatment methods has failed to substantiate the claims made for them and most have been abandoned.

In spite of the identification of facial migraine syndromes and appreciation of the psychological aetiology of atypical facial pain, many patients with facial pain syndromes are still subjected to extensive, ineffectual dental surgery and sinus drainage procedures, indicating that these discredited theories of facial pain mechanisms die hard and that belief in their existence is not confined to the general public.

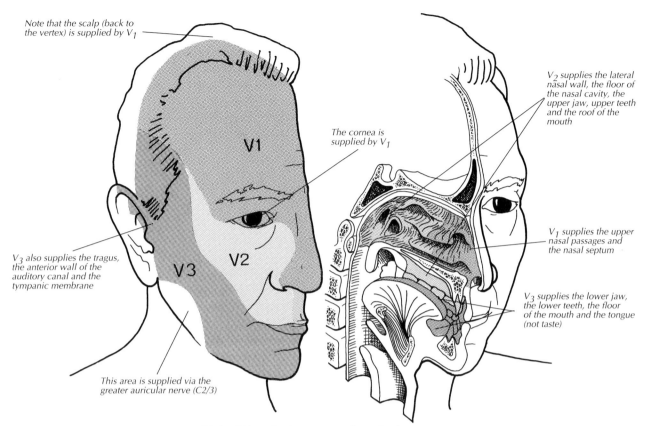

Note that the scalp (back to the vertex) is supplied by V₁

The cornea is supplied by V₁

V₂ supplies the lateral nasal wall, the floor of the nasal cavity, the upper jaw, upper teeth and the roof of the mouth

V₃ also supplies the tragus, the anterior wall of the auditory canal and the tympanic membrane

V₁ supplies the upper nasal passages and the nasal septum

V₃ supplies the lower jaw, the lower teeth, the floor of the mouth and the tongue (not taste)

This area is supplied via the greater auricular nerve (C2/3)

21.1   Trigeminal nerve supply to the face.

Trigeminal Neuralgia (Tic Douloureux)

Although great emphasis is rightly placed on the fact that the pain of trigeminal neuralgia never extends outside the anatomical territory supplied by the fifth nerve, it is not sufficiently appreciated that it is unusual for the pain to involve a whole division, let alone the entire territory of the nerve, and in most cases the pain runs along the line demarcating the third from the second division and the second from the first division respectively (Figs 21.2 and 21.3). It is also notable that the first (ophthalmic) division is involved in less than 5% of cases. An important practical point that emerges from this is that one of the least likely causes of pain in the eye or forehead is tic douloureux. The commonest cause of pain in this area is migraine. Symptomatic tic douloureux due to underlying causes is extremely rare and its recognition and illustrative case histories are included in Chapter 6.

Location of the Pain

The pain occurs in two zones. These are the mouth–ear zone, affected in some 60% of cases and the nose–orbit zone, affected in 30% of cases.

Pain in the mouth–ear zone (Fig. 21.2) spreads from the region of the lower canine tooth back to a position deep in the ear or, less frequently, the pain may radiate in the reverse direction from the ear to the jaw. Quite often the pain also spreads around the hinge of the temporomandibular joint and into the upper jaw. It therefore runs along the line of the boundary between the second and third divisions and is not confined to the third division.

Pain in the nose–orbit zone (Fig. 21.3) typically shoots up from the nostril to the inner and/or outer orbit. The eyeball itself is not involved in the pain, but may seem to be surrounded by it. Patients often describe this pain as the feeling of a 'red-hot poker pushed up the nose' and note that the eye seems quite painless but is bathed in 'a rim of agony'. It is only from such graphic descriptions that an idea of the severity of this pain can be appreciated. It will be noticed that in these cases the pain starts in the second division but spreads into the first division as high as the eyebrow. It very rarely extends above it. At the height of an attack the patient may find it difficult to locate the pain so precisely but the preliminary jabs of pain occur in the zones described above and can usually be accurately localized.

Quality of the Pain

The pain of tic douloureux is characteristic. It starts as a feeling, like 'electricity', 'red-hot needles' or 'a machine-gun firing red hot bullets' into the affected

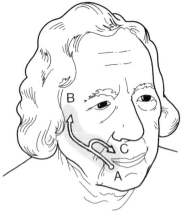

The pain radiates from A to B and is a deep sensation like a series of hot needle jabs, followed by a searing sensation. It may also involve C at the heights of the pain. Less frequently it may shoot from B to A or C. Chewing, talking, smiling or hot and cold fluids in the mouth are the main triggering factors. The ophthalmic division (V_1) is involved in less than 5% of cases

21.2 Mouth–ear zone trigeminal neuralgia. This is the distribution of pain in 60% of cases.

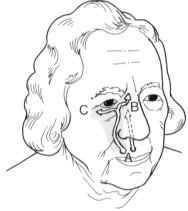

The pain shoots from A (the upper canine or the upper lip) to around the eye to B or C. The areas B and C may also be trigger points. The main areas triggered by touch for this distribution are the alar of the nose, and the outer third of the upper lip. Hot and cold fluids in the mouth will also trigger if the teeth are sensitive.

21.3 Nose–orbit trigeminal neuralgia. This is the distribution of pain in 30% of cases.

zone. This rapidly builds up into an excruciating pain that is felt deep in the face, and is confined to the areas described above. It only lasts for a few seconds, but is then replaced by a very unpleasant ache or a burning sensation as if a red-hot poker had been dragged across the face. The pain is not continual, although at the height of a bad attack episodes may recur so rapidly that the patient is never entirely pain-free. Attacks may vary from one every few minutes to one or two a day.

Triggering of the Pain

The third major feature of the condition is the phenomenon of 'triggering'. The severity of an attack is judged by the frequency with which attacks occur and this in

turn bears a close relationship to how easily attacks can be triggered.

Attacks affecting the mouth–ear zone are particularly triggered by motor activity, therefore chewing, smiling and yawning are major provocative factors. Pain in this zone is less often triggered by cutaneous stimuli, but hot or cold fluids touching the lower canine tooth or lower lip may also be provocative.

In contrast, pain in the nose–orbit zone is typically provoked by cutaneous trigger points. These are found at the alar of the nostril, the outer third of the upper lip and at the medial end of the eyebrow. Hot and cold fluids in the mouth are also effective stimuli, as is blowing the nose or attempting to clean the teeth. At the height of a very severe attack cutaneous sensitivity may be so great that a draught on the face from turning the page of a book, eye movement, a stumble or a sudden noise may be sufficient to provoke a burst of pain.

Diurnal Variation

One of the more remarkable features of trigeminal neuralgia, and another important distinguishing feature from migrainous neuralgic pain, is the rarity of attacks of pain during the night. Unless the patient inadvertently turns on to the affected side their sleep is usually undisturbed. It is hard to attribute this solely to reduced triggering stimuli. Attacks during the day are the rule and patients who are seen at the height of an attack are almost impossible to examine. The involuntary startle if any attempt is made to touch the affected side of the face is diagnostic of the condition. So is the distraught, unkempt haggard appearance caused by the inability to wash, shave or clean the teeth. In an attack the patient may be unable to speak, or if they attempt to do so they speak like a ventriloquist, trying not to move the lips or tongue.

Natural History and Treatment

The natural history of the condition is for attacks to occur with increasing frequency, although initially there may be periods of months to years between episodes and the accuracy of the diagnosis made in the first attack may be questioned if a second episode is long delayed. The tendency to prolonged remissions governs the therapeutic approach. It is inevitable that the condition will recur and usually, as the recurrences become more frequent, triggering becomes more pronounced and the attacks therefore more disabling. This certainly means that definitive treatment has to be considered as soon as the diagnosis is established. It is thought that the reason that this very characteristic and very painful condition was not clearly recognized until the 1600s, was because of its occurrence in the elderly, and prior to that time too few people lived long enough to develop it. It can occur in childhood, but with the exception of its occurrence in patients with multiple sclerosis, which accounts for only some 3% of cases, most patients are over 60 years of age.

In patients under 60, intracranial nerve root section or neurovascular decompression should be considered as definitive treatment. In patients over 60 and those reluctant to consider intracranial surgery, stereotactic thermocoagulation of the ganglion is a less hazardous alternative. The disadvantages of surgical treatments are a degree of anaesthesia, which may be disabling in its own right, or an even more unpleasant condition, a dysaesthetic pain syndrome in the numb area known as anaesthesia dolorosa. Because of these strictures medical management of the condition is not only desirable but often perfectly satisfactory, and surgery need only be considered in a small proportion of patients where pharmacological treatment fails.

Although carbamazepine is regarded as the drug of choice it may have serious drawbacks in these very elderly patients. It is often forgotten that phenytoin was a highly successful treatment before the advent of carbamazepine and still has a useful role in management. It is much less likely to cause disabling cerebellar side-effects.

The major advantage of carbamazepine is its speed of action. A 100 mg dose may produce significant relief within 2 hours: indeed, if it does not do so a higher dose must be tried. The effective dose should be repeated three or four times daily, ideally taken about an hour before meals for maximum effect. Very few elderly patients can tolerate more than 200 mg q.d.s. Once an effective dose of carbamazepine has been established, and particularly if nausea and giddiness prove to be a problem, the parallel use of phenytoin may have considerable advantage. It should be introduced in a dose of 100 mg t.d.s. and will take 5–7 days to achieve therapeutic levels. Unless the carbamazepine dose is reduced at about that time even more marked toxic effects will become apparent. It is usually possible to halve the dose of carbamazepine after 5 days, and after 1–2 weeks it may be possible to use it on an 'as necessary' basis to supplement the background effectiveness of the phenytoin. Using this technique, even 90-year-old patients can be treated effectively. It is at this stage that the final disadvantage of both phenytoin and carbamazepine may become apparent, and that is cutaneous allergy. A very severe skin rash may occur at any time between 3 weeks and as late as 6 months after starting either medication, and requires immediate withdrawal of the drug. If neither drug can be used surgical measures have to be considered. There are no other established pharmacological treatments but in the future, when oxcarbazepine, a carbamazepine derivative which has less risk of causing skin rash, is introduced an effective alternative treatment will become available.

Psychologically Based Facial Pain Syndromes

Referring back to the two psychologically determined types of headache, there are two analogous types of facial pain. These are the conditions known as atypical facial pain and psychotic facial pain. Both conditions occur predominantly in females.

Atypical Facial Pain (Fig. 21.4)

Atypical facial pain is usually misdiagnosed in the first instance as being due to dental or sinus disease, and many patients are edentulous and have undergone numerous surgical procedures by the time they are referred for a neurological opinion. The mistake is made because the first symptom is almost always pain in one or other maxillary region, and is first identified as toothache. The pain is described as deep, burning and continual. There is no jabbing onset as occurs in tic douloureux. In spite of patients' insistence that the pain is unbearable, their affect is often inappropriate and their facial appearance is quite unlike that of the patient with tic douloureux.

The pain usually extends in three directions, as shown in the figure. It radiates back behind the ear, down on to the neck or across to the opposite maxillary area. All these sites of extension of the pain immediately exclude tic douloureux, and ought to relieve any concern that the pain has an organic basis, as it clearly transgresses the anatomical boundaries of the fifth

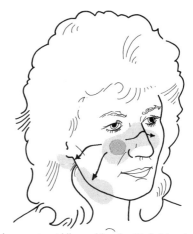

Mainly young to middle-aged females. Underlying depressive illness is usually present. The pain usually starts in the upper jaw and maxilla. Early spread is to the other side and back to below and behind the ear. Finally spread onto the neck and entire half head may occur. May sometimes be similar to migrainous neuralgia, which is the main differential diagnosis

21.4   Atypical facial pain.

cranial nerve. The main differential diagnosis is migrainous facial neuralgia. Eventually the pain may involve the whole head and neck bilaterally, and patients may even complain that it sometimes spreads down into the arms or trunk.

The longer the history the more bizarre the quality and distribution of the pain. As some patients take several years to reach a neurologist some very florid symptoms may be present by the time they are seen. At that stage delusional overtones often appear in the description of the pain, with complaints such as 'the bone is going rotten', or large transient 'swellings of the face' being reported. The patients often clutch their face, unlike the patient with tic douloureux who shields their face but is very careful not actually to touch it. Sometimes in extreme cases there is a dramatic arrangement of towels or scarves around the face, ostensibly to protect it but rather, one suspects, to act as a badge of courage. It is also a notable feature that these patients always bring a friend or relative with them to explain how bad the pain has become. This scenario is almost diagnostic in its own right.

Psychotic Facial Pain

Psychotic facial pain may be an extension of this condition (just as psychotic headache may supervene in a patient with tension headache) or it may occur acutely in pure form. It is psychotic in the sense that, despite the duration of the symptoms and all evidence to the contrary, the patient is totally convinced that there is a sinister underlying cause that only time will reveal. This is probably the reason that surgical treatment is avidly sought and attempts at medical treatment are always abandoned within days, often on the pretext of florid and unbelievable side-effects. In psychotic facial pain the pain is typically confined to a single area (the tongue is a favourite site) and delusional symptoms appear early. In addition to the usual pain and non-existent swellings or discolorations of the tongue or face, an underlying cancer phobia is always present. The patient is almost always female and no amount of reassurance or negative investigation will convince them otherwise, even when the symptoms have been present for 10–15 years, which is not at all unusual.

Treatment of Psychologically Based Facial Pain

In atypical facial pain, if the condition is correctly diagnosed early, a good response to combinations of tranquillizers and antidepressants may be anticipated. Once the delusional overtones appear the chances of significant alleviation of the symptoms rapidly diminish. The same is true of psychotic facial pain, although in this instance no blame for failure can be attributed to a delay in referral as patients seem not to respond to any

treatment! The temptation to advise surgical denervation of the face must be avoided: the pain is not relieved and is often replaced by anaesthesia dolorosa, a painful numbness of the denervated area. Psychiatric referral is unrewarding and often starts a new round of referrals to a new group of surgeons.

Facial Migraine Syndromes (Fig. 21.5)

Reference has already been made to the many eponymous autonomic neuralgias that are all variants of migraine affecting the facial vasculature. They include the condition known as cluster headache, discussed in the previous chapter. Nasal congestion and pain deep in the eye are features of that condition. This is also true of all the facial migraine variants, and stabbing pain in the ear or a sensation as if the mastoid bone had been inflated may also be noted. Patients should be closely questioned as to the presence of any of these symptoms during episodes of facial pain.

Sluder's Lower-Half Headache

Sluder's lower-half headache, although quite rare, is perhaps the most typical of these conditions. The pain is described as dull and bursting, with an occasional throbbing component. It often has a hot or burning quality and the face in the affected area may become flushed. It may be located at the base of the nose, in the cheek or eye, and especially in the ear or in the region of the mastoid. In the ear the pain may have an acute lancinating quality, as if a dagger had been thrust into the ear and twisted. In the mastoid region it is often described as a sensation as if the ear had been pumped up with a bicycle pump. There is usually pain deep behind the eye although nasal congestion is variable, as indeed it is in cluster headache. The pain may radiate down into the side of the neck, on to the cheek and into the jaws or tongue. It shows a distinct tendency to start during the night and may wake the patient from sleep, although it is rarely as intense as cluster headache. Unlike cluster headache it can also occur throughout the day, but may also recur in a clockwork pattern at special times. Sluder's lower-half headache is probably unique to females and may represent a female variant of cluster headache, showing a similar tendency to occur in clusters, demonstrate a seasonal variation and a favourable response to the methysergide maleate and lithium carbonate combination discussed in the previous chapter.

Other Migraine Variants

Migraine affecting the temporal artery may be accompanied by visible swelling and tenderness of the artery.

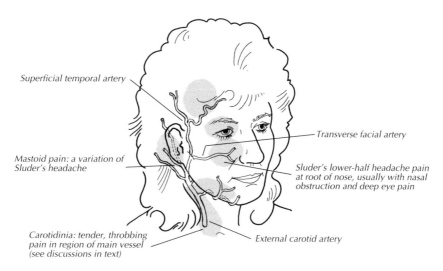

Superficial temporal artery

Transverse facial artery

Mastoid pain: a variation of Sluder's headache

Sluder's lower-half headache pain at root of nose, usually with nasal obstruction and deep eye pain

Carotidinia: tender, throbbing pain in region of main vessel (see discussions in text)

External carotid artery

21.5 Facial migraine syndromes.

This may be readily misdiagnosed as temporal arteritis unless the age of the patient is taken into account: 30-year-old women do not suffer from cranial arteritis!

Carotidynia is a former diagnostic term for an episodic throbbing pain in the side of the neck due, it has been postulated, to swelling and tenderness of the carotid artery caused by migraine. Similar symptoms may occur during the course of an otherwise typical migraine headache, and pain in this distribution is often described in Sluder's headache. Slight pressure on the vessel causes pain but firm pressure may transiently completely relieve the symptoms, as may pressure on the superficial temporal artery in ordinary migraine.

In all the facial migraine syndromes the important clues are retro-orbital pain of a stabbing, throbbing type or a dull bursting feeling in the ear. These syndromes occur mainly in women between the ages of 25 and 50. It is not uncommon for female patients who have had typical migraine all their life to develop more localized neuralgic migraine in the eye, nostril, jaw or ear at the menopause. This often causes considerable alarm, as it is so different from their previous attacks and tends to be much more persistent. It is a pattern of headache that also seems to be common in patients recently started on HRT (hormone replacement therapy), and a trial of HRT withdrawal is advisable before starting the patient on methysergide and lithium carbonate, which is likely to prove the most effective treatment.

Postherpetic Neuralgia (Fig. 21.6)

This rarely presents a diagnostic problem as the causative attack of shingles is usually obvious. However, in the 3–5 days between the onset of the initial pain and the eruption of the vesicles, at the onset of herpes zoster, there is a considerable diagnostic problem. Ophthalmic herpes occurs in the elderly and the initial pain in the forehead may mimic cranial arteritis. The ESR is not too helpful as it may well be elevated, even when the subsequent diagnosis proves to be herpes zoster.

Daily examination until the vesicles appear in the eyebrow or over the forehead is the best way of confirming or excluding the diagnosis. They usually appear on the fourth or fifth day and as they erupt the pain may diminish. If the pain fails to improve it is essential to use the strongest analgesics necessary to control it, as there is a strong suspicion that inadequate pain relief at this stage may predispose to the subsequent development of the postherpetic neuralgia syndrome. The use of acyclovir may reduce the number of vesicles and subsequent scarring, but there is no evidence that its use or the use of steroids reduces the risk of developing postherpetic neuralgia.

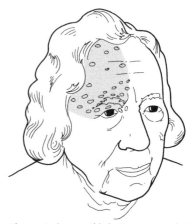

Most frequently seen in the very elderly. It occurs mainly following first-division herpes zoster; although the whole zone hurts, the pain in the eyebrow and around the eye is especially severe. The residual thin papery white scars are anaesthetic. The tender areas are the patches of intact skin between the scars. The pain is continual and burning, with severe pain provoked by touching the eyebrow or brushing the hair. The condition shows a tendency to a modest spontaneous remission after several years

21.6 Post-herpetic neuralgia.

As the patients are often old and lonely the early administration of anti-depressants with the analgesics, to prevent a depressive reaction, probably has some merit, and amitriptyline or imiprimine, with their beneficial effects on neural pain syndromes, may have a special place in early management but must be used cautiously in low dosages in the elderly.

Treatment

If postherpetic neuralgia develops, as it will in some 30% of patients with ophthalmic herpes, the initial pain alters to a continual dull burning sensation, with exacerbations provoked by touching the eyebrow or brushing the hair. It is not the scars that are sensitive, it is the normal skin between them: the scars are actually anaesthetic. The pain may remit after 12–18 months, but this is by no means certain, and those patients with persistent pain present a distressing and formidable therapeutic problem. The suicide risk is high, and in the absence of effective therapy the use of narcotic analgesics may be necessary.

Where there is a considerable degree of triggered pain, provoked by touch, phenytoin 100 mg t.d.s. may prove helpful and further improvement may be achieved by combining it with amitriptyline 10 mg t.d.s. Elderly patients do not tolerate higher doses. The use of capsaicin 0.025% cream rubbed into the affected area for 28 days has been suggested and its use continued if successful. Unfortunately the cream is highly irritant and very few patients can achieve satisfactory application. The worst pain is often in the eyelid and the eye itself, and as special efforts have to be made to avoid getting the cream in these areas, complete success is impossible. It is difficult to see that this treatment will ever achieve acceptable results in postherpetic neuralgia in the ophthalmic division.

Temporomandibular Osteoarthritis (Costen's Syndrome) (Fig. 21.7)

Whether Costen's syndrome is a true entity is much disputed, but certainly osteoarthritis affecting the temporomandibular joint occurs and produces pain which is maximal and often only present when the patient is chewing. The joint itself is usually tender to palpation, although it is possible to mistake this for tenderness of the temporal artery. The pain may radiate forward into the face or upwards into the temporalis muscle. The condition can be relieved by prosthetic devices that prevent overclosure of the bite. As with tooth and sinus disease, the problem arises when it is assumed that disease of the joint can cause pain in the face without the joint itself being painful. Patients with atypical facial

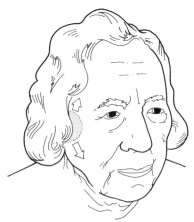

Pain is obviously in the temporomandibular joint, spreading towards on to the face and up into the temporalis muscle. The joint is tender to touch and pain is provoked by chewing or just opening the mouth. The pain ceases almost entirely if the mouth is held shut and still

21.7   Costen's syndrome (temporomandibular arthritis).

pain and the migrainous facial pain syndromes are often suspected of having this condition, and may be subjected to a great many unsuccessful dental and maxillofacial procedures on the basis of this diagnosis. The world record for unsuccessful surgical procedures in one patient with atypical facial pain is 122 separate operations over a 20-year period.

Other Causes of Facial Pain

Temporal arteritis has already been mentioned several times, and of particular interest in the context of facial pain is the situation where the arteries to the muscles of mastication, including the tongue, are involved in the process. In these cases the patient may present with 'intermittent claudication' of the masseter muscles, the facial muscles or in the tongue. The age of the patient is always a clue to this condition, and the diagnosis must always be considered in any patient over the age of 60 who has headache or face pain.

Anginal pain is known to radiate up into the neck and lower jaw, in addition to the more typical radiation down the arm.

CASE REPORT I

A 73-year-old woman was seen with quite severe bilateral pain in both upper and lower jaws which came on while walking, especially on cold days. Shortly after the onset of this pain a gripping feeling in the chest was noticed. The pain in the jaws was the presenting symptom and the seat of the worst pain. Cardiological advice was sought and the diagnosis of cardiac pain referred to the jaws was confirmed by subsequent investigation.

Malignant disease in the skull base, often due to direct extension from a carcinoma of the nasopharynx, tends to involve the first and second divisions of the

Table 21.1 Questionnaire approach to facial pain

	Trigeminal neuralgia	Atypical facial pain	Migrainous facial pain	Postherpetic neuralgia	Costen's syndrome
Age/sex	Over 50 F > M 3 : 1 R > L 5 : 1	F > M 30–50 years (rare in men)	M = F Typically 40–50 age range	F > M Over 70 years	Elderly females
Site	Lower jaw – ears Upper lip – nose **Strictly** unilateral	Maxillary area Whole face Often **both** sides involved	Anywhere Deep eye pain or feeling of swelling in mastoid, sinus pain or toothache	Over V_1 nerve distribution Most severe in eyebrow	In or anterior to temporo- mandibular joint
Nature of pain	Like hot needles for seconds, followed by severe pain	Described only as 'continual' 'unbearable' or 'intolerable'	Throbbing or pulsatile Lacrimation or conjunctival injection	Very severe Non-stop burning and itching	Severe aching pain in joint Radiating forwards
Special features	Unilateral Isolated attacks Even when severe each pain is an individual attack	Extensive bilateral Continual Interferes with sleep and life	Sporadic attacks Patient well between attacks Often nocturnal or early morning	Tender areas between white scars of herpes eruption	Over TM joint Pain **when eating**
Aggravating factors	Hot/cold fluids in mouth or chewing Blowing nose Smiling or talking	None, but may complain of triggering after many consultations	Alcohol HRT Often seasonal Cold > warm	Touching affected area Cold draughts	Chewing Yawning Talking
Relieving factors	Carbamazepine Phenytoin Surgical treatment: microvascular decompression or stereotactic thermocoagulation	Antidepressants Tranquillizers Limited success if syndrome well established	Prevention: Methysergide with lithium carbonate Acute attack: Ergotamine Sumatriptan (inj.)	Phenytoin Antidepressants may be necessary Imipramine Amitriptyline most effective	Maxillofacial opinion Bite correction or surgery

fifth nerve. Facial pain or a patch of numbness in these divisions should be regarded as being due to nasopharyngeal carcinoma until proved otherwise. Painless numbness over the chin is particularly ominous and, unless there is known trauma to the mandible, is likely to be due to malignant disease. The surprising fact that numbness rather than pain may occur with malignant infiltration of the fifth nerve was emphasized in Chapter 6, with illustrative cases.

Tumours in the cerebellopontine angle will usually distort the root of the fifth nerve but a pain resembling tic douloureux is rare. Careful examination in such a case will usually reveal other signs, such as a depressed corneal response or deafness, which are incompatible with the diagnosis of tic douloureux. However, tic douloureux may complicate two structural conditions in the cerebellopontine angle and skull base. These are Paget's disease and basilar impression due to senile osteoporosis. Both these conditions alter the anatomy of the tip of the petrous bone, which may irritate the trigeminal nerve root. Both may be diagnosed by plain skull x rays.

Aneurysmal dilatation of the carotid artery in the cavernous sinus will damage the first division of the fifth nerve, causing severe pain in the forehead and eye. This is accompanied by multiple extraocular nerve palsies and a bloodshot eye and the diagnosis should be quite obvious. It occurs mainly in hypertensive elderly women (see Chapter 5).

Ectasia of the basilar artery occurring in elderly hypertensive patients may produce considerable brainstem distortion and may present as trigeminal neuralgia (see Chapter 11).

The evaluation of a patient with facial pain depends on a very clear description of the location, quality and behaviour of the pain. With very few exceptions investigations will be normal, and in those cases where investigations will be of assistance, definite physical signs will usually be found. Therefore it is important to take a detailed history and carefully examine all the cranial nerves in a patient with facial pain. This can be a time-consuming exercise and for a proper assessment at least 40 minutes should be allowed. A snap diagnosis is likely to be incorrect.

22. Attacks of Altered Consciousness

This deliberately all-embracing title has been used to emphasize the fact that altered consciousness is not synonymous with epilepsy. From the patient's point of view the diagnosis of epilepsy has far-reaching implications, both for employment and social activities, and in some instances the inability to drive a motor vehicle may lead to loss of employment. In some countries there are still laws denying an epileptic patient the right to marry and have children, based on Victorian concepts as to the cause and nature of epilepsy. While the protection of the patient and the public implicit in the restrictions placed on an epileptic patient have to be accepted, the serious consequences of an incorrect diagnosis are obvious. There is only one thing worse than failing to correctly diagnose epilepsy and that is an incorrect diagnosis of epilepsy when the patient is suffering from another condition or may only have fainted.

Some patients are on anticonvulsant drugs quite unnecessarily because of overreliance on the significance of an EEG. Often the EEG has been allowed to act as a final arbiter in cases of clinical uncertainty, with diagnostic errors in both directions. The diagnosis must be firmly based on the history, and particularly on any eyewitness accounts that are available. It is worth going to any lengths to get such an account if there is any chance of locating the eye-witness to an attack. A long-distance phone call or even a detailed letter answering specific points may completely alter the diagnosis.

As epilepsy is such an enormous subject coverage will be confined to fairly classic identifiable attacks, and a neurological opinion is suggested for borderline cases. The alternative possibilities will be covered in greater detail than is usual in a textbook on neurology, as the alternatives lie in the field of general medicine and will often be diagnosed without recourse to neurological advice.

Epileptic Phenomena

Epileptic phenomena have been reclassified in recent years and a very complex international classification system now exists which, although clarifying various epileptic types based on clinical phenomena and associated EEG findings, has done little to clarify the situation for the neurological novice and general physician. As this book is mainly intended for these audiences, a more traditional framework in which to discuss epilepsy has been adhered to because, even using this simple classification, frequent errors are made in identifying the type of epilepsy and the most appropriate treatment, which are now accepted as the two main pillars of successful epileptic diagnosis and management.

Traditionally, epileptic attacks are classified into three main groups: petit mal attacks, complex partial seizures (previously called psychomotor seizures or temporal lobe attacks) and grand mal epilepsy (loss of consciousness with or without motor activity). There are considerable misconceptions about the exact meanings of these terms and serious therapeutic errors may result from mistaken diagnosis. The single most important error is an almost universal belief that the term 'petit mal' is a literal translation and merely means any short-lived attack, or any attack in which the patient falls but does not actually jerk or become incontinent.

Petit Mal (Generalized Absence Seizure)

Petit mal describes the single most easily identifiable and constant variant of epilepsy. It is very uncommon and accounts for less than 2% of all epilepsy cases. Attacks usually begin in childhood, between 5 and 10 years of age. It is very unusual for attacks to start after the age of 12. Episodes last 1–10 seconds and consist of a brief suspension of awareness. The motor activity may consist merely of some fluttering of the eyelids or a brief jerk of the hands. The facial expression may remain quite normal and facial colour does not alter. There is no confusion at the end of the episode and conversation or play will resume as if nothing had happened. The child is unaware that an attack has occurred. If there is any awareness it is normally because of the reaction of bystanders, and the child learns to sense that something must have happened. Attacks may occur at the rate of several per minute or even hundreds a day. The first evidence may be failing ability in the classroom, and a previously attentive and skilled child may start to fall behind their peers. The attacks themselves may be so brief that they pass unnoticed, and because the child is not aware of the events they are equally baffled as to what is going wrong. It is often the brothers and sisters who eventually draw attention to the absences.

The EEG is diagnostic. The abnormality consists of generalized runs of 2–3 Hz spike-wave activity, **always** associated with an observed attack. These may occur during the resting record and are particularly likely to be provoked by overbreathing, which is best achieved in small children by asking them to blow a handheld windmill on a stick. The technician recording the EEG will always write that an attack was observed, such as 'staring', eyelid fluttering', 'stopped counting' or 'stopped overbreathing' on the record during each attack. If the technician writes 'nil seen' opposite such a discharge the diagnosis of petit mal is **not** confirmed. This is the most common cause of misdiagnosis and may compound the error of an incorrect clinical suspicion of seizure type. In **any** epileptic patient the most frequent event seen on an EEG is a short run of spike-wave activity. This does not mean that the patient has petit mal unless the EEG technician **always** notes a clinical attack of petit mal at the same time. Non-neurologists reading an EEG factual report note that spike-wave activity at 2–3 Hz was seen and immediately conclude that the diagnosis is petit mal. This is a serious mistake because of the therapeutic problems that may follow.

The drug of choice for the treatment of petit mal is ethosuximide in a dose of 250–500 mg t.d.s. The response is dramatic and immediate, and often as little as 250 mg b.d. (morning and mid-afternoon) will suffice. If an incorrect diagnosis has been made and the episode is an atypical absence attack or a complex partial seizure, ethosuximide may actually be provocative and lead to a worsening of the epilepsy or the advent of major seizures, further compounding the diagnostic error. For this reason sodium valproate has achieved popularity as a treatment for petit mal, as it does not carry the risk of worsening other seizure types.

In a correctly diagnosed case there is very little risk of other seizure types supervening and most children are seizure free by puberty, and the medication can then be safely withdrawn. However, if the diagnosis was incorrect it is not uncommon for puberty to herald the onset of major epilepsy, supervening on what were actually complex partial seizures and totally altering the benign prognosis given to the parents when the incorrect diagnosis of petit mal was originally made.

In the UK there can also be a socially based diagnostic inaccuracy. In some circles the very benign-sounding 'it is only petit mal' is more acceptable than a diagnosis of 'epilepsy', and patients in their 20s still having unequivocal major epilepsy are sometimes encountered who have continued in the belief that their attacks do not constitute 'epilepsy' in the socially unacceptable sense of the word, and some have even obtained driving licences in the belief that they are not suffering from epilepsy.

Complex Partial Seizures (Temporal Lobe or Psychomotor Epilepsy)

A bewildering range of epileptic phenomena arise in the temporal lobe. Brief episodes of this type are those most often mistakenly diagnosed as 'petit mal'. There are many features to distinguish these 'minor' attacks, not the least being that petit mal is an unlikely diagnosis in a anyone over 20 years of age.

In a child the differentiation may present some difficulty but a careful history will usually elicit the following pointers:

1. The child will become pale and obviously distressed.
2. They may complain of abdominal pain or nausea, or funny sensations in the perineum.
3. They may just run and hold on to their parent in an alarmed and frightened way, but are unable to describe what is happening.

There is no doubt at all that the child is **aware** that something is wrong. This is totally different from true petit mal, where the child is the last person to be aware that anything unusual is happening to them. The episode may be very brief, perhaps 5–10 seconds, or may last several minutes. It is often followed by a period of confusion and drowsiness. They will not resume their previous conversation or play activity, where they left off. Sometimes uncontrolled laughter may occur as part of the attack. This is called 'gelastic' epilepsy.

In older patients an epigastric sensation, often described as if something were 'rising up' inside the abdomen or chest, may be followed by pallor, lip-smacking or chewing movement, and more complex 'zombie-like' activity. Recurrent irrelevant sentences may be uttered but no formal conversation can be carried on with the patient. These sentences may always be the same: one patient said 'what a funny place to put a carpet' as a prelude to all her documented attacks!

Afterwards the patient is usually aware that an attack has occurred, as they feel confused, 'washed out' or sleepy, but they are amnesic for any events that occurred while consciousness was impaired. The patient may recall that just before the onset a sense of familiarity with the situation (déjà vu) or, conversely, failure to identify their own room or surroundings (jamais vu) had occurred. Sometimes it is familiarity with the words that are being spoken (déjà entendu) or even the feeling that they know exactly what is going to be said next that may precede the onset.

In other instances a sudden unpleasant taste in the mouth (gustatory aura) or a sudden unpleasant smell (olfactory aura) may be noticed. These phenomena are extremely brief: the patient does not have the opportunity to identify the smell or taste with certainty, only that it is always unpleasant. These latter phenomena are thought to arise in the uncus and are sometimes known as 'uncinate' fits.

Sometimes patients notice alterations in their perception of time: either everything will seem to be happening in slow motion or everything seems speeded up. This may be one of the reasons that the patient's own view of the duration of an attack may differ from that of observers. The patient's feeling that he felt 'funny' and 'nodded off for a second' may in fact encompass several minutes of frankly peculiar behaviour and complex repetitive motor activity for which they have no memory. Because of the amnesia and the complex motor activity the patient may find themselves in a different room or, if the attack occurs in the street, several hundred yards from their intended destination.

Patients may experience episodes of this sort for months or even years without realizing their significance. They may only come to light when an episode proceeds to a major convulsion or perhaps a nocturnal fit is observed, and in questioning the patient as to other episodes a classic history of previous attacks of this sort emerges.

Complex partial seizures are without doubt both the most frequent type of episode occurring in adulthood and the most difficult to control with medication. Nearly all the advances in the therapeutics of epilepsy in recent years have evolved from attempts to control this particular seizure type but unfortunately, although all drugs prove similarly effective against major seizures, there is still no universally effective drug that will control complex partial seizures.

The currently accepted drugs of choice are carbamazepine in a dose of 100–400 mg t.d.s. or sodium valproate 200–1000 mg t.d.s., the doses being titrated against seizure control and, to a lesser extent, serum levels of the anticonvulsant. Phenytoin 300–600 mg daily, monitored by blood levels, can be successful but may sometimes worsen complex partial seizures. These three agents are the front-line drugs and in the last 3 years three additional agents have become available, used in conjunction with one of the above. These are lamotrigine, in a dose of 50–200 mg b.d., vigabatrin

in a dose of 500–1000 mg b.d. and gabapentin in a dose of 300–600 mg t.d.s. All may produce a significant reduction in episodes but rarely achieve complete control. Two diazepam-derivative drugs, clonazepam in a dose of 0.25–2.0 mg t.d.s. and clobazam in a dose of 10 mg nocte to 10 mg t.d.s., can be extremely effective, but it is claimed that the effect wanes rapidly. This view is currently subject to further investigation.

Tonic–Clonic Seizures (Grand Mal or Major Seizures)

These epileptic events are those most generally immediately recognized as 'fits'. The main requirement is that the patient completely loses consciousness, and if unsupported will fall to the ground. There may be a brief warning (the aura), which is often one of the features noted in complex partial seizures, and the collapse may or may not be associated with involuntary movements or incontinence.

Under the definition tonic–clonic fits a sequence of involuntary movements is required, but using the more general definition of major epilepsy, one of the variants that is most difficult to distinguish from a syncopal attack is the type known as an 'akinetic seizure'. In these episodes the patient suddenly falls forwards on to the face and then, after a brief period of rigidity, consciousness is regained. The absence of prodromal symptoms and the tendency to injury, particularly to the nose and brows, are useful pointers to the diagnosis of this type of epilepsy. It is a particularly common pattern of epilepsy in seriously brain-damaged patients and a clear indication for the wearing of a suitable crash helmet by sufferers. These patients are readily identified by multiple scars on the eyebrows and lips, a broken nose and the absence of front teeth.

Classic major attacks with tonic–clonic movements leave little doubt as to their nature. They most often occur during sleep or first thing in the morning, the bathroom being a favourite venue. Attacks during the day are much less frequent. If the patient is awake the attack may occur without warning: the patient suddenly stares, may appear to look around the room and stiffens. The contraction of the chest muscles may sometimes lead to a groan or a shout, and the patient then crashes to the ground and may sustain injury. The seriousness of this will depend entirely on the situation and attacks in the bathroom are particularly dangerous, whereas attacks occurring in bed carry little hazard. During this time the patient will become progressively anoxic and pass through a phase of being bright red in the face and appearing to be straining, to an increasingly dusky hue. By this time they may have bitten their tongue or been incontinent of urine. Suddenly the patient will go limp, and after a further period of 15–30 seconds will resume breathing but in a stertorous way.

If their mouth is damaged they will blow frothy bubbles and an alarming gush of blood from the now relaxed mouth will occur.

Traditional attempts to force the mouth open with a variety of metal or wooden implements during the tonic phase is unhelpful. It will not facilitate breathing because the patient is not breathing anyway, will usually damage the teeth, and if the tongue has not already been bitten, may open the teeth sufficiently for the tongue to sustain damage if the mouth clamps shut again. For similar reasons, the application of an oxygen mask is unavailing, although reassuring to bystanders. If possible – and this is sometimes difficult to achieve – the patient should be rolled on to their side or face into an approximation of the recovery position.

The patient will then start to jerk rhythmically, which may have a focal onset in one limb, and if so this is important to note. Typically, it will be of generalized onset, rhythmic and symmetrical. The movements tend to occur with the patient in a flexed posture and forced extension of the back should be regarded with some suspicion (see later), although backward jerking of the head against a wall or floor may be sufficiently forceful to cause further injury. It is best not to restrain the patient at this stage but to make sure that they are not sustaining further injury against hard objects. Any purposeful or resistive movements at this stage should again arouse suspicion. This clonic phase may last several minutes and is followed by the patient becoming completely limp, continuing to breath deeply and going into a deep unrousable sleep. If they are wakened they will usually be extremely confused, a situation further compounded when they find that their bedroom is filled with neighbours, ambulancemen or policemen – a scenario which is repeated all over the country every night of the year!

Because the majority of patients have their attacks in bed on awakening or shortly thereafter, neurologists see surprisingly few actual seizures, so much so that when a patient has a convenient attack in the clinic one immediately wonders whether it is organically based!

Although incontinence of urine and injury are thought to be diagnostic of epilepsy, both can occur in other types of unconsciousness, including 'simple faints', especially if the faint occurs in a dangerous situation such as a bathroom or a public toilet. These are common locations because the premonitory symptoms of a faint prompt the patient to seek privacy and somewhere to vomit. These symptoms should always be very carefully assessed. Less than half the patients with epilepsy have ever been incontinent in an attack and relatively few have ever sustained a serious injury, but patients who faint with a full bladder can be incontinent of urine and if they faint in a dangerous situation may sustain injuries similar to those occurring in a fit. Although great significance is always placed on the epileptic aura, the premonitory symptom of a pending fit is often a very brief peculiar sensation which may be unique to that patient or no more than an awareness that it is about to happen again. It never consists of a prolonged period of feeling increasingly peculiar and ill, and almost never will the patient say 'I think I am going to pass out'. If the patient has time to involve bystanders in what is about to happen it is infinitely more likely to be a faint than a fit.

Another common variant of major epilepsy that it is important to identify is preceded by morning myoclonus. This may only be discovered in response to a direct question, as the patient may not have realized its significance. The patient will have noticed that when they first awaken, while cleaning their teeth, putting on make-up or eating their breakfast, brief uncontrolled jerks will intrude causing injury or spillage. The term 'messy breakfast syndrome' finds immediate recognition in these patients. They will often realize in retrospect that major episodes have only ever occurred as the culmination of a series of such jolts and if there have been no early morning myoclonic jolts there is no risk of them having a fit later in the day. There are often specific EEG changes and effective treatment exists for this variant, which will be discussed later.

The diagnosis of epilepsy does not mean that the patient has a cerebral tumour, in fact the risk of this is extremely low. Even in the peak decade for cerebral tumours (45–55 years of age) prospective studies have shown that less than 10% of this highly selected group presenting with a first epileptic seizure eventually prove to have a cerebral tumour.

Cerebral tumours can present as epilepsy in all age groups. Very rarely, children under 15 may have gliomas but the order of risk ranges from 0.02% below 15 years of age to 10% at 50 years of age. Careful history-taking and physical examination is important in selecting tumour suspects. In any age group a focal onset, residual weakness or numbness after an attack, or a focal abnormality on EEG should certainly be taken into consideration. In children, however, focal onset attacks, focal EEG abnormality and a postictal Todd's paralysis occur so often that these findings rarely prove to be of ominous significance.

In the adult residual weakness after an attack has very ominous implications, and it is perhaps wrong to use the expression 'Todd's paralysis', with its benign connotation, in this group. If an appropriate focal EEG abnormality is found further investigation is indicated. At this stage non-neurologists are usually quite happy if cerebral scanning reveals no abnormality. The neurologist is not so readily reassured. 'Once a tumour suspect, always a tumour suspect' is a useful rule. Several examples of this problem will be found in Chapter 8. In the past, patients often developed neurological signs some 5–15 years after initial negative investigation, and reinvestigation then revealed the tumour that had been there throughout. Some might regard this as a serious diagnostic failure, but when one considers the possible consequences of cerebral surgery, if a patient can conceal their tumour for 15 years it is very much to their advantage.

There are two case reports in Chapter 8 (Case report XXXII on page 126 and XXXVI on page 131) that are striking examples of the need to continually reconsider the diagnosis of epilepsy, and indeed the possibility of an underlying lesion, however long the history and however reassuring or misleading the EEG. This is worth emphasis because for 50 years the EEG has been regarded as a critical diagnostic tool and final arbiter in the field of epileptic diagnosis and the management of collapse. To the non-neurologist it is accorded the status of an oracle, and patients who have clearly had a fit may be allowed to resume driving because the EEG was normal. Conversely, a patient who had merely fainted and was unfortunate enough to have a 'precautionary' EEG that showed minor abnormalities might find themselves banned from driving, with consequent loss of employment. The EEG should only constitute a small part in the overall assessment of patients with 'funny turns' and collapses.

If a patient is found to have a cerebral tumour, it is surgical accessibility and the potential physical defects resulting from surgery that governs operation, not the mere demonstration of the tumour. There is also a widely held view that uncontrolled epilepsy indicates the presence of a tumour, but this is certainly not the case and one of the disarming features of epilepsy associated with cerebral tumours is that it is often easy to control. The only exception to this is the tendency for frontal tumours to cause status epilepticus (see Chapter 9).

Treatment of Tonic–Clonic Seizures

The three standard drugs, phenytoin, carbamazepine and sodium valproate, have been shown to have equal efficacy and will completely control tonic–clonic seizures in some 70% of cases. If the first drug used fails, the use of an alternative drug, an additional second-line anticonvulsant such as lamotrigine, vigabatrin or gabapentin, or a combination of two of the major drugs, should be considered. There is increasing emphasis on using a higher dose at night to minimize sedative side-effects, but this also effectively targets the most vulnerable time, which is during sleep or first thing in the morning. Where fits have always occurred at these times, smaller holding doses may be sufficient during the day.

The identification of morning grand mal attacks preceded by myoclonic jerking is therapeutically important. Sodium valproate may prove extremely effective used overnight. Alternatively, clonazepam 0.5–2 mg overnight may be completely effective and prove a simpler regimen, if very few major fits have ever occurred. If either of these agents fails, methsuximide 300 mg nocte may prove effective. Unlike ethosuximide, a closely related agent, this does not seem to carry the risk of provoking major episodes and can be dramatically effective for this variant of epilepsy.

The drug which is finally chosen and the exact dosing schedule will depend on the individual patient. Monitoring blood levels has almost become an article of faith in some quarters, but its value lies mainly in establishing that the patient is indeed taking the medication and is metabolizing it normally. Very rarely does forcing the drug levels into the so-called 'therapeutic range' suddenly control the epilepsy. In some patients complete control is established without the patient ever achieving these standard levels. It is important to recognize that the object of the exercise is to prevent fits occurring rather than achieving an 'ideal' blood level.

Uncontrolled Epilepsy

It is a sad fact that where epilepsy is a consequence of brain damage sustained in infancy, following brain trauma or after cerebral vascular accidents, complete control may prove impossible. However, the use of appropriate medication will almost always achieve some small improvement to justify the effort. If all attempts are unavailing, before accepting that this is truly uncontrollable epilepsy there are some important questions to ask. Perhaps surprisingly, the first is 'is it really epilepsy?' and this is the subject of the next section. In specialist centres other causes of collapse or pseudoseizures are responsible for some 30% of uncontrolled 'epilepsy'.

'Has the type of epilepsy been correctly identified?' If complex partial seizures are misidentified as petit mal, the use of ethosuximide may not only increase the number of attacks but may also provoke major seizures. Conversely, the use of phenytoin in a patient with true petit mal may provoke petit mal status. It is for this reason that sodium valproate is such a popular drug in paediatric practice, as it is effective for both types of epilepsy.

In the occasional patient almost all major anticonvulsant drugs will make the situation **worse**, and even provoke status epilepticus. If the addition of a new drug to the regimen is accompanied by worsening of attacks, this possibility should always be considered.

The possibility that toxic levels of any major anticonvulsant drug may **cause** convulsions is also often overlooked. This situation may occur in complex multiple anticonvulsant drug regimens, or when other drugs are used without allowing for metabolic interactions.

Finally, the possibility that the patient is taking excess alcohol or has been given other drugs that may be epileptogenic should be considered. These include antidepressants, major tranquillizers, antimalarials and amantadine hydrochloride. The group most frequently inadvertently used, sometimes in 'over-the-counter medications', are the antihistamines. These may be taken for allergic phenomena or gastrointestinal upset while on holiday, unless epileptic patients are specifically warned of this risk.

Pseudoseizures (Non-Organic Epileptic Events)

It is source of surprise to relatives and other doctors that patients should wish to simulate events which have such a dramatic impact on their social acceptability and other activities, but there is no doubt that pseudoseizures are very much more common than is generally appreciated. For this reason they are also underdiagnosed by non-specialist physicians. This difficulty is compounded if a patient with genuine epilepsy chooses to supplement their genuine attacks with pseudoseizures for effect, or to avoid difficult situations. This is particularly common in the institutional situation.

There are several very strong pointers to non-organic events.

1. They tend to occur randomly and in public: indeed, the vast majority of events occurring in the waiting area of the neurology outpatients department tend to be of this variety.

2. The posture adopted is usually diagnostic and is a hyperextended or frankly opisthotonic type with the back arched, which can only be achieved by the patient lying on their side. This particular posture has been referred to 'hysteroid epilepsy'.

3. Typically the eyes are held tightly shut; in genuine epilepsy the eyes are open and usually roll up. Attempts to open the eyes for examination are firmly resisted and, if successful, the eyes will be seen to come down from below the lids to stare straight ahead, demonstrating a normal Bell's phenomenon. When a conscious patient shuts their eyes they automatically roll up into the head, but in an unconscious patient the eyes will stare straight ahead and are obviously doing so the moment the eyelids are pulled open. This finding alone should preclude the need for the aggressive demonstration of an intact corneal reflex, which in the unconscious patient is depressed or absent.

4. Any limb movement tends to be jerky and irregular and may become semipurposive. If a bystander attempts to move the patient, a punch or a kick towards the person concerned is diagnostic! Similarly, attempts to elicit the plantar responses will provoke a dramatic withdrawal of the legs or an equally dramatic kick in the direction of the would-be examiner.

5. Later, when the patient is just lying still and apparently unconscious, eyelid fluttering may be a prominent feature and the patient may be amenable to suggestion. For example, telling a nurse that the patient 'will usually turn on to their left side' at that stage will usually be rewarded by the patient doing just that. Even more dramatically, on one occasion I was called back to the bedside when a patient had 'recovered' to be told that if I ever talked about him like that again while he was 'unconscious' he would punch me on the nose! All I had done was to demonstrate to the attending nurses those features that indicated that the episode was not an epileptic event.

CASE REPORT I

A 22-year-old female university student in her first term was transferred to be nearer her home from a hospital in the north of England. She had been under the care of her uncle, a consultant physician, in status epilepticus for 1 week. She arrived on a diazepam infusion, continuing to have what were clear-cut non-organic epileptic events during which a standard 16-channel EEG remained normal. She was confronted with the situation and promised that she would be allowed to resume driving in the near future if she stopped. This proved more effective than the intravenous medication. She subsequently admitted that she had had a crisis of confidence as to whether she had chosen the correct degree course, and 3 years later wrote a letter of thanks for the way she had been handled and to confirm that she had obtained a first-class honours degree.

This case also emphasizes the disadvantage of being looked after by a relative. No-one had dared to suggest the possibility of non-organicity because of the family relationship of the original attending physician.

Nursing staff who choose to behave in this way may present further difficulties by using mydriatic eyedrops, self-administered insulin or thyroid hormone, or even by producing factitious septicaemia. They may also be deliberately incontinent of urine or faeces to further dramatize events. It is important to regard such patients as ill and in need of help, and not to allow the situation to become adversarial. It is vital that, having established the correct diagnosis, appropriate psychological and medical help is provided.

Electroencephalography (EEG)

The EEG has the considerable advantages of being harmless, inexpensive and easily repeatable. Unfortunately, EEG findings are relatively non-specific and their value depends on careful correlation with the history and physical findings. For this reason any physician ordering an EEG should have a clear idea as to what information he expects it to provide. The EEG can give both false negative and false positive results and serious errors can only be avoided if these limitations are recognized.

Technique

The patient sits in a comfortable chair in a quiet room and either saline-soaked pads or stick-on electrodes are applied to the scalp in internationally agreed positions. Considerable technical skill is involved in assuring good electrical contact to avoid artefacts. Recordings are made on a multichannel machine using special arrangements of electrodes, known as montages, in anterior–posterior and transverse positions to provide a grid of information. This enables the technician to isolate an abnormality in two planes.

The resting record is taken with the patient sitting quietly and opening and closing their eyes on command. This reveals the basic alpha rhythm, which normally 'blocks' (i.e. attenuates or disappears) on eye opening. The resting record may be normal. The first provocative procedure then begins. The patient is asked to hyperventilate for 3 minutes, which is best achieved by breathing out fully at the end of each breath rather than trying to take deep breaths. This normally causes a slowing in rhythms and an increase in amplitude and may be enhanced by hunger, and this is the reason that the time of the patient's last meal is always documented on the EEG. This accentuates any abnormalities and may provoke frank epileptic discharges in epileptic patients. Finally, a flickering strobe light is placed in front of the patient and the flicker rate varied. Many normal people show a following response, producing phasic potentials over the occipital pole at the same rate as the flicker. In photosensitive epilepsy epileptic discharges and even an epileptic fit may be provoked.

When the clinical suspicion of epilepsy or an intracerebral lesion is high and the routine EEG is normal, further provocative measures can be used coupled with special electrode placements. The inner and inferior surfaces of the temporal lobe are inaccessible to normally sited electrodes. An electrode in the pharynx or, more commonly, a wire inserted under the base of the skull through a special needle, a sphenoidal electrode, can used to detect abnormalities in this area. This special recording technique may be coupled with a sleep-deprived and a sleep recording. If non-stop seizure bursts are seen, the use of intravenous diazepam during the recording can be very instructive and typically the abnormal activity ceases immediately.

Interpretation

A full discussion of EEG abnormalities would require several chapters; only a brief mention of the most significant wave forms is possible here.

Alpha Rhythm

The alpha rhythm consists of cyclic activity at a rate of 8–12 Hz, most easily seen in the posterior leads and apparent when the eyes are closed. The voltage is normally slightly lower over the dominant hemisphere. Unilateral absence of the alpha rhythm could indicate a lesion in that hemisphere.

Beta Rhythm

A beta rhythm consists of fast activity at rates of 20–22 Hz, usually maximal in the frontal leads. It is increased in anxious patients and markedly increased by all sedative drugs and tranquillizers. Asymmetry of beta activity may indicate an underlying lesion on the side of the reduction, but this is less reliable than asymmetrical alpha activity. If prominent in patients not known to be on sedative drugs possible sedative drug abuse may be suspected.

Theta Rhythm

Theta waves occur at rates of 5–7 Hz and are responsible for most diagnostic confusion. They are normally present in childhood but diminish with maturation of the EEG in adolescence. They often reappear during overbreathing and a minor symmetrical 'increase in theta activity' in the temporal leads is of dubious significance. As with other rhythms, marked asymmetry is significant and suggests a lesion in the temporal lobe on the side of the theta activity. Quite marked theta rhythm changes are often found in the absence of any subsequent CT or MRI scan abnormality.

Delta Rhythm

Delta waves are the most significant and ominous abnormalities seen in the EEG. They consist of slow waves of very low to extremely high voltage at rates of 1–4 Hz. In children delta activity is often seen in the resting record, and is greatly accentuated by overbreathing. This is not pathological in children but is grossly abnormal in the adult. A focal delta wave abnormality nearly always indicates a serious lesion in the underlying brain.

The use of the EEG in the investigation of attacks of unconsciousness was discussed earlier. The importance of careful clinical evaluation of the attack must again be emphasized. The EEG cannot confirm whether someone is epileptic or not, and if a syncopal attack is certain an EEG is unnecessary. Conversely, if the patient had an unequivocal epileptic convulsion a normal EEG cannot alter the diagnosis. Overinterpretation of minor abnormalities may condemn a patient who has only fainted to years of unnecessary restrictions and anticonvulsant drugs. Even worse, an epileptic patient may remain untreated and be allowed to continue normal activities because the EEG was normal.

The potential value of the EEG varies in different types of epilepsy. In petit mal the EEG is invariably diagnostically abnormal, with spike-wave discharges at 2–3 Hz always accompanied by an observed episode. In grand mal epilepsy the initial EEG is normal in 40% of patients, although a positive yield may be increased if several further EEGs are done in the ensuing months. The 'false negative' rate may be even higher in patients with nocturnal epilepsy and akinetic grand mal. When akinetic grand mal or grand mal is preceded by myoclonic jerking, a characteristic 'poly-spike wave' pattern may be found. This consists of several high-voltage spikes preceding a slow wave occurring across all leads, somewhat similar to the abnormality seen in petit mal but not necessarily accompanied by an observed attack.

The EEG is of limited value in the follow-up of epileptic patients unless, in spite of normal scanning, an underlying lesion is still suspected. The EEG may become normal as children with epilepsy mature, in spite of continuing attacks. Conversely, a grossly abnormal EEG may persist in patients who have been attack-free for years. In such cases the risk of recurrence is high if treatment is discontinued.

The only clear indication for repeating EEGs is where the diagnosis of epilepsy remains uncertain, where the seizure type remains unclassified or where entirely new symptoms appear which would justify an EEG in their own right. The introduction of simultaneous video monitoring of the patient has increased the value of the EEG in determining seizure type, and is particularly useful where prolonged recording is necessary to pick up an attack.

The use of more sophisticated graphic displays of EEG data produces impressive presentations but has not dramatically improved the diagnostic ability of EEG. The advent of 24-hour EEG monitoring with a portable six-lead machine is of more value, especially if a documented episode is witnessed during the recording period. Unfortunately, the machine may be damaged during a seizure and one patient suspected of having non-organic episodes chose to disconnect his tape and smash the recording machine in anger. Twenty-four-hour recordings are of particular value in patients suspected of suffering non-organic pseudoseizures. They usually continue to have their episodes with abandon, and even allowing for the inevitable movement artefact it is quite clear that there are no accompanying epileptic discharges.

In the investigation of suspected intracranial lesions there are several problems. Quite substantial extracerebral lesions may fail to produce any EEG abnormality, whereas small intrinsic tumours may produce subtle or even generalized EEG abnormalities for many years before further investigation confirms the presence of a tumour (see Case reports in earlier chapters). When there are obvious clinical findings the EEG usually merely confirms the location of the lesion but cannot provide conclusive evidence of its nature; for example, an EEG cannot distinguish a recent cerebrovascular accident from a tumour.

In the investigation of headache there are difficulties due to the wide range of abnormalities that have been reported in association with migraine, abnormalities that might even suggest a neoplastic lesion in a 'non-migrainous' subject.

Having stressed the limitations of EEG in diagnostic neurology it is only fair to reiterate the immense value of the test as a simple, safe and inexpensive screening procedure. It remains an extremely useful investigation in patients with atypical psychiatric disorders and dementia, and is the first investigation indicated in suspected epilepsy.

Status Epilepticus

The most feared potentially lethal complication of epilepsy is major status epilepticus. This occurs when convulsive fits follow one another **without** recovery of consciousness between episodes.

Absence status and complex partial seizure status produce a confused 'twilight' state in which the patient partially rouses, the eyes appear to stare then glaze over, the head drops and the mouth drools. The patient may moan and then appears to lighten and may start to lift the head up again, and then the whole process is repeated. This state can last for several days and is particularly common in severely brain-damaged epileptic patients. Minor status epilepticus of these types does not threaten the patient's life but may inflict further damage on the already compromised brain.

Major status epilepticus is life-threatening and immediate effective treatment is obligatory. The death rate approaches 60% untreated, and even with skilled management the death rate is 10%. There is some evidence that the longer the status continues the harder it becomes treat, so that skilled advice should be sought the moment it is clear that the attacks are not coming under control.

Management

1. If possible identify the cause. This may include missed medication, provocative drugs or alcohol, intercurrent infection (including meningitis), metabolic

abnormality (including hypoglycaemia) or new cerebral pathology in a long-standing epileptic patient.

2. Full cardiorespiratory support should be established with intravenous access. Blood for routine haematological, biochemical and drug level studies is taken.

3. An infusion of dextrose–saline supplemented with vitamin B$_1$ should be started.

4. Diazepam should be given intravenously. Care should be taken to establish whether intravenous or rectal diazepam had already been given prior to admission. In UK a 10 mg bolus repeated once within the first 60 minutes is usually given. In the USA an infusion at the rate 2 mg/min up to 20 mg maximum is preferred. Either regimen is effective in 80% of patients and there is no doubt that the effectiveness of diazepam has transformed the management of this condition.

5. If the patient has for some reason missed their normal medication, when blood levels are available their normal drugs should be reinstituted, via nasogastric tube if necessary. If this simple precaution is neglected, the risk of further status when the acute drugs are discontinued is high.

6. If the patient is not a known epileptic or is not on oral phenytoin, intravenous phenytoin may be used next if diazepam fails. In such cases 50 mg/min up to 250 mg should be given. It is worth monitoring the ECG during this as phenytoin may cause heart block. Another 600 mg may be given orally over the next few hours. The total loading dose (i.v. + oral) should not exceed 15 mg/kg, which is approximately 900 mg in the adult. If the patient is already on phenytoin only the 250 mg intravenous loading dose should be used until blood levels are available.

7. If these measures fail (convulsions continue 60 minutes after these measures are completed), in the UK chlormethiazole is infused at a rate of 0.7 G/hr. This is given intravenously as a 0.8% solution infused at 60 drops/min until convulsions cease, and then reduced gradually to 10 drops/min while other anticonvulsants have time to take effect. This treatment seems not to be used in the USA.

8. Before diazepam, paraldehyde was a widely used and effective agent. Its mode of action remains uncertain. The drug must be fresh and administered **only** via a glass syringe (it dissolves plastic). The loading dose is 10 ml, given as 5 ml into the upper outer quadrant of each buttock. A dose of 5 ml 4-hourly may be repeated over the next 24 hours. It may cause sterile abscesses and produces an unpleasant garlic-like smell that permeates the ward for several days but it can be life-saving. Paraldehyde is no longer readily available in the USA but its demise is hard to understand. It is extremely safe and would be the author's preferred next choice should diazepam fail. Perhaps the effectiveness of diazepam has led to a whole generation of neurologists who are no longer aware of its value?

9. Patients who respond initially to diazepam and then relapse may be maintained by a diazepam infusion, but in some cases clonazepam 0.1 mg/kg intravenously per 24 hours may be more effective in maintaining control, and either of these two measures is also the treatment of choice in minor, partial status epilepticus.

10. The use of intravenous barbiturates is not recommended. If the patient has already had diazepam the risk of respiratory depression is high, and the wearing-off effect of barbiturates can actually provoke further seizures.

11. If all measures fail general anaesthesia, with muscle relaxants and positive pressure respiration, may be used. Unfortunately this only shelves the problem and there is concern that permitting continuing uncontrolled cerebral activity causes further damage to the brain, in spite of the reassuring absence of convulsive phenomena and accompanying anoxia achieved by this strategy. It should only be used when it is anticipated that the treatment initiated for intercurrent problems and newly introduced anticonvulsants are going to be effective in due course, and that the patient will not promptly resume status when the anaesthesia is discontinued.

It is very important to seek expert advice **quickly** for any patient in status epilepticus. A differential diagnostic guide to epileptic events is provided in Table 22.1.

Syncopal Attacks

Syncopal attacks, vasodepressor syncope, vasovagal attacks or simple faints are the main differential diagnosis in a patient who has had an attack of unconsciousness, or more colloquially a 'black-out'. A careful history should reveal the diagnosis. Diagnostic problems are commonly created when a bystander with presumed medical knowledge confidently diagnoses an epileptic fit. Elderly retired nurses are particularly likely to rush to this diagnosis and it can be very hard to undo the harm that acceptance of their opinion produces. Frequently patients who have collapsed in a dentist's chair, or following a blood test at a doctor's surgery, find themselves in the same situation simply because medical personnel misinterpret what they are seeing and are more inclined to make a diagnosis than document exactly what they witnessed. The circumstantial evidence surrounding the attack may be much more important than eye-witness diagnosis.

The attack is often postural, and indeed it is very unusual for an attack to occur in any position other than sitting or standing.

There are two major requirements:

Table 22.1 Differential diagnosis of epileptic variants

Epilepsy	Petit mal	Complex partial seizures	Major convulsions	Akinetic grand mal
Age	5–15 years	Any age	Any age	Any age
Onset	Instantaneous	Prolonged prodrome	Very brief warning if any	None at all: suddenly crash forwards
Duration	5–10 seconds	From few seconds to hours or days	2–5 min	30–60 seconds
Type of attack	Brief suspension of awareness then resume previous activity	Prolonged altered behaviour: may culminate in major attack	Period of rigidity with cyanosis (tonic phase) then generalized jerking (clonic phase) then sleep	Unheralded sudden fall Very brief attack. Little or no jerking but injury risk high
Facial features	Eyelids may flutter or 'day dreaming'	Pallor, anxious bewildered look Lip-smacking or chewing movements Looking round room	Unconsciousness Eyes may roll up or to the sides	No particular features Facial features are always coarse due to repeated trauma: brow, nose & teeth all damaged
Limbs	Slight jerking movements of arms but unusual to have any movement	Rather ponderous 'zombie' activity or fiddling with clothing	Generalized jerking Look for **focal** jerking at onset or focal weakness after	Initially rigid then quite still Breathing stertorous
End of attack	Abrupt No confusion	Confused and amnesic	Confused, drowsy Headache	Often severe headache
Continence	Very rarely incontinent	Rarely incontinent	Occasionally incontinent	Occasionally incontinent
EEG	Invariably abnormal and diagnostic Always associated with clinical attack with each seizure burst	Often abnormal: sphenoidal record may increase value	Normal in 40% patients in interictal phase	May be normal or show generalized abnormalities

1. The patient is often primed to collapse by an ongoing or sudden stressful emotional situation.
2. For the actual episode to occur, the physical circumstances must be provocative.

A very hot day, prolonged standing, hot stuffy rooms, a hot bath or severe abdominal pain may all predispose to a sudden drop in blood pressure. If the patient is already under emotional stress an attack is more likely. If there have been multiple attacks over a relatively short period it is almost guaranteed that the patient is in the middle of some emotional crisis, although at first they may conceal this. Even when small children start fainting regularly at school, background family pressures often underlie a series of collapses.

Most patients who are prone to syncope have a history of fainting in school assembly, at church, during their periods or when in stressful situations already established by their early teens. Girls and boys seem equally vulnerable at this age, although attacks in girls are more predictable and are sometimes period related due to dysmenorrhoea. Boys tend to be less likely to carry the tendency into adulthood, whereas girls who have fainted regularly in their teens will often continue to do so as an adult. In males at any age 'fainting' is usually associated with emotional pressures in provocative circumstances.

In some cases a faint may be almost instantaneous. This is often in situations that are obviously dramatic and include the sight of blood, severe emotional shock or extreme fear, when the circumstances would automatically lead to the presumption that a faint has occurred. Unfortunately, in a very sudden attack of this type there are no classic prodromal symptoms and an increased likelihood that some convulsive movements may be noted at the height of the attack. In such cases the circumstantial evidence should be regarded as diagnostic. Surprisingly often people learning first aid faint when shown videos of injuries, and in spite of the obvious provocation are invariably diagnosed by other members of the group as having had a fit.

In a typical syncopal attack there is quite a long prodromal period of 'feeling faint'. This is often described as a feeling of hunger, coldness with 'goose-pimples', or suddenly feeling very hot, light-headed and clammy. Speckles of light with gradual misting or blacking out of vision accompany the dizzy sensation. Noises seem to become louder until a sudden silence, which is the usual prelude to the actual loss of consciousness. This often happens as the patient unwisely gets to their feet to 'get some fresh air' or in an attempt to get to a toilet. They may manage to reach a more dangerous location before they actually collapse, converting what would have been a faint into a head injury.

It is generally believed that as soon as the patient falls to the ground they become conscious, as cerebral blood flow is restored, but in many instances they will not become fully conscious for several minutes, and if this is not appreciated a more serious cause of collapse will be suspected. As the patient is in the process of collapsing they go deathly white and start to sweat profusely. This is a response to adrenaline outpouring and is absolutely the reverse of an epileptic event, where the patient's colour will remain normal or they may even flush or become slightly blue in the face, as if straining.

In a faint the 'deathly white' appearance suggests that the patient is dead, and this view is compounded because their pulse is barely perceptible. It seems likely that many apparently successful resuscitations performed by the public have been an incorrect interpretation of the natural history of a severe faint. Perhaps the most diagnostic feature that can be obtained from the patient's own history is that as they are coming round they feel as if they are wakening from a deep sleep and can hear voices talking about them or to them, as in the distance. There is a distinct gap before vision returns, and they then see faces staring down at them. At that stage they are often aware that they feel cold and shivery, having felt extremely hot just before the collapse, and nausea and even vomiting may rapidly ensue.

If the patient attempts to get up immediately they may well collapse again, and if this is clearly documented it is further definitive evidence of syncope. Fainting can only occur in the supine position in a few rare pathological states. These include diabetic autonomic neuropathy, tabes dorsalis, Shy–Drager syndrome (autonomic neuropathy and parkinsonism), late pregnancy and during severe blood loss.

Cerebral anoxia occurs during a faint because of impaired cerebral blood flow, which is the cause of the loss of consciousness. If the patient is deliberately held in an upright position or is not allowed to lie flat, an epileptic event may ensue. Attempts by bystanders to get the patient upright cause more problems than they solve. Probably the most public demonstration of how not to manage a syncopal attack was recently seen on television when President George Bush fainted during a banquet in Japan: instead of being allowed to lie flat he was immediately hauled to his feet by an army of attendants! There is little doubt that with increasing age

there is a greater risk of a simple syncopal attack terminating in an epileptic seizure.

It is accepted that in some 15% of otherwise classic syncopal attacks the patients eyes will roll up and some generalized jerking of the limbs, which is perhaps best described as shivering or jactitation, rather than convulsing, is observed. Even if a more definite epileptic event supervenes on what clearly started as a syncopal attack, based on circumstances, the patient's own history and the observations of bystanders, the patient need not be regarded as suffering from epilepsy even for driving licence purposes. During a syncopal attack the prolonged warning usually allows the patient to fall fairly gracefully, the collapse resembling a sack of potatoes collapsing to the ground. Occasionally the patient will injure themselves. This is particularly likely if they are out in the street, in a toilet or a bathroom, and urinary incontinence may occur if the patient has a full bladder at the time.

An EEG is rarely of help in this situation. Most neurologists, if they are certain that a faint occurred, would not arrange an EEG. This is because some 20% of nonepileptic patients have minor EEG abnormalities and such findings might cause diagnostic confusion. It is best to rely on clinical judgement in this situation and to arrange for the patient to report any further attacks and go to some lengths to obtain eye-witness accounts.

Specific Types of Syncopal Attack

There are several varieties of syncopal attack that are likely to occur in males. These are carotid sinus hypersensitivity (also known as vasodepressor syncope), cough syncope, micturition syncope and cramp syncope.

Carotid sinus hypersensitivity causes abrupt fainting whenever the patient touches the side of their neck. This may occur when turning the head, wearing a tight collar, or while shaving, and may easily be mistaken for arterial disease such as a carotid artery thrombosis or a vertebrobasilar ischaemic attack. The condition is extremely rare.

Cough syncope occurs at the end of a protracted bout of coughing, which is in effect a prolonged Valsalva manoeuvre, impairing venous return and reducing the cardiac output. This is common in emphysematous patients.

CASE REPORT II

A 29-year-old man had been referred to another hospital for exclusion of epilepsy and he was offered an appointment 12 months later. Two attacks had occurred 3 days apart and he had been told not to drive while awaiting the appointment. An earlier appointment was arranged at another hospital some months later. The delay had unfortunately already cost him his job. He was seen 6 months after the original referral.

The day before the first attack his sister had died from toxic shock syndrome within 4 hours of the onset of symptoms. He had had influenza and, while coughing protractedly that evening, reached the stage where he could not exhale any further, went blue in the face and collapsed. An exact repetition occurred 48 hours later while lying in bed. This was clear-cut cough syncope, with devastating consequences for employment. He was possibly primed to faint by the impact of his sister's death.

Micturition syncope is an unpleasant and potentially dangerous syndrome. The attacks occur when the patient has had to get up from a warm bed to pass urine. It is unique to males who, while standing and straining against a hypertrophied prostate gland, inadvertently perform the Valsava manoeuvre. There is also speculation that the sudden emptying of the bladder has a reflex effect. In any event, syncope is the result and in a toilet or bathroom this can be disastrous. What started as a faint may end up as a serious head injury. Elderly males with nocturia are well advised to pass urine in a sitting position.

Cramp syncope is another condition to which males seem particularly prone. The patient is wakened by severe cramps in one or other calf. The instinctive reaction is to leap from the bed to stand on the affected leg. The combination of suddenly standing upright and the excruciating pain will cause a precipitate drop in blood pressure and a syncopal attack which readily culminates in epileptic features. The circumstantial evidence should be diagnostic, but these patients are frequently misdiagnosed as nocturnal epilepsy because the exact circumstances were not taken into account.

CASE REPORT III

A 63-year-old man was referred because of personality change 8 years after a diagnosis of epilepsy. It was noted that he had had two normal EEGs and a normal CT scan shortly after the original diagnosis. The recent personality change included irritability, poor concentration, loss of interest in work and hobbies, sleep disorder, impotence and flattening of affect. He seemed to have a typical depressive illness. When asked about the epilepsy, he said that it was strange that all the attacks had occurred when he was in pain. Further questioning revealed that the first attack occurred after he had shut a finger in the car door, and the nine subsequent episodes all occurred in the middle of the night, when he had leapt out of bed with leg cramp. On a few occasions he had been incontinent of urine. Further enquiry revealed that he had always been the boy in his class who fainted in assembly at school, and both his father and sister had similar histories. He had been on phenytoin 300 mg daily since the original diagnosis and his wife attributed the dramatic change in personality, mood, and particularly his impotence, to the drug. He had not had any hint of repitition after withdrawal of his anticonvulsant and his depression has lifted without medication.

Hyperventilation Attacks

These episodes are also called hyperventilation syncope, although it is almost unknown for the patient actually to lose consciousness. These episodes are well recognised in the USA but are very underdiagnosed in the UK. Many anxious patients referred with attacks of 'dizziness' are suffering from this condition. Once the patient is in an ENT clinic there is a tendency to embark on a full investigation of vertigo, even though the patient is merely complaining of a 'woozy' 'floaty' head. It seems likely that very considerable sums of money could be saved by avoiding unnecessary investigation in this group of patients.

The patient is usually anxious and in a great many cases a phobic situation exists that provokes episodes, and the first question to such patients should identify whether there is any specific location in which attacks occur.

CASE REPORT IV

A 38-year-old woman was seen for the first time in a follow-up clinic. She had been attending the hospital for 10 years with a diagnosis of epilepsy, which had continued on a regular basis in spite of many modifications to her treatment. The episodes were typical of light-headed 'woozy' anxiety attacks. When asked about the timing of her attacks she related that they were always in the day, out in the street and, on further questioning, always at the same place. It transpired that this was where her mother has been run over and killed while crossing the road a few years prior to the onset of her attacks. Withdrawal of anticonvulsant drugs, the use of a mild tranquillizer and reassurance led to cessation of attacks.

This patient had been attending a neurological hospital diagnosed as suffering from epilepsy for over 10 years before she was asked the question that unearthed the real nature of her episodes.

The condition occurs almost exclusively in females, and attacks occurring in supermarkets or crowded shops are such a constant feature that the term 'supermarket syndrome' would seem appropriate. The patient typically develops the attack while queueing at the checkout desk. Patients relate either placing everything back on the shelves or just leaving their trolley and hurrying from the shop. In the less common cases in males, episodes while driving seem surprisingly frequent and many of these patients are brought in by ambulance from lay-bys where they have parked after suffering an attack. Several patients in this situation have noticed a sensation as if the road were running up a bank as the first symptom of pending trouble, but breathlessness and eventually chest pain are their major symptoms and a heart attack is always the suspected diagnosis.

Daytime attacks may be coupled with true panic attacks which, for reasons that are obscure, often occur in the night. The patient typically wakes already feeling breathless, with tightness in the chest, apparently gasping for breath, a situation rapidly progressing to generalized paraesthesiae, light-headedness and even visual obscuration. Such episodes seem to end when the patient becomes too exhausted to continue the overbreathing that underlies the condition. Incorrect diagnoses of asthma, myocardial infarction, gastrointestinal haemorrhage and epilepsy are often entertained.

Patients whose attacks always occur in various phobic situations seem to respond well once the mechanism of their attacks is explained to them, often after long periods of ineffectual psychotherapy. A major problem seems to be that the patients understand that because their symptoms have a psychological basis they must therefore be imaginary. They know that they are not, and any reassurance therefore falls on deaf ears. Although the attacks are determined by anxiety, the severity and frightening nature of the physical symptoms should not be underestimated. The fully developed picture can only develop in a state of anxiety with elevated blood catecholamines. It is impossible to reproduce a full-blown attack merely by hyperventilating.

In a typical episode the patient will suddenly feel light-headed and often describe a feeling as if their head were 'floating off their body', sometimes reaching the situation of depersonalization where they feel as though they are watching themselves acting in a play. The surroundings will suddenly become oppressive and threatening. As they walk they feel as if they are treading water and weaving from side to side. Their legs feel very heavy and their hands, and feet, and often their face, will start to tingle and feel numb. They become petrified by the thought that they will collapse and make a fool of themselves. Accompanying friends advise taking deep breaths, which is the worst thing they can do as this merely aggravates and perpetuates the situation.

The physicochemical mechanism of the condition is that subconscious hyperventilation, often no more than a series of resigned sighs, reduces the alveolar $p\text{co}_2$. As the blood becomes alkalotic the ionized calcium falls, producing fine tingling sensations in the limbs and around the mouth. The muscles become weak and the patient nearly always uses the expression 'my legs turn to jelly'. By this stage the chest muscles become tired and ache and the resultant pain in the chest adds to their fears. In males this invariably leads to the suspicion that they are having a myocardial infarct. The patient complains that they feel as if the chest were in a vice and that 'deep enough breaths' cannot be taken. By this time the parallel rise in $p\text{o}_2$ tension leads to cerebral vasospasm, causing further light-headedness – but **not** vertigo – and little black spots in front of the eyes. The classic tetanic posture of the hands usually illustrated as a diagnostic feature of the condition is in fact surprisingly rare. This may be one of the reasons why this diagnosis is so often missed.

In some cases of chronic mild anxiety a steady state is reached in which the patient always feels slightly light-headed and gets 'dizzy' whenever the anxiety increases. The importance of excluding this group of patients from those with vertigo has been discussed in Chapter 7. If this symptom is coupled with peripheral paraesthesiae a misdiagnosis of multiple sclerosis can be made. Every time there is a newspaper or magazine article describing multiple sclerosis there is an epidemic of patients with these symptoms, convinced they have the condition. Sometimes patients who actually have multiple sclerosis are identified in this way, but more often patients who will not accept reassurance have their lives irreversibly blighted, and many self-diagnose so-called ME syndrome as an alternative that is more acceptable to them than anxiety. This is very much the 'downside' of media attempts to educate the public. Considerable reassurance, and sometimes only the passage of time, is necessary before the patient's symptoms eventually subside.

A very dangerous and well known schoolboy trick is to combine forced hyperventilation with a Valsalva manoeuvre in a squatting position. This leads to loss of consciousness, and occasionally the combined metabolic and anoxic insult causes an epileptic seizure. Furthermore, during EEG recording one of the ways of accentuating an abnormality is hyperventilation for 2–3 minutes. This will occasionally provoke an epileptic event on the EEG. This may be a predisposing factor in some epileptic patients who insist that their attacks are related to stressful situations.

Drop Attacks

This is another condition that is almost exclusive to females. Attacks may occur at any age but are more common in the elderly. Some patients may relate isolated episodes at 5–10 year intervals since their 20s. The aetiology is uncertain and there is no evidence that it is caused by epilepsy, transient ischaemic attacks or any identifiable pathological state. The attacks occur without warning and typically while the patient is actually walking. They may liken the sensation to that experienced when chopped behind the knee with the heel of a hand. There is no dizziness or confusion and no impairment of consciousness.

The patient is almost thrown forwards, first on to their knees and then on to the face and chin. If they manage to put their arms out in front of them, a Colles fracture is often the result. The knees and nose are invariably grazed and bruised, but provided any injury permits the patient can get up immediately with no risk of a repeat attack. They always describe the feeling as one of considerable embarrassment as bystanders help retrieve their shopping from the pavement. A search for an uneven paying stone follows, and if nothing is found the shoes are blamed. One patient had 20 pairs of shoes that she would not wear again that were innocent victims of this conclusion. One elderly lady assaulted the man who attempted to help her up, convinced that he had pushed her from behind and was responsible for the original fall!

The attacks may occur fairly frequently for a few weeks or months and then stop, or may occur as infrequently as once a year for several years. There is no doubt that plump patients wearing high-heeled shoes seem particularly vulnerable, but thin patients in sensible shoes are not exempt.

Careful enquiry often reveals that the patient was looking from side to side, either while crossing the road or looking into shop windows, at the moment of the fall and advice not to do this would seem wise. Holding a companion's arm is of limited help and frequently the companion and the patient both fall over because of the unanticipated violence of the fall. Reassurance that the attacks appear to be without ominous significance and will eventually cease seems wholly justified by the natural history of this peculiar disorder.

Although sudden falls without loss of consciousness have been described in patients with pineal tumours and intraventricular cysts there is no justification for extensive investigation in a female patient with a classic history of drop attacks.

Cerebrovascular Disease

Although 'little strokes' are popularly supposed to cause brief episodes of unconsciousness in the elderly, the evidence for this is sparse. In fact, other than in massive cerebral haemorrhage or cerebral embolism, loss of consciousness during a cerebrovascular accident is unusual. Therefore, it seems unlikely that a 'little stroke' without observable sequelae would be capable of causing unconsciousness. The majority of patients who have had a stroke and are not rendered dysphasic are able to describe in great detail the sequence of events that occurred. One must therefore always be alert to the other causes of loss of consciousness in the elderly, and avoid the 'ragbag' diagnosis of a 'small stroke'.

Transient Global Amnesia

This is another relatively rare and intriguing condition that occurs in the middle-aged of either sex. It consists of episodes of total amnesia lasting minutes to many hours, during which time the patient behaves perfectly normally for ongoing physical activities but if engaged in conversation will keep asking the same question over and over again, and will have clearly forgotten the answer within a typical time span of 15–30 seconds. This particular observation is virtually diagnostic of the condition but the ability of the patient to continue with a sequence of activities is quite extraordinary.

Patients have been known to drive 50 miles or more, usually to some destination they know, but for no clear reason. Others have arrived home with shopping they did not intend to buy and some have reported a series of complex tasks, such as towing a caravan across France, completing a business deal or keeping a hairdressing appointment involving traversing Cairo twice, without recollection and without incident. Some of the earliest cases reported followed immersion in cold water, but several following hot showers and three occurring during intercourse, have been seen by the author in recent years.

In a personal series of over 100 patients, 70% gave a history of migraine and 17% of them were known to have a migraine at the onset of the amnesia. Several other reported series have noted this association and it seems likely that it is due to bilateral medial temporal lobe ischaemia caused by migrainous vasospasm in the posterior cerebral arteries. This is further supported by the frequent association with migrainous attacks, starting with bilateral migrainous visual phenomena of cortical type in several instances (see Chapter 3).

It is worth presenting in detail one of the most dramatic examples of this condition as it exemplifies so many of the important diagnostic features. This patient did **not** have a history of migraine.

CASE REPORT V

A 50-year-old businessman was due to have a sales meeting in London and went up the day before to reconnoitre a parking space at the venue; he noted a small restaurant where he proposed to have a meal before returning home the next day. On the day of the meeting he completed an hour's negotiating and recollected saying that he would go down and collect some more samples from his vehicle. Two hours later he found himself in the fast lane of the major trunk road out of south London, with no recollection of the intervening period. Somewhat shaken, he drove to his factory, who confirmed that they had telephoned the meeting and discovered that he had left but had in fact completed the contract that was the subject of the meeting. He found some loose change in his pocket which he knew had not been there that morning, and surmised that he might have gone into the restaurant as he had intended. He returned the next day by train (he was too frightened to go by car) and went to the restaurant. He waited for a quiet moment and sheepishly asked if he had been in the restaurant the day before. To his surprise they confirmed that he had – twice! They related that he seemed slightly remote and when he paid his bill asked them whether he had paid it already. They were concerned enough to watch him go to his car, get in and then get out again, and come back over to the restaurant to ask if he had just been in there! There has been no repetition in the 4 years since this episode.

The extent of both mental and physical activity performed without recollection in this particular case is amazing. In recent years it has also emerged that during the episodes it is not only immediate memory that is lost for some 15–30 seconds, but there may also be a retrograde memory loss extending back months or years during the episode which recovers completely to normal afterwards. During the attack, the patient may be unable to identify the house they are currently living in, the car in the drive outside, or even recently acquired friends, and in one instance the husband who was with them at the time. As an example of retrograde memory loss in an attack the following case is worthy of note.

CASE REPORT VI

A 47-year-old female estate agent left home at 7.15 p.m. to go to an aerobics class after a light meal. She had no recollection of events from halfway along the 7-mile drive to the venue until she awakened the following morning. During that time she attended and completed the aerobics class without arousing comment. She arrived home an hour later than usual and her husband noted peculiar behaviour. She did not seem to know where she had been and kept asking who had put all the plant bulbs on the window ledge, even though she had done it herself the previous evening. Every 30 seconds she asked who was responsible for the bulbs. Her husband then asked her about her daughter. She thought that her daughter was still living in an apartment she had vacated many months before, and had no recollection that she was due to complete the contract on her daughter's new flat the next day or the amount of the deposit. Her husband persuaded her to go to bed. When she awakened the next morning he immediately asked her how much she had to pay for the deposit on her daughter's flat and she instantly answered correctly, and went on to ask him why on earth he had asked her such a silly question. She had returned completely to normal and had no recollection of the previous evening. She had a clear-cut history of previous migraine episodes with visual phenomena, of bilateral occipital ischaemic type.

The prognosis is excellent. Some 10% of patients may have further episodes but the vast majority do not repeat, although they live in dread of a repetition because the attack makes almost as dramatic an impact on them as does the period of amnesia in patients following head injury, and they anguish constantly about the missing period in their life and how they behaved during the episode.

Migraine and Loss of Consciousness

There is considerable and renewed interest in the occurrence of attacks of altered consciousness occurring in association with migraine, and the association with transient global amnesia has been detailed above.

There are three other variants: a pathologically drowsy state resembling narcolepsy; prolonged syncopal episodes possibly due to spasm of the basilar artery with brainstem ischaemia; and epileptic events associated with migraine. Although migraine and epilepsy are common conditions, some series show a 10% prevalence of epilepsy in migraine sufferers as opposed to 0.8% in the general population. Many patients with migraine have fainted at the height of an attack without there being any suspicion that this was an epileptic attack. This is particularly common in patients with severe vomiting, abdominal pain and diarrhoea. The possibility of epilepsy occurring in association with migraine should always be considered in patients who have both headaches and attacks of loss of consciousness. Patients have been reported who have only ever had fits at the height of a migraine attack. It is also noteworthy that the headaches that follow an epileptic fit have many features in common with migraine in both quality and location.

Severe drowsiness amounting to an irresistible desire to go to sleep may occur as a migrainous prodrome, and some sufferers are fortunate enough to be so drowsy during an attack that they are able to get off to sleep. This is particularly true in childhood migraine and may account for the brevity of attacks in this age group.

Patients with evidence of vasospastic vertebrobasilar ischaemia in migraine find that in addition to the visual disturbance, slurred speech, unsteadiness and generalized paraesthesiae, they feel giddy, disorientated and drowsy. If combined with vomiting, splitting headache and neck stiffness, the distinction from subarachnoid haemorrhage and meningitis can test the most experienced clinician.

Meniere's Disease and Loss of Consciousness

In the original description of the syndrome that bears his name, Menière included 'a fainting state' as part of a typical attack. Certainly the tendency to fall during the severe vertigo is understandable, but some patients do appear to lose consciousness during the attack. Differentiation from a temporal lobe epileptic attack preceded by vertigo (a rare but well recognized variant) or migraine affecting the basilar artery, with vertigo and unconsciousness, must be made. The typical auditory phenomena of Menière's disease are an important clue to the diagnosis (see Chapter 6).

Narcolepsy

Narcolepsy was fully discussed under sleep disorders in Chapter 10. In the present context it is important to note that it consists of an abrupt irresistible desire to go to sleep, but the patient can be easily roused. It would be incorrect to regard the episodes as attacks of unconsciousness, although from a driving regulation aspect it is regarded as a disabling condition. The current regulation states that the patient may resume driving when their episodes are controlled. Implicit in this is a presumption that the condition has been distinguished from mere tiredness at the wheel and that appropriate treatment over a suitable period has prevented its recurrence.

In reality patients often only come to attention as a consequence of an accident, and treatment is usually immediately successful. The problem really requires a greater public awareness of the condition, but because effective treatment involves the use of amphetamine there is often a surprising reluctance to entertain the diagnosis even when the patient has sought advice. Even though the condition is lifelong, it is not uncommon for patient and their general practitioner to repeatedly ask the neurologist whether the patient can now stop their drugs because they are 'better'. Treatment must be continual once the condition has been diagnosed and it would seem advisable, as in the case of epilepsy, to ask the patient to stop driving if for any reason they discontinue their treatment.

Cardiac Disease

If the heartbeat ceases for longer than a few seconds, consciousness is lost. The most frequent cause is a Stokes–Adams attack occurring in patients who have complete heart block. The slowly beating denervated ventricle may stop beating for 5–30 seconds, leading to an abrupt loss of consciousness without warning, the patient often being unaware that anything has happened.

CASE REPORT VII

A middle-aged extremely obese man was admitted following a fall from a ladder; he had no idea why he had fallen. While the history was being taken he had six Stokes–Adams attacks, at the end of each apologizing for 'dropping off'. He had complete heart block caused by a recent silent myocardial infarction.

CASE REPORT VIII

A 98-year-old semiretired construction engineer (he now only went to his firm in the city of London on 2 days each week!) was referred with a diagnosis of epilepsy. He was not quite sure what had happened, and said that as far as he was concerned he had merely 'nodded off', but friends told him that

he looked as if he was going to die during the attack and suggested that he sought advice. While being examined he suddenly fell back, went deathly white and was in asystole. Perhaps bravely, assuming that this was one of his attacks, no action was taken and in about 30 seconds he suddenly flushed and apologized for losing concentration and asked what he had to do next. His resting pulse was 42, his blood pressure was normal and there were no other abnormalities. Three more episodes occurred during the examination and he was transferred immediately for cardiac pacing. He died at the age of 104.

In these attacks the patient becomes abruptly unconscious and extremely pale. As the attack continues there is rapidly increasing cyanosis until the heart starts beating again, when the patient suddenly flushes as the bright red hyperoxygenated arterial blood that has been lying in the pulmonary vascular bed suddenly recirculates. The patient then regains consciousness abruptly.

Patients with valvular disease, especially aortic stenosis, are prone to have syncopal attacks. Paroxysmal arrhythmias are responsible in some cases and careful cardiac evaluation is indicated in all cases of syncope, even in those cases that at first sight would appear to be straightforward vasovagal episodes.

CASE REPORT IX

A 73-year-old woman presented with most peculiar episodes. Over 4 weeks she had had five episodes of transient weakness in her right leg, which felt like a 'lump of lead'. This only lasted 2–3 minutes and had always recovered fully. The episode that prompted referral occurred while she was crossing the road at speed. She suddenly found herself flying forwards on to the road. A car was approaching and as she tried to get up she found that both legs were weak, so that she crawled on all fours to safety. It was 5 minutes before she was able to stand. She was fit enough the next morning to give a practical demonstration in the consulting room. She had had a hysterectomy for carcinoma of the uterus 4 years previously, followed by radiotherapy. On physical examination the only findings were the residuals of a Bell's palsy that she had suffered at the age of 28. An uncertain diagnosis of transient ischaemia was made, uncertain because the arms had not been involved and in this latest attack both legs had been affected without other symptoms to suggest brainstem involvement. Cervical spine X-rays to exclude instability or disease of the upper cervical spine revealed no abnormality. Over the next 3 weeks she developed some ankle oedema and intermittent attacks of quite severe dyspnoea, so severe that she was unable to speak. Cardiovascular examination by both a neurologist and a cardiologist was normal. The cardiologist thought that multiple pulmonary emboli were the most likely cause of her recent episodes of breathlessness. However, further investigation revealed a pedunculated tumour in the right atrium, which at operation proved to be metastatic uterine carcinoma in the inferior vena cava extending up into the atrium. Her collapses were presumably due to intermittent blockage of the tricuspid valve. She died 6 months later after partial excision of the tumour and radiotherapy.

Autonomic neuropathy may cause syncopal attacks by an admixture of altered cardiac rate and rhythm and loss of peripheral vascular control. Routine evaluation of elderly patients with possible cardiac syncope should include the response of the pulse rate to the Valsalva manoeuvre and testing for postural hypotension as they stand up. Failure of the heart to speed up after a Valsalva and a significant drop in both the systolic and diastolic pressures indicates an autonomic neuropathy and requires further investigation.

Hypoglycaemia

Although special charts distinguishing between diabetic and hypoglycaemic coma are included in many texts the differentiation is usually straightforward. The patient going into a diabetic coma becomes progressively obtunded over a period of hours, whereas hypoglycaemia can be truly 'syncopal' in onset. It can occur in patients on oral agents or insulin and may be sufficiently severe to cause epileptic fits. In spite of the obvious connection diabetologists seem surprisingly reluctant to recognize the association, and demand electroencephalographic studies. When the human insulins were first introduced a surprising number of diabetic patients were suddenly referred with nocturnal epilepsy, and in spite of previous experience with epilepsy under these circumstances in patients on long-acting insulins, there was an initial reluctance to accept hypoglycaemia as the cause. This dilemma was further compounded when blood sugars, taken after an episode, were satisfactory or even high. It was only when regular sugar levels during the night were estimated that hypoglycaemia was identified. In the last 10 years not a single insulin-dependent diabetic patient referred to the author with newly acquired epileptic events proved to have epilepsy. On careful evaluation, all were found to be suffering from unrecognized hypoglycaemia.

CASE REPORT X

A 19-year-old know diabetic woman on human insulin was referred because of the advent of nocturnal seizures. These had all occurred around 2.30 a.m. and the parents had been very assiduous in checking the blood sugar after each episode, and had found levels between 5 and 7 m.mol on all occasions. She had already been assured that this could not be due to hypoglycaemia but the regularity of attacks and the timing was distinctly unusual for epilepsy. The parents were enthusiastic enough to follow the suggestion to wake her up at 1.45 a.m. and check her blood glucose level, and within a few days levels as low as 1.5 m.mol were detected. The attacks ceased the moment diabetic therapy was adjusted.

Primary hypoglycaemia is extremely rare, although frequently suspected. The prodromal symptoms in the patient who is becoming hypoglycaemic are very similar to the prodrome of a syncopal attack. In both situations these symptoms are produced by adrenaline release in response to falling blood pressure and falling blood sugar respectively. In the premonitory phase of hypoglycaemia there is often a personality alteration, with aggression as a common feature, which may be severe. Increasing pallor, sweating and finally yawning are the major physical clues to the diagnosis. Any pathologically drowsy patient who yawns continually or demonstrates unusual or inappropriate behaviour should be regarded as hypoglycaemic until proved otherwise. Failure to identify the condition can have tragic or fatal consequences.

CASE REPORT XI

A 30-year-old woman was referred to the neurology unit after admission to a general hospital in coma. The blood glucose on admission there was recorded at 3.5 m.mol. The history started 3 years earlier, with episodes of inappropriate and uncommunicative behaviour lasting only minutes and occurring up to ten times a day. Her father had died of malignant thymoma in his 40s and this was thought to be one of the reasons for her anxiety. She had been seen by a consultant neurologist who thought that these were panic attacks, and treatment with chlorpromazine was recommended. On the day before this admission she had her worst ever episode, lasting 2 hours. During this her GP administered 50 mg chlopromazine intramuscularly. She woke several hours later, spoke to her husband and went to the toilet. She returned to bed and appeared to sleep. Twelve hours later she was found to be unrousable and was taken to the first hospital. On referral to the neurology unit, with the exception of generally decreased tone, depressed reflexes and a right extensor planter response, there were no abnormalities. As the blood tests had been done only 2 hours previously they were not repeated on admission. Following a normal CT scan a lumber puncture was performed. The glucose levels in both CSF and blood were less than 1.00 m.mol and the serum calcium level was 3.15 mmol/l and the phosphate was 0.84 mmol/l. This suggested the presence of both an insulinoma and a parathyroid tumour and the diagnosis of multiple endocrine adenoma type I was made. Her blood glucose was maintained in the normal range with considerable difficulty, but after 5 days it was quite clear that she had suffered irreversible brain damage. Her family refused postmortem examination.

This case is an object lesson in the importance of the family history and the dangers of a psychological diagnosis when the patient has 'action-replay' episodes. Anxious patients usually have a constellation of symptoms that vary continuously and often occur in specific situations.

Once a hypoglycaemic patient loses consciousness there is a real risk of progressing to an epileptic fit. Immediate intravenous injection of glucose is indicated. When hypoglycaemia is complicated by a severe epileptic fit there is a considerable risk of brain damage. In spite of adequate replacement, if the coma has been prolonged and particularly if a fit has occurred, the patient may take several hours to regain consciousness due to the combined metabolic and anoxic insult. If this diagnosis is suspected and there is likely to be delay in getting the patient to hospital, it is essential to give intravenous glucose or glucagon even though biochemical confirmation may be prevented. The considerable dangers to the nervous system of prolonged hypoglycaemia should never be underestimated. Hypoglycaemic episodes often remain unidentified when transient neurological phenomena without loss of consciousness occur. In a younger patient hypoglycaemia may readily enter into the differential diagnosis but in the older patient more common conditions such as transient ischaemic episodes may be incorrectly diagnosed. The following case report is a typical example of this situation.

CASE REPORT XII

A 22-year-old woman was referred because of frequent syncopal attacks and had been admitted in coma to several hospitals over 4 years. She had gradually developed a spastic dysarthria and a spastic tetraparesis and a diagnosis of multiple sclerosis had been suspected, although the attacks of coma were regarded as unusual. When her blood sugar was eventually checked on her first admission to a neurological unit during an attack, it was found to be 0.5 μmol. She was subsequently shown to have an islet-cell tumour. Her blood sugar had not been estimated on any of her previous admissions.

Table 22.2 Differential diagnosis of non-epileptic attacks

Attacks	Vasovagal	Hyperventilation	Drop attacks	Stokes–Adams	Hypoglycaemia
Age/sex	Young M > F Usually teens M – isolated attack F – often repeat	F > M	Middle-aged or elderly females	Any age M&F	Any age M & F
Situations	Church Dances Public houses Queuing	Crowded shops Supermarkets Lifts/escalators Men: often in cars	Always while walking: in mid-stride	Any time Not exertional	Missed meals Drug abuse Misuse of insulin (? deliberate)
Prodromal symptoms	Faint hot 'swimmy' or clammy feeling Vision blurred Hearing fades	Prolonged 'dizziness' Paraesthesiae in limbs and round mouth Legs 'like jelly'	None Typically very sudden	None Very sudden onset	Personality change Confusion Aggression Hunger Sweating Yawning
Consciousness	Briefly unconscious Often recall falling	Very rarely become unconscious	Conscious throughout Embarrassed	Unconscious briefly. Think they have 'nodded off'	Unconscious and may convulse
Duration of attack	Seconds, unless propped or held upright, then can last longer	Prolonged attack ends when exhausted	Seconds only	Up to 30 secs. or fatal arrest	Mins–hours if undiagnosed Convulse or fall Can sustain injury
Colour change	Very pale Deathly white and sweating	Pale and often sweating with fear or exertion of overbreathing	Normal	Pale initially Cyanosed during attack Flushed after	Pale and sweating ++
Recovery	Abrupt but often vomiting supervenes	Slowly ceases due to exhaustion	Abrupt and complete	Abrupt and complete	Slow and confused for some hours after
Precipitating features	Anxiety Pain (esp. visceral) Blood loss Heat/excitement Fear, ghoulish event or film	Anxiety and phobic states, especially in situations where it happened before	Unknown Almost all occur while walking along	Complete heart block with ventricular standstill	Excess insulin dose Hypoglycaemic drugs Islet-cell tumour Retroperitoneal sarcoma
Special types	Micturition syncope Cough syncope Carotid sinus hypersensitivity Cramp syncope	'Supermarket' syndrome			

In this patient the clue to the diagnosis was present in the coma, but the insidious development of neurological findings, it would seem, had been regarded as the possible cause rather than the effect of these episodes.

Patients who prove to have islet-cell tumours often run surprisingly low resting blood sugars and it is only when the levels become profoundly reduced that symptoms occur.

A superb example of hypoglycaemia with focal neurological phenomena is to be found in Case Report I in Chapter 9 on page 141. This was a classic diagnostic error and in this particular instance first-hand observation confirmed that there really were none of the typical outward manifestations of hypoglycaemia.

As an appropriate reminder at the end of this chapter devoted to what are sometimes called 'fits, faints and funny turns', the following brief case report is of particular interest. It emphasizes the importance of estimating the blood sugar and serum drug levels in **any** unconscious patient, however unlikely the possibility of hypoglycaemia or drug intoxication may seem to be.

CASE REPORT XIII

In 1961 a 30-year-old civil servant collapsed by a postbox. When the ambulance arrived he was dead. He was resuscitated in the ambulance and admitted to the intensive care unit, and as full haematological, biochemical cardiological and neurological investigations as were available at that time were performed to determine the cause of his collapse. All were normal. Three days later the hospital was contacted by his brother, who had just received the suicide note that the patient had presumably posted just as he had collapsed.

Even at 72 hours a very high barbiturate level was found! At no stage, in view of the circumstances of his collapse, had the possibility of a drug overdose even been considered. Unfortunately, in spite of intensive care the patient subsequently died from irreversible brain damage.

This case came to mind several years later, when the neurosurgical team asked for advice as they were about to perform angiography on a man found unconscious in an hotel room with the DO NOT DISTURB sign on the door. He had depressed reflexes but normal pupil responses. It was suggested that a drug screen was performed first and a very high barbiturate level was confirmed. He made a full recovery.

One of the most frequent reasons for referring a patient to the neurological clinic is for the investigation of an attack of altered consciousness. There are usually no detectable physical signs between episodes and the EEG will rarely give diagnostic information. The diagnosis depends entirely on the detailed history and the eye-witness account. It is worth going to considerable lengths to obtain such an account if there is any uncertainty based on the patient's own history and the second-hand accounts of what he was told that bystanders had observed. The referring doctor can make a very helpful contribution if, whenever such a patient is sent for an expert opinion, the patient is advised to find, question and if at all possible bring the witness to the clinic with him. This will often prevent incorrect diagnosis and save time and unnecessary investigation.

To aid history taking and evaluation a table is included to facilitate differential diagnosis (Table 22.2).

23. Trauma and the Nervous System

Head Injuries and Their Complications

Accidents accompanied by head injuries are an increasingly significant cause of death and morbidity in children and young adults. The complications and sequelae of head injuries present many problems of management, some of which may require lifelong medical supervision. As many of the accidents occur while the patient is on holiday, indulging in dangerous pastimes or in road traffic accidents, the primary evaluation of the situation may become the responsibility of a doctor who has no special experience in the management of head injuries. The need to get the patient to specialist care may result in the continued observation being performed by a series of doctors. This makes for poor continuity of assessment, which is so vital for the early detection of impending disaster in head injury management. Finally, the patient may return home to his GP's care many hundreds of miles away. Subsequently, if an event such as an epileptic seizure occurs the full significance or importance of this is hard to assess unless a full report of the original injury is available. If the injury occurred abroad it may prove difficult to obtain such details.

The above is the original introduction to this chapter and has been left unchanged as the basic points remain the same. It serves as a useful starting point to review those changes that have occurred in the last 20 years in the evaluation and management of the head-injured patient, which have altered the prognosis for survival but unfortunately done little to alter the outcome, and have produced two new problems, the persistent vegetative state and the concept of brainstem death.

Seatbelt legislation, crash-helmet laws, better car design and better protective equipment in the recreational fields such as horse riding and cycling have produced marked improvements in safety, a striking reduction in serious head injuries and a dramatic decline in maxillofacial injuries. Unfortunately, children still fall out of windows, climb on to unsafe structures and run out into roads and sustain severe trauma. To this we must now add serious trauma inflicted by parents, boyfriends and siblings on children. A subdural haematoma in an infant is highly likely to be due to shaking trauma inflicted by a 'carer'.

The documentation for patients injured abroad has improved markedly and patients now usually arrive with their X-rays and CT scans, making the ongoing management more securely based than was often the case in the past. In this respect, the debt owed by both patients and doctors worldwide to the pioneering work of the Glasgow neurosurgeons is enormous. Their work in establishing the basic standards of head injury assessment and ongoing management and the almost universal adoption of the Glasgow Coma Scale has been an outstanding advance, permitting inter hospital transfer with greater certainty as to the continuing progress of the patient. This scale was introduced before CT scanning was readily available and served to indicate those patients who required contrast studies to detect intracranial collections of blood. At present the use of the Coma Scale has its main value in ongoing assessment, rather than its previous critical role in detecting the early signs of deterioration requiring instant investigation.

The availability of CT scanning has allowed early recognition of the potentially fatal acute extradural haematoma and the diagnosis of the later insidiously developing chronic subdural haematoma. The so-called 'acute' subdural haematoma was always known to carry a poor prognosis because of coexisting underlying brain damage, and CT scanning has confirmed that the subdural collection is secondary to the haemorrhage from the 'burst lobe' syndrome, usually affecting the frontal pole or the temporal lobe. The prognosis is really that of the underlying brain injury rather than the subdural collection, and the prognosis for this group has been little altered by more precise early recognition. The dramatic improvements in intensive care that have ensured the survival of patients who only 20 years ago would have died of their injuries, have unfortunately produced very severely brain-damaged patients requiring long-term care, and two newly identified problems: the persistent vegetative state and brainstem death.

Later in this chapter the important differences between head injuries in the child and the adult will be considered separately as there are some differences in the clinical features and the outcome. In all age groups the general management is the same and this will be dealt with in detail and the important age-related differences will be highlighted.

Initial Assessment of the Unconscious Patient

Severe head injury often occurs in the setting of other major trauma. There are almost no **survivable** complications of head injury that will kill the patient within the first few hours, but many general surgical conditions such as cardiac tamponade, torn lung hilum, ruptured liver, spleen or kidney, or major haemorrhage from fractures may kill the patient within the hour unless promptly recognized and treated. Yet often the surgical team are so concerned because the patient is unconscious that they may be allowed to deteriorate and die of other injuries while what proves to be an inappropriate and unhelpful CT scan is carried out. A CT scanner used in this way in a district general hospital may operate to the patient's disadvantage. Unfortunately, in many hospitals the possession of a CT scanner has come to be regarded as a substitute for an immediate neurological or neurosurgical opinion.

The immediate management must involve establishing an airway by endotracheal tube, or even an immediate tracheostomy if maxillofacial injuries indicate the need for an alternative airway. Anoxia at this stage is possibly the single most important factor in the pathophysiology of cerebral oedema. Blood pressure must be stabilized and the simple rule to be remembered is that a **falling blood pressure** is a prime indicator of surgical shock and surgical shock is almost never the consequence of haemorrhage from head wounds, except in a young child, where serious blood loss from a scalp injury can occur.

The signs of rising intracranial pressure with the possibility of fatal brain displacements are RISING BLOOD PRESSURE, SLOWING PULSE and SLOWING OR PERIODIC RESPIRATION.

The signs of concealed internal bleeding and the development of surgical shock are FALLING BLOOD PRESSURE, RAPID THREADY PULSE and RAPID RESPIRATION.

This ought to be easy to recall, but within the last 2 years a patient nearly died in a CT scanner of massive blood loss from pelvic and femoral fractures because the signs noted in the second section above were interpreted by an orthopaedic team as indicating 'coning'. The scan was completely normal.

Whenever a patient has sustained a head injury, particularly if there are maxillofacial injuries, the possibility of a coexisting neck injury – which occurs in some 10% of such cases – must be immediately addressed and the head immobilized in a neck brace until cervical spine instability or fracture has been excluded. This can often make intubation difficult but is an essential consideration before intubation is attempted.

Surgical emphysema in the neck and chest wall indicates a ruptured trachea, oesophagus or lung. Fractured ribs or a flail chest with paradoxical respiration, if associated with falling blood pressure and a rapid pulse, all point to a major intrathoracic lesion such as lung avulsion, pneumohaemothorax or cardiac tamponade.

Blunt trauma to the abdominal cavity may be obvious from external bruising but the girth at umbilical level should be documented routinely on arrival and the tape left in position for repeat measurement. Increasing girth, absent bowel sounds or evidence of surgical shock with no other obvious cause may indicate a ruptured liver, spleen or kidney. Abdominal paracentesis is not foolproof and laparotomy may be required. Immediate urinary catheterization will enable careful fluid balance measurements to begin and haematuria may indicate damage to the kidney or bladder from the trauma.

While these initial assessments are being made, one member of the team should be trying to establish as much detail as possible about the nature of the accident and the patient's status when found and during transportation to hospital. Whether they have regained consciousness, lost consciousness in transit, have convulsed, whether they were walking or talking at any stage, whether they had been drinking or taking drugs or whether they are known to be epileptic or diabetic, can all be very important additional factors at this stage of evaluation.

Many simple neurological observations can be made from the end of the trolley while others are establishing the airway, putting up drips and assessing the thorax and abdomen. The patient's responsiveness to pain during these manipulations may be obvious and it may be apparent that one limb, or the limbs on one side or either leg, fails to move during these activities. This might indicate the possibility of a plexus injury, a developing hemiparesis or paraplegia. Spontaneous eye movements, moaning or attempting to speak, and coughing on the tube indicating an intact gag reflex are easily observed reassuring signs. When the patient's immediate condition is stable a more formal neurological examination can be attempted.

The Head

External examination of the head and palpation with gloved hands will reveal areas of bruising, bogginess and lacerations and possibly even palpable deformity of the skull. Small important lacerations may be missed if the patient's head and hair are blood-soaked from nasal or facial haemorrhages, and this initial palpation is very important in establishing the nature and angle of the blow or blows to the head. Any lacerations should be explored in theatre under general anaesthetic if necessary before suturing, unless there is uncontrolled haemorrhage.

The Eyes

Inspect the patients eyes. Is there evidence of local trauma to the brow or lids? Is the cornea abraded? Are the pupils symmetrical and round? Do the eyes open spontaneously to command or pain? If the eyes are open is either eyelid ptosed? Is either eye proptosed? If there is haemorrhage into the conjunctiva which comes forwards from the back of the eye this would indicate a middle cranial fossa fracture.

Are the eyes roving or deviated to one or other side? Is one eye clearly deviated into an unusual position? These observations may indicate a brainstem injury or extraocular nerve lesion. If one pupil is already fixed and dilated, the possibility of local trauma, third nerve palsy or optic nerve avulsion exists, but it is important to identify this abnormality immediately as the later development of this finding might indicate a progressive tentorial herniation. For this reason, no mydriatic drops should be put into the eye to facilitate fundal examination, which should be performed merely to confirm that the retina is undamaged and that the optic discs at that stage show normal appearances.

The Nose

Any nasal discharge should be inspected. Is it watery or like blood mixed with water? Either finding might indicate CSF rhinorrhoea due to an open fracture of the floor of the anterior cranial fossa or through the frontal or ethmoid sinus. If continuous haemorrhage occurs a major venous sinus injury may be the cause and require urgent surgical intervention.

The Ears

Examine the ears. Direct trauma to the external ear or blood running back off the face may enter the ear canal and simulate bleeding coming from inside. Clean the external meatus carefully and watch for watery discharge, which may be CSF otorrhoea. This constitutes an open fracture of the skull. If blood is coming through a torn drum, a fractured petrous bone is certain. If the drum is intact it may be bulging and dark in colour, indicating haemorrhage into the middle ear with the same implications. Over the next 24 hours bruising may

appear over the mastoid region, indicating a middle cranial fossa fracture. This is called Battle's sign.

The Face

If facial injuries permit, the symmetry of the face should be examined. If there are spontaneous movements nothing more need be done. If not, and the patient's level is light enough, a grimace may be provoked by pressing the supraorbital nerve. An acute lower motor neuron paralysis on one side will usually indicate a transverse fracture of the petrous temporal bone and a serious skull base injury. The position of any lacerations, particularly over the bony prominences, may indicate the possibility of local nerve trauma to motor branches of the seventh nerve or sensory branches of the fifth nerve. If there is evidence of damage to either nerve, particularly if the eye will not close or the cornea appears insensitive, measures to protect the cornea should be instituted immediately.

The Limbs

The limbs should be assessed individually. By this stage this may be technically extremely difficult because of splints, to protect intravenous access or fractured limbs. Is the tone normal? If one arm is floppy and the other shows normal tone a plexus avulsion injury may be present, a particularly common complication of head injury in motorcyclists. This suspicion may be confirmed by absent reflexes in the affected limb. If the tone is increased in a limb, or both limbs on one side, this may be early evidence of a pyramidal lesion and, appearing this soon after the injury, usually indicates damage at brainstem level. The reflexes on the affected side may well be enhanced. If the patient is unconscious, both plantar responses are almost bound to be extensor. If both lower limbs are floppy and areflexic and there is no plantar response, the possibility of a paraplegia due to an injury of the thoracolumbar spine is extremely high. The response of individual limbs to pain should be noted. Pinching the upper chest wall or pressing a pen into the nailbed is the preferred method for the upper limbs and pinching the skin of the leg or eliciting the plantar response for the lower limbs. Whether the provoked responses are semipurposive or merely a flexion or extension response of the limb should be noted. If there is no response to painful stimuli down one side or in the lower limbs, the possibility that this is due to sensory deficit must also be borne in mind.

All these observations should permit an immediate conclusion as to whether there is any evidence of focal injury to the brain, spinal cord or the major nerve plexuses. They also provide much of the basic information for the Glasgow Coma Scale chart, which over the next few days will give an excellent guide as to whether, from a neurological perspective, the patient is improving or deteriorating. This will be detailed later.

Neurological Investigations

Provided the patient's condition is stable, X-rays of the skull, cervical spine and thoracolumbar spine should be taken. There is considerable advantage in taking the cervical spine films first to exclude instability or fracture dislocation of the neck, before attempting to X-ray the skull, which requires careful positioning involving neck extension. Skull-base views present particular problems in the presence of possible neck injury and are only successful in detecting a basal fracture in 50% of cases at best. A CT scan will give much more precise views of the skull base.

Skull films should include a straight lateral, a straight anteroposterior (A/P) and a Towne's view. The latter is particularly important to detect fractures extending from the occipital area into the foramen magnum and petrous temporal bone fractures. The straight A/P view is very useful for detecting orbital fractures and fluid levels in the sinuses. The lateral view is the best for detecting vault fractures, particularly those traversing the middle meningeal arteries, and the presence of air in the skull or fluid levels in the sphenoid or ethmoid sinuses provides confirmation of an open skull fracture with communication through the dura to the nasal passages. An expert opinion on skull films is important. Skull fractures are demonstrable on X-ray in 80% of fatal head injuries.

Whether to proceed to an immediate CT scan is debatable. If the patient has steadily deteriorated since the injury and all other causes of deterioration have been excluded, a CT scan should be performed on the possibility that the deterioration is due to a very rapidly collecting extradural haematoma. This is unlikely in the absence of a visible fracture on the plain films. In most instances very little will be seen on the scan. There may be some effacement of surface markings, some blurring of the grey/white interface and some small haemorrhages in the region of the corpus callosum and upper brain stem, but the appearances may be misleadingly reassuring. A CT scan at 12–24 hours may be quite different and much more informative. There may be clear evidence of diffuse or focal cerebral oedema, with reduced ventricular size and displacement, loss of grey/white differentiation and surface markings and often several areas of intracerebral haemorrhage that were not apparent on the original scans. Blood and fluid levels in the sinuses, particularly the ethmoids and sphenoids, may be apparent and any intracranial air is readily detectable as small jet-black bubbles. Unfortunately, these findings do not indicate treatable lesions and if the patient continues to deteriorate may

well indicate the likelihood of a fatal outcome. The timing of further scanning will depend on the patient's subsequent progress, but after 24 hours it is unlikely that any new collection of blood that could be surgically evacuated with advantage will appear. After 2–3 days, sudden deterioration in the cerebral status may well be the result of traumatic fat embolism, pulmonary embolism or disseminated intravascular coagulation, rather than indicating new intracranial pathology.

Other less common problems can cause dramatic changes in brain function. These include electrolyte disturbances and post-traumatic inappropriate secretion of antidiuretic hormone, which may cause hyponatraemia predisposing to further cerebral oedema or diabetes insipidus, which may be particularly severe if steroids are also in use. Both conditions should be quickly detected on the fluid balance chart and by twice-daily electrolyte studies and treated by fluid restriction or the use of Desmopressin respectively.

The Glasgow Coma Scale

The Glasgow Coma Scale is shown in Table 23.1. It has proved effective with observers at all levels of sophistication and produces comparable results from different centres. It is based on three major functions: eye opening, the best motor response and the best verbal response. The presence of severe maxillofacial or ocular injuries can interfere with the eye observations and the best motor responses may be modified by fractures and paralysis. The verbal response is obviously severely influenced by the presence of an endotracheal tube or possible aphasia due to the injury. Clearly, under any of these circumstances the scale has to be modified but should still provide valuable information. The worst possible score is 3, where the patient is unable to do anything, and the maximum score is 15, where for all purposes the patient is regarded as normal. Some neurosurgical units have adopted the scale with such enthusiasm that even patients admitted for lumbar disc surgery are coded out with a Glasgow Coma Scale of 15 on their discharge summary! The best response is charted as a dot in the square on the appropriate line, allowing 'at-a-glance' detection of the general trend of observations.

Traditional Head Injury Observations

Prior to the advent of the Glasgow Coma Scale, head injury observation consisted of monitoring pupillary size and reactions, abnormality of doll's-head eye movements and the development of new signs in the limbs. The pulse, respiration rate and blood pressure were also considered in parallel. The objection to these parameters is that they do not indicate a worsening of the situation but only become clearly abnormal when the

Table 23.1 Glasgow Coma Scale chart

	Name:											
Date: Time:												
Eye opening												
spontaneous E4												
to speech only E3												
to pain only E2												
none E1												
Best motor response												
obeying commands M6												
localizing to pain M5												
withdraws to pain M4												
abnormal flexion M3												
extensor response M2												
none M1												
Verbal response												
totally orientated V5												
confused conversation V4												
using inappropriate words V3												
incomprehensible sounds V2												
none V1												
Total score (3–15)												

patient has been allowed to deteriorate to a near-terminal state. By the time the patient has a fixed dilated pupil and an obvious hemiplegia they are already close to death, rather than in the process of deteriorating. However, most units do continue to monitor these findings in parallel, and particularly during the first 24 hours the detection of altering pupil size on one side has continued to prove a reliable indicator of pending trouble at a time when other observations may not have altered significantly. In situations where there is no access to sophisticated investigations this still remains the single most reliable physical sign in the management of head injury.

Pupil Reactions

Provided the pupil responses have initially been established as equal and reactive, and are not modified by local trauma or medication and are not becoming obscured by progressive oedema of the eyelids, **any** change in pupillary symmetry or reduction in reactivity to light on one side is a valuable physical sign. It is very rarely false lateralizing and, until proved otherwise, indicates tentorial coning on that side. Of course, this may not necessarily be due to a removable clot. It may be due to progressive oedema in a severely traumatized hemisphere, but as an indicator of the need to reconsider the situation it probably has no equal. Hundreds of lives have been saved in the past by this one observation and it would seem unwise to forget its value in the future.

Abnormal Eye Movements

Deeply unconscious patients lie with their eyes open, staring straight ahead, and the use of tape to hold them closed to protect the cornea is important. Roving eye movements, particularly if always to the same side, usually indicate unilateral brainstem damage and are an unfavourable prognostic sign. If the eyes are immobile and it is certain that the neck is not injured, doll's-head eye movement testing can demonstrate the integrity of brainstem mechanisms at mid-pontine level. If the patient's head is held between the hands and rotated 45° side, to side, the eyes should remain fixed straight ahead if the brainstem function is normal. Up and down movements can be tested in the same way and demonstrate the integrity of the upper brain stem. It is loss of eye movement on one or all of these movements that is pathological. An alternative test is to inject 20 ml of iced water into the external auditory meatus provided the ear drum is intact. This will drive the eyes towards the cold ear. This can then be repeated on the opposite side. This is the safest test to perform in patients with neck injuries.

The Limbs

Limb tone and movement assessment is a more subjective test and is only really of value if performed by the same observer on every occasion. The passive tone in the limb, the degree of withdrawal to pain and whether the response is flexion or extension, the briskness of the reflexes and any change in the plantar responses, may all indicate a measurable improvement or deterioration. Sometimes one side clearly improves faster than the other, indicating the possibility of a hemiparesis on one side as the patient slowly recovers consciousness.

A clearly deteriorating situation, increasing tone or a decrease in movement on one side should indicate a progressive lesion of the opposite hemisphere. This can be a **false lateralizing sign**. If the brain is being pushed across, for example from the right to the left side, the left cerebral peduncle may be squashed against the hard tentorial edge, which will produce a hemiparesis on the **same** side as the lesion. Pupillary dilatation will occur on the same side, as the lesion and is almost never a false localizing sign. This information is of vital importance to doctors forced to manage head injuries without the advantage of CT scanning to guide their every move.

Vital Signs

The importance of the correct interpretation of a rising blood pressure and slowing pulse in the unconscious patient has already been stressed. At one time changes in the pattern of respiration were advanced as an important indicator of the level of neural damage in the brain and brain stem, but this has not proved practical and is not widely used for monitoring head-injured patients.

All the foregoing discussion has dealt with the management of the immediate life-threatening effects of trauma and the observations necessary to detect the development of treatable delayed complications affecting the nervous system. For practical purposes this is the detection of the development of intracranial collections of blood producing brain displacement.

Intracranial Haematoma

Sixty per cent of patients with fatal head injuries die before reaching hospital. This is usually due to massive basal fractures with laceration of the major venous sinuses or the intracranial portion of the carotid artery. Of the survivors who eventually die, 70% do so within the next 24 hours, 80% within 7 days and 90% within 1 month.

Eighty per cent of the fatal injuries are related to skull fractures, and the presence of a skull fracture increases the risk of a treatable haematoma developing 400-fold. Of the patients who survive to reach hospital, 75% die as a consequence of intracranial haemorrhage. Extradural haemorrhage is responsible in 25% of cases and, when detected and treated, 75% of patients make an excellent recovery. Intradural haemorrhage (previously called acute subdural haematoma), associated

with severe underlying brain damage, accounts for 50% of the deaths and most survivors are left with severe neurological disability.

Skull fractures are present in 90% of adults who develop a haematoma. Children, however, may develop a fatal haematoma without a fracture, so that although a fracture indicates a very definite risk, normal skull X-rays cannot be regarded as totally exclusory, particularly in children. Because of these observations all patients with skull fractures should be admitted for observation even if there was **no** definite history of loss of consciousness. Any patient who **has** lost consciousness should be admitted for observation, even if they seem to have fully recovered by the time they are seen and there is no skull fracture on X-ray. This is the group who are occasionally allowed home and subsequently die (Fig. 23.1).

In the past a great deal has been made of the so-called 'lucid interval', in which a patient who has been knocked unconscious comes round and is apparently back to normal and then slips into coma and dies. This sequence occurs in less than 15% of patients who have an extradural haematoma. Most go from coma into deeper coma and death, unless the responsible haematoma is identified and removed. Patients in the 'lucid interval' sometimes demonstrate inappropriate and belligerent behaviour, particularly if they have been drinking or have had a convulsion, and later have no recollection at all of their 'lucid period'. Attributing such behaviour to the effects of drink or an unpleasant personality and arranging for the patient to be placed in custody rather than under observation is a serious mistake.

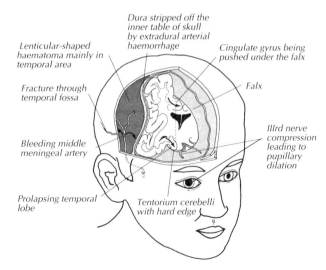

Lenticular-shaped haematoma mainly in temporal area

Dura stripped off the inner table of skull by extradural arterial haemorrhage

Cingulate gyrus being pushed under the falx

Fracture through temporal fossa

Falx

Bleeding middle meningeal artery

IIIrd nerve compression leading to pupillary dilation

Prolapsing temporal lobe

Tentorium cerebelli with hard edge

23.1   Acute extradural haematoma.

When identified, evacuation of extradural haematomas, massive subdural haematomas and sometimes even resection of the underlying damaged brain, can be life-saving. Occasionally evacuation of a single large deep intracerebral haematoma following trauma is justified where its size alone is life-threatening.

Since the advent of CT scanning in district general hospitals it is surprising how few patients actually need neurosurgical intervention. Although intracranial collections of blood are the preventable causes of fatalities, the majority of patients just have cerebral oedema and multiple small intracerebral haemorrhages that are not amenable to a surgical approach. Many of these patients die and the survivors are often left with residual neurological disability. The management of this group of patients remains the biggest challenge in the field of head injury.

Management of a Deteriorating Situation NOT due to a Haematoma

Uncontrolled cerebral oedema is the cause of death and disability in a majority of serious head injuries. A variety of treatments have been tried and some are still in use in spite of little evidence of their value.

Intravenous mannitol may produce short-term benefit and permit a patient to survive long enough to reach a CT scanner or neurosurgical unit, but unless a treatable clot is subsequently identified the benefit is short-lived as mannitol enters the extracellular fluid in the brain and the osmotic effect diminishes. Long-term administration with pressure monitoring has not demonstrated long-term effectiveness or benefit.

Shortly after the dramatic beneficial effect of glucocorticoids in cerebral oedema due to tumours was demonstrated, their use in head injuries enjoyed a vogue, sometimes in heroic doses – up to 48 g of dexamethasone in 24 hours. Steroids have never been demonstrated to be of benefit and cause numerous other problems – hypertension, diabetes, gastric erosion and electrolyte disturbances – which further jeopardize the patient's condition.

Hyperventilation, so successful during neurosurgical anaesthesia in acutely reducing intracranial pressure, is ineffective in trauma-associated oedema and because of the vasoconstrictive effect of hyperoxygenation may actually aggravate the brain damage. To achieve hyperventilation the patient must be paralysed, preventing proper neurological observation. No benefit has been demonstrated.

Barbiturate narcosis has been used on the basis that animals subjected to cranial trauma when pretreated with barbiturates have a higher chance of survival. This is hardly mirrored in the clinical situation and there is no evidence of benefit, and as with hyperventilation proper clinical evaluation becomes impossible the moment the patient is deeply anaesthetized by the barbiturate.

Sadly, the prognosis in these patients has not been altered by any of these techniques and improvement in the outcome awaits new methods of treatment.

Communicating Hydrocephalus

One of the major advances in management resulting from CT scanning is the detection of communicating hydrocephalus as a delayed complication of serious head injury. It occurs in patients who have had considerable haemorrhage into the subarachnoid space as a consequence of skull fracture, torn blood vessels or brain injury. At any time from 10 days to several weeks after the acute injury, a relatively rapid generalized deterioration in alertness, altered behaviour or the development of new bilateral physical signs may occur, and CT scanning may demonstrate marked enlargement of the ventricular system. This is due to CSF circulation block at the arachnoid granulations. The same condition may occur following meningitis or following very high spinal fluid protein levels as a consequence of Guillain–Barré syndrome or spinal tumour.

Ventriculoperitoneal shunting can produce a gratifying improvement, often to a situation better than before the sudden deterioration. A routine CT scan 3 weeks after the injury in any patient with heavy bloodstaining of the CSF would seem a wise precaution to detect the earliest evidences of this condition. Unfortunately, shunting brings with it the further complications of post-shunt subdural haematoma and the risk of epilepsy and infection, but these risks have to accepted and anticipated when the indications for shunting are clear-cut.

Fatal Outcome

It is obvious from the foregoing discussion that in spite of skilled management and major advances in intensive care medicine, may patients with severe head injury and multiple injuries still die. Modern supportive skills have created two new clinical conditions: the persistent vegetative state and brain death in the presence of a beating heart, the criterion previously used to define death.

Persistent Vegetative State

The patient may at first appear to be recovering. The eyes may open and even appear to look around. Some occasional limb movements may be observed and blood pressure and respiration are maintained without support. Unfortunately, no further improvement occurs and no evidence of a sentient state emerges, the patient demonstrating no response to their surroundings or to speech. This was thought to be due to damage in the upper brain stem but pathological evidence from the longest-known survivor in this state has demonstrated diffuse thalamic damage as the likely cause.

Brain Death

This situation has achieved prominence because of transplant surgery. What had previously been a straightforward clinical decision to withdraw ventilatory support when it was clear the irreversible brain damage had occurred, was suddenly regarded as a situation causing diagnostic difficulty and an ethical dilemma. This reflects the traditional belief that if the heart is still beating the patient is alive. To demonstrate irreversible brain damage, it has to be shown that brainstem reflex activity maintaining respiration and protective reflexes has completely ceased. The pupils are dilated and fixed to light, the corneal reflexes are absent, doll's-head eye movements are absent, there is no protective gag reflex and no spontaneous breathing. Most of these signs are readily demonstrable by standard clinical testing, including cold-water irrigation of the ear. To demonstrate cessation of respiratory reflexes without producing hypercapnia requires oxygenation of the lungs via a catheter down the endotracheal tube while the pump is disconnected for 5 minutes. If no respiratory effort is made during that time, the test is positive. A second repeat of these tests within the next 24 hours is required to permit withdrawal of respiratory support.

Other Complicated Outcomes

Some patients present problems short of the conditions described above. They also present ongoing management problems.

Locked-In Syndrome

This is a particular problem of lower brainstem cerebrovascular disease or damage due to atlantoaxial dislocation. The patient is rendered tetraplegic and unable to swallow or speak, but may demonstrate that they have intact sensation. The only movements that they can make are blinking and eye movements, and a code of 'Yes' and 'No' answers may be devised using eye movements, enabling the patient to demonstrate intellectual capacity. With good nursing care these patients may survive for years.

Coma Vigil

This state may follow bilateral frontal lobe damage or upper brainstem lesions due to trauma or following neurosurgery. The eyes move, the patient may eat, swallow and breath spontaneously and even occasionally move, but they show no evidence of the ability to speak or perform anything other than these primitive tasks. They may follow carers around the room with their eyes but no purposeful movement or attempt at communication is witnessed. This condition may persist for years with good nursing care.

Post-Traumatic Aphasia

If the patient has suffered extensive damage in the dominant parietal region, often evidenced by right-sided motor signs, they may have motor and receptive aphasia and their inability to communicate or obey simple commands with anything other than blank stares and lack of comprehension may indicate complete aphasia. Once again, with good nursing care prolonged survival is possible.

Late Complications of Head Injury

If the patient is fortunate enough to survive the original injury, not develop a haematoma and recover from complicating general surgical and orthopaedic injuries, it is highly likely that they will be subject to a variety of longer-term complications of practical and medicolegal importance.

Amnesia

There are two types of amnesia associated with head injury and they have long been regarded as reliable indicators of the severity of **diffuse** brain damage.

Pre-Traumatic Amnesia

This consists of amnesia for the event itself and a variable period prior to the injury, which is obligatory for the definitive diagnosis of 'head injury' and the main defining factor of so-called 'concussion'. The amnesic period is often surprisingly brief: the patient may recall events occurring only a few hundred yards before the accident. Conversely, they may have no recollection of the purpose of their journey and sometime no recall of events of that day. Very long periods of pre-traumatic amnesia extending back months or years can occur and are usually associated with very severe damage in the temporal or frontal lobes, and sometimes on return home from hospital the patient may not recognize the house that they have perhaps lived in for the last 5 years. This memory is never retrieved and is always a source of great anguish to the patient.

Post-Traumatic Amnesia

This period of amnesia shows a closer correlation with the severity of the injury and is defined as the period prior to the patient establishing full orientation and continual memory. This end point may be very difficult to define. It is not uncommon for patients to go home with everyone confident that they are now fully recovered, only to discover in the follow-up clinic that they cannot identify the doctors who looked after them or recognize the ward that they were in for several weeks prior to their discharge, and have no recollection of their time in hospital.

The duration of post-traumatic amnesia correlates with the following definitions of severity of injury:

5 minutes or less duration – very mild injury

5–60 minutes, duration – mild injury

1–24 hours, duration – moderate injury

1–7 days, duration – severe injury

7–30 days, duration – very severe injury

30 days or more duration – extremely severe injury.

Epilepsy

There are important differences between early- and late-onset epilepsy complicating head injuries which sometimes causes confusion. Children are particularly likely to suffer fits closely related to the injury that subsequently prove to be isolated epileptic events.

Early Epilepsy

Early-onset epilepsy is defined as occurring within 7 days of the injury. At this early stage some of the episodes reflect metabolic abnormalities due to anoxia or electrolyte disturbance and the effects of other injuries, such as severe sepsis and fever, rather than the brain injury itself. Only 5% of patients suffer early fits and of these only 25% go on to have further episodes. Furthermore, the prognosis is good, with relatively few of these patients showing a continued tendency to seizures requiring long-term medication.

Late Epilepsy

Late epilepsy is defined as starting after 7 days. This usually does reflect brain damage and occurs in 15% of severely brain-damage patients, nearly all of whom will manifest their epileptic tendency by the end of the first year. Unfortunately, 75% of these patients will have ongoing epilepsy still requiring medication 10 years later.

There is some merit in not starting anticonvulsant medication after a single early fit, especially in children,

provided the risk of another episode would not jeopardize the outcome of the head or other injuries. For example, if the patient is unconscious and on ventilatory support treatment is obligatory, but if the patient is conscious and recovering well treatment could safely be withheld and may ultimately prove unnecessary. Conversely, the development of late-onset epilepsy not only requires immediate treatment but the patient should be advised that it is highly likely that the treatment will need to be lifelong. There is no convincing evidence that the immediate prophylactic use of anticonvulsants in all head-injured patients prevents the development of early or late-onset epilepsy, and there are disadvantages attached to the high loading doses recommended if the patient is in poor clinical condition. Routine anticonvulsant prophylaxis has not been universally adopted.

Headaches

Although to the general public headache would seem to be an obvious and inevitable consequence of head injury, it is surprising how rarely headaches follow severe craniocerebral trauma. Some mildly injured patients develop a vascular type of headache even in the absence of a previous history of migraine, and this seems to be particularly likely to be triggered by injuries to the brow and facial skeleton. As a general rule the patients who claim that their lives are totally destroyed by intractable headache are the survivors of unpleasant and frightening accidents in which the trauma was minimal. These headaches usually have the features of a tension headache and are probably of psychogenic origin. Usually the patients run out of superlatives to describe the severity of the pain but are surprisingly vague on detail as to the exact location and behaviour of the headache, and often become quite angry if probing questions are pursued in an attempt to get a clearer description.

'Dizziness' and Vertigo

The important distinction between the complaint of 'dizziness' and vertigo was discussed at length in Chapter 6. Following head injury the distinction is again of considerable importance. Following severe blows to the head, particularly to the occipital area or in association with petrous fractures, severe ongoing vertigo which slowly recovers, through a phase of benign positional vertigo, is a very common and readily explicable complication. Non-specific but severely disabling 'dizziness' tends to follow relatively trivial trauma and frequently coexists with intractable non-specific headaches, as described above.

Poor Concentration

Patients who have severe amnesic problems following head injury have considerable difficulty with immediate recall and short-term memory, which becomes very apparent as soon as they return home. They also tend to anguish continually about the gap in their memory. It is as if there is a giant wall that they have to leap to access their remote memory and they never quite learn to cope with this problem. Poor concentration without memory impairment is a problem of apparently trivial trauma and is the third component of the triad known as the post concussional syndrome.

Post concussional Syndrome

This is a highly controversial syndrome of considerable medicolegal significance. It is undoubtedly the commonest sequela to head trauma and is encountered in its most severe form in patients who by all other criteria have suffered minimal trauma: many have not even lost consciousness but have merely been 'stunned' in the most trivial of accidents. The triad consists of 'terrible' headaches, ongoing 'dizziness' and 'poor concentration'. It is much debated whether this is purely a psychological consequence of head trauma or represents a genuine syndrome indicating brain damage. Careful psychometric testing may help detect evidence of brain injury in some cases, but the overwhelming consensus view is that this syndrome is psychogenic in origin. In some cases this view is reinforced by the presence of frankly non-organic physical findings, as detailed in

other chapters. It is perhaps advisable to label such symptoms as 'functional' rather than using the more concrete sounding but pejorative 'hysteria' or 'malingering', terms which defy strict definition.

Anosmia

Loss of sense of smell with associated impairment of taste sensation complicates 7% of head injuries and most often follows blows to the occiput. It is presumed that the fore-and-aft motion of the brain shears off the fine nerve filaments in the cribriform plate. Incomplete damage may produce dysosmia, where all sensations are modified by pervasive scents or unpleasant smells. This does not recover and presents some potential hazard to the patient in the event of failure to detect fire, burning cooking, leaking gas or petrol fumes.

Visual Defects

It is only after full recovery from major trauma that the full extent of visual pathway or extraocular nerve damage becomes apparent. Either visual field defects or disabling diplopia may cause problems. It should be relatively easy to localize the damage using the information in Chapters 2 and 4.

Facial Palsy

An upper motor neuron facial weakness may be part of a residual hemiparesis following hemisphere damage.

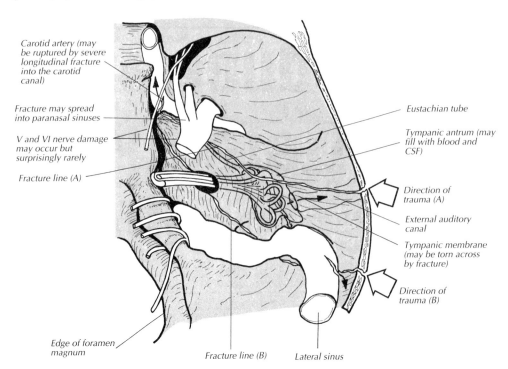

23.2   Longitudinal fractures of the petrous temporal bone.

Lower motor neuron facial nerve palsy complicates petrous fractures. Transverse fractures due to a blow on the occiput are responsible for 20% of cases, usually of immediate onset, and only 50% recover. Longitudinal fractures due to a direct blow to the side of the head are responsible for 80%. These typically appear several days after the trauma and the prognosis for recovery is excellent. It has been claimed that the use of steroids in these cases is beneficial, but this is doubtful and the risk of steroids in the likely presence of an open fracture is an obvious disadvantage (Figs 23.2 and 23.3).

Personality Change and Dementia

Following head trauma a very frequent complaint from the relatives, and sometimes the patients themselves, is that their personality has altered, usually for the worse. The patient may be described as short-tempered, irritable, aggressive and unpleasant. An association with complex partial seizures due to temporal lobe damage can present special problems, as some of the behavioural change is the result of the limitations that the epilepsy places on the patient resuming their former lifestyle. Severe frontal lobe damage may produce striking loss of social graces and alienation of friends and relatives, making the patient even more isolated and bad-tempered. These changes can be totally life-destroying and yet are hard to define and quantify, and are often handled less than sympathetically because there is no visible disability such as a hemiplegia to invoke a more sympathetic response. There is also increasing evidence that some of the survivors of severe head trauma over the last 20 years, as they approach late middle age, are showing intellectual decline possibly related to loss of neuronal reserves as a consequence of their injury. Some of these patients have never been scanned previously and on scanning have evidence of extensive atrophy, and some show changes suggestive of long-standing unrecognized communicating hydrocephalus, presumably a consequence of their original injury.

Special Features of Head Injuries in Childhood

Head injuries account for some 15% of childhood admissions to surgical wards. There are several special features of head injury in childhood.

Children may initially appear to be more ill than the adult. Even quite minor trauma may cause drowsiness, confusion and vomiting without there necessarily being serious implications. The rules for admission and observation still apply.

The potential for recovery from serious craniocerebral injury is very much greater in the child than in the adult. In addition to the usual causes of head injury at any age, there are certain special risks in children. Falls from balconies of high-rise flats, injuries from swings and roundabouts and, increasingly recognized,

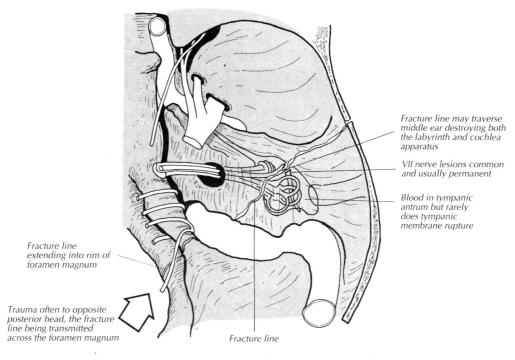

Fracture line may traverse middle ear destroying both the labyrinth and cochlea apparatus

VII nerve lesions common and usually permanent

Blood in tympanic antrum but rarely does tympanic membrane rupture

Fracture line extending into rim of foramen magnum

Trauma often to opposite posterior head, the fracture line being transmitted across the foramen magnum

Fracture line

23.3   Transverse fractures of the petrous temporal bone.

trauma inflicted on the child by the parents or other carers.

Another easily overlooked form of potentially lethal injury in children is the penetrating type of lesion around the orbit, from knitting needles, sharp sticks or pencils. A small skin laceration or perhaps a wood splinter may mark the entrance of a track leading through the skull and dura into the brain. This type of injury often occurs without loss of consciousness and it is not until meningitis or brain abscess occurs a few days later that the seriousness of the original injury becomes apparent.

Following head trauma children develop cerebral swelling very easily, rapidly leading to confusion and drowsiness. This must be carefully distinguished from an intracranial collection of blood, and CT scanning (if available) is indicated if there is any suspicion of a developing focal abnormality.

Epileptic seizures occur very easily in the child and a fit may occur within minutes of any injury severe enough to produce loss of consciousness. In this situation there is a double danger; either the head injury will be thought to be more severe than it really is, the postictal state being mistaken for cerebral swelling, or the whole situation may be thought to be a fit and its sequelae, and the developing complications of the unrecognized head injury be missed. The child who is apparently 'sleeping it off' may be going into coma.

The apparent severity of the injury, as judged by the distance fallen or the speed of the vehicle, does not bear a reliable relationship to the risk of complications. The elastic skull of the child is less easily fractured than that of the adult, and basal fractures occur much less frequently in the child. There is a much greater risk of an intracranial haematoma developing in a child who has not sustained a skull fracture than in the adult. Conversely, even a mild knock without loss of consciousness can cause a skull fracture and a fatal extradural haematoma, whereas the same injury in another child may cause alarm because of drowsiness and vomiting but be followed by full recovery in a few days. The admission and observation rules are the same as in the adult.

All children who have lost consciousness must be admitted. A skull fracture or the possibility of a puncture type of injury both require admission whether or not the child has been unconscious. Other serious injuries to the cervical spine, thorax or abdominal contents should also be excluded. It is very important to remember that even in childhood head injuries **rarely** cause surgical shock.

Some children go through a period of confusion and irritability just before becoming unconscious, and this should be regarded as an ominous sign even if at first sight the child appears to be more active than previously.

Assuming no specific complications have occurred, following any injury with a prolonged period of unconsciousness the child will inevitably go through a period of confusion. The presence of the parents at this time will hasten full recovery. Strange faces in a strange building will tend to worsen the confusion and make this period more distressing for the child. Early discharge to the more familiar home situation hastens recovery but during this time weekly follow-up is reassuring to both the parent and the doctor.

As in the adult, chronic subdural haematoma may occur in the weeks following head injury. Any deterioration in school performance, headaches, drowsiness, unsteadiness of gait, double vision or vomiting should raise suspicion. In the infant vomiting is a notable early sign and tense fontanelles are usually found. In the older child the symptoms are more subtle, especially as children do not seem to notice or complain of headache in the way that adults do. In these cases, although there are no fontanelles to bulge the head can expand and either the skull sutures separate or a bulge may appear on the skull, usually in the temporal fossa overlying the haematoma.

CASE REPORT I

A 12-year-old boy fell 12 feet on to concrete. He did not recall losing consciousness but remembers striking his head. He did not tell his parents. Several weeks later he complained of failing vision and some mild headache. He denied drowsiness and there had been no decline in his schoolwork. On examination there was a bulge in the skull above the left ear, severe bilateral papilloedema and increased reflexes on the right side. He had a very large subdural haematoma in the left temporal fossa.

Although seizures occurring immediately following trauma are more common in the child, the ultimate risk of post-traumatic epilepsy is no greater than in the adult. Immediate seizures may indicate an increased risk of further seizures, but in many cases early fits prove to be of no long-term significance. In general, the longer after the injury the first attack occurs the more likely it is that the child will have further attacks. The first attack will usually occur within the first 18 months after the injury. The risk of seizures occurring later, even if none occur during the acute phase of the injury, is greatly increased if there has been a depressed fracture, a haematoma requiring evacuation (especially an acute subdural haematoma), or infection following a penetrating injury. There is probably a case for putting children in these categories on prophylactic anticonvulsants for the first 2 years after the injury.

The postconcussional syndrome is fortunately not a feature of childhood head injuries. However, there is some similarity in that children who suffer from behavioural problems following a head injury usually do so after a relatively mild injury. Furthermore, careful evaluation often reveals that their premorbid behaviour was poor. Very often the incident that led to the head injury occurred under circumstances that raise suspicion of the child's normal behaviour. Often the home circumstances are unsatisfactory and the difficulties presented in the management of such a child are formidable.

At the other end of the scale are overprotective parents and teachers who create a difficult situation for the child by prolonging the period away from school, making special concessions and preventing the child from resuming normal activities, especially games. As the latter provide the only light relief in a week at school this restriction is rarely appreciated by the child. It is essential to allow the child to resume normal activities as soon as possible. Even if the head injury was serious, the potential for recovery is very high and will not be fully realized if the child is unnecessarily restricted.

Special Features of Head Injuries in the Adult

As the majority of adult head injuries occur in road traffic accidents or industrial accidents it is essential that very complete and accurate medical records are kept for medicolegal purposes. If the patient had been drinking, it is very dangerous to assume that drowsiness, confusion or ataxia are purely due to alcohol. A classic example of this problem follows.

CASE REPORT II

A 38-year-old man, a known epileptic, went drinking every Friday evening. He usually became drunk and this often brought on an epileptic seizure. Because he was not supposed to drink with his medication he was also in the habit of stopping his drugs to avoid problems! One evening, as he returned home with his brother from such an outing, he had a fit on the stairs and fell some 8 feet back into the hall. His brother, following his usual practice, put him into bed to sleep it off. He became alarmed when he could not rouse him the following morning. The patient's pupils were widely dilated, asymmetrical and fixed to light. Both legs were spastic, with bilateral extensor plantar responses. There was a palpable fracture right across the vertex. He was neither postictal or postalcoholic, but suffering from large bilateral extradural haematomas.

It is also very important to remember that because of impaired clotting mechanisms the heavy drinker has a greatly increased risk of developing subacute or chronic subdural haematomas following head trauma.

CASE REPORT III

A man, 67 years of age in 1960, was in hospital for the investigation of a gastric ulcer. On the day following a barium meal he was noticed to have a right facial weakness. Further examination revealed a mild right hemiparesis which had appeared overnight. His CSF was examined and showed an elevated protein. The pressure was normal. He gave a history of having been unconscious after being run over by a car 7 years before. Investigation by carotid angiography revealed an enormous left-sided chronic subdural haematoma. At operation the capsule of the haematoma was nearly half an inch thick.

The reason for the sudden onset of physical signs with a lesion that had clearly been the same size for many years is not apparent. If this had not occurred while he was in hospital it would undoubtedly have been regarded as a mild stroke. On the other hand, he would not have been subjected to the undoubted risks of a lumbar puncture, which fortunately passed off without incident. The management of this case reflects the paucity of available investigational techniques at that time very accurately. A lumbar puncture was regarded as less hazardous than carotid arteriography, which in those days was performed by a direct needle puncture under general anaesthetic.

Occasionally patients are seen when the history and signs do indicate the classical sequence of events to be anticipated, if only all patients were this typical!

CASE REPORT IV

A 71-year-old man fell while boarding a cruise ship. He fell on his left shoulder and cut his head. He resisted attempts to get treatment as he did not want to miss the cruise and apart from pain in the left shoulder, the trip went off uneventfully. He was sure he had not been unconscious at any stage. Seven weeks later while in church, he had a series of jerks in the left arm, almost certainly focal epilepsy, lasting for 60 seconds. In the next 7 days he repeatedly dropped objects from his left hand and while driving, kept veering to the left, towards the kerb and parked vehicles. He felt that this was due to the pain in his left shoulder. In the three days before he was seen, further weakness had developed in the left arm, he had become increasingly drowsy and for the first time in his life he had some headache on the right side. He was fully orientated for time and place but preferred to let his wife give the history. On examination, he had a left hemiparetic gait. There were no eye signs. He had a clear-cut left upper motor neurone facial weakness and he had left sided pyramidal weakness and a L extensor plantar. There was very dramatic left sensory extinction. He was in sinus rhythm with no bruits and a blood pressure of 170/80. The CT scan was diagnostic of a large subdural haematoma. This was successfully evacuated. Scans on next page.

This history was so suggestive of a subdural haematoma that it seemed too good to be true, and in the letter dictated to the GP before the scan was seen, it seemed reasonable to comment that it might well prove to be a glioma – fortunately for once a classical history **did** indicate a classical lesion!

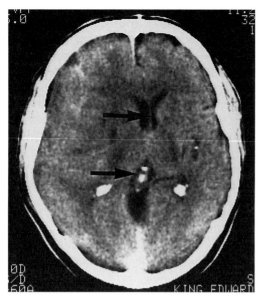

Marked displacement of midline but edge of subdural not visible.

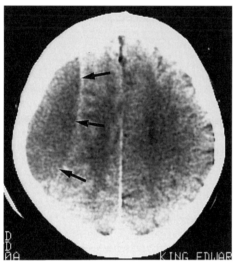

Edge of subdural haematoma clearly seen, pushing hemisphere down and across to the left.

CRIV.   *Subdural haematoma of two months duration.*

Chronic Subdural Haematoma

Although it is appropriate to consider chronic subdural haematoma in the chapter on head trauma, it should be stressed that in a majority of patients the responsible head trauma cannot be identified with certainly. There are several striking peculiarities.

1. Chronic subdural haematoma is quite unusual after serious head trauma. Patients tend to have either an acute extradural haematoma or an acute subdural haematoma (now called an intradural haematoma) associated with underlying brain damage.

2. In over the half of patients no trauma can be identified, although the ubiquitous history of 'standing up under a cupboard door' or 'walking into a doorframe' is often cited but often of uncertain significance.

3. Even when more suspicious trauma, such as swimming into the wall of a swimming pool (as detailed in case history below) or a blow from an up-and-over garage door, can be identified, the patient is usually insistent that they were not knocked unconscious or even stunned by the experience and at the time did not think the injury was significant.

CASE REPORT V

A retired 75-year-old woman presented with a possible left-sided epileptic fit, which was sufficiently atypical that a transient ischaemic attack was also suspected. The only physical sign was a left extensor plantar response. A CT scan revealed a large chronic subdural haematoma. One year previously she recalled swimming backstroke into the swimming pool wall. The haematoma was evacuated through a burr hole, with disappointingly little change in the CT scan appearances. Just prior to discharge, routine haematological studies included an ESR of 37. She was asymptomatic (without headache) at that time. Three weeks later she was admitted with very severe right-sided headache and blurred vision and recurrent haematoma was suspected. The CT scan was unaltered but the sedimentation rate was 116. The headache cleared within hours of the use of prednisolone, even though a subsequent biopsy of the temporal artery was negative. A diagnosis of cranial arteritis seems certain as the cause of the subsequent events. A repeat CT scan 6 months later was completely normal showing complete resolution of the haematoma.

4. Underlying disorders may predispose the patient to the condition. Alcoholism combining both the risk of frequent head trauma with impaired clotting mechanisms is a notable example, but anticoagulants and blood dyscrasias carry the same risk. The elderly atrophic brain is particularly vulnerable and the developing symptoms of the condition are more likely to be mistaken for vascular disease or dementia in this age group.

CASE REPORT VI

A 78-year-old woman underwent a hip replacement procedure and was given subcutaneous heparin for 3 days prior to full mobilization. Her postoperative course was uneventful and she went home. Three weeks later she presented with a 10-day history of brief episodes of right-sided weakness, with features entirely compatible with transient ischaemic attacks, and was started on soluble aspirin by the admitting physicians. A CT scan revealed an extremely large subdural haematoma which required surgical evacuation.

5. The characteristic feature of the condition is that there is **no** characteristic feature. The onset may be very abrupt, as noted in a previous example, and mimic a cerebro-vascular accident. It can be very insidious and mimic a tumour. It may produce epileptic events or even simulate transient ischaemic attacks.

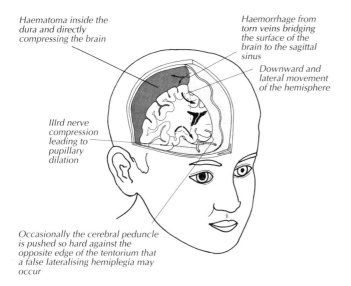

Haematoma inside the dura and directly compressing the brain

Haemorrhage from torn veins bridging the surface of the brain to the sagittal sinus

Downward and lateral movement of the hemisphere

IIIrd nerve compression leading to pupillary dilation

Occasionally the cerebral peduncle is pushed so hard against the opposite edge of the tentorium that a false lateralising hemiplegia may occur

23.4 Chronic subdural haematoma.

May be acute, sub-acute or chronic depending on several factors (see text) Usually high parietal in position

The typical site for these haematomas is shown in Fig 23.4. The leak is a low-pressure venous ooze resulting from tearing of the veins bridging the veins of the cortex to the sagittal sinus. Why there is such a variation in the rate of development of the various types and the exact mechanism by which the contents change from blood to a thin yellow fluid in the chronic type is unknown. The latter are often called 'subdural hygromas', as the evidence of previous bleeding is minimal or absent.

Traumatic Lesions of the Spinal Cord

Although the cervical and lumbar spine are the least supported parts of the spinal column their mobility to some extent protects them from damage. The majority of serious spinal injuries occur in the dorsal area, particularly between T6 and T12. In the absence of any pathological abnormality of the vertebra (osteoporosis due to steroids, metastatic cancer), considerable force is needed to fracture the thoracic spine. This may be either compressive, i.e. falling from a height on to the feet, or due to hyperflexion, when a weight falls on to the back. The force needed is so great that these fractures are frequently accompanied by cord transection. Cervical cord injuries, although less frequent, account for the majority of early deaths, due to respiratory paralysis.

Cervical Spine Injuries

1. The mechanisms and results of fractures of the cervical spine are indicated in Figs 25.5 and 23.6. These may result from trauma to the front or back of the head, as shown.

2. Atlantoaxial dislocation may also occur in patients with rheumatoid arthritis due to ligamentous degeneration or absorption of the odontoid peg. This usually, but not always, occurs in those patients on steroids.

CASE REPORT VII

A 71-year-old woman was admitted under the care of orthopaedic surgeons with a 4-week history of progressive generalized weakness. This had started with a sensation as if she were standing on stinging nettles, and after 2 weeks

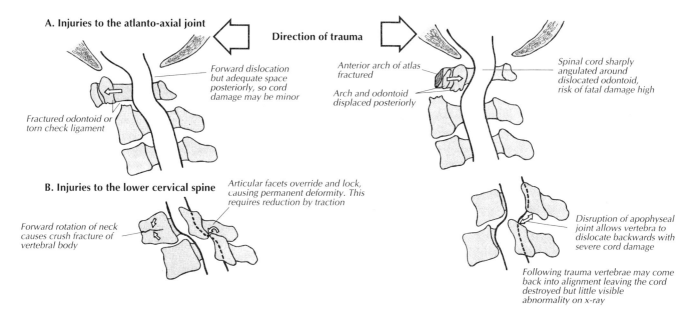

A. Injuries to the atlanto-axial joint

Direction of trauma

Forward dislocation but adequate space posteriorly, so cord damage may be minor

Fractured odontoid or torn check ligament

Anterior arch of atlas fractured

Arch and odontoid displaced posteriorly

Spinal cord sharply angulated around dislocated odontoid, risk of fatal damage high

B. Injuries to the lower cervical spine

Articular facets override and lock, causing permanent deformity. This requires reduction by traction

Forward rotation of neck causes crush fracture of vertebral body

Disruption of apophyseal joint allows vertebra to dislocate backwards with severe cord damage

Following trauma vertebrae may come back into alignment leaving the cord destroyed but little visible abnormality on x-ray

23.5 Mechanism of cervical spine injury: posterior blow

23.6 Mechanism of cervical spine injury: anterior blow

similar symptoms had started in the hands. By that time she was unable to walk and then developed increasing weakness of both arms. There were no cranial nerve symptoms. She had had multiple joint replacements and orthopaedic procedures for severe rheumatoid arthritis and was on prednisolone 5 mg daily. Neurological examination was very difficult because of joint deformity. All reflexes were absent and no clear plantar responses were detectable. The motor weakness was consistent with a pyramidal distribution. All sensory modalities were intact in spite of the sensory symptoms. MRI scanning revealed gross atlantoaxial subluxation, with the odontoid peg through the foramen magnum and into the posterior fossa. In spite of her age and frail condition, following a transoral removal of the odontoid peg and posterior stabilization of the cervical spine she was discharged home 8 weeks later walking on sticks with a left foot drop.

This patient had originally been admitted as a possible peripheral neuropathy due to rheumatoid arthritis, because of the absent reflexes. This demonstrates the subtlety of examination required when the patient has other severe disabilities, the possible diagnostic catch of absent reflexes for other reasons and the paucity of sensory findings even in patients with prominent sensory symptoms.

3. Atlantoaxial dislocations occurring in childhood may produce an unusual delayed myelopathy. The injury often results from a fall on to the back of the head from a swing. An acute transient tetraparesis lasting less than 30 minutes may occur with complete recovery. Some 20 years later the patient develops a progressive tetraparesis punctuated by acute episodes of tetraparesis while flexing the neck, sneezing, or when slapped on the back. This is presumably due to repeated mild trauma inflicted by the sliding dislocation on neck flexion. (The anatomical features of the foramen magnum region are shown in Fig. 23.7.)

CASE REPORT VIII

A 38-year-old man was referred because of increasing clumsiness of gait due to a spastic tetraparesis. He was partially sighted due to retrolental fibroplasia. At the age of 4 he had fallen from a swing and been unconscious and totally paralysed for about 20 minutes. Following recovery he was completely deaf, suggesting bilateral temporal bone fractures. He was otherwise well until 4 years before referral. Over that period he had developed stiffness of the limbs and clumsiness. He frequently played touch football (the American game) and his friends found that if he was running with the ball he could best be stopped by a sharp push into the middle of his back. This made him drop the ball and fall to the ground, temporarily tetraplegic. It was these repeated insults that probably led to his spastic tetraparesis. He was found to have sliding atlantoaxial dislocation.

4. Cervical spine fractures between C1 and C3 level are usually fatal, as they inevitably interfere with respiration. The following are two extreme examples.

CASE REPORT IX

A 9-year-old girl was struck by a slow-moving vehicle. She was deeply cyanosed but breathing spontaneously when picked up by the ambulance crew. On admission she was unconscious and apnoeic. Following stabilization she was demonstrated to have a fractured right femur, fracture dislocation of the right shoulder and wide angulation of the spinous processes of C1 and C2, indicating disruption of the posterior spinal ligament at this level. The clinical signs in the limbs were those of a flaccid quadriplegia. CT scan revealed haemorrhage around the brain stem and upper spinal cord. She was ventilated but 12 hours later developed a profound bradycardia leading to cardiac arrest.

CASE REPORT X

A 17-year-old boy attempted suicide by leaping from a staircase with a rope around his neck. The drop was estimated to be about 12 feet. His father had severe Parkinson's disease and his mother had committed suicide by walking into the sea a few months earlier. When cut down he was still breathing and indeed continued to breath spontaneously for over 20 minutes until some 300 yards from A and E department. He was deeply cyanosed on arrival and endotracheal tube insertion proved extremely difficult. This was subsequently shown to be due to the trachea being detached from the lower end of the larynx. Cervical spine X-rays revealed a typical hangman's fracture of the pedicles of the C1 vertebra. Following surgical repair of the trachea and oesophagus he recovered consciousness but was totally tetraplegic and required ventilation. He was able to indicate by eye movements and blinking that he was in full possession of his intellectual faculties. He lived for 5 weeks on a respirator before being overwhelmed by a chest infection.

5. Mid-cervical fractures at C3/4 level are potentially more serious as there is less room for the spinal cord to ride the blow and the risk of respiratory paralysis is maximal at this level. Fragments of vertebra are more likely to break off and compress the cord, and fractures of the transverse process may damage the vertebral artery. This may cause brainstem signs or further vascular damage to the cord below the level of the fracture (see cord blood supply, Chapter 14).

CASE REPORT XI

A heavily built 70-year-old male huntsman was thrown from his horse and landed on his head. He picked himself up and, in accordance with hunting tradition, got back on the horse and continued riding for another 10–15 minutes before increasing discomfort in his neck prompted him to dismount and summon help. He was then transported across country in a Land Rover for several miles until he could be transferred to an ambulance where he was fortunately put into a collar. Cervical spine films in the A and E department revealed a fracture dislocation at C3/4 level and skull traction was applied. There were no neurological signs at that stage. Forty-eight hours later he developed a right homonymous hemianopia due to an infarct in the distribution of the left posterior cerebral artery. This was thought to be due to vertebral

(a) Foramen Magnum – bony structure (anterior)

Articular surface for occipital condyle

Transverse process of atlas perforated by vertebral artery

Altanto-axial joint Note. There is no disc between C and C2 – these are synovial joints

Note. It is possible that the anterior spinal artery is damaged by lesions here, and the cord damage is partly due to ischaemia and not entirely direct trauma

Very thin anterior atlas (the odontoid peg of the axis being its separated body)

Left vertebral artery

(c) Foramen Magnum – soft tissues (anterior)

Basilar artery

Vertebral artery

Dura – firmly attached to the rim of the foramen magnum – site of meningioma

Single anterior spinal artery– note its origin opposite the odontoid – in addition to the cord supply down to T1, it supplies the ventral medulla and the pyramids

(b) Foramen Magnum – bony structure (lateral)

Hypoglossal canal (XII)

Odontoid peg (also called the dens)

Absent spine to allow neck extension

Massive spine of axis for extensor muscle insertion

Articular surface for occipital condyle

Arch of atlas – thin and weak

Vertebral artery – note course on upper surface of the atlas to gain access to the cranial cavity

Axis – very strong arch

(d) Foramen Magnum – soft tissues (lateral)

Note. Lower medulla and pyramids opposite odontoid

Fourth ventricle

R. vertebral artery and cut orifice of L. vert. artery

Apical ligament

Synovial joint

Dural sheath of cord with sleeves for roots

Cerebellar tonsil

Cisterna magna

Atlanto-occipital ligament

Ligamentum flavum

Extradural fat (venous plexus)

Posterior longitudinal ligament (continous above with tectorial membrane and vertical part of the cruciate ligament

Anterior spinal artery descending to T1 level

23.7   Anatomical features of the foramen magnum

artery damage and probably embolic, as there were no other brainstem signs. Two years later he developed epilepsy, usually provoked by heavy alcohol intake. Ten years after these events he celebrated his 80th birthday, his only complaint being inability to drive because of his visual field defect and epilepsy.

Clinical Features of Cervical Spine Injuries

The clinical features of damage at any level are dominated initially by the stage of spinal shock, with a total flaccid paralysis below the level of the lesion. At this stage the sensory findings provide the best evidence of the extent and severity of the damage. As soon as the cord settles down (the nature of spinal shock is not understood) tone returns to the limbs below the level of the injury and the extent of local damage becomes obvious, as the residual weakness and wasting of the supplied muscles becomes apparent.

Central Cord Syndrome

Taking a mid-cervical fracture as an example, a flaccid tetraparesis occurs acutely but the patient may show a flicker of movement in the feet and have some preservation of pinprick sensation in the sacral dermatomes. This picture is typical of the central cord syndrome, the signs being rather similar to an advanced case of syringomyelia. As time passes, power in the legs will improve in the extensor groups and the reflexes become brisk. Some finger movement may reappear but wasting and weakness will remain in the muscles supplied by C4, C5 and C6. Sensation tends to improve but some slight loss of joint position sense in the feet usually remains. An unpleasant central pain syndrome may be a permanent feature when recovery has occurred. The following is an excellent example of this condition.

CASE REPORT XII

A 58-year-old boiler engineer slipped off the top of a boiler, sliding some 9 feet on to his head and shoulders. He was immediately unable to move his arms or legs and had no sensation below shoulder level. Breathing was unaffected and on arrival at hospital he seemed remarkably 'undistressed'. On examination he had flaccid tone in all four limbs, the arm reflexes were absent, the leg reflexes quite brisk but there was no plantar response due to sensory loss. He could move both legs slightly, only just able to flex the hips and extend the knees, but was unable to move his feet or toes. He was unable to sense the movement in his legs. His arms were totally paralysed, he had lost all sensory modalities to T1 level and there was a zone of hypersensitivity over the cervical dermatomes. A chest X-ray revealed paralysis of the right hemidiaphragm and a fractured spinous process at C5. There was no spinal instability. Over the next 24 hours increasing burning sensations over the cervical dermatomes indicated damage to the central spinal cord at cervical level. Recovery was extremely slow, but 6 months later he was able to walk with a frame and had regained continence. His major residual disability was impaired joint position sense in the legs and impaired pain and temperature sensation over the shoulders.

Another not uncommon mechanism of cervical spine fracture results from the patient tumble-diving into the shallow end of a swimming pool, striking the forehead on the bottom and fracturing the cervical spine at mid to lower cervical level. The following is a classic example of this mechanism and demonstrates the entire history and results of such an injury, as the accident happened in 1976 and the patient was followed until 1990.

CASE REPORT XIII

A 30-year-old man dived into a hotel swimming pool that was marked as 5 feet deep at that point. He recalled hitting the bottom with the top of his head. He then discovered that he was lying on the bottom, fully conscious but quite unable to move. He was able to look around and kept his mouth firmly shut. A gardener noticed that he failed to surface and pulled him out. He lay on the edge of the pool, able to breathe but unable to move either his arms or legs, and was numb to shoulder level. He was taken to hospital and put in skull traction for a fracture dislocation at C5/6 vertebral level. He was unable to move for 3 weeks, when his legs started to move and slight contractions could be seen in the proximal arm muscles. The sensory level dropped to the upper thorax and he specifically noted that the sensation in the axilla and down the inner aspect of both arms remained abnormal. He was also surprised to discover that the saddle area, including his penis and scrotum, felt normal compared to the rest of his body, and was aware of frequent erections while he was still catheterized. He started walking with aids at 5 months. When first seen for a medicolegal opinion 2 years after the accident, the findings were as follows: there was severe wasting and weakness of all muscles innervated by C7, C8 and T1; both legs showed increased tone, with minimal pyramidal weak-

ness, all reflexes were extremely brisk and both plantars were flexor. Sensory testing revealed a level to pinprick at C6 bilaterally with complete preservation of the sacral dermatomes. Dorsal column sensation (vibration and joint position sense) was intact in both arms and legs. Over the last 12 years he has continued to make some slight further improvement and continues to work as a motoring journalist.

This is a particularly good example of sacral sparing due to preservation of the peripheral spinal cord, which is also reflected in the intact dorsal column sensation and ultimate minimal pyramidal deficit in the legs. The brunt of the injury has fallen on the central grey just below the level of the lesion.

Management

As long as the neurological state is static or improving, treatment is aimed at maintaining reduction of any fracture dislocation using skull callipers and whatever weight is necessary to maintain the reduction. If the reduction remains unstable after 6 weeks, fixation may be required.

The main indications for surgical intervention are progression of neurological signs or radiological evidence of a fragment of the vertebral body or the arch still compressing the cord.

Thoracolumbar Injuries

Simple crush fractures of the upper lumbar vertebrae are quite common in the elderly patient, and a crush fracture with cord compression may be the presenting symptom of metastatic malignant disease, particularly of the prostate gland or primary malignancy of the vertebra in myelomatosis. Crush fractures may also occur during the tonic phase of a major epileptic seizure. In the majority of instances the spinal cord is not damaged and symptomatic treatment is all that is required.

In severe fracture dislocation of the vertebra with complete shearing of the ligaments and fractures of the articular facets, total cord destruction occurs. The very unstable fracture will often reduce spontaneously by the time the patient reaches hospital. In these cases cord damage is complete and irreversible and the immediate aim must be the prevention of urinary tract infection and bedsores while awaiting the recovery of reflex tone. The position in which the patient is nursed can be critical in determining whether they develop a paraplegia in flexion or a paraplegia in extension. From a rehabilitation point of view the latter is more desirable.

Fracture dislocations below L1 level damage the cauda equina and as these are peripheral nerves there is considerable potential for recovery. Complete reduction is necessary and operative fixation may be required to prevent further damage to the cauda equina. Burst fractures of the L1 vertebra are particularly devastating in the male, producing impotence due to damage to the hypogastic sympathetic plexus, which lies on the front of this vertebra.

Sometimes an unusual mechanism of injury may lead to an incorrect diagnosis, especially if the X-rays taken in A and E are not sufficient to adequately demonstrate the lesion. The following case demonstrates the importance of not making value judgements about a patient's personality and behaviour at first sight.

CASE REPORT XIV

A 20-year-old fine art student was taken to A and E after falling off a toboggan on to his lower back. He was in severe pain when seen and the X-rays performed only demonstrated the spine from L1 downwards. These were normal and he was discharged. Continuing pain and the development of a bilateral foot drop led to his admission. In retrospect he realized that he had difficulty with bowel movements, had dribbling incontinence of urine and was impotent at that time, but was not asked about these functions and was in such pain that he paid little attention to these symptoms. Unfortunately, the notes made it clear that he was regarded as a 'strange boy' from the Arts faculty, who was elaborating his symptoms. He was also refused analgesia because it was incorrectly suspected that he might have a drug problem. He took his own discharge. It was several weeks before further X-rays were taken because of continuing symptoms and an exploded fracture of the body of T11 was demonstrated. At this stage, in spite of clearly documented upper and lower motor neuron signs and continuing sphincter disturbance, he was told that nothing more could be done. A year later, an orthopaedic surgeon who was asked for a second opinion demonstrated bone fragments within the canal damaging the cauda equina, which were removed. Unfortunately, when examined 5 years later for a medicolegal opinion, he still had a combination of upper and lower motor neuron difficulties typical of damage to the terminal spinal cord and cauda equina. He had residual bladder problems and was unable to ejaculate.

This combination of physical symptoms and findings is diagnostic of cauda equina damage, and in view of the high potential for good recovery the failure to quickly identify and appropriately treat the responsible fracture was a serious error.

Delayed Complications

In recent years it has been increasingly recognized that a syringomyelic syndrome may complicate spinal cord trauma. This may occur after periods varying from 1 to 15 years when the previously static neurological state alters. The first symptom is usually pain above the level of the lesion, followed by the development of further lower motor neuron signs in the same area. Myelography, and latterly CT and MRI scanning, has confirmed that this syndrome is due to a syringomyelic cavity developing in and extending from the damaged area. It has also been shown that a similar syndrome may follow apparently trivial trauma, particularly to the cervical spinal cord. Sometimes the later development of physical symptoms may occur when the severity of the original injury has not been fully appreciated.

CASE REPORT XV

A 6'5" tall, 33-year-old man was referred because of progressive clumsiness, difficulty walking and a sensation when he coughed like an electric shock radiating up towards his neck and down both legs, followed by transitory weakness and numbness of both legs. This had been particularly distressing as he was a keen amateur basketball player. Four years previously he had attempted to prevent seven off-duty soldiers from gatecrashing his sister's 21st birthday party. He was severely beaten around the head by both punches and kicks, and knocked unconscious. His left shoulder was fractured and his left arm had been weak since that time. He was seen by an orthopaedic surgeon 3 months after the injury who documented that both triceps jerks were absent. Those responsible were convicted of criminal assault. On physical examination he had increased tone in the right arm with extremely brisk biceps and supinator reflexes and an absent triceps jerk. In the left arm the biceps and supinator jerk were depressed and the triceps jerk was absent. The finger jerks were brisk bilaterally. There was no focal weakness or sensory loss. Both legs were spastic with clonus, more marked on the right, and the plantar responses were extensor. There was loss of vibration sense in the left leg and impairment of pinprick on the right to C7 level. Plain X-rays and CT myelography revealed severe cord compression at C5/6 and C6/7 by a combination of disc fragments and bone hypertrophy. Surgical removal of all disc fragments and osteophytes produced an excellent result but he was unable to resume playing basketball.

This was undoubtedly an undetected consequence of the original injuries and the symptoms took 4 years to evolve, in spite of unusually provocative physical activity.

Spinal injuries are generally managed by orthopaedic surgeons as the neurological consequences are usually immediate and irreversible. The potential for making neurological damage worse during the initial management places immense responsibility on bystanders, ambulance crew and casualty departments. If spinal damage is suspected immense care in moving the patient is vital until spinal instability has been excluded.

24. Neurological Complications of Systemic Disorders

Throughout this book great emphasis has been placed on the importance of detecting systemic diseases that may present as a neurological illness. In a general hospital setting the neurological department has an important role in the evaluation of patients already diagnosed as suffering from a specific condition who have subsequently developed a neurological problem. The potential neurologist therefore requires an extremely good knowledge of general medical and surgical disorders and their potential for causing neurological problems. Although many of these conditions have been mentioned elsewhere, it was felt that a final chapter in which some of these problems were grouped together would be helpful. The material is considered in eight main sections:

Pregnancy and labour

Diabetes mellitus and glucose metabolism

Collagen vascular disease

Endocrine and metabolic diseases including alcoholism

Cardiovascular diseases

Neoplastic diseases

Infectious diseases

The neurocutaneous disorders and dermatological manifestations associated with neurological disease.

Neurological Complications of Pregnancy and Labour

Eclampsia

This is the most serious complication of pregnancy. It is the ultimate expression of uncontrolled hypertension in pregnancy and is thought to be due to immunological mechanisms, even though an abnormally large uterus is the major feature in many cases. It is best avoided by skilled management of the pre-eclamptic state, which is indicated by rapid weight gain, proteinuria and a rising blood pressure. It occurs most often in the first pregnancy, in hydramnios, in patients with a multiple pregnancy, and in patients with preexisting diabetes mellitus or renal disease. Eclampsia is heralded by a sudden uncontrollable rise in blood pressure, chest pain, confusion, drowsiness and the onset of focal or generalized seizures. Following the seizures the patients may remain unconscious due to cerebral oedema or multiple petechial haemorrhages in the brain. In this situation the mortality rate is 10%.

In most patients the onset of eclampsia occurs immediately before or during labour and the danger rapidly diminishes as soon as the uterus is evacuated. In some women the onset may occur several days after delivery, so that continued observation is necessary in any patient who has had preeclampsia.

Seizures should be controlled with intravenous diazepam or barbiturates, and in comatose patients cerebral oedema should be reduced with dexamethasone or mannitol given intravenously.

CASE REPORT I

A 21-year-old primigravida with a twin pregnancy became eclamptic at the onset of labour, having three major seizures. Immediate caesarean section controlled the blood pressure but 48 hours later the patient had not recovered consciousness. An EEG showed symmetrical high-voltage delta activity, although the physical response to deep painful stimulation suggested that the patient had a right hemiparesis. She was treated with intravenous dexamethasone and recovered consciousness some 72 hours after delivery, and left hospital without sequelae.

Cerebrovascular Accidents

Less specific forms of cerebrovascular disease than eclampsia may be associated with the pregnant state. Cerebral aneurysms and cerebral angiomas may rupture during pregnancy due to changes in blood pressure or altered circulatory dynamics.

Cerebral venous thrombosis is a specific delayed complication of pregnancy and is especially likely to occur in patients with sickle-cell anaemia. The thrombosis usually occurs 2–3 weeks after delivery. The clinical picture depends on the site and extent of thrombosis. Localized cortical vein thrombosis may produce focal deficits such as a flaccid monoplegia, but thrombosis of the sagittal or lateral sinus will produce drowsiness, coma and papilloedema and may prove fatal. Even in the milder cases considerable residual deficit occurs and there is a high incidence of epilepsy in later years. In recent years many cases that would have previously been identified as cerebral venous thrombosis have proved to be arterial vascular lesions. If the diagnosis of **venous** thrombosis is certain, anticoagulants may be indicated.

Embolic cerebrovascular accidents may occur during labour, when either air or amniotic fluid may be forced into the uterine veins. This will usually result in pulmonary embolization. Occasionally cerebral embolization may occur from these sources. It is thought increasingly likely that this is due to paradoxical embolization through a potentially patent foramen ovale which becomes patent when right atrial pressure is raised.

Another very rare disorder that is likely to occur during pregnancy and the puerperium is thrombotic thrombocytopaenic purpura. This produces fever, renal failure, haemolytic anaemia and multiple vascular lesions of the brain. A simple haematological profile is usually diagnostic (see section on collagen vascular disease).

Cerebral and Spinal Tumours

Certain cerebral tumours tend to be aggravated by pregnancy owing to either increased vascularity or hormonal changes. Vascular tumours such as meningiomas and tumours of the pituitary gland, which has a natural tendency to increase in size during pregnancy, are particularly affected.

CASE REPORT II

A 26-year-old primigravida suffered a series of focal seizures affecting the right arm during the third trimester of pregnancy. Full investigation after delivery revealed a large left parasagittal meningioma, which was successfully removed after delivery.

CASE REPORT III

A 30-year-old woman had suffered a mild paraparesis during two previous pregnancies and multiple sclerosis had been suspected. During her third pregnancy the paraparesis was more severe and worsened following delivery. Investigation and exploration revealed an extensive mid-dorsal lipoma.

CASE REPORT IV

A 36-year-old woman developed a partial right third nerve palsy during pregnancy and failed to establish lactation or menstrual periods following delivery. She was referred for a
neurological opinion 2 years later when her vision became impaired. On examination, in addition to the partial third nerve palsy there was a bitemporal hemianopia and optic atrophy. Investigation and exploration revealed a very large cystic pituitary adenoma.

It is also important to remember the tumour that specifically complicates pregnancy; the hydatidiform mole or chorioncarcinoma. The diagnosis is clear-cut when the pregnancy is confirmed as a hydatidiform mole; what is less well appreciated is that chorioncarcinoma may follow an apparently normal pregnancy in some 15% of cases. The following is an example.

CASE REPORT V

A 25-year-old housewife from Yorkshire was visiting her in-laws. She had completed a normal pregnancy 4 months earlier. Since the pregnancy her appetite had been poor, she had lost a lot of weight, but continued breast feeding six times daily. During the drive down she had felt slightly nauseous and developed a mild headache. This had become severe over the previous 36 hours and she started vomiting. She had developed diplopia in the 18 hours prior to admission. On physical examination there was bilateral papilloedema and disconjugate eye movements. There were no long tract signs and the plantar responses were flexor. A CT scan revealed numerous cerebral metastases in the hemispheres, brain stem and posterior fossa. The chest X-ray revealed multiple metastases. Abdominal ultrasound revealed four discrete lesions in the liver. The uterus was thought to be bulky, although the gynaecologist was uncertain as to whether this was pathological 4 months post partum. An hCG level of 188,000 units left no doubt as to the diagnosis. She was referred to a specialist unit for chemotherapy but succumbed to her disease 4 days later.

Epilepsy

It is important that females of child bearing age using oral contraceptives are aware that a high-dose formulation is necessary if they are taking enzyme-inducing agents such as phenytoin, carbamazepine or any barbiturate derivative, as enzyme induction reduces the effectiveness of the pill. There is no evidence that the pill itself is provocative of epilepsy.

Epilepsy is usually not seriously affected by pregnancy, although some patients may suffer a slight increase in attacks in the later stages. The main risk occurs in the few days following delivery, when patients may suffer their first attack for months or years. It is therefore very important to continue medication during labour.

Anticonvulsant serum levels fall during pregnancy, but unless this leads to further attacks it would seem inappropriate merely to treat the blood level. Following pregnancy, breastfeeding is only a problem with highly sedative drugs such as barbiturate derivatives. All anticonvulsants are secreted in breast milk and may cause skin rashes if the infant is allergic to the agent in use.

Because of concern about the teratogenic potential of anticonvulsants it is sometimes suggested that drugs should be withdrawn during pregnancy. This has little to commend it. If the indications for continuing treatment with anticonvulsants were clear-cut before the pregnancy, then is it is vital that the drugs are continued during pregnancy because of the increased risk of attacks both during the pregnancy and after delivery. With this in mind, it is perhaps appropriate to use the agent least likely to cause problems and this is generally accepted to be carbamazepine. Both phenytoin and valproate have definitely been shown to produce fetal syndromes and are best avoided if carbamazepine proves to be an effective alternative.

After delivery the risk to the baby if the mother has an attack while changing or bathing it should be emphasized. It is advisable to change the baby on the floor and never to bath the baby unless accompanied. This might seem unnecessarily alarmist, but once a patient has been seen who came round in her bathroom to find her 2-year-old standing in the bath crying with the 6-month-old drowned in 3″ of water, the realization that this **is** essential advice is both immediate and lasting.

Multiple Sclerosis

Multiple sclerosis occurs in women of child bearing age and therefore a chance association with pregnancy is highly likely. The disease may have its onset in pregnancy, and occasionally patients are seen who have only had attacks during pregnancy. This is in striking contrast to the normal tendency for established MS to remain quiescent during pregnancy but with a high risk of relapse in the 3 months following delivery. Widely differing figures for the degree of risk exist, with risk levels as high as 25% in some series. It is difficult not to lean towards advising against pregnancy when two patients who have died as a consequence of a relapse provoked by a pregnancy remain vividly in mind. For all these reasons it is very difficult to advise patients in this situation, and one must weigh the risk against the desire to have children and also the future possibility that progress of the disease may render the mother unable to care for a young family.

CASE REPORT VI

A 36-year-old woman developed an acute attack of multiple sclerosis while breastfeeding her 3-month-old baby. She had visual blurring, poor concentration, difficulty word finding, generalized weakness and ataxia, urinary retention, difficulty swallowing and inability to write. The symptoms started to improve and 6 months later she had slurred speech, mild ataxia, brisk reflexes and extensor plantar responses. Later that year even these physical signs appeared to have fully recovered. The neurologist who was looking after her in Italy

advised strongly against a further pregnancy, but in 1989 she became pregnant. Within weeks she became severely ataxic, being barely able to walk, and her plantar responses were again extensor. She had a miscarriage. MRI scanning at that time showed typical white matter lesions and she was given ACTH (adrenocorticotrophic hormone), with minimal improvement. She was then given intravenous methylprednisolone, again with little or no response, by which time she was unable to stand without support and had suffered a remarkable deterioration in intellectual function, being unable to do calculations or converse coherently. She returned to her home in England, where she was found to have evidence of bilateral pyramidal involvement, severe ataxia and unequivocal evidence of dementia. The MRI scan at that stage revealed severe generalized white matter demyelination, with minimal involvement of the cerebellum and brain stem in spite of her signs. She was admitted to a nursing home where she became progressively confused, failing to recognize her husband or her son, and required total nursing care. She died 18 months after the onset of her second attack of MS which was almost certainly triggered by the second pregnancy.

It is likely that most neurologists have seen a case of this sort and it is very difficult, faced with such a tragedy, to remain an unbiased adviser when the question of further pregnancies is raised. The evidence that there is a risk is overwhelming: it is only the degree of risk that is in question and personal experience suggests that attacks that occur under such circumstances are particularly malevolent, as in this case.

Myasthenia Gravis

Myasthenia gravis also occurs in young women. In many patients the myasthenia tends to improve during pregnancy and relapse within 3 weeks of delivery. The child may be born with a transient myasthenic state or cholinergic blockade, either situation requiring considerable skill in management. The neonatal myasthenic state usually clears within a week. If thymectomy is considered necessary this should be carried out before the patient embarks on a pregnancy. The modern management of myasthenia gravis with steroids and immunosuppressant drugs has also added the risk of fetal abnormality due to treatment, and pregnancy is inadvisable if the patient is on such treatment.

Chorea Gravidarum

Chorea gravidarum has become an uncommon disorder with the decline of rheumatic fever as it usually represents a recrudescence of previous Sydenham's chorea during pregnancy. The movement disorder may respond well to diazepam or clonazepam and in resistant cases haloperidol has been recommended, but this introduces further worrying possibilities such as acute or tardive dyskinesia. Cases provoked by the oral contraceptive pill have been increasingly recognized and

and the following example documents pill-induced chorea followed by severe chorea gravidarum during a subsequent pregnancy.

CASE REPORT VII

An 18-year-old woman was admitted with a 2-week history of distressing twitching of the right face and tongue rapidly followed by the onset of choreiform movements of the right arm and leg. This was sufficient to interfere with speaking and swallowing. Clinically there was a diffuse choreiform movement disorder, although the bulk of the movements were right-sided. There was no previous history of any form of rheumatic fever, no confirmatory evidence of recent strepto-coccal infection, and it was thought likely that this was related to the recent use of the oral contraceptive pill. This was discontinued and within 3 weeks the movements completely subsided. Two years later she became pregnant and this progressed normally until 17 weeks. She then very rapidly developed severe generalized chorea, particularly of the bulbar muscles, sufficiently severe to prevent speaking and swallowing and she required tube feeding. She was on no other medication and there were no other signs. Haloperidol 5 mg t.d.s. gave good control of the movements. Two months later she became extremely unwell; intrauterine death was diagnosed and a fetus with multiple developmental defects was removed. All medication was withdrawn and the choreiform movements did not recur.

This case is not only a good example of the hormonal relationships of chorea but also indicates the life-threatening severity of the condition in a severe case. As no medication was given until after 17 weeks of the pregnancy, it is uncertain whether this was the cause of the fetal malformations, but treatment was obligatory.

Peripheral Nerve Lesions

Carpal tunnel syndrome is the commonest neurological complication of pregnancy. It may be very severe indeed during the night and remit completely in the day; even at the height of an attack nerve conduction studies may be normal. It may respond to diuretics or night splinting and usually remits following delivery. Operative decompression during pregnancy is very rarely justified.

Low back pain and lumbar root radicular pain are quite common and have been attributed to ligament laxity, sciatic nerve compression by the baby's head and lumbar root lesions. The symptoms usually remit following delivery and it seems certain that simple mechanical causes are the explanation.

Meralgia paraesthetica due to compression or traction of the lateral cutaneous nerve of the thigh may occur either during the pregnancy as the abdomen protrudes or even after pregnancy, when the abdomen suddenly flattens. Although the obturator nerve is vulnerable during obstetric procedures damage is actually

quite rare. These conditions are discussed in greater detail in Chapters 16 and 17.

Neurological Complications of Diabetes Mellitus and Glucose Metabolism

There are a large number of neurological complications of diabetes, most based on the accompanying vascular disease, particularly the changes in the small arterioles.

Peripheral Nerve Lesions

Diabetic peripheral neuropathy occurs most frequently in patients with late-onset diabetes rather than in juvenile diabetics. Whether this form of symmetrical damage is due to vessel disease is uncertain.

Mononeuritis multiplex is very common and is undoubtedly due to pressure on a nerve which is rendered vulnerable to compression damage by impaired microcirculation. Included in this category is infarction of the femoral nerve or upper lumbar nerve roots, the condition known as 'diabetic amyotrophy'.

Evidence of diffuse autonomic dysfunction has been defected in 90% of diabetic patients but fortunately significant clinical symptoms occur in relatively few patients. Disorders of potency and postural hypotension are the main problems. Although nocturnal diarrhoea is always quoted as a specific pointer to the diagnosis there is considerable doubt as to the validity of this observation and no theoretical basis for its occurrence.

Extraocular Nerve Lesions

Isolated extraocular nerve palsies are a common complication and have been shown to be due to infarction of the extraocular nerves. These are fully discussed in Chapter 5. The following case history provides a good example of this condition occurring in a diabetic patient.

CASE REPORT VIII

A 50-year-old Hispanic American presented with a painful right third nerve palsy. This was thought to be due to his known diabetes and angiography was not performed, but diagnostic confidence was somewhat shaken when a fourth nerve palsy occurred on the same side a week later. Within days the left third and fourth nerves also became affected and the diagnosis seemed more certain. This was confirmed by complete recovery of all the affected nerves over the next 6 weeks.

Visual Defects

Visual problems in diabetes are common and diabetes remains one of the major causes of blindness. This is usually due to retinal arterial or venous disease and cataracts. Because diabetic patients are prone to coronary artery and cerebrovascular disease, amaurosis fugax due to carotid or cardiac originating emboli is common and progressive ischaemic optic neuritis may occur. Acute optic neuritis related to the diabetic state has been reported but is rare.

Cerebrovascular Disease and Spinal Vascular Disease

Diabetics are particularly prone to suffer a wide range of cerebrovascular accidents with much greater frequency than the general population. The diabetic patient is also particularly subject to some of the specific vascular problems related to small-vessel disease affecting the internal capsule, basal ganglia and the spinal cord. These include the pseudobulbar palsy syndrome (Chapter 9), the atherosclerotic rigidity syndrome (Chapter 12), and anterior spinal artery thrombosis (Chapter 14).

Metabolic Syndromes

Diabetic Ketotic Coma

The management of diabetic coma is the province of the general physician and this section will be confined to recognition of the condition. Neurological units must be continually on the alert for patients in diabetic coma. In the past there were occasions when the diagnosis was not made until the CSF glucose was found to be grossly elevated. The CT scan in diabetic coma will also be normal. With the ease of immediate serum glucose determinations the risk of missing diabetic or hypoglycaemic coma is now very small, but in the past glucose levels were not always routinely determined and the most extreme example seen was a patient transferred from a district general hospital to a neuro-surgical unit, where the diagnosis was not made until the glucose level in the CSF, obtained at burr hole ventriculography, was determined by the biochemist! In general, the onset of diabetic coma is subacute and usually complicates an intercurrent disorder such as a urinary tract infection or pneumonia, often present for several days before the patient becomes comatose. A careful history of the mode of onset of the coma is essential. In spite of this the diagnosis can present enormous problems. The following case is a good example.

CASE REPORT IX

A 30-year-old man who had been diabetic for many years was in normal health when his wife left to visit her mother on a Friday evening. She returned on the following Sunday afternoon to find him comatose. On arrival in hospital he was pale, sweating and comatose with a low blood pressure. The clinical appearance was suggestive of hypoglycaemia and intravenous glucose was given as soon as blood had been taken for glucose and electrolyte determination. Shortly after admission he started having focal and generalized seizures. He was pyrexial but had no detectable neck stiffness. The blood sugar on arrival was 1200 mg%. He died within 20 minutes of admission and at post mortem was found to have miliary tuberculosis and tuberculous meningitis, presumably the infective factors that triggered the diabetic coma.

Hyperglycaemic, Hyperosmolar, Non-Ketotic Coma

This increasingly recognized condition is of greater neurological importance as the clinical presentations embrace a wide range of neurological phenomena. These include focal or generalized epileptic seizures, transient or progressive 'stroke-like' pictures, a 'tumour-like' course, an extrapyramidal syndrome or a comatose state of subacute onset. The dominant metabolic features are gross hyperglycaemia and hypernatraemia and a considerable increase in serum osmolarity. The ketosis that is the feature of diabetic coma does not occur and the condition is not necessarily a complication of overt or subclinical diabetes. In fact, the primary cause is not understood and following recovery there is often minimal evidence of diabetes. The major clinical clue to the diagnosis is dramatically severe clinical dehydration in a patient who has been unwell for only a few hours.

CASE REPORT X

A 68-year-old retired hospital matron was admitted to hospital in a comatose state. She had normally reactive pupils and bilateral extensor plantars and was markedly dehydrated. She had been perfectly well earlier in the day but had been noted by relatives to be excessively thirsty, and had been drinking unusually large quantities of Coca Cola. She then developed slurring of speech, dysphasic difficulties and a mild right hemiparesis, and lapsed into coma during the drive to the hospital. To complicate matters she was and had been in atrial fibrillation for some months and diabetes had been excluded by full investigation a few months previously. She continued to deteriorate and both pupils became dilated and fixed to light. At that stage a serum glucose of 860 mg% and a serum sodium of 158 mmo/l were found. At that time the serum osmolarity could not be determined. There was no ketosis. Overnight she was given a total of 11 litres of hypotonic saline and 5% dextrose in water intravenously. By the following morning she had recovered consciousness and within 24 hours was completely normal with no residual physical findings. The original referral diagnosis had been a cerebral embolism with subsequent cerebral oedema.

The main clues to the diagnosis were the extreme thirst and fluid intake in spite of which she was severely dehydrated on admission.

Hypoglycaemic States

Hypoglycaemia has many important neurological features:

1. It may produce altered or psychotic behaviour.
2. It can produce focal neurological signs mimicking a cerebrovascular accident.
3. It can cause focal or generalized seizures leading to coma.
4. It can produce progressive neurological disease if unrecognized.

Although hypoglycaemic coma is widely discussed the important clinical states short of coma are rarely given the attention they deserve, and are easily missed unless this possibility is given equal consideration.

1. Hypoglycaemic pre-coma may produce altered behaviour, often resulting in aggression or antisocial behaviour. In diabetics on insulin this usually results from missing a meal or from unanticipated exercise. In patients with autonomous insulin-secreting tumours hypoglycaemia is more likely to occur during the night, when dietary intake ceases and insulin production continues unaltered. Any patient with a history of severe nocturnal confusion should be regarded as an insulin-secreting tumour suspect.

2. In patients with impaired cerebral perfusion hypoglycaemia may cause focal signs such as transient hemiparesis, dysphasia or dyspraxia. Animal experiments have shown that if one carotid artery is ligated focal signs develop in the poorly perfused territory when hypoglycaemia is provoked. Because of this, transient ischaemic attacks in a diabetic patient might be due to hypoglycaemic episodes with poor cerebral perfusion on one side, rather than cerebral embolic events. This possibility is worth considering in insulin-dependent diabetics when the evidence for carotid artery embolic disease is minimal and treatment with aspirin or anticoagulants is unsuccessful.

3. In some hypoglycaemic patients purely focal or generalized seizures may occur. Hypoglycaemia as a possible cause should always be urgently considered in any patient who has a first seizure. Unfortunately autoregulatory mechanisms will have often produced a normal blood sugar level by the time the patient reaches hospital, and a normal sugar should not be regarded as totally exclusory if the clinical picture suggests that hypoglycaemia is a real possibility. The Case Report X in Chapter 22 (p. 396) is an excellent example even when the possibility seemed to have been excluded.

Failure to identify the nature of these attacks might have led to progressive brain damage as a result of repeated hypoglycaemic insults. It is also likely that the combination of seizure activity in cerebral cells, while they are deprived of their main metabolite, is doubly damaging. Following restoration of the blood sugar to normal, the recovery of consciousness is not always as prompt as might be expected. It is not unusual for a patient who has had a severe hypoglycaemic fit to take 12–24 hours to make a full recovery.

4. Repeated episodes of hypoglycaemia may cause irreversible damage to the basal ganglia, cerebellum, cortex and hippocampus. Progressive dementia, spasticity with dysarthria, extrapyramidal syndromes and ataxia may result. A syndrome resembling motor neuron disease has been reported in patients with chronic hypoglycaemia, although this would seem to be exceptionally rare.

In recent years many insulin-dependent diabetics have been referred to the author for neurological advice with a diagnosis of nocturnal epilepsy. On further investigation not one has proved to be epileptic and all have been demonstrated to be hypoglycaemic due to insulin. Because the greatest risk of this happening is during the night, and because most idiopathic epileptic events also occur during the night, it is very easy to dismiss the possibility of hypoglycaemia. Determined efforts must be made to prove or disprove this possibility. (See also section in Chapter 22 on altered consciousness during hypoglycaemia)

Neurological Complications of Collagen Vascular Diseases

The collagen vascular diseases include a diverse range of disorders which have a common pathological basis in diffuse inflammatory changes in the connective tissue, and particularly in the connective tissue of the blood vessels. The aetiology of these disorders is due to altered immunological mechanisms. Quite often features of the different conditions overlap and all tend to become even more potentially lethal when complicated by widespread arteritis. Usually the neurological complications of these disorders reflect the extent and severity of the vascular changes.

Systemic Lupus Erythematosus

This disorder usually affects females (85% of cases). Neurologists should be particularly aware that some cases are provoked by drugs used in the treatment of neurological disorders. These include hydrallazine (used to treat acute hypertensive cerebrovascular disease), procaineamide (used as a muscle relaxant), and trimethadione and diphenylhydantoin (anti convulsants). The pathological lesion consists of fibrinoid degeneration of the walls of small arteries and arterioles. Involvement of the joints, skin, heart and kidneys are the main non-neurological problems.

Focal or generalized seizures or episodes of acute psychosis may complicate up to 30% of cases: 50% of patients with systemic lupus erythematosus have abnormal EEGs. Microvascular lesions are responsible for these cerebral manifestations and also predispose the patient to cerebrovascular accidents, choreiform movement disorder, extraocular nerve palsies, peripheral neuropathy, mononeuritis multiplex, polymyositis and Guillain–Barré syndrome. Retinal vascular lesions may cause visual symptoms and fundal appearances resembling papilloedema.

Rheumatoid Arthritis

In this disorder the brunt of the connective tissue damage falls on the periarticular tissues, but in the majority of cases there is also evidence of a systemic disturbance. The commonest neurological complications are carpal tunnel syndrome due to the soft tissue changes around the wrist joint and ulnar nerve compression palsies due to the use of elbow crutches or prolonged periods of bed rest, with consequent weight bearing on the elbows.

In very severe cases a diffuse peripheral neuropathy or mononeuritis multiplex may occur. It was originally suspected that the use of steroids caused the neuropathy, but it is likely that the use of steroids merely parallels the severity of the disease and the overlap into more serious disorders. The use of high-dose steroids also makes the patient more liable to steroid psychosis, steroid myopathy and odontoid peg resorption or fracture. These latter conditions may be incorrectly regarded as progression of the disease rather than neurological complications of treatment.

The use of penicillamine in the treatment of rheumatoid arthritis has produced new complications. A myasthenic syndrome and inflammatory myopathy complicate the use of the drug (see Chapter 19).

Considerable muscle atrophy occurs in long-standing cases and although much of this results from disuse, evidence of inflammatory muscle disease is found in 5% of cases. This has to be distinguished from steroid myopathy, which may complicate very prolonged steroid use even in relatively low dosage.

The most serious neurological complication is due to avulsion or absorption of the odontoid peg. This may happen acutely during a sneeze or a fall, or be found on routine X-ray in patients complaining of neck pain. An acute or progressive spastic tetraparesis results and may prove fatal. This complication may produce insidious worsening of the patient's disability, which is easily mistaken for progression of the disease (see Case Report VII in Chapter 23).

Polyarteritis Nodosa

This is the most lethal of the collagen vascular diseases and unlike systemic lupus erythematosus and rheumatoid arthritis occurs more frequently in males (80% of cases). The age incidence is similar, the majority of cases occurring in the 20–40 age group. A very similar disorder has been described as a reaction to sulphonamides, penicillin and diphenylhydantoin.

The main pathological lesion is a panarteritis with destruction of all layers of the arterial wall, with local thrombosis and occasionally rupture of the vessel with microhaemorrhages.

The common neurological manifestations are due to peripheral nerve and nerve root infarction. The disease is one of the commonest causes of mononeuritis multiplex, but equally often infarction of multiple nerve roots occurs particularly affecting nerve roots C5–C7 and L2–L4. Once the patient becomes disabled by such lesions, the risk of further compression palsies is extremely high.

Although cranial nerve palsies and cerebrovascular accidents may occur they are uncommon.

The most dangerous complication of the condition is due to renal arteriolar disease, often leading to uncontrollable hypertension. A few patients also develop polymyositis and the use of high doses of steroids to control the underlying disease may cause a steroid myopathy, adding to the diagnostic problems.

CASE REPORT XII

A 48-year-old aeronautical draughtsman had suffered from unexplained asthma for several years. Over a period of a few weeks he lost weight and felt very ill. Over a period of days he developed bilateral ulnar and median nerve palsies. His ESR and eosinophil count were elevated. He was given steroids, with complete remission of the systemic systems and a slow recovery of the nerve lesions. A few weeks later he became unable to walk because of the rapid development of gross weakness of both hip flexor muscles and the quadriceps. EMG evidence confirmed an acute inflammatory myopathy. The dose of steroids was increased, with a rapid improvement in muscle strength. During this time the late-onset asthma that he had had for 4 years prior to the onset of the neurological syndrome remitted completely and he remained under good control for 18 months. He then developed an acute unilateral internuclear ophthalmoplegia with severe giddiness and ataxia due to a brainstem vascular accident. Further evidence of extensive disease affecting both the lungs and kidneys appeared and he died 6 months later of renal complications.

In this case, the onset with pulmonary disease and asthma suggests that this may be a variant of polyarteritis nodosa known as Churg–Strauss syndrome, but such severe renal involvement is relatively unusual. The following case is a definite example of this condition in a 36-year-old man.

CASE REPORT XIII

A 36-year-old man had suffered from episodic asthma for 4 years, requiring up to 60 mg prednisolone daily for control. Between episodes, which were usually triggered by virus infections, he was completely well and no other diagnosis had been considered. The day before flying to Australia he developed slight numbness over the outer border of the left foot. On arrival he had developed a complete left sciatic nerve lesion. Two days later he developed severe abdominal pain and signs of intestinal obstruction. At laparotomy he was found to have multiple areas of bowel necrosis due to vasculitis. A diagnosis of Churg–Strauss syndrome was made and he was treated with high-dose steroids and immunosuppressants. While still in hospital he developed a right peroneal nerve lesion and a left radial nerve lesion. He had lost 4 stone in weight over 3 weeks, and these may well have been compression palsies because they recovered rapidly. When first seen by a neurologist in the UK, 3 months after these events, he had a complete left sciatic nerve lesion. He subsequently developed diabetes requiring insulin due to the steroids, and had nocturnal epileptic events that proved to be due to hypoglycaemia. The sciatic nerve lesion slowly improved and 4 years later recovery is almost complete. His renal function was carefully monitored throughout and remained satisfactory. During the aggressive treatment of the vasculitis his asthma remained under complete control.

Another unusual form of this disorder, which occurs in young patients, is known as Cogan's syndrome. This consists of a combination of interstitial keratitis, bilateral vestibular symptoms and deafness.

CASE REPORT XIV

A 26-year-old housewife developed right-sided headache, felt increasingly unwell and lost weight. The headache was associated with vertigo. These symptoms partially remitted and then recurred on the left side. The clinical findings and otoneurological studies suggested a left-sided cerebellopontine angle lesion and the systemic illness suggested this might be due to metastatic malignant disease. During neurosurgical investigations she developed bilateral keratitis, the ESR rapidly rose to 140 mm and the eosinophil count rose to 40%. High-dose steroids led to a prompt remission of all the symptoms, although she remained partially deaf.

Although the ESR is widely regarded as an old-fashioned and unreliable test, it remains an important investigation for the neurologist. The speed with which the result is obtained and the almost invariable gross elevation in patients with collagen vascular disease cannot be matched by any other test.

Polymyositis

This acute inflammatory disease of muscle may complicate any of the collagen vascular diseases already discussed. It also occurs as a primary condition and is sometimes a remote complication of malignant disease. It is discussed in detail in Chapter 19.

Scleroderma

Scleroderma is characterized by thickening of the collagen in the skin, producing the typical skin changes of the disorder and similar changes in the bowel, which may result in malabsorption. The condition can also occur in association with systemic lupus erythematosus and dermatoamyositis.

Clinical presentations include Raynaud's phenomenon and rarely muscle weakness and evidence of cutaneous nerve damage in the thickened skin. Steroids are not helpful in this condition.

Sjögren's Syndrome

Sjörgren's syndrome is discussed in the final section of this chapter on dermatological disorders and the C.N.S.

Polymyalgia Rheumatica

This disorder is also discussed in Chapter 19. It occurs in the elderly and is characterized by severe nocturnal muscle pain in the limbs and girdle regions, usually associated with systemic symptoms and an elevated ESR. Some of these patients later develop temporal arteritis. The response to steroids is dramatic and diagnostic.

Thrombotic Thrombocytopenic Purpura

This is an extremely rare and ultimately lethal condition dominated by acute haemolytic anaemia and thrombocytopenia. The onset is usually acute, with abdominal pain, fever, vomiting, headache and jaundice, quickly complicated by confusion, delirium and coma, with seizures, hemiplegia and almost any other acute cerebrovascular event.

The main pathological lesions are due to severe acute inflammatory changes in arteriolar walls, with thrombosis and multiple petechial haemorrhages throughout the substance of the brain, but particularly in the cortex. Very rarely the disorder may run a relapsing course over several years but is almost always eventually fatal. Steroids may prove helpful.

The frequency with which collagen vascular diseases present as acute neurological emergencies places considerable responsibility on the neurologist to recognize this group of diseases. The value of the ESR as a screening test has been emphasized but it may be normal in some instances.

Neurological Complications of Endocrine and Metabolic Disease

Although there are some specific complications associated with changes in hormonal levels per se, in many instances the neurological involvement in endocrine disorders is really a reflection of alterations in electrolyte metabolism. These problems are discussed in greater detail in the chapters on muscle and peripheral nerve disease. Discussion here will therefore be extremely brief and references to more detailed discussions are given.

Thyrotoxicosis

In thyrotoxic exophthalmos with ophthalmoplegia (see Chapter 5), the exophthalmos is probably due to excessive thyroid-stimulating hormone production or long-acting thyroid-stimulating hormone effects, but the diplopia is not purely due to displacement of the globe. In many instances frank weakness of the superior rectus or lateral rectus muscles may be present and this has been shown to be due to inflammatory changes in the affected extraocular muscles.

Thyrotoxic myopathy occurs more frequently in men, even though thyrotoxicosis is much more common in women. It may occur in the absence of more dramatic evidence of the disorder and this is sometimes called 'masked thyrotoxicosis'. The rapid onset of upper limb weakness and wasting with brisk reflexes may mimic motor neuron disease (see Chapter 19). The muscle weakness usually recovers surprisingly rapidly once the euthyroid state is restored. Thyrotoxicosis also occurs in some patients with periodic paralysis, particularly in Asians, and also occurs in 10% of patients with myasthenia gravis.

Acute thyroid crisis, with fever, delirium, epileptic seizures and coma, has become rare now that immediate control of the peripheral effects of thyroid hormone can be achieved with ß-blockade.

In addition to the classic tremor of the hands that occurs in thyrotoxicosis, a rare but more dramatic complication is the acute onset of choreiform movements due to the hormonal effect on the basal ganglia (Chapter 12).

Another important group to consider are those patients in whom auricular fibrillation secondary to thyrotoxicosis has caused cerebral embolism. This may be a presenting symptom of thyrotoxicosis.

Myxoedema

Carpal tunnel syndrome is a frequent complication of myxoedema (see Chapter 16). Proximal muscle weakness is quite common in cretinism and adult myxoedema (see Chapter 19). Although myxoedema madness is often stressed as a complication of myxoedema it is extremely rare. Complete mental apathy and physical inertia usually dominate the clinical picture. Acute cerebellar dysfunction may also complicate myxoedema but it is also exceedingly rare (see Chapter 12).

Hyperparathyroidism

The complications of hyperparathyroidism directly reflect the elevation of serum calcium. This may produce a variable proximal muscle weakness (see Chapter 19) or profound personality change, occasionally amounting to an acute psychotic state (see Chapter 10). It can also produce a dramatic choreiform disorder (see Chapter 12).

Hypoparathyroidism

It is presumed that the low serum calcium level causes the complications although the exact mechanism is far from clear. In children hypocalcaemia may present as convulsions and papilloedema, which may prompt investigations along purely neurological lines unless this unusual presentation is recognized. Extrapyramidal disorders may occur, usually choreiform movements associated with the deposition of calcium in the basal ganglia. Tetany may be provoked by minor hyperventilation or occur spontaneously. Proximal muscle weakness may occur (see Chapter 19). Psychotic changes in personality have been reported but are much less frequent than in hypercalcaemia. In adults cataracts are a common complication of unrecognized chronic hypocalcaemia.

Cushing's Syndrome

In the active stages of this disease mental changes due to high endogenous steroid levels may precipitate a 'steroid psychosis'. Similarly, a proximal 'steroid myopathy' occurs and this, combined with the deposition of fat over the back of the neck and shoulders, produces the 'buffalo hump' shape of the patient who has the fully developed syndrome.

Where the disease is due to a functional tumour of the pituitary gland bitemporal field defects (see Chapter 3) or extraocular nerve palsies (see Chapter 5) may occur. Following adrenalectomy pituitary hypertrophy may cause similar problems, usually combined with dramatic hyperpigmentation.

Addison's Disease

The physical symptoms of this disorder are dominated by mental and physical lethargy and inertia. A mild proximal myopathy with easy fatiguability occurs and exertion is often accompanied by muscle cramping. The disorder is readily dismissed as being due to anxiety or depression unless the clinical clues of hyper-pigmentation and syncope due to the associated hypotension are recognized.

Acromegaly

In the early stages of this disorder there is a consider-able increase in muscle strength which parallels the dramatic changes in facial appearance and the increase in size of the hands and feet. As the pituitary gland is damaged by the enlarging eosinophil adenoma, proximal weakness ensues as panhypopituitarism develops. The tumour may compress the optic chiasm, causing a bitemporal hemianopia. The overgrowth of the hands frequently leads to carpal tunnel syndrome, and peroneal nerve entrapment has also been reported. Diabetes mellitus with all its neurological con-sequences occurs in some 20% of patients with acromegaly.

Hypopituitarism

The features of panhypopituitarism, including the visual problems caused by pituitary tumours, are described in Chapter 3. The problems presented by the tumour itself may be combined with features of both myxoedema and Addison's disease.

Inappropriate Secretion of Antidiuretic Hormone

Hyponatraemia may occur for many reasons, but a variety of special interest to the neurologist is due to inappropriate secretion of antidiuretic hormone (ADH). The term 'inappropriate' has been applied because nor-mally when serum sodium and osmolarity are falling a hypotonic urine is secreted as ADH production falls. If ADH continues to be secreted a hyperosmolar urine is produced and the renal excretion of sodium continues, further compounding the situation. This is a very simple and incomplete explanation of an extremely compli-cated metabolic situation.

The neurological importance of the condition stems from the fact that the syndrome itself may produce symptoms and signs suggesting intracranial disease, and a variety of intracranial conditions such as cerebral metastases and other neurological diseases such as Guillain–Barré syndrome may actually **cause** inappro-priate secretion of ADH. The neurological manifesta-tions are due to water intoxication and typically include

confusion, headache, nausea and vomiting. Later the patient may become comatose and epileptic seizures can occur. There may be considerable fluctuation in the symptoms on a day-to-day basis.

Many cases are due to an underlying oat-cell carci-noma of the lung and in some instances the tumour itself secretes ADH. The difficulty in distinguishing the clinical picture from that produced by multiple cerebral metastases is obvious, but simple if the importance of an abnormally low serum sodium is recognized.

Meningitis, subarachnoid haemorrhage, cerebral tumours, Guillain–Barré syndrome and head injury may all be complicated by the condition. Myxoedema and acute porphyria have also been implicated and the pos-sibility of the cerebral symptoms being ascribed to the underlying disease rather than to the potentially fatal disturbance of salt metabolism is obvious.

The condition is relatively easily treated by fluid restriction to less than 1000 ml daily. Salt loading does not help and is only indicated in patients who are comatose or convulsing in an immediate attempt to reduce the water intoxication. Routine electrolyte studies in confused, comatose or convulsing patients are of considerable importance.

CASE REPORT XV

An 18-year-old university student was admitted to hospital after a motorcycle accident. He was conscious on arrival but was remarkably confused. He insisted he was drunk and that it was 10 p.m. He was actually quite sober and it was 4 in the afternoon. He was bleeding from both ears but no fracture was seen on X-ray. Far from improving, he became increas-ingly confused over the next 12 hours and his serum sodium fell to 119 mmol/l. He was still secreting a concentrated urine (specific gravity 1030). An EEG showed a slow wave distur-bance over the left frontal region, indicating contrecoup bruis-ing of the left frontal lobe. Fluids were restricted immediately and osmolarity studies revealed a low serum osmolarity of 252 mmol/l and a urine osmolarity of 723 mmol/l. Within 24 hours he became rational and the EEG became com-pletely normal. He made an uncomplicated recovery.

The remarkably rapid onset of confusion in this patient suggests that he had cerebral bruising with oedema, rapidly compounded by the simultaneous development of inappropriate ADH secretion with water intoxication. Sometimes the possibility of this condition is not even considered in spite of suspicious electrolyte abnormalities.

CASE REPORT XVI

A 56-year-old man was referred for investigation of presenile dementia. This was of recent and rapid onset and the unusual feature in the history was that on two occasions his behaviour returned to normal for several weeks. On admis-sion his serum sodium was 112 mmol/l. A check with the referring hospital revealed that during his two admissions with an acute confusional state, the serum sodium level had been less than 120 mmol/l. A chest X-ray and bronchoscopy was normal but bronchial washings demonstrated cells diagnostic of oat-cell carcinoma. His symptoms were controlled by fluid restriction and he was transferred back to the referring hospital, where he subsequently died of metastatic disease several months later.

Alcoholism

The neurological complications of alcoholism are considered here because they basically represent metabolic effects rather than a direct toxic effect of alcohol. In the UK this problem presents a minor, but unfortunately increasing, part of neurological practice. In the USA these complications are extremely common.

Alcoholic peripheral neuropathy, the complication most directly related to altered niacin metabolism, is the most common complication. It is described in Chapter 18. Acute compression palsies caused by the inebriated patient lying on the vulnerable nerves are common. The radial and peroneal nerves are usually affected (see Chapters 16 and 17).

Acute and chronic muscle changes due to alcohol have been reported. The symptoms of the acute form resemble the effects of sudden exertion on untrained muscles, with pain and tenderness on movement, and may be accompanied by myoglobinuria. This usually follows a period of high alcoholic intake. The chronic form consists of a mild generalized myopathy (see Chapter 19). Cerebellar degeneration may also occur in an acute partially reversible form and a chronic irreversible form with massive degeneration of the anterior lobe of the cerebellum (see Chapter 12).

Acute haemorrhagic polioencephalitis or Wernicke's encephalopathy is invariably associated with damage to the hippocampal–mamillary body complex, causing the abrupt memory deficit known as Korsakoff's psychosis. The brainstem features are described in Chapter 11. The immediate administration of massive doses of vitamin B_1 may reverse the potentially lethal brainstem lesion but recovery of the memory disturbance is variable and always incomplete.

One very unusual and almost specific complication of alcohol abuse is acute auditory hallucinosis. In this condition a pure auditory hallucination, often musical in content, is associated with paranoid thoughts. Acute auditory hallucinosis and delirium tremens are alcohol **withdrawal** syndromes. Both are common in alcoholics who have been admitted to hospital for other reasons. Any patient having an epileptic fit 2 or 3 days after admission to hospital should be suspected of alcohol abuse as this is the typical timing of an alcohol withdrawal fit, unless alcohol is being smuggled in to the patient to maintain their intake. Delirium tremens often begins in this way as a series of epileptic fits followed

by severe confusion and agitation, sympathetic overaction and vivid visual hallucinations.

Alcohol or sedative drug abuse should be suspected in any patient who has a fit in the first few days after admission to hospital for other disorders or elective surgery.

Neurological Complications Associated With Cardiac Disease

The most frequent cardiac disease is myocardial infarction. Because this is only one manifestation of diffuse vascular disease it is hardly surprising that some 40% of patients who suffer a cerebrovascular accident subsequently die of a myocardial infarct.

During and following acute myocardial infarction there are the immediate risks of impaired cerebral perfusion during the shock phase and the later risk of cerebral embolism when the circulation recovers and a mural thrombus becomes detached from the damaged heart wall. In some series as many as 30% of cerebral emboli were found to originate in the heart. Attempts to prevent this complication with anticoagulants may lead to subarachnoid haemorrhage. Fortunately, anticoagulants no longer play a major role in the management of myocardial infarction, but the use of thrombolytic agents has produced a new risk of cerebral haemorrhage.

Congenital cardiac disease carries many risks. Coarctation of the aorta is associated with a high incidence of cerebral aneurysms – almost certainly a direct consequence of the associated hypertension. The risk of subarachnoid haemorrhage is high and subarachnoid haemorrhage in children under 15 should always suggest this possibility.

Congenital cyanotic heart disease may cause complications due to chronic cerebral anoxia, polycythaemia or cerebral abscess as the blood bypasses the normal filtering effect of the pulmonary circulation.

CASE REPORT XVII

A 29-year-old man who had long outlived his prognosis had truncus arteriosus, atrial septal defect and ventricular septal defect with a compensatory polycythaemia of 24 g/l. He had severely limited exercise tolerance. While on holiday, he had a series of focal fits affecting the left hand. His cardiologist thought this was due to the polycythaemia and he was venesected. He went on to have a grand mal fit with postictal weakness of the left arm. Staphylococcus aureus was isolated in a blood culture and an isotope scan showed a right parietal lobe lesion. He was transferred for neurological care and a CT scan (see below) revealed appearances typical of a cerebral abscess. Because of its location the neurosurgical view was that this should be treated with intravenous antibiotic therapy. Only one further focal fit occurred. A

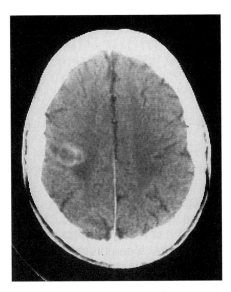

CRIII. *Cerebral abscess 2° to congenital cyanotic heart disease*

sequence of scans demonstrated satisfactory resolution of the lesion. He was back to his usual state of health when last reviewed a year after these events.

Congenital and acquired disease of the aortic and mitral valves predispose to subacute bacterial endocarditis. This may cause cerebral embolism, cerebral abscess or mycotic aneurysms, which typically develop at the trifurcation of the middle cerebral artery and may reach considerable size.

The modern surgical treatment of valvular disease, although now much safer using cardiac bypass and an open heart approach, carried the risk of operative or postoperative clot or air embolism causing a cerebrovascular accident.

The evaluation of patients who have suffered syncopal attacks always requires careful auscultation of the heart to detect aortic or mitral valve lesions, and in patients complaining of syncope occurring on exertion evidence of atrial septal defects and pulmonary valve disease should be sought. The stethoscope remains an important part of the neurologist's diagnostic equipment. In older patients the possibility of underlying arrhythmia may require ambulatory ECG monitoring.

Neurological Complications of Neoplastic Disease

The neurology of malignant disease is a subject in itself and it is only possible to make some broad generalizations here.

In spite of many extremely interesting but very rare remote complications of malignant disease the fact remains that the majority of patients with malignant disease who develop a neurological disorder prove to have metastatic deposits or a complication of the surgical, radiotherapeutic or oncological treatment of their condition. The rare remote complications have been mentioned elsewhere and include peripheral neuropathy (Chapter 18) polymyositis (Chapter 19), Eaton–Lambert syndrome (Chapter 18), limbic encephalitis (Chapter 10), cerebellar degeneration (Chapter 12) and inappropriate secretion of ADH (see above). A suggested relationship between motor neuron disease and visceral malignancy has not been substantiated.

Surprisingly, in view of their widespread nature and chronic clinical course, the malignant lymphomas produce relatively few neurological complications other than by direct spread. Mid-thoracic spinal cord compression due to Hodgkin's disease and meningeal infiltration in the leukaemias are probably the most frequent problems encountered. Fungal meningitis due to *Cryptococcus neoformans* (cryptococcal meningitis) may occur in conditions compromising the immune system. This is best demonstrated by an indian ink preparation of the CSF. Progressive multifocal leukoencephalopathy was previously a very rare condition due to an opportunist virus infection of the CNS in patients with chronic diseases, particularly those leading to altered immune mechanisms. Since the advent of AIDS this has become quite a common disorder, but it remains an important complication of chronic malignant disease that is extremely difficult to diagnose antemortem. It produces a rapidly progressive illness in which brainstem and cerebellar signs are coupled with confusion and drowsiness. All patients with this condition have died, usually within a few months of onset.

An altered immune state may also predispose to the development of severe or even generalized herpes zoster, and this condition may complicate malignant lymphomas and chronic lymphatic leukaemia.

In addition to metastases (the sources and locations of the common metastases to the CNS are described in Chapters 8 and 15) there are the additional problems posed by the neurological side-effects of cytotoxic drugs and radiation damage to the spinal cord, particularly following thoracic radiation (Chapter 14) to the cauda equina (Chapter 15) and the brachial plexus (Chapter 16).

As a cautionary note it is important to remember that just because a patient has had malignant disease in the past it does not follow that any new disorder is necessarily a complication of that malignancy. An open mind is necessary until the diagnosis is established beyond doubt.

CASE REPORT XVIII

A 42-year-old woman who had had a mastectomy for carcinoma of the breast 4 years previously developed diabetes insipidus and a bitemporal field defect. A metastasis seemed certain as this condition is a recognized complication of carcinoma of the breast, and steroids and other hormonal therapy were used without effect for several months. Further investigation and exploration were eventually undertaken and revealed a cystic craniopharyngioma, which was successfully resected. (This patient was seen in 1961, long before scanning, which would have made the diagnosis simple.)

Infectious Diseases and the Nervous System

In general, infection of the nervous system is a complication of infection elsewhere. For example, meningococcal meningitis can be regarded as a complication of meningococcal septicaemia, tuberculous meningitis is a complication of a breaking down tuberculous lesion or miliary tuberculosis, and herpes zoster, *Listeria monocytogenes* and cryptococcal meningitis are opportunistic nervous system infections in the presence of debilitating disease or altered immune status.

The meninges and subarachnoid space may be infected by viruses, bacteria, spirochaetes and fungi. The relative incidence of these causes varies enormously in different areas of the world and viral and bacterial infections sometimes show a seasonal variation.

A classic case of meningitis is unmistakable but there are many subtle presentations that may lead to a fatal delay in diagnosis. There are also several common disorders that can mimic meningitis to the extent that an immediate lumbar puncture seems desirable. These situations may include any febrile illness in childhood, acute influenza, a severe migraine attack or subarachnoid haemorrhage. In all these situations a CT scan is desirable (if available) before performing the lumbar puncture. This is because of the very dangerous situation in which neck stiffness in a drowsy patient is actually due to coning. In these patients a lumbar puncture may prove fatal. The decision to do a lumbar puncture should always be taken after very careful consideration as to what information will be obtained and whether there seems to be any hazard. It has been estimated that up to 100 patients a year in the UK die as a result of unwise lumbar punctures (see also Chapter 15).

The diagnosis of meningitis may prove difficult to make in infancy and senescence and tuberculous meningitis may produce a 'tumour-like' clinical picture in any age group. In infancy the child may become unusually quiet or utter only occasional brief cries. Neck stiffness may be difficult to detect and the child may be merely a pyrexial, quiet, listless, limp infant. An epileptic fit is a common early feature of meningitis in infancy and may provide a clue to the diagnosis.

In senescence the features that make the diagnosis difficult may include an apyrexial course or neurological symptoms dominated by confusion and delirium, or focal signs due to cerebral venous thrombosis, mimicking a cerebrovascular accident.

At any age local inflammation of the brain, venous sinus thrombosis, cerebral arterial occlusions, blockage of CSF circulation or cranial nerve palsies may result in misleadingly focal presenting signs. If these complications develop later in the course of illness, they may prompt reconsideration of the diagnosis and require definitive treatment in their own right. Many of these complications occur in incorrectly or inadequately treated meningitis.

Classic Features

In typical acute meningitis the clinical features include a pyrexial onset, severe headache with photophobia and the rapid development of neck stiffness and backache. The signs known as Kernig's sign and the Brudinski sign only add further evidence of meningeal inflammation and do not dramatically alter the significance of neck stiffness. The similarity of the headache and generalised myalgia to prodromal influenza is immediately obvious. If left undiagnosed and untreated drowsiness, vomiting and eventually coma may ensue. Different types of meningitis affect different age groups and produce some specific features which may have diagnostic value.

Meningococcal Meningitis

Neisseria meningitides remains the commonest infecting organism, showing a seasonal variation (January to June) and an association with overcrowding. The illness invariably starts as a meningococcal septicaemia, and this may prove to be the main problem and cause death. In some cases a chronic meningococcal septicaemia without meningitis may occur. The disease usually affects the under-12 age group and starts as an acute pharyngitis with fever, which may rapidly worsen to include a petechial rash and in some cases a florid purpuric rash. In this group massive intravascular coagulation may occur with shock and circulatory collapse. This is known as the Waterhouse–Frederichsen syndrome. The collapse was previously attributed to adrenal haemorrhage and high-dose steroids were recommended as treatment, but it is now clear that endotoxic shock, the vasculitic component and myocarditis combine to produce this potentially lethal situation. Skilled intensive care and appropriate antibiotics have markedly improved the survival rate. Steroids now appear to have no value.

The onset of the meningitis is often associated with a herpes simplex eruption around the mouth. Metastatic infection of the eyes, joints and bones may occur and complicate the later course. Late complications occur relatively rarely in correctly diagnosed and treated meningococcal meningitis.

Penicillin is the drug of choice, although sulphonamide-sensitive organisms are still responsible for the majority of cases in the UK. The dosage is 20 million units/24 hours in adults and 250,000 units/kg/24 hours in children, always given intravenously. There is no indication for intrathecal penicillin in this condition. If the patient is penicillin sensitive chloramphenicol 100 mg/kg/day is effective.

Haemophilus Influenzae Meningitis

Haemophilus meningitis occurs almost exclusively in children under 5 years of age. It tends to have a slower onset and initially the signs of meningitis may be minimal. The child may be merely drowsy and febrile. The special complication of *Haemophilus influenzae* meningitis is the tendency to produce a subdural collection of pus. This may lead to an apparent relapse or the later development of focal neurological signs. This is often the result of inadequate treatment with ampicillin. A high association with inappropriate secretion of ADH has also been identified: fluid overload should be avoided and the serum sodium closely monitored.

Chloramphenicol remains the drug of choice in a dose of 75 mg/kg/24 hours for at least 10 days. If ampicillin is used a very high dosage is necessary: 400 mg/kg/24 hours should be given by intravenous infusion. Ampicillin-resistant strains are found in 10%–20% of patients and ampicillin alone is no longer recommended treatment.

Pneumococcal Meningitis

Pneumococcal meningitis is relatively uncommon. It is most often seen in extremely young children and elderly men, often complicating a pulmonary infection. It is the organism most often implicated when the dura is damaged by a skull fracture, middle ear disease or sinus infections. The organism may also reach the brain via the bloodstream in patients who have pneumococcal pneumonia. It is potentially the most lethal form of meningitis, a somewhat paradoxical situation considering that the organism is extremely penicillin sensitive. The danger arises from the rapid development of a thick basal exudate, cortical venous thrombosis and cerebral oedema. Total eradication may prove difficult and frequent recurrences may occur in patients with underlying sources of infection such as a basal skull fracture. Inappropriate ADH secretion is a common complication and persistent deafness a frequent sequela.

Penicillin in adequate dosage is the treatment of choice. The dose is 12–20 million units/24 hours (150 mg/kg/day) in the adult and 250,000 units/kg/24 hours in children, given intravenously. Chloramphenicol is recommended in patients who are allergic to penicillin in a dose of 100 mg/kg/24 hours.

Other Organisms

Other Gram-positive and Gram-negative organisms may cause meningitis. For this reason it was traditional to use a triple therapy regimen in those patients who did not have clinical evidence to suggest a specific organism and where the Gram stain of the CSF was uncertain. The traditional regimen included penicillin, chloramphenicol and sulphadiazine, all three drugs being used until the organism was identified. Recently regimens which include kanamycin and gentamicin combined with penicillin have been suggested, and many use wide-spectrum antibiotic such as ampicillin and cephalosporins. Most hospitals now have an antibiotic policy where the bacteriologist recommends the antibiotics to be used in meningitis when the organism is not immediately identifiable. The old regimen was remarkably successful, utilized readily available and inexpensive antibiotics and may still have some merit where more exotic agents and skilled bacteriological advice is less readily available.

The currently recommended empirical treatments where a free choice of antibiotics is available are an aminoglycoside with ampicillin or a cephalosporin in neonates, chloramphenicol plus ampicillin or a cephalosporin up to age 6 years, and penicillin plus a cephalosporin in all others. These regimes are calculated to have maximum bactericidal activity against the most likely organisms found in these age ranges.

The most important point in the management of meningitis is that once the diagnosis has been made, an **adequate** dose of the appropriate antibiotic must be given. Therapeutic failures result from the use of inadequate doses of appropriate antibiotics or the use of specialized antibiotics such as cloxacillin or cephalosporin alone, in the mistaken presumption that the meningitis is due to a rare or antibiotic-resistant organism.

Intrathecal therapy is rarely indicated in the treatment of meningitis: therapeutic disasters have occurred as a result of the incorrect use of intrathecal injections of antibiotics. The correct dose of penicillin used intrathecally is 20,000 units in aqueous solution. This should be prepared by a pharmacist and no other dilution or diluent should be used. It is not recommended for routine use. The intrathecal use of streptomycin is discussed in the next section.

Tuberculous Meningitis

Tuberculous meningitis is one of the most serious complications of tuberculosis. It results from haematogenous spread of the organism

Although tuberculous meningitis can occur at any age the peak incidence is between 2 and 5 years. The onset may be heralded by listlessness, lethargy, poor appetite and weight loss. The meningitic phase may occur very abruptly, with acute extraocular nerve palsies, vomiting, headache and epileptic seizures progressing to coma.

In the adult all these symptoms may occur but the onset can be extremely gradual and is sometimes dominated by intellectual and personality changes. Tuberculous meningitis should always be suspected in any vaguely ill patient with headache and personality change.

The diagnosis may be suggested by the CSF findings. The fluid is usually mildly pleocytic, containing 50–300 cells (main lymphocytes), a slightly raised protein and a normal or slightly reduced glucose level. This type of fluid may occur in several other conditions discussed below, but unless an alternative diagnosis can be established it should be standard practice to start antituberculous therapy on suspicion alone while the result of CSF culture is awaited.

The following case report is an excellent example of this situation, although unfortunately the diagnosis was made too late for a successful outcome.

CASE REPORT XIX

A 38-year-old woman was admitted to a district general hospital with her 10-year-old daughter, both suffering from an acute respiratory illness confirmed as mycoplasma pneumonia. The daughter quickly recovered and was discharged home, but the mother failed to respond to treatment and continued to produce purulent sputum, and over 3 weeks became progressively confused and drowsy. On the day before neurological referral she developed diplopia and became semiconscious. When first seen she could only just be roused long enough to complete one test at a time. There was no papilloedema and the only physical findings were a left sixth nerve palsy and a left extensor plantar response. She was immediately transferred to the neurological unit, where a CT scan demonstrated hydrocephalus and CSF examination produced a fluid containing 2.4 g/l of protein, 45 lymphocytes/mm³ and a glucose level of 0.9 mmol/l (blood glucose 7 mmol/l). This was entirely consistent with the clinical diagnosis of tuberculous meningitis and she was started on quadruple antituberculous therapy. The hydrocephalus worsened and required shunting, serial CT scanning revealed extensive basal and upper brainstem infarction. She remained wheelchair-bound and intellectually severely impaired. Mycobacterium tuberculosis *was isolated from the CSF at 10 days.*

This case is a typical example of the difficulty of diagnosis in a condition that has become extremely rare, and the role of the mycoplasma infection in this case is uncertain: it certainly masked the onset of the condition. There would appear to be no typical presentation of tuberculous meningitis and it is only by always con-

sidering this diagnostic possibility in any confused or drowsy patient with headache, particularly if cranial nerve signs appear, that incorrect diagnosis will be avoided.

Treatment is with a combination of three or four agents selected from streptomycin, isoniazid, ethambutol, pyrizinamide and rifampicin. All penetrate the inflamed meninges adequately. Intrathecal streptomycin is rarely indicated but if the decision to use intrathecal therapy is taken, the dose used is only 50–100 mg diluted in saline and CSF in the syringe and then reinjected slowly. In severe cases the use of corticosteroid drugs has been recommended but this remains controversial. To some extent the agents used initially will depend on the known antibiotic resistance of local strains of bacteria. Streptomycin is normally used initially in a dose of 1 g daily for 4–6 weeks and then 1 g twice weekly thereafter 6 months. Isoniazid in a dose of 8–10 mg/kg daily in divided doses is given with pyridoxine 50 mg daily to prevent neuropathy. Rifampicin is used in a single dose of 600 mg/day. Ethambutol is used in a dose of 15 mg/kg/day for 6 weeks and the patient's colour vision should be carefully monitored. Pyrizinamide is used in a dose of 30 mg/kg/day.

The exact regimen and combination used will vary from patient to patient and may subsequently be altered by the culture sensitivity to the various agents and the development of side-effects requiring withdrawal of one or more of the drugs. The duration of treatment is also variable. The response is often quite dramatic and patients are reluctant to continue treatment when they feel well. It is generally recommended that the final regimen, which will usually consist of only three drugs, should be continued for 1 year.

Benign Aseptic Meningitis (Viral Meningitis)

The enteroviruses and the mumps virus are the main causes of this condition. The illness usually starts with an influenza type of prodrome with fever, muscle pains and headache. The onset of neck stiffness heralds the meningitic phase. Clinically it is unusual for the patient to appear particularly ill, although photophobia and malaise are prominent symptoms.

The CSF usually contains between 30 and 300 cells, almost all lymphocytes, although in the first 24 hours of the illness up to 10% of the cells may be polymorphs. The other constituents are usually normal and a significant increase in the protein or decrease in the glucose should raise serious doubts as to this diagnosis.

No specific treatment is necessary and the condition usually subsides within 7–10 days. With the exception of the variant known as lymphocytic choriomeningitis recurrences are unusual, although a mild headache may persist for some weeks. Patients should be made aware that this is a very benign condition and it is likely that the majority do not actually go to hospital. The word 'meningitis' holds such terror that it is not unusual to see patients 20 years later, still unnecessarily concerned that they have suffered brain damage as a result of viral meningitis.

Lymphocytic choriomeningitis is quite rare and is due to a virus transmitted by mice. It is characterized by a very high cell count, which may rise to 5 000 lymphocytes, and a rather more protracted course.

It is important that special care is taken with any patient who has a 'sterile' meningitis, especially if they have been given antibiotics before admission to hospital. If the CSF contains any polymorphs, if the protein is significantly elevated or the glucose is low there are several other conditions that must be considered. These include partially treated bacterial meningitis, tuberculous meningitis, cerebral abscess, cerebral tumour, cerebrovascular accident or malignant infiltration of the meninges. Fungal meningitis, which is extremely unusual in the UK, should also be considered especially in patients with known malignant lymphomas.

The CSF should always be cultured for tuberculosis and unusual organism such as *Listeria monocytogenes* and stained with indian ink for *Cryptococcus neoformans*. It is also useful where there is a very high cell count and a low sugar to examine a cell block for malignant cells. Carcinomatous meningitis may be mistaken for bacterial meningitis unless this policy is adopted.

Careful follow-up is indicated in such cases and a repeat CSF examination should be made before the patient is discharged. This is usually unnecessary in patients who have a typical aseptic meningitis, although a convalescent serum should always be obtained in an attempt to identify the causal virus.

Neurocutaneous Disorders and Dermatological Manifestations Associated With Neurological Disease

Throughout this text there have been several references to neurofibromas occurring in a setting of neurofibromatosis and the high association with other malignant and benign CNS tumours. Tuberous sclerosis has also been mentioned. It is appropriate to discuss the other conditions in this group of inherited disorders, and in particular the dermatological markers of these conditions. There are also some characteristic cutaneous manifestations associated with underlying infectious disorders, some rare skin diseases that

have been shown to be complicated by neurological disorders, and finally, many of the drugs used in neurology produce a variety of skin rashes, some unique to that agent. An attempt has been made to summarize much of this material for reference purposes in this section.

The Neurophakomatoses

These are five disorders due to genetically based dysplasia of neuroectodermal tissue affecting the skin, the retinae and the underlying neural tissues. The are neurofibromatosis, tuberous sclerosis, angioblastomatosis, craniofacial naevus and ataxia telangiectasia.

Neurofibromatosis

This condition is inherited as an autosomal dominant with a prevalence of 35/100 000. The defect is on chromosome 17. It is now classified in eight forms as NF I–VIII. Mutations account for 50% of new cases. NF V is restricted to one segment with a cutaneous pigmentary lesion and an underlying vertebral or neural defect; NF VI consists of café au lait patches with no underlying lesion; NF VII is a late-onset variant and NF VIII is an uncertain grouping with less classic features. The important variant are NF I and NF II.

NF I (Von Recklinghausen's Disease) The cutaneous components consist of café au lait patches, cutaneous nodules, freckles in the axillae and Lisch nodules (small hamartomas in the iris). The neural components are spinal root and peripheral nerve neurofibromas, plexiform neurofibromas of the fifth nerve, cervical plexus and lumbar plexus (with a high risk of malignant transformation) and piloid astrocytomas of the optic nerve or pons. Acoustic nerve tumours are extremely rare, but cerebral astrocytomas in other sites and neurofibromas on other cranial nerves are found.

In some patients the condition may be associated with mental retardation, short stature and multiple bony malformations. There is a 5% incidence of phaeochromocytomas.

If parents have an affected child and neither has any evidence of the condition, the risk of a further affected child is 1:10 000 (the standard population risk). If one parent is affected the risk of further affected children is 50%.

The following example of this condition emphasizes some of its clinical and genetic features (see also Case report V in Chapter 6, an extraordinary example of the extent of intracranial tumours that may occur in this condition).

CASE REPORT XX

A 3-year-old girl was noted to be walking into things and was unable to pick up her toys or reach for offered objects. She was found to be blind, with bilateral optic atrophy. On general examination she had widespread café au lait patches but no obvious skin nodules. When explaining to her mother, who was 6 months' pregnant, that it was likely that her condition was associated with the brown patches, the mother said 'what like these?' and pulled up her skirt to reveal that her entire left thigh was covered by one large café au lait patch. Investigation confirmed an extensive bilateral optic nerve and chiasmal glioma in the child. The second child was unaffected.

NF II (Bilateral Acoustic Neuromas)   This is inherited as an autosomal dominant; the genetic defect has now been identified on chromosome 22 and predictive testing is available. The associated café au lait patches tend to be very pale and relatively few. Cutaneous nodules are few and tend to be on the back. Spinal root neurofibromas are common but other CNS tumours are rare. An excellent example of this condition will be found in the Case report IV in Chapter 6 (p. 71).

Tuberous Sclerosis (Bourneville's Disease)

This condition was also first identified by Von Recklinghausen but the first full description was credited to Bourneville. It is transmitted as an autosomal dominant with low penetrance and variable expression. This makes for very atypical clinical pictures and the prevalence rate is therefore difficult to establish, but is thought to be 1–2/100 000.

There are numerous types of skin lesion. The hardest to detect, but the one that is usually present at birth, is the depigmented naevus or ash-leaf macule. These are usually found on the trunk using a Wood's light. The second skin lesion is the shagreen patch, an area of thickened yellow skin in the lumbar area (a hamartoma) detected later in childhood, and the classic lesion, adenoma sebaceum, may not appear until the teens or later. This consists of small yellowish-red lesions over the nasolabial folds and cheeks. They are angiofibromas and are usually mistaken for acne unless they are strikingly reddened. Café au lait patches may occur. Subungual fibromas are fleshy lesions that are found under or alongside the nails and are diagnostic.

Ophthalmoscopy may reveal multiple retinal hamartomas that look like mulberries, and close examination of the iris may reveal areas of hypopigmentation.

The neurological complications are related to the presence of subependymal hamartomas in the ventricular system, which may become sufficiently large in later life to block CSF circulation. The condition is frequently associated with mental retardation but patients with normal intellect are now being increasingly recognized. A good example of this is given below. The commonest complication is epilepsy and in infancy tuberous sclerosis is the commonest identifiable cause, associated with hypsarrhythmia (salaam attacks). A CT scan demonstrating these lesions in infancy, associated with this condition, is shown in Chapter 12, page 201. Some patients may not become epileptic until later in life.

CASE REPORT XXI

An 11-year-old boy presented with epilepsy consisting of both complex partial and major seizures. He was highly intelligent and on routine examination no abnormality was noted. His EEG showed generalized epileptic features. Complete control of his epilepsy was established and he was followed yearly. He developed normal teenage acne. AT the age of 16, over a 3-week period, he developed headaches, vomiting and papilloedema. CT scanning revealed not only a substantial tumour blocking the CSF circulation but multiple subependymal lesions diagnostic of tuberous sclerosis. Examination with a Wood's light demonstrated ash-leaf macules. One subungual fibroma was found and some of his facial lesions were slightly reddened and thought to be minimal evidence of adenoma sebaceum. He made a full recovery following surgery and his epilepsy remained controlled. No lesions were demonstrated elsewhere.

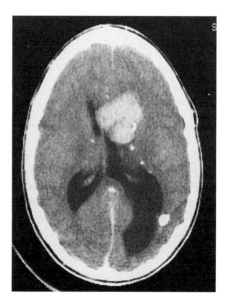

CRXXI. *Undiagnosed tuberous sclerosis presenting as hydrocephalus due to intraventricular tumour.*

Hamartomas of the kidney, lung, heart, liver and spleen can occur, and in particular the rhabdomyomas of the heart may cause arrhythmias or intracardiac masses. Syncopal collapses in patients with tuberous sclerosis should prompt careful cardiac evaluation.

Angioblastomatosis (Von Hippel–Lindau Disease)

This is a very rare autosomal dominant disease with variable penetrance. The retinal haemangioblastomas may cause visual failure and the cerebellar haemangioblastomas may cause acute posterior fossa haemorrhage (see Chapter 11). Rarely are the two lesions associated in the same patient. Cysts may occur in visceral organs. The importance of recognizing the familial incidence of this condition is shown in the following case.

CASE REPORT XXII

A 56-year-old man was admitted as an emergency after collapsing at a funeral. He related that he had suddenly become extremely giddy, developed a severe headache and started vomiting. He and the congregation assumed that this was emotionally based but vomiting continued, the headache became worse and he started to become drowsy and sought medical advice. On examination he had nystagmus and cerebellar signs. He was asked whose funeral he was attending and it transpired that it was that of his sister, who had died of a cerebral tumour. He could not remember what it was called until offered the expression 'haemangioblastoma', which he immediately identified. Investigation revealed that he had an intracerebellar haemorrhage from a cerebellar haemangioblastoma which in this case was quite unequivocally familial!

Craniofacial Naevus (Sturge–Weber Syndrome)

This is a rare and sporadic condition. The affected patient is born with a port-wine stain over the trigeminal nerve distribution. This may range from a small strawberry-sized blemish to a large indurated and purple-coloured arteriovenous malformation occupying the whole side of the face. Bilateral involvement can occur but is rare.

If the lesion involves the eye, blindness due to glaucoma may occur. The commonest neurological complication is epilepsy due to maldevelopment of the cerebral cortex, usually in the parieto-occipital region on the same side. This can often be identified by 'tramline' calcification in the cerebral gyri on straight skull films. The epilepsy may be difficult to control and the cerebral lesion may be associated with hemiparesis or visual field defects. An X-ray demonstrating the typical calcification is included below.

Ataxia Telangiectasia (Louis–Barr Syndrome)

This is an autosomal recessive condition with a prevalence of 1/40,000. The cutaneous manifestations are many but the most striking and diagnostic feature is the telangiectasia of the conjunctivae, the eyelids, the ears and face, the flexor aspects of the limbs and the dorsum of the hands. Lesions may also be found on

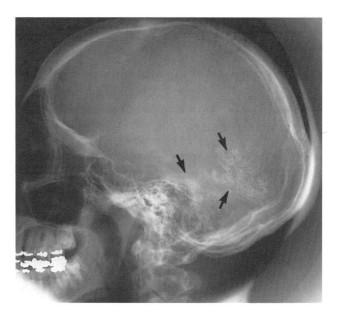

Tramline calcification in cortical gyri in Sturge–Weber syndrome.

the palate. Premature ageing changes (progeria) occur in the skin and hair with alopecia, in contrast to hirsutes of the limbs. Café au lait patches may be found and increased pigmentation occurs in the warm areas of skin. Vitiligo may be a later feature.

The neurological components consist of degeneration affecting the cerebellum, brain stem and extrapyramidal system, with ataxia, gaze disturbances and extrapyramidal features causing severe progressive disability.

Death is usually due to recurrent chest infection related to immunological deficiency. Some 10%–15% of the patients develop reticuloendothelial malignancies in childhood or epithelial malignancies if they survive into adulthood.

Cutaneous Manifestations Associated With Neurological Diseases

Sjögren's Syndrome

This disorder is included here because the dry eyes, dry mouth and dry mucocutaneous areas (the sicca syndrome) are the major manifestations. A wide variety of neurological and other organ involvement may occur but those of major neurological significance are peripheral neuropathy, entrapment syndromes, mononeuritis multiplex, spinal cord inflammatory lesions, low-grade proximal myopathy and meningoencephalitis. The behaviour of the central nervous system lesions and the MRI scan findings are remarkably similar to multiple sclerosis. The condition is probably under-recognized.

Dermatomyositis

This condition may occur in isolation, complicate other collagen vascular diseases or be associated with underlying malignant disease. It is discussed in detail in Chapter 18. The cutaneous manifestations consist of a purple discoloration (usually described as 'heliotrope') of the eyelids and thickened red patches over the nailbeds and extensor aspects of the fingers. These are called Gottron's papules. They may also be found on the extensor aspects of the limbs. Telangiectasia of the nailbed may be seen on close examination. The neurological lesion is an inflammatory proximal myopathy.

Hartnup Disease

This rare condition is characterized by a pellagra-like rash on exposed areas associated with intermittent cerebellar ataxia. It is described in Chapter 12.

Behçet's Syndrome

This is a very rare disorder in Europeans characterized by recurrent severe orogenital ulceration and occasionally erythema nodosum. It is associated with a relapsing neurological picture of recurrent meningoencephalitis or multiple sclerosis-like attacks. Cases with neurological involvement were said to carry a poor prognosis but more extensive studies have not confirmed this. The most dangerous lesions appear to be bowel ulceration, with a risk of perforation and venous thrombosis. The mechanism and nature of the condition remains obscure and treatment with prednisolone, colchicine and thalidomide is currently under investigation.

Incontinentia Pigmenti

This is a very rare genetic condition of dominant inheritance but only manifest in females. It is thought that males affected by the gene die in utero. It is characterized by a bullous eruption in infancy with progression to scaly areas of hyperpigmentation which have a whorled appearance. Affected areas on the scalp may produce patches of woolly hair of different colour. It is associated with abnormal dental development and a variety of ocular abnormalities. Nervous system involvement occurs in 80% of patients and includes mental retardation, seizures and the development of a spastic paraparesis.

Infectious Diseases of the CNS Associated With Skin Lesions

Neonatal infections with herpes simplex, *Listeria monocytogenes*, *Candida albicans* and Rubella all occur and produce cutaneous manifestations and neonatal neurological problems but are beyond the scope of this book. In childhood all the viral exanthemata may be associated with neurological complications, usually an encephalopathy or meningoencephalitis.

The two exanthemata of special interest are measles, causing an acute encephalitis or the delayed complications of subacute sclerosing panencephalitis, and the rare complications of varicella, which can produce an acute, potentially fatal encephalitis or the fully reversible acute transverse myelitis or acute cerebellar syndrome that typically occur in the weeks following the initial infection.

Both Coxsackie and Echoviruses may cause skin rashes associated with aseptic meningitis and meningoencephalitis.

Meningococcal meningitis is typically associated with a maculopapular rash, which may become petechial or even purpuric in severely affected patients. The characteristic rash usually enables the correct bacterial diagnosis to be made before the CSF is even examined.

Pneumococcal and meningococcal meningitis may both be associated with a perioral herpes simplex eruption as a diagnostic clue to the underlying organism.

Lyme disease (*Borrelia burgdorfii*) is due to a tick bite and the classic skin lesion is known as erythema chronicum migrans. This is a erythematous rash which extends out from the original site. Facial weakness is the commonest neurological manifestation but radiculopathy and peripheral neuropathy have also been identified.

Herpes zoster may affect any nerve root or be generalized in patients who are immunocompromised. The classic locations are in the first division of the fifth nerve, which may be associated with extraocular nerve palsies, or the geniculate ganglion, associated with Bell's palsy. Brainstem involvement may complicate herpes zoster affecting either of these nerves. Transverse myelitis may complicate thoracolumbar nerve root involvement. Cervical or lumbar sacral root involvement is frequently associated with motor root deficit, and careful inspection of the thoracic myotomes will often reveal segmental weakness accompanying herpes zoster affecting a thoracic root.

Vogt–Koyanagi–Harada syndrome is a rare disorder thought to be immune based and virus triggered. The cutaneous lesions consist of patchy depigmentation of the hair and eyelashes and alopecia areata. It is associated with retinal detachment and meningoencephalitis.

Leprosy (Hansen's disease) has many cutaneous manifestations and is discussed in Chapter 19. The protean cutaneous manifestations of syphilis are beyond the scope of this text, but in view of the recrudescence of this disorder may well assume significance in the future.

Drugs Used in Neurology Associated With Skin Rashes

There are four mechanisms of skin hypersensitivity, accounting for reactions ranging from mild skin irritation through to serious desquamation and potentially lethal anaphylaxis.

Patients often announce that they are 'allergic' to all drugs. They usually mean that they are allergic to the thought of taking drugs, and can be guaranteed to phone within hours of the first dose to report a list of real and imagined side-effects. It would seem a good general policy to advise patients of the common anticipated effects of drugs, such as sedation, to mention other dose-limiting side-effects and to indicate any symptoms that should lead to immediate withdrawal, such as wheezing with ß-blocking agents or skin irritation with anticonvulsants. If no warnings are given some patients will continue taking the drug in spite of serious side-effects and others will stop after a single dose and only report the failure of the medication to help them, in review some weeks later.

Skin rashes are potentially the most serious side-effect of many agents used in neurology. The commonest rashes are symmetrical itching and reddened, macular or papular eruptions over the flexor aspects of the limbs or on the trunk. If the rash becomes rapidly generalized the drug should be stopped immediately. Any reaction involving blistering is potentially the most dangerous and rechallenge with the drug could prove fatal. Erythema multiforme, a spreading reddened patch which may have a raised or bullous centre, is potentially serious and, if blistering of the orogenital areas occurs, may require treatment with steroids. The entire skin may subsequently blister and peel, with a possible fatal outcome. This is called Stevens–Johnson syndrome.

Anticonvulsants

Barbiturates

Barbiturates and barbiturate derivatives such as primidone frequently cause skin reactions with widespread erythema or recurrent local irritation (a fixed drug eruption). They may cause photosensitivity and in rare patients trigger the bullous eruption of porphyria.

Phenytoin

Phenytoin may cause a simple allergic skin rash but can also cause an extremely complicated condition mimicking collagen vascular disease or reticuloendothelial malignancy, with skin rash, fever, joint pain, hepatosplenomegaly and haematological changes. Whether phenytoin is responsible for acne-like skin lesions in epileptics is still disputed, but it is certainly responsible for the skin thickening and coarsening of the facial features and gingival hypertrophy in long-term use.

Carbamazepine

Carbamazepine may cause severe skin reactions, usually within weeks of starting or sometimes after many months of uncomplicated use. Many patients seem to cross-react to phenytoin as well, making the treatment of trigeminal neuralgia particularly difficult in such cases.

Valproate

Generalized skin reactions may occur but seem to be less frequent than with other agents. However, hair loss and changes in hair texture have been noted in some patients.

Lamotrigine

Some 2% of patients taking lamotrigine develop a skin rash, usually within days of starting treatment. The incidence may be reduced by using very low initial doses.

Antidepressants and Tranquillizers

Amitriptyline

Amitriptyline, widely used in neurology as an antidepressant, migraine prophylactic or as adjunctive therapy in pain control, may rarely cause skin rashes.

Benzodiazepines

As a group of these drugs very rarely cause skin rashes, and therefore clonazepam and clobazam may be of particular value in epileptic patients who have reacted to barbiturate-derived agents and carbamazepine.

Phenothiazines

Severe generalized exfoliative reactions may occur to phenothiazines. Photosensitivity is common and in some patients a lupus-like syndrome may occur.

Jaundice occurs in patients who develop intrahepatic cholestasis.

Lithium

Lithium carbonate may produce an acne-like eruption and hair loss. Pre-existing skin disease characterized by dry skin may be exacerbated, particularly psoriasis.

Antimigraine Drugs

Propranolol

Although skin reactions are uncommon a generalized eczematous rash may occur and psoriasis may be worsened.

Nifedipine

Although calcium channel blocking agents seem not to cause skin rashes, unacceptable flushing of the face, hands and feet may limit their use.

Methysergide Maleate

Cutaneous reactions are rare but hair loss may occur.

Antiparkinsonian Drugs

Amantadine

This agent produces a specific cutaneous lesion called livedo reticularis, a blotchy red rash associated with ankle oedema, particularly affecting the lower legs and rarely the arms. It can occur even after 6–9 months of use and if the patient is not too distressed by it, does not worsen if the drug is continued.

Dopamine

Skin rashes have not been reported but alopecia may occur and it has been suspected that malignant transformation of benign melanomas may be provoked by the use of dopamine.

Agents Used in Cerebrovascular Disease

Anticoagulants

Heparin and coumarin anticoagulants may both cause alopecia. Coumarin drugs have been associated with cutaneous vasculitis, with serious skin ulceration. This occurs particularly in fatty areas of the trunk, within days of starting treatment, and is a very serious complication which may require surgical debridement.

Aspirin

Aspirin may cause a variety of skin rashes, including erythema nodosum and exfoliative dermatitis. It may exacerbate lupus erythematosus and urticarial rashes.

NSAIDs

Several of these agents have caused skin eruptions, some serious, with anaphylactic reactions. Psoriasis may be improved in some cases and worsened in others.

Corticosteroids

Steroids are often used to treat severe skin reactions due to other drugs. It is often forgotten that steroids, particularly in the doses used in neurological disease, may cause serious skin problems. In the elderly, thinning of the skin with severe bruising and loss of skin from minor trauma, is a major problem. At any age, bacterial or fungal infection of the skin is a continual risk and acne may be markedly exacerbated.

The above discussion of the cutaneous complications of neurological diseases and their treatment is by no means exhaustive, but again emphasizes that the neurologist requires a considerable knowledge of general medicine and surgery to practise effectively in what is often regarded as a rather circumscribed and erudite specialty.

Throughout the entire text attention has been given to the importance of assessing the whole patient, including their personality and reaction to their disease, as well as always considering the possibility that their neurological symptoms are a direct or remote complication of disease elsewhere. There are very few medical or surgical conditions that have no associated neurological connections or complications, and it is often the recognition of the underlying disorder by the neurologist that enables effective treatment to be given. This is sadly not the case with many of the classic neurological disorders, which are often incorrectly regarded as the only interest and province of the neurologist.

Neurologists should be regarded as general physicians who have chosen to specialize in the effects of **all** diseases on the nervous system and its functioning, and not merely as the custodians of a vast list of rare, untreatable, eponymous syndromes.

Suggestions for Further Reading and Study

The failure to include numerous references to justify every statement in this volume may at first sight seem to indicate ignorance or immense conceit, but I hope that it is seen as neither, for several reasons.

This is intended as a primer, a 'how to do it' approach to the intimidating subject of neurological disease. The text cannot flow if it is punctuated by references that the undergraduate reader will be unlikely to consult, even if only superscript numbers are used. Anyone with access to a library or a computer can instantly obtain every current reference. This is the reason that many volumes now contain reference lists longer than the actual chapters.

The information covered here is core material, gained from lecturers, discussions with colleagues and personal experience in the field over 35 years, and is widely accepted as the basis of clinical diagnosis. The text attempts to put this in a setting of the anatomy and physiology of the nervous system, using readily available knowledge. I hope that none of it is controversial or even academically novel. It is intended as a practical guide which broke new ground in the original edition by including the basic preclinical knowledge needed to understand clinical neurology.

Subject-based review journals now include such detailed citations that the need for extensive reference lists in undergraduate textbooks is increasingly inappropriate. It is pertinent to point out that anyone can become an instant expert in any disease once they have thought of the diagnosis and conducted a literature search. The tricky part is thinking of the diagnosis in the first place. The aim of this text is to facilitate the first steps along that road.

In Great Britain, the first move made by many students who have passed what they often regard as the unimportant hurdles of anatomy and physiology, is to sell their skeleton and all their basic textbooks. This is the first mistake. All this information suddenly assumes lasting significance in the clinical setting, and retaining these books, lecture notes and the skeleton will prove valuable.

While still an undergraduate, if time permits, it is worth developing an interest in the history of medicine, not only to marvel at the clinical skills demonstrated for centuries, but also to be aware of just how much of our present knowledge has been filtered down and distilled from such shaky beginnings. The biographies of the 'names' attached to many syndromes also make interesting reading, and in recent years many books have appeared characterising the person behind the name that has become a medical household word.

For the anatomical basis of clinical practice, the standard giant tomes of anatomy are still the place to look for detailed information. For better understanding, these can be supplemented by the excellent photographic anatomical texts which have now replaced the old coloured-diagram illustrations of 30 years ago.

Books that encourage thought, like *Grant's Method of Anatomy* and Sodeman's *Pathologic Physiology*, can lighten the hard work of learning factual material. Subspeciality texts on the anatomy of peripheral nerves, embryology, neuroanatomy and neurophysiology are all 'next step' volumes in expanding core knowledge.

Once clinical studies are underway, the limited time available for studying neurology would at first sight suggest that small quick-reference volumes are best, but these require either rote learning or considerable tutorial back-up before the information can be used. It is more profitable to read round a topic in one of the major texts, especially if you have seen a patient with the condition to act as a coat-hanger for the information. Unfortunately, a brief attachment to the neurology service will permit only a small snapshot of the subject. When attached to other services, always be alert to the patients who have co-existent neurological disease or a neurological complication of the disease or its treatment which will emphasise the broad spread of the subject into all specialities.

The modern major textbooks of neurology are now much better written and illustrated than the older pedantic and often boring volumes available in the 1950s and 1960s, but still use a traditional layout of subject material and often fail to indicate how a neurological diagnosis is arrived at in the first place. Once a diagnosis is established in any patient you have seen, these texts will provide an overview of the topic, and comparing the approach from two or three major texts will be even more helpful in obtaining a balanced view.

Because textbooks are inevitably out of date within a couple of years, the next step is to take advantage of the excellent review journals which in most instances are absolutely up to date on publication. Outstanding volumes for this purpose are the *Medical Clinics of North America* and *Neurological Clinics*, the editors often choosing to deal with current and controversial topics from an unusual standpoint which is both provocative and instructive. *Seminars in Neurology* provide topic-related volumes which are brief, but perhaps more helpful for quick review for the undergraduate preparing a case for presentation. It is also worth searching the other 'Clinics' volumes covering critical care, orthopaedics, infectious diseases and radiological diagnosis, which all contain occasional articles on neurologically related topics that give a different point of view and arouse further interest.

Finally for up-to-date access to the literature with brief review articles, the *Current Topics* series has provided both a regular review every year of all major topics in specific fields in their six volumes, and has built a database that can be accessed via the journal reference list or disk. It has become an invaluable part of every neurologist's library.

It should not be forgotten that the best way of learning is to see and discuss cases with one's colleagues and teachers, who should be able to give a balanced approach to the clinical problem at hand. Do not assume that the only truths are written down and that everything written down is necessarily true. Those journals that include a correspondence section are adequate testimony to the uncertainty and continuing controversy that may surround even published peer-reviewed papers. When looking up specific references in such journals it is important to scan the correspondence columns in the subsequent 2–3 months to see whether any strong feelings were expressed about the validity of the data presented and the conclusions drawn. Several journals now include regular review sections on controversial topics with proponents for both sides presenting their views and supporting data. These are mainly of value to experienced workers in the field and are not necessarily the best source of information for the undergraduate but do serve to emphasise the shifting nature of clinical certainty.

To understand the origin of clinical skills, the old volumes of neurological journals in all languages between 1920 and 1960 are a source of excellent papers, many of which are now regarded as classical descriptions of signs and diseases. In those days the correlation of clinical skills, with neuropathology, were frequent subjects simply because there were no other diagnostic skills available at that time. If time is taken to seek out these papers, both information and pleasure in equal measure are guaranteed. These old volumes are a much under-utilised resource.

In the seemingly esoteric but fascinating field of neurology, maximum enjoyment of the speciality can be best achieved by finding out what happened before and how the present level of skill was attained, and then to consider what the present level of skill is, and how much will still be valid in 10 years time. CT scanning itself remains the biggest leap in imaging and this was only 20 years ago, and 15 years ago the level of imaging now achieved by MRI scanning seemed like science fiction.

I have been told by many young consultant neurologists that reading the first edition of this text when they were undergraduates made the subject less intimidating and aroused the enthusiasm that led them to embark on a career in neurology. If this is so, I hope they will keep alive the spirit of attention to detail both in history-taking and clinical skills that still form the basis of the speciality, to guide their use of the sophisticated investigational tools that they now have, which were only just on the horizon when the first edition was written and published.

Index